Practical Guide for
Clinical Neurophysiologic Testing · EEG

SECOND EDITION

Thoru Yamada, MD
Professor Emeritus, Department of Neurology
Carver College of Medicine
University of Iowa
Iowa City, Iowa

Elizabeth Meng, BA, R. EEG/EP T.
EEG Technologist-Department of Neurology
Abrazo Maryvale Campus
Phoenix, Arizona

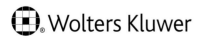 Wolters Kluwer

Philadelphia · Baltimore · New York · London
Buenos Aires · Hong Kong · Sydney · Tokyo

Acquisitions Editor: Chris Teja
Development Editor: Sean McGuire
Production Manager: Bridgett Dougherty
Senior Manufacturing Manager: Beth Welsh
Marketing Manager: Rachel Mante-Leung
Design Coordinator: Holly McLaughlin
Production Service: SPi Global

Second Edition

Library of Congress Cataloging-in-Publication Data
Names: Yamada, Thoru, 1940- author. | Meng, Elizabeth, author.
Title: Practical guide for clinical neurophysiologic testing. EEG / Thoru Yamada, Elizabeth Meng.
Other titles: EEG
Description: Second edition. | Philadelphia : Wolters Kluwer Health, [2017] | Includes bibliographical references and index.
Identifiers: LCCN 2017029420 | ISBN 9781496383020
Subjects: | MESH: Nervous System Diseases—diagnosis | Electroencephalography—methods | Neurologic Examination—methods
Classification: LCC RC386.6.E43 | NLM WL 141 | DDC 616.8/047547—dc23 LC record available at https://lccn.loc.gov/2017029420

To electroneurodiagnostic technologists/students, neurology residents, and clinical neurophysiology fellows, and the patients whom they serve

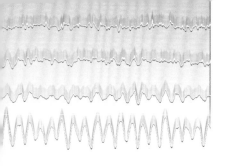

Contributing Authors

MICHAEL CILBRERTO
Assistant Clinical Professor, Department of
  Pediatrics-Neurology
Carvers College of Medicine
University of Iowa
Iowa City, Iowa

ELIZABETH MENG, BA, R. EEG/EP T.
EEG Technologist-Department of Neurology
Abrazo Maryvale Campus
Phoenix, Arizona

PETER SEABA, MS
Senior Engineer, Division of Clinical Electrophysiology
Department of Neurology
University of Iowa Hospital and Clinics
Iowa City, Iowa

THORU YAMADA, MD
Professor Emeritus, Department of Neurology
Carver College of Medicine
University of Iowa
Iowa City, Iowa

MALCOLM YEH, MD
Associate Clinical Professor, Department of Neurology
Carver College of Medicine
University of Iowa
Iowa City, Iowa

Foreword

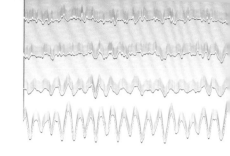

It is with pleasure that I prepare this foreword to a work by a couple of my friends in Iowa, whose professional accomplishments I have witnessed firsthand for the past 40 years. Dr. Yamada, as Director of the EEG Laboratory, has proven his proficiency in clinical neurophysiology with his insatiable desire to learn and to teach. Elizabeth Meng excelled as the chief EEG technologist and a principal instructor for our EEG technology course cosponsored by the University of Iowa and Kirkwood Community College. Their joint collaboration early on culminated in the publication of the book entitled "*Practical Guide for Clinical Neurophysiologic Testing*" which was received well by the EEG community. The first edition, though originally intended for use by EEG technologists, enjoyed a very favorable reception from neurology residents and clinical neurophysiology fellows, who prepare for the qualification examination by American Board of Clinical Neurophysiology (ABCN).

I welcome the timely publication of the second edition with the addition of a new chapter, Continuous EEG Monitoring for Critically Ill Patients, to meet the current trends and increasing demands to use EEG in this developing field. The book now includes video-EEG recordings, which show various types of seizures and artifacts as well as changing EEG patterns in real time sequence. The readers, regardless of the prior experience, will enjoy the visually alluring EEG recording and the corresponding patient's behavior that serve as a simple guide to correlate clinical and neurophysiological abnormalities. Both novice and expert will benefit from the numerous aids to the examination of waveform abnormalities. The new edition also incorporates the current EEG terminologies recently proposed by American Clinical Neurophysiology Society (ACNS), which should prove handy for those needing a quick access to proper description in formulating an EEG report.

This book meets the practical needs of physicians who perform EEG, evoked potentials, and bedside monitoring, providing a commonsense approach to problem solving for frequently encountered cortical lesions. Thoughtful, expert comments pertinent to EEG patterns will help ease the beginner's anxiety about performing EEG monitoring. The more experienced electroencephalographer will appreciate the well-organized, practical outlines of clinical conditions and electrodiagnostic features. I have no doubt that the second edition will receive as favorable reception as the first by technologists and practitioners alike. I anticipate that the book will gain an excellent reputation as a standard guide in electrodiagnostic medicine. I take great pride in knowing that the volume is the product of my colleagues in Iowa and hope that its use will not only enhance the electrodiagnostic evaluation but also encourage research and teaching in the field of clinical neurophysiology.

Jun Kimura, MD
Professor Emeritus
Kyoto University, Kyoto
Professor Emeritus
Department of Neurology
University of Iowa Hospitals and Clinics
Iowa City, Iowa

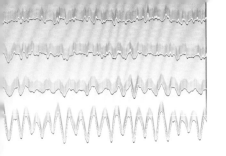

Preface

Our involvement in teaching both NDT (electroneurodiagnostic technology) and Neurology residency programs since the 1970s has enabled us to experience the evolution and progression of electroencephalography (EEG) and related fields. It is to that end that we have seen the need for a second edition of *Practical Guide to Clinical Neurophysiologic Testing – EEG*. In recent years, a new subspecialty has evolved in Neurodiagnostics called Continuous Critical Care EEG (CCEEG) monitoring. There has been a tremendous call for this long-term recording especially since the advent of digital EEG equipment. In this second edition, we included many video-EEG recordings since EEG of any type is a very dynamic science, therefore, to view it as a "moving picture" rather than as a time limited, static presentation is important. Studies have documented that many patients in the ICU, both comatose and awake, have intermittent neurologic events that can be captured with this new technology, thus improving patient outcomes. We hope this new chapter will be useful as you begin to delve into CCEEG.

The second edition of the textbook also gave us an opportunity to add new nomenclature and new standards recommended by The American Clinical Neurophysiology Society (ACNS). You will be able to access about 60 videos on topics from artifacts to seizures. The videos are on line, and you have the access code under the scratch off tag inside the front cover.

Initially, the first edition of this book was intended primarily for education of EEG/NDT technologists, but we realized that the book was also useful for neurology residents, clinical neurophysiology fellows, and also general neurologists because any physicians who interprets EEGs should also know the technical aspects of the recording in order to provide accurate and appropriate interpretation and to avoid misinterpretation of EEG data.

We would like to thank Malcom Yeh, MD, the late Peter Seaba, MS, and Michael Ciliberto, MD, who provided their expertise and experience in particular chapters. Additionally, the book would be nothing if not for the EEG samples recorded by the very talented University of Iowa neurodiagnostic technologists: Marjorie Tucker, CNIM/CLTM/R.EEG T./EP T., Deanne Tadlock, R.EEG T./CLTM, Jada Frank, R.EEG T./CNIM, Prairie Seivert, R.EEG T., CNIM, Tom Wiersema, R.EEG T./CNIM, Kassy Jacobs, R.EEG T./CNIM, Sara Davis, R.EEG T., Holly Heiden, R.EEG T., Lori Grant, R.EEG T.

We are also indebted to our patients who provided important and useful data which we use for teaching and the advancement of clinical neurophysiological science.

Lastly, we would like to acknowledge our spouses, Patti and John, whose love and support allowed us the time we needed to work on this project.

Thoru Yamada, MD

Elizabeth Meng, BA, R. EEG/EP T.

Contents

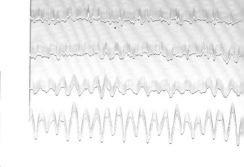

Online Videos: Practical Guide for Clinical Neurophysiologic Testing · EEG

Chapter 4

Video 4-1 For a more dynamic view of alias signals, view the video that demonstrates how analogue signals are recorded and represented in digitized form.

Chapter 7

Video 7-1A An example of unusually prominent and frequent Lambda waves in 30-year-old woman when she was reading a brochure. Note repetitive sharply contoured positive discharges at O1 and O2 electrodes (channels shown with red tracings)

Video 7-1B This is the same patient as in Video 7-1A, showing frequent POST in stage 2 (N2*) sleep. Note the similarity of Lambda in awake and POST in sleep.

Video 7-2 An example of K-complex triggered by click noise during stage 2(N2*) sleep.

Chapter 9

Video 9-1 Subject is a normal 25 year old woman. Hyperventilation produced prominent delta build-up, which is a normal finding, although the degree of build-up was more prominent than usually seen for this age subject.

Video 9-2 An 8-year-old otherwise healthy girl presenting with staring spell noted by teacher and parents. Technologist asked her to hyperventilate. She started to hyperventilate (frame 12:42:55). Within 20 seconds of the start of hyperventilation, EEG started to show 3 Hz, generalized rhythmic spike-wave bursts (frame 12:42:12). This is typical EEG feature for absence seizure. She then stopped hyperventilation and her eyes were open with a staring gaze. Technologist asked the patient to remember the word "butterfly" during the episode. The spike-wave burst lasted about 20 seconds and the patient quickly returned to a normal state but she was unable to recall the correct word (butterfly) given during the episode.

Video 9-3 Patient was a 12-year-old female with a history of generalized shaking since the age of 15 months. Her older sister was diagnosed with absence seizures. EEG showed photoparoxysmal discharges with generalized spike-wave burst at 9 Hz photic stimulation. The photic stimulation was quickly stopped after the discharges. Note slow-wave discharges continued after the cessation of photic stimulation. The photoparoxysmal discharges were repeatedly produced by 9 Hz photic stimulation. No other EEG abnormality was found.

Chapter 10

Video 10-1 Patient was a 30-year-man with a diagnosis of complex partial epilepsy (focal seizure with impaired awareness) since age 14. MRI showed right hippocampal sclerosis. The ictal discharges started with rhythmic sharply contoured delta of about 3 Hz arising from right temporal region. Within a few seconds, the patient was aware of impending seizure (aura) and pushed the event button. By then the rhythmic delta activity was more widely spread, yet still right>left. The EEG technologist came in and asked several questions to which the patient seemingly responded correctly but his behavior was not quite normal.

Video 10-2 Patient was a 62-year-old woman presenting with episodes of confusion which started about 3 years ago. She was amnestic for these episodes. MRI was unremarkable. Interictal discharges consisted of well-defined spike discharges from right temporal region, maximum at the anterior temporal electrode (see Fig. 10-9). Seizure started while she was talking on the phone. The ictal discharges started with rhythmic, sharply contoured theta bursts from right hemisphere (frame 16:55:24). The theta bursts progressively became larger toward the end of seizure. The seizure ended at frame 18:55:50. During the event, she continued to talk on the phone carrying on a seemingly normal conversation.

Video 10-3A&B Patient was 35-year-old woman with a long history of complex partial seizure. MRI showed left hippocampal atrophy (shown by circles; compare left and right), consistent with mesial sclerosis (Video 13A). EEG showed ictal discharges started with beta activity, maximum at left posterior temporal region (first frame) with subsequent spread along with bilateral diffuse rhythmic sharp discharges from parasagittal region (2nd frame). This was followed by left>right rhythmic sharply contoured delta activity (middle of 3rd frame to 5th frame). The ictal event stopped at 6th frame (Video110-3A). The same patient had another seizure while in sleep (Video 110-3B). The ictal event started shortly after the interictal spike from <u>left</u> temporal region (middle of 2nd frame) with beta activity from <u>right</u> hemisphere. This was followed by rhythmic spikes involving mainly right hemisphere (3rd frame) when the patient raised right arm with repetitive hand motion (automatism). Subsequently the ictal discharges evolved to right>left rhythmic delta/theta pattern. The ictal event stopped at 7th frame.

Video 10-4 Patient was a 16 year old boy presenting with episodes of body stiffening, staring and lip smacking which started about 2 years ago. The spells usually occurred during sleep. The seizure captured during this EEG started shortly after arousal from N3 sleep. The ictal discharges started with 2.5 Hz rhythmic delta of frontal dominance, along with increased tonic muscle artifact (the patient was not moving during the onset of ictal delta activity). Then the patient showed rhythmic axial body shaking. Although EEG was partly contaminated by movement and muscle artifacts, the rhythmic delta activity was not artifacts because the delta frequency was not synchronous with movements. The delta discharges became progressively slower toward the end of seizure t artifacts. The seizure lasted about 30 seconds and postictal EEG showed diffuse slow delta (~1Hz) which was slower than expected for N3 sleep. About ~1 minute after the seizure, the EEG seemed to return to N3 sleep. This type of seizure cannot be differentiated from a type of parasomnia such as body rocking without capturing the spell by video EEG recording.

Video 10-5A Patient was a 53-year-old man with a history of traumatic brain injury in childhood. The first seizure was 7 years ago with apparent tonic–clonic convulsion. Most of his seizures were preceded by visual hallucination. MRI was unremarkable. EEG showed mild delta slowing at the occipital region, left>right. When EEG started to show small spikes from left occipital region, he felt the sensation of seizure and pushed the event marker (frame 17:00:55) and he prepared himself by lowering the head of bed for impending seizure. Recurrent spike discharges from left occipital region became clear when muscle artifacts decreased (frame 17:01:29). The nurse's appropriate questions and interaction with the patient helped to recognize his seizure semiology. He stated to the nurse "Light show is going" pointing the right lower visual field (frame 17:01:38). He was able to describe clearly what he was seeing. Also, he was able to follow the nurse's commands while repetitive recurring spikes continued. Up to this point, the seizure can be classified as simple partial seizure or focal seizure with awareness*.

Video 10-5B This is continuation of the same seizure of Video 10-5A (3 minutes and 16 seconds after the last frame). EEG now changed to slower and larger spike-wave bursts associated with the more generalized theta/delta slow waves. The patient then became confused and did not respond to the nurse's questions. Along with increased generalized rhythmic spike-wave bursts, his face started twitching (not seen) (frame 17:07:56). This case shows an example of simple partial seizure (focal seizure with awareness**) changing to complex partial seizure (focal seizure with impaired awareness**).

Video 10-6 Patient was an 11-year-old boy with initial presentation of tonic–clonic convulsion at school. His mother also noted occasional spells of staring which started about 6 months ago. She stated that he could speak through these spells and continues his activities with eyelid fluttering. Shortly after hyperventilation, EEG started to show generalized rhythmic polyspike-wave bursts with initial frequency of 4 to 5 Hz, which progressively slowed down to 2 to 3 Hz spike-wave bursts. This pattern is characteristic for juvenile absence and different from classical absence seizures (compare with Video 9-2). Also, the patient was not totally out of contact during this episode. Note also, occipitally predominant RDA* or OIRD just before (frame 09:08:34) and right after (frame 09:08:51) the spike-wave bursts.

Video 10-7 Patient was a 7-year-old boy with spells of unresponsiveness which can be self-induced by looking at flashing light or interrupting bright light by shaking hand with spread fingers in front of him. The parents also noticed eyelid fluttering, especially with eye closing. EEG showed episodes of bifrontally dominant polyspike-wave bursts, which were consistently exacerbated by photic stimulation. Immediately after the 5 Hz photic stimulation, there was a brief generalized polyspike-wave burst, which was followed by slight arm jerking. With continued photic stimulation, generalized 2.5 Hz spike-wave burst appeared, which was associated with eyelid twitching (not shown). These features were characteristic for Jeavons syndrome.

Video 10-8 Patient is a 47-year-old man with a long history of tonic–clonic convulsions since the age of 14. MRI was normal. EEG for seizure onset was totally obscured by tonic muscle artifacts. The patient vocalized with tonic limb posturing, which was followed by clonic movement. In-between the muscle artifacts, EEG appeared to show diffuse slowing. Postictally, the patient was unresponsive with some background slowing.

Video 10-9 Patient was a 10-month-old baby girl presenting with episodes of "tenses up her whole body" noted by her parents. MRI showed diffuse cortical atrophy and delayed myelination. Prior to seizure, EEG showed high amplitude and diffuse irregular delta slow waves (frame 13:35:59). There were large delta slow waves followed by sudden flattening EEG pattern (electrodecremental seizure) when baby showed sudden forward motion with arm bending posturing (Salaam spasms) at frame 13:36:07.

Video 10-10 Patient was a 44-year-old woman presenting with a history of generalized tonic–clonic convulsions which started at the age of 22. Patient denies any warning sign (aura) before seizure. MRI was unremarkable. Prior to seizure, EEG showed bilaterally diffuse, frontal dominant polyspikes which are slightly right>left (note phase reversal at FP2 in frame 09:57:26). With seizure onset, the patient vocalized with head turning to right and right arm jerking (frame 09:57:37). EEG was then obscured by clonic then tonic muscle artifacts. During clonic phase (frame 09:58:34), diffuse delta/theta slowing was evident, seen during artifact free moments. Postictally, EEG showed marked flattening. This is likely focal onset secondary generalized tonic–clonic convulsion.

Video 10-11 Patient was a 20-year-old man who had first seizure 2 years ago, presenting with initial dizziness followed by loss of consciousness and generalized tonic–clonic convulsion. MRI was unremarkable. The seizure started when the technologist was present. Just prior to the onset of seizure, EEG showed right>left frontal dominant generalized spikes (frame 08:58:28). The ictal onset was sudden generalized flatting, which was followed by generalized spike-wave bursts (right>left) and somewhat irregular diffuse delta slow waves (frame 08:58:33). This was followed by rhythmic right>left sharp delta bursts. At this moment, the astute technologist noticed that the patient started having seizure and asked questions (frame 08:58:39). The patient was unresponsive, and EEG was showing generalized rhythmic spike-wave bursts (frame 08:58:56), which became progressively more prominent subsequently, changing to polyspike-wave bursts (08:59:02). His head started turning to right (frame 08:59:07), which was followed by generalized tonic–clonic convulsion (frame 08:59:13) and then tonic posturing (frame 08:59:30). EEG was then totally obscured by muscle artifacts. Postictally, EEG changed to burst suppression pattern with bursts consisting of generalized irregular polyspike waves. This case is an example of partial complex seizure (focal seizure with impaired awareness**) with secondary generalized tonic–clonic convulsion.

Video 10-12 Patient was a 22-year-old woman with a long history of seizure since the age of 2 when she had an intraparenchymal hemorrhage. CT scan showed scattered areas of increased attenuation consistent with old calcifications likely from her intraparenchymal hemorrhage at age 2. Ictal EEG captured while the patient was sleeping showed the onset of ictal event with gamma range fast activity initially arising from left frontotemporal region (frame 13:18:21). This was followed by beta activity then evolving to repetitive spikes with wider spread. The ictal discharges quickly generalized but maintained left>right prominence. Toward the end of seizure, the ictal pattern changed to repetitive spike-wave bursts, left>right, which progressively slowed down (frame 13:18:38). The ictal event lasted less than 30 seconds. Despite ictal discharges becoming generalized, the patient showed no observable clinical change. The patient moved slightly after the seizure ended (frame 13:18:46).

Video 10-13 Patient was a 22-year-old male with history of focal onset secondary generalized tonic-clonic convulsions. In addition, the patient has brief but frequent partial seizures consisting of giggling and laughing with some confusion or unresponsiveness. These spells occur either in sleep or in awake state. Neurological examination and Brain MRI were normal. The ictal event captured in awake state showed the onset of bifrontal dormant beta with progressive slowing in frequency. The seizure lasted only about 10seconds. The patient showed smiling with giggling sound.

Video 10-14   Patient was a 52-year-old man with a long history of intractable epilepsy, with mostly generalized tonic–clonic convulsions. MRI was unremarkable except for mild cortical atrophy. EEG showed intermittent brief episodes of sudden onset of generalized beta activity followed by rhythmic, sharply contoured theta discharges changing to rhythmic sharp-wave bursts (frame 01:29:35) before ending the ictal discharges (frame 01:29:44). EKG rate was 60/minute (1/1 second) before the ictal event which progressively slowed to 20/minute (1/3 seconds). The ictal event lasted about 10 seconds, and EEG quickly normalized with recovery of EKG rate (frame 01:29:44).

Video 10-15   Patient was an 18-year-old female presenting with syncopal episodes often preceded by dizziness. These episodes tended to occur while standing up. About 1½ minutes after tilting table raised up, EKG rate started to drop from approximately 100 beats/minute to 30 beats/minute (with 2 seconds asystole) when her head dropped (frame 11:11:15). EEG then started to show diffuse, bifrontal dominant delta. The prominent delta activity continued for about 25 seconds, and then EEG activity started to recover, though EKG rate remained bradycardia (~60/second) for a while as compared to the rate before syncope.

Chapter 11

Video 11-1A   An example of EEG changes due to cerebral ischemia shown by ligation of internal carotid artery during endarterectomy surgery. The right internal carotid was clamped at the mark "Clamp on" in the first frame 10:46:28. Within 20 seconds after the clamp, EEG started to be depressed on the right hemisphere (frame 10:46:48).

Video 11-1B   The surgeon placed a shunt in at frame 10:50:28 to restore the carotid circulation. EEG then gradually recovered and returned nearly to baseline at frame 10:52:05.

Video 11-2   An example of EEG changes after Propofol injection for induction of anesthesia. EEG started with waking record. In the middle of first frame (09:47:13), anesthesia staff started IV injection of Propofol. Within a few seconds of the injection, EEG started to show slowing and prominent diffuse delta slow waves (middle of frame 09:47:21). Delta waves became progressively slower (from 3 to 0.5 Hz) (frame 09:47:21 to 09:47:47), and then EEG changed to burst suppression pattern (frame 09:47:55). It took only about 40 seconds after the injection to achieve burst suppression.

Chapter 13

Video 13-1   Patient was a 69-year-old female presenting with shortness of breath and mental status changes. CT scan showed multiple scattered infarctions in the posterior fossa as well as left and right middle cerebral and anterior cerebral artery territories, consistent with embolic infarcts. EEG started on the same day of admission. While the patient remained in coma, EEG showed continuous, generalized sharp discharges without evolution or significant incidences (GPD*).

Video 13-2A   Patient was a 78-year-old male with a history of left middle cerebral artery aneurysm clipping 20 years ago with subsequent right hemiparesis, expressive aphasia, and seizure disorder. Prior to this admission, he was found to be confused and had generalized tonic–clonic convulsion. EEG recording started on the day of admission. EEG showed periodically recurring bursts of irregular polyspike-waves from left hemisphere (PLEDs/LPD+F*) with greater prominence in the temporal region. Occasionally, the bursts had a longer duration, becoming close to a BIRD pattern (frame 03:31:21). The ictal events started with continuously recurring polyspike-wave bursts from left temporal region (03:31:38). This evolved to a greater degree of polyspike-waves, involving also the parietal region (frame 03:31:55). Subsequently, the ictal discharges faded, first at the parietal discharges (frame 03:32:29) and then at the temporal region (frame 03:32:37). There was no observable

clinical change, and therefore, this was consistent with nonconvulsive seizure.

Video 13-2B   Patient was a 57-year-old male found unconscious at home. He was found to have left intraparenchymal hemorrhage. EEG started after surgical evacuation of hematoma. EEG showed continuous PLEDs/LPD+F* pattern from left hemisphere. Periodic discharges from parietal and temporal regions were asynchronous but time locked between the two discharges with temporal discharges consistently leading parietal discharges by 200 to 500 msec. The ictal event started with serial polyspike-wave discharges from left temporal region while the parietal discharges maintained a periodic pattern (frame 15:39:43). When temporal discharges started to slow down, parietal discharges changed to an ictal pattern with serial polyspike-wave bursts (frame 15:40:00). As temporal ictal discharges further slowed down, parietal discharges also slowed down and ended at almost the same time (15:40:51). There was no observable clinical change, and therefore, this was consistent with nonconvulsive seizure.

Video 13-3A   Patient was a 63-year-old female with a history of high-grade follicular lymphoma admitted with mental status changes and possible seizures. The diagnosis was chemotherapy (Ifosfamide)-induced encephalopathy. EEG started on the second day of admission. Before SIRPID started, EEG showed diffuse slow (0.5 to 1 Hz) delta with intermittent low-voltage theta waves (frame 18:01:10). With the increased muscle artifact and arousal (frame 18:01:27), EEG started to show more theta background activity. Subsequently, diffuse and intermittent triphasic sharp-wave discharges appeared. Unlike the patient in Video 13-3B, the triphasic discharges remained sporadic and never became fully rhythmic or continuous. The triphasic discharges progressively decreased, and eventually, EEG returned close to baseline with the decrease of muscle artifact (after frame 18:04:09).

Video 13-3B   Patient was an 89-year-old female presenting with confusion and was found to have intraparenchymal hemorrhage. EEG started on the same day of admission. EEG showed diffuse theta/delta slowing with some interspersed scattered minor sharp transients when the patient was resting quietly. Whenever she was aroused by others or spontaneously evidenced by an increase in muscle artifact, EEG showed initially brief generalized suppression, followed by recurrent generalized triphasic sharp-wave discharges (frame 22:59:05). These triphasic discharges became progressively more prominent, rhythmic and continuous as the patient became more aroused evidenced by seemingly purposeful movement (adjusting pillow at frame 22:59:48). The triphasic waves became more "spiky" consisting of spike-wave bursts and could be considered to be nonconvulsive seizure (frame 23:00:30 to 23:01:01). As the muscle artifact decreased, the paroxysmal discharges subsided (after frame 23:01:13).

Video 13-4   Patient was a 52-year-old male presenting with a problem in speaking and found to have intracranial hemorrhage in the left frontal lobe. EEG showed semirhythmic delta from the left frontal region, which became progressively more rhythmic and higher amplitude with wider spread (LRDA). The focal delta activity became more sharply contoured and eventually evolved to a sharp and wave complex. Since the patient did not show any motor sign, the pattern was consistent with nonconvulsive focal seizure.

Video 13-5   Patient was a 57-year-old male presenting with confusion and difficulty with complex tasks and found to have a brain tumor in the right temporal region originating from the right sphenoid. EEG was started one day after surgery. The EEG showed frequently recurring irregular polyspike-wave bursts from the right central and mid-temporal region. Each burst lasted 2 to 4 seconds (BIRD). The similar discharges became intermittently more prolonged and more rhythmic, consistent with electrographic seizure. Note that DSA indicated numerous BIRDs interspersed by true ictal events expressed by thicker lines during a 4-hour segment. There was no observable clinical change associated with ictal discharges and therefore it is consistent with nonconvulsive seizure.

Video 13-6A&B Patient was a 65-year-old man with a history of brain tumor resection from the left temporal lobe about 30 years ago and subsequent seizures. He was admitted with acute encephalopathy and the EEG showed recurrent electrographic seizures. Initially, 2 to 5 ictal events were recorded every 4 hours. Each ictal discharge started with sharply contoured rhythmic theta bursts from the left temporal region, maximum at the anterior temporal electrode. Shortly after the onset of ictal discharges, apparently there was a change in respiration giving an alarm signal. After the alarm signal, there was an increase of muscle artifact, and the EEG started to show increased slower theta slow waves bilaterally. Each ictal event lasted about ½ to 1 second, and the sequence of each event was similar from one seizure to another (A&B). In this case, the only clinical signs of seizure were a change in respiration pattern and increase of muscle tone.

Video 13-7 Patient was a 61-year-old male who had cardiac arrest following cervical trauma. EEG showed burst suppression pattern with prolonged suppression period lasting 20 to 50 seconds. The burst was associated with vigorous head jerking; thus, it was not possible to differentiate EEG bursts from the movement artifacts. A paralyzing agent (Rocuronium) was given at the frame of 10:43:02. After muscle artifacts were completely eliminated, the bursts consisting of generalized polyspike and spike-wave continued without muscle artifacts, verifying that the patient was having myoclonic seizures associated with burst suppression pattern.

Video 13-8 Patient was a 65-year-old male with a history of stroke in the left hemisphere 2 years ago who presented with right arm twitching. EEG showed diffuse slowing in the background activity and intermittent, nearly periodically recurring well-defined focal spikes from the left hemisphere, maximum at the parietal region. Associated with each spike, right arm jerking occurred, consistent with epilepsia partialis continua. The events continued for hours.

Video 13-9 Patient was a 50-year-old female presenting with shaking spells. The patient had multiple shaking spells captured by video EEG. With rhythmic shaking of body and head, EEG showed rhythmic diffuse theta bursts, synchronous with the shaking frequency. Close scrutiny of the waveform distribution, however, showed double and triple phase reversal at F3, C3, and P3 (frame 19:19:03), supporting that these theta bursts were artifact. This event was detected falsely as a high probability seizure by computer program (see Fig. 13-4B).

Video 13-10A This is the patient from case 4. EEG started to show small periodically recurring small sharp transients from the left hemisphere. These small sharp discharges evolved to periodic spikes, maximum at the left parietal/posterior-temporal region, which progressively grew to higher amplitude and wider spread spikes. Eventually, spikes became spike and polyspike-waves toward the end of this ictal event. There was no clinical change associated with the ictal event, thus it was consistent with nonconvulsive focal seizure.

Video 13-10B In another occasion, the same patient seen in Video 13-10A (case 4) showed more prominent epileptiform/ictal activity. This started with periodic spikes arising from the same location as of Video13-10A. The spike discharges became polyspikes at frame of 05:10:14. The ictal discharges progressively became more polyspikes with higher amplitude, wider spread and faster frequency (frame 05:10:48). At frame of 05:11:22, repetitive muscle twitch artifacts appeared, and subsequently, there were visible muscle twitches of right hand and mouth, synchronized with spike-wave discharges. Poetically, there was EEG flattening, left>right.

Video 13-11 This is the same patient shown in Figure 13-14. Prior to the ictal event, EEG showed diffuse theta/delta slowing with slightly higher amplitude on the left hemisphere than the right. There were intermittent sharp discharges from left hemisphere, maximum at the parietal region. These discharges gradually increased in amplitude and incidence with recruiting beta activity. The ictal event consisting of polyspike waves progressively became rhythmic with increased amplitude and wider spread. Toward the end of seizure, the frequency of spike-wave bursts slowed down. The patient showed no movement, consistent with nonconvulsive seizure.

Video 13-12 Patient was a 61-year-old female with a past medical history of end-stage liver disease with cirrhosis secondary to hepatitis C. She presented with acute mental status change and generalized tonic–clonic convulsions. By the time ccEEG was started, she was in a comatose state and EEG showed recurrent electrographic seizures without visible clinical changes. The ictal events started with increased beta activity with interspersed spikes from the left posterior head region. As the seizure progressed, beta activity increased in incidence and amplitude (frame 09:06:48). With the increase of beta activity from the left, sporadically and independently occurring sharp and spike discharges from the right hemisphere (maximum at temporal electrodes) started to increase (frame 09:07:02) but remained as an interictal pattern. When the beta activity from the left posterior head region started to fade (frame 09:09:14), beta activity appeared from the left anterior temporal region, which was followed by increased spike and sharp discharges from the right hemisphere. The left-sided seizure ended at frame 09:09:43, when recurrent sharp discharges from the right continued and intermittently increased. Starting around frame 09:10:56, interictal spike and sharp discharges occurred independently from left and right hemispheres. Then the beta discharges started to appear from the right posterior head region as an independent ictal event (frame 09:11:10), while left-sided sharp and spike discharges became a more frequent and periodic pattern (PLEDs/LPD*). The right-sided beta progressively became more prominent with wider spread and higher amplitude. This ictal event started to fade becoming more polyspike-wave burst at frame 09:14:35. Immediately at the end of the right-sided ictal event, beta ictal pattern started again from the left posterior head region. This "see-saw game" continued intermittently for several hours until more vigorous treatment was started. There was no clinical change associated with these ictal events (nonconvulsive seizures).

Chapter 15

Video 15-1A Vertical eye movement monitors with eyes open and closed (*blink*): with eyes closing or blinking. Fp1/Fp2 electrodes (*black*) show positive (downward) deflection (due to eyeballs moving upward) (see Fig. 8-16), while infraorbital electrodes (X1, X2, Pink tracings) show negative (downward) deflection. Opposite to these deflections is true for eye opening. Note that left and right lateral cantus electrodes, one above (PG1) and one below (PG2) the eye level (shown by) brown tracings, show opposite polarity between left and right either eyes opening or closing.

Video 15-1B Lateral eye movement with left and right lateral gazing: with looking to the left, F7 becomes positive (downward) deflection and F8 becomes negative (upward deflection). Opposite to this deflection is true for looking to the right. Left and right lateral cantus electrodes show opposite polarities between the two either for right or left gazing.

Video 15-2A This subject (one of our EEG technologists) has a special talent, capable of blinking very rapidly (eyelids fluttering) to the alpha frequency range. With fluttering, Fp1/Fp2 electrodes record alpha frequency activity, while maintaining the same polarity rules for eye blinks (same as shown in Video 15-1A), indicating eye balls go upward with each blink.

Video 15-2B This subject is even able to control the frequency of eye blinking from slow to fast.

Video 15-3 An example of glossokinetic potential created by vocalizing "la,la,la…". This shows 4 Hz frontal dominant activity with greater amplitude at infraorbital electrodes (X1, X2) than Fp electrodes. Note that the blink artifacts show opposite polarities between Fp and infraorbital electrodes. Also left and right outer canthus electrodes (Pg1/PG2) register opposite polarity for eye blinking but the same polarity for glossokinetic potential.

Video 15-4 Difference between glossokinetic potential and frontal delta activity. At the frame of 15:48:27:35, this patient swallowed a few times associated with diffuse delta slow waves (glossokinetic potential) with almost equal amplitude between Fp1/Fp2 (*green*) and infraorbital electrodes (PG1/Pg2 *red*). Toward the end of this video (15:49:09), there were diffuse frontal dominant delta slow waves with the greater amplitude at FP1/Fp2 than at infraorbital electrodes. This was frontal delta activity. Note that the patient did not swallow with this event.

Video 15-5 Pulse artifacts stopped by body/head movement. At the frame of 05:55:42, there was rhythmic delta frequency activity coinciding with ECG rate at F7 and Pg2 (or A2) electrode, indicating pulse artifacts. In the next frame, the patient moved and pulse artifact at F7 electrode disappeared but not at Pg2 (or A2) electrode. This indicates that the pulse artifacts may alter depending on the head position in relationship with electrode locations.

Video 15-6 Respiration artifacts associated with gasping in a comatose patient on ventilator. This was obviously due to vigorous head movement.

Video 15-7 The respiration artifact consisting of complex and various waveforms with each respiration. Careful observation showed each abdominal movement coincided with frontal dominant sharply contoured theta/delta bursts. The waveforms were not exactly the same and could be easily mistaken as the periodic EEG discharges. The respiration artifacts were verified by disconnecting the ventilation tube temporally, observing the disappearance of the periodic artifacts. Because there was no notable head or body movement associated with respiration, it is unlikely that the artifacts were due to head movement. It is more likely due to movement of water bubble accumulated in the ventilation tube.

Video 15-8 These respiration artifacts may be created by bubbling water in ventilation tube. Note that the water bubble was moving back and forth with respirations. Also note that the waveform of each respiration artifact differed from one to the other. The last portion of frame at 06:57:13 showed that artifact disappeared when the ventilation tube was moved.

Video 15-9 The artifacts by Parkinson tremor with head shaking at about 5 Hz associated with muscle artifacts. Note that delta activity showed double phase reversal at F4 and C4 (see also Fig. 15-22).

Video 15-10 The artifacts produced by body/head shaking. The rhythmic 3.5 Hz delta from right parasagittal region can be verified to be artifacts by finding the triple double reversal at F4 and C4 electrodes, supporting that these slow waves were not EEG activity.

Video 15-11 The artifacts produced by hands tapping showing at left parasagittal region. The artifact was more involved at F3 electrode, which was likely due to higher impedance evidenced by 60 Hz artifacts at F3 electrode. The artifacts can be verified by double phase reversals at F3 and P3.

Video 15-12 The artifacts produced by nurse attempting to stimulate the patient's respiration by patting the chest. This produced rhythmic theta bursts, which showed double phase reversal at F3 and P3, supporting these were artifacts.

Video 15-13 The artifacts produced by mother rocking baby's right temporal electrodes. The artifactual waves showed triple phase reversal at F8, T4, and T6.

Video 15-14 The artifacts produced by bed shaking for respiratory stimulation in semicomatose patient. The artifacts occur with the same frequency as the bed vibration and appeared mainly on T5, O1, and O2 electrodes with intermittent double phase reversal at T5 and O1 electrodes. The same artifacts were seen at ECG (X1-X2) electrodes. When the frequency of bed shaking became faster (frame 04:45:56), only ECG channel picked up the artifacts.

Video 15-15 The artifacts induced by unknown medical device, which produced a squeaking noise. With the onset of noise, 4 Hz artifacts were induced to the channels with high impedance (channels 6, 7, 13, and 16 evidenced by the presence of 60 Hz artifacts). Unlike the movement-induced artifacts, there was no double or triple phase reversal (check channels 6, 7, and 8).

Video 15-16 The artifacts induced by dialysis device. This produced regularly recurring electrode "pop"-like artifact at a rate about 1.5 Hz ain channels 3 and 6 shown in red tracings. (This cannot be electrode "pop" because of two channels with synchronous occurrence). At the end of frame 12:04:12, there was a click sound indicating that dialysis was switched off when the artifacts stopped. The switch box was placed back on the patient's bed by nurse, seen at the end of the last frame.

Video 15-17 Sixty Hz interference artifacts induced by the cell phone being charged. When the patient was holding the cell phone that was being charged in his hand, 60 Hz artifacts were introduced, mostly to the channels with high impedance. The artifacts disappeared when the patient disconnected charging power cable.

Chapter 16

Video 16-1 Patient was a 36/37 weeks (gestational age) baby girl presenting with respiratory failure and respiratory acidosis. Neurological examination revealed normal muscle tone and strength with symmetrical movement of all extremities. EEG recording started one day after birth. Along with EEG recording, vital signs of SaO_2 (%, *blue line*), heart rate (bpm, *pink*), and respiration rate (rpm, *green*) were simultaneously measured. Resting EEG included awake and active and quiet sleep were appropriate for age. Seizures occurred mostly in quiet sleep showing trace alternant. Prior to the onset of ictal discharges, baby showed some wiggling leg movements. The ictal event started with repetitive sharp discharges arising from left occipital electrode (frame 08:37:17). The discharges became progressively faster with greater amplitude and wider spread to left temporal and also right occipital electrode (frame 08:37:28). As spike discharges spread more widely, the ictal discharges became rhythmic spike-wave bursts with progressive slower frequency. Up to this point, SaO_2 remained above 95%, heart rate above 150 bpm, and respiration rate above 30 rpm. As seizure progressed, respiration rate and heart rate progressively slowed down and SaO_2 started to fall below 90% (frame 08:38:01). As the ictal discharges started to fade, SaO_2 dropped below 80%, and bag mask ventilation was started (frame 08:38:12). SaO_2 dropped to 74% and reparation rate fell to 11 rpm (frame 08:38:35). Toward the end of ictal event, SaO_2, heart rate, and respiration rates started to recover (frame 08:38:46) and seizure ended at frame 08:38:57. But after the ictal event was over, SaO_2, respiration rate, and heart rate started to drop again, which required another bag mask ventilation, when EEG showed relative suppression possibly due to postictal phase (frame 08:39:08 to 08:39:30). At the frame 08:39:53, SaO_2 and respiration rate returned to above 95%, 150 bpm and 40 rpm, respectively.

Introduction: History and Perspective of Clinical Neurophysiologic Diagnostic Tests

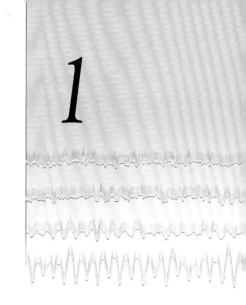

THORU YAMADA and ELIZABETH MENG

Early History of Electroencephalogram and Related Fields

In 1875, Richard Caton (Fig. 1-1), a physiologist from the Royal Infirmary School of Medicine, Liverpool, England, successfully recorded electrical activity from an animal brain.[1] He reported his experiments in the *British Medical Journal*.[2] His paper stated that "…the galvanometer has indicated the existence of electrical currents. The external surface of the gray matter is usually positive in relationship to the surface of section through it…." This was the first description of electrical activity from animal brains. After Caton's discoveries, electroencephalogram (EEG) work shifted to Eastern Europe. Caton's work remained unrecognized for the next 25 years because at that time, communication in the scientific world was extremely slow. In 1890, Adolf Beck, from the Jagiellonian University in Krakow, Poland, found oscillatory potentials when recording between two electrodes placed on the occipital cortex of a rabbit. Unaware of Caton's earlier work, he claimed to be the first to discover animal brain electrical activity. Interestingly,

there was another twist to the EEG history. There was another physiologist, Fleischl von Marxow, from the University of Vienna, who also described similar brain electrical activity in animals and deposited his findings in a sealed envelope at the Imperial Academy of Science of Vienna in 1883. Depositing a sealed envelope containing scientific discoveries pending confirmation was a common custom in the European scientific community at that time. Obviously, he was also unaware of Caton's work.

When Beck's article appeared in the German journal, *Centralblatt*, in 1890,[3] it caught von Marxow's eye and allowed him to open the sealed envelope deposited in 1883. Beck and von Marxow then started to argue, each claiming to be the first to discover brain electrical activity. Noticing the argument of these two esteemed physiologists, Caton settled the argument with a letter that stated: "In the year 1875, I gave a presentation before the Physiological Section of the British Medical Association in which electrical currents of the brain in warm-blooded animals were demonstrated and…. May I be permitted to draw your attention to the following publication (*Br Med J*. 1875; 2:278)…. I have published this, so I think it must be conceded that I am already an earlier discoverer." This letter settled the argument, and Caton was accepted as the first to discover brain electrical activity in animals.

After this discovery, more than 50 years had passed when Hans Berger (Fig. 1-2) first described electrical activity from electrodes placed on the human scalp. Berger was a psychiatrist from Jena, Germany, and was interested in objective measures of human brain function and the mind.[1] He postulated that there would be localized increase of blood flow and increased heat by chemical breakdown in the cortex in response to movement or sensory stimulation of extremities. Using crude techniques, such as plethysmography and thermometry, he attempted to demonstrate these changes. His hypothesis turned out to be amazingly correct and can be now demonstrated by positron emission tomography (PET), single photon emission computerized tomography (SPECT), and functional magnetic resonance imaging (fMRI). When he began to use electrical recordings, he was able to successfully record oscillatory potentials of around 10 hertz (Hz), which he called "alpha rhythm" (Fig. 1-3). He also found that alpha rhythm was best seen in an awake subject with closed eyes and it attenuated when the subject's eyes opened or the subject performed a mental task. His first paper appeared in 1929 and was titled "*Electroenkephalogram*

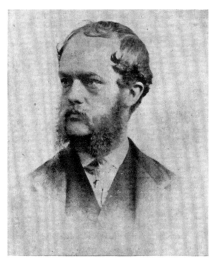

RICHARD CATON IN HIS THIRTIES—AT THE PERIOD OF HIS WORK ON THE ELECTRICAL ACTIVITY OF THE BRAIN

FIGURE 1-1 | Richard Caton, who first reported electrical activity from the animal brain in 1875.

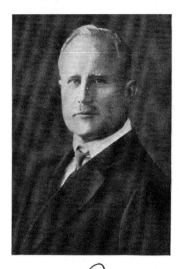

HANS BERGER (1873–1941), WHO FIRST RECORDED THE ELECTRICAL
ACTIVITY OF THE BRAIN IN MAN IN 1925
(From: Kolle, *Grosse Nervenärtze*)

FIGURE 1-2 | Hans Berger, who first reported electrical activity from the human brain in 1929.

des Menschen."[4] His "*Electroenkephalogram*" is now referred to as electroencephalogram in English. He subsequently found that the frequency of EEG activity slowed down during sleep or in disturbed consciousness. He postulated that electrical activity travels from one area to another through the process of mental activity, predicting the activity of the corticocortical network system during various brain functions. Berger's pioneering discoveries were at first received with skepticism, primarily because such a slow oscillation like alpha rhythm [having a duration of about 100 milliseconds (ms)] could not be explained by known electrical activity of the nervous system (i.e., action potentials, which have a duration of 1 to 2 ms). In 1935, however, prominent physiologists Adrian and Mathews, from England, finally approved Berger's work and apologized for their long disbelief, and called the EEG waves as "Berger rhythm."[5] Subsequently, the interest in EEG research

quickly spread all over the world. In 1936, there were six EEG laboratories in the United States. They were Brown University (H. Jasper), University of Iowa (J. Knott), Tuxedo Park in New York (A. Loomis), Boston University (W. Lennox), Harvard University (H. Davis), and Mayo Clinic (L. Yeager and D. Klass). As early as 1935, Gibbs et al.[6] discovered 3-Hz spike-wave discharges in association with absence seizures. In 1936, Jasper[7] found focal spikes in focal seizure. In the same year, Walter[8] found focal slowing corresponding to the site of a brain tumor. Since then, research and clinical application of EEG in various neurological diseases has made rapid progress and EEG has become an essential diagnostic tool in the field of clinical neurology, neurosurgery, and psychiatry.

Development of Evoked Potentials

The next major step forward in the diagnostic utility of clinical neurophysiology was the development of the evoked potential (EP) recording. The EP is an electrical potential recorded in response to an external stimulus: visual, auditory, or somatosensory. The amplitude of most EPs detected from scalp electrodes is usually very small [<10 microvolts (μV)] and considerably smaller than the ongoing spontaneous EEG activity (generally from 30 to 100 μV or more). The EP is thus buried under the ongoing activity and is not readily visible. An innovative method of extracting the EP from the ongoing EEG activity was first introduced by George Dawson[9] from London, England. He, at first, used a "photographic summation" technique by superimposing a number of photographed waveforms (which included both EP and ongoing EEG) in response to repeated external stimuli. This brought out the overall configuration of an EP waveform by minimizing the ongoing EEG activity. Later, he used an electronic summation technique (Fig. 1-4), which subsequently became the principle of the summation/averaging technique used today with computer technology. The smaller the EP response and the larger the noise (ongoing EEG activity or artifacts not related to the stimulus), the greater the number of summations required to extract a measurable and reliable response. Data gained from the various EPs, namely, visual (VEP), auditory (AEP), and somatosensory (SSEP), advanced the clinical applications of

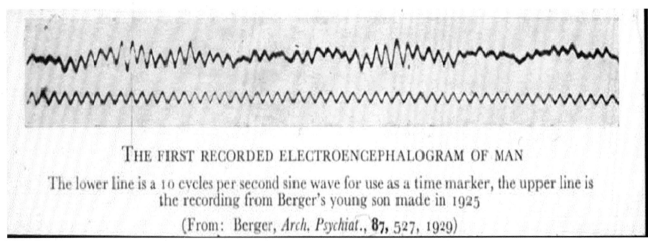

THE FIRST RECORDED ELECTROENCEPHALOGRAM OF MAN

The lower line is a 10 cycles per second sine wave for use as a time marker, the upper line is the recording from Berger's young son made in 1925

(From: Berger, *Arch. Psychiat.*, **87**, 527, 1929)

FIGURE 1-3 | The first photographic EEG recording in human by Hans Burger published in 1929. This showed sinusoidal 10-Hz rhythm, which he called "alpha rhythm."

PROCEEDINGS OF THE PHYSIOLOGICAL SOCIETY
19 MAY 1951

A summation technique for detecting small signals in a large irregular background. By G. DAWSON. *Neurological Research Unit, Medical Research Council, National Hospital, Qu Square, London, W.C.*1

The cerebral responses to nerve stimulation which can be picked up from the scalp in man small in relation to spontaneous activity of scalp muscle and brain. They have been detected superimposing a number of records; this emphasizes regular features, while the irregu background appears as a diffuse thickening of the whole trace (Dawson, 1947, 1950). I

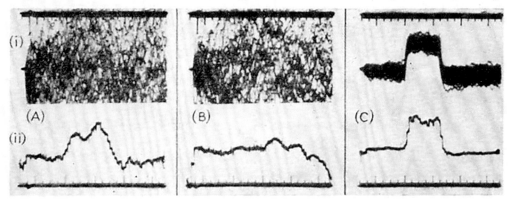

FIGURE 1-4 | This is first somatosensory-evoked potential after stimulation of ulnar nerve using electronic summation technique by George Dawson in 1951. There was clear difference between contralateral **(A)** and ipsilateral **(B)** responses to the side of stimulation.

EPs for various neurological disorders. EPs have been especially useful in the diagnosis of multiple sclerosis (MS). In MS, EPs tend to show abnormalities even if there are no clinical signs or symptoms relating to the examined EP modality. Also, EPs have become important tools for monitoring peripheral as well as central nervous system functions during surgery (intraoperative monitoring). The clinical applications of EPs were further facilitated by the introduction of the far-field potential (FFP).

Discovery of the Far-Field Potential

The concept of FFP was first developed by Jewett[10] who successfully recorded the small amplitude activity (<1 µV when recorded from the scalp) in response to auditory stimulation. The response consisted of several wavelets occurring within 10 ms following an auditory click. Because the latency of the response was so short, it was not understood at first as to how this response could be recorded from the scalp. Jewett then proposed that the multiple wavelets of the auditory response were generated at the brainstem. He postulated that the impulses passed through the various structures of the brainstem auditory pathway and they were picked up at the scalp via a volume conduction spread, rather than being transmitted via the anatomical auditory pathway within the brain. In other words, the scalp electrodes detected the potentials that were generated at a distance; thus the term "far-field potential" was introduced. The concept of FFP was revolutionary because up to that time, the potential recorded from a given electrode was assumed to be generated directly under or nearby that electrode (so-called

near-field potential). The short-latency auditory response was at first called the "Jewett bump" and is now referred to as the "brainstem auditory-evoked potential (BAEP)" or "auditory brainstem response (ABR)." With the use of FFP recording techniques, it became possible to measure the potentials arising from distant sites or deep within the brain tissue which were otherwise not accessible by a noninvasive recording technique.

The FFP was thought to represent the widely spread volume-conducted potential reflecting the advancing field of positivity when the traveling impulse (near-field potential) approaches the pickup electrode. When the BAEP was introduced, each wavelet of the BAEP was thought to be generated at a specific anatomical site, for example, wave I from the auditory nerve, wave II from the cochlear nucleus, wave III from the olivary nucleus, wave IV from the lateral lemniscus, and wave V from the inferior colliculus.[11] Although the above-presumed generator sources turned out to be not quite correct, BAEP reflects various levels of auditory pathway within the brainstem and allows us to evaluate brainstem functions noninvasively by surface electrodes. FFPs were also discovered in *somatosensory-evoked potentials*,[12] which have enabled us to examine the functions and integrity of the spinal cord, brainstem, and thalamus in the sensory system. Discovery of FFP is indeed a revolutionary step forward for neurophysiologic diagnostic testing.

The Digital Era

In the early 1970s, computerized tomography (CT) scan brought a revolutionary method for detecting and localizing brain lesions noninvasively. Until that time, EEG and brain scan were the only noninvasive methods of detecting brain lesions, but both are relatively poor in precisely localizing lesions. With the appearance of the CT scan, some thought that CT would replace EEG and eventually clinical EEG would vanish as a neurological diagnostic test. This prediction was incorrect, because there is a fundamental difference between an EEG and a CT scan. The EEG primarily reflects brain function, while CT represents anatomical brain structures. In order for EEG to compete with CT, however, the effort was made to improve the anatomical accuracy in localizing lesions by topographic mapping based on EEG or EP data. Topographic mapping is accomplished by measuring the amplitude values of given waves and interpolating values where there are no electrodes from the known values of neighboring electrodes. Mapping becomes more accurate with a greater number of available electrodes. Topographic mapping with quantified EEG data gave a false sense of hope that EEG might be able to compete with CT scan or the newly emerging magnetic resonance imaging (MRI) in both anatomical and functional brain disturbance. This hope was not easily fulfilled primarily because electrical activity recorded from the scalp was greatly attenuated and distorted by the intervening tissues, such as cerebral spinal fluid (CSF), skull, and scalp existing between the brain and the electrodes. Additionally, the scalp-recorded electrical activity might reflect not only cortical activity but also subcortical activity. The effects of FFP might further complicate the issue. It was necessary to take these factors into account before the scalp-recorded electrical activity could accurately predict the anatomical source of a given wave and understand the clinical significance of dynamic changes in brain electrical activity. Recent advances in computer applications for recording and analyzing EEG data have moved research one step closer to achieving these goals.

Digital EEG

Paper written analog EEG tracings have become obsolete, and most of the EEG laboratories now routinely use digital recording systems. Fast computer processors and improved video screen resolution have made it possible for digital EEG tracings to parallel paper written analog EEG tracings in quality. Moreover, there are many advantages of digital EEG over analog EEG. The first advantage is that EEG stored in digital format allows for changing the display of the recorded activity (i.e., montages, filter settings, sweep speed, the amplitude scale, etc.) as an off-line procedure as needed upon EEG interpretation.

The second advantage is the capability of recording continuously at the bedside without the attendance of an EEG technologist. Long-term bedside EEG monitoring, especially in the intensive care unit (ICU), allows detection of episodic events such as intermittent or clinically unrecognizable seizures. It also allows the monitoring of progressive brain function changes in comatose patients. The computer programs for detection of spikes or seizure events are not as accurate as one would hope and register many false-positive events. Nonetheless, the programs are useful by reducing the vast amount of EEG data to be analyzed by visual inspection within a reasonable time period. Continuous EEG monitoring, which instantaneously reflects dynamic changes of brain function, is one of the major merits of digital EEG. No other functional testing such as PET, SPECT, or fMRI can compete.

The third advantage is the capability of transmitting data instantaneously to a distant review site. If needed, digital video images, along with EEG data, can be transmitted. This allows for smaller clinics or hospitals to consult with skilled electroencephalographers (EEGers) anywhere in the world.

The fourth, and potentially promising application for further advancing EEG technology is computerized data analyses using topographic mapping, advanced statistical and quantitative analysis, dipole localization, etc., which may disclose findings not readily recognized by visual inspection and may eventually lead to a more accurate assessment of the dynamically changing brain function, including cognitive function.

Dipole Localization

It is possible to estimate an electrical source with inverse calculation by measuring the potential field (i.e., dipole field distribution), which spreads between the electrical source and the pickup electrode via volume conduction.[13] Dipole localization is based on the following two principles. One is that the current flows from a positive source to a negative source, creating positive and negative fields on the electro-conductive media. Assuming that the electro-conductive media are homogeneous and of a spherical shape, measuring the current values at a minimum of three sites in three-dimensional spheres can estimate the location of the current source by the inverse calculation. In cases of scalp-recorded potentials, however, the measured activity is attenuated and distorted by intervening tissue between the electrode and cortex (CSF, skull, and scalp). Furthermore, the head shape is not exactly spherical and has individual variations. Under these conditions, an attempt to improve the accuracy of source localization is in progress by quantifying the homogeneous volume conductions and by taking individual head shapes into account by MRI and other measures. This can be accomplished by MRI or CT scan, which reconstructs the individual head and face shapes in three dimensions. Electrode placements are measured by a stereotactic sensor device onto the MRI. With further refinement of methods and technologies, it may become possible to determine precise anatomical locations of electrical sources of a given activity within the brain, which in turn will improve the diagnostic utilization of EEG or EP studies. In EEG, for example, finding the accurate anatomical location of interictal or ictal epileptic discharges will eliminate the necessity of invasive intracranial recording for presurgical evaluation of seizure surgery. For EP studies, finding the sensory cortex before surgery using SSEPs would be useful in planning surgical strategy in patients having a brain tumor near the sensory or motor cortex.

Magnetoencephalography

As was discussed previously, electrical current detected from scalp electrodes is attenuated and distorted due to the intervening tissues between the cortex and scalp. This problem can be overcome by using magnetic fields that are not affected by these tissues. *Magnetoencephalography* (MEG) detects magnetic fields created by current flow over the cortex.[14] Because magnetic fields appear vertically in relation to the direction of current flow, magnetic sensors placed over the head can detect magnetic field created by the tangentially directed current flow over the cortex but not by the radially oriented current flow. This characteristic can be an advantage or a disadvantage over conventional EEG recording. It can be advantageous because MEG selectively detects tangentially oriented current, avoiding the various mixtures of tangentially and radially oriented current components inherent in EEG recording, which makes isolating and analyzing a given component of interest more difficult. Conversely, a disadvantage is that MEG is poor to detect radially oriented current sources. Another major disadvantage is the cost of the equipment, which is 100 times greater than a digital EEG system. The cost of maintenance is also high. Additionally, MEG cannot be used for long recordings, and it is almost impossible to record a clinical seizure. Even if MEG happens to be recorded at the time of a clinical seizure, slight head movement impairs the recording. Despite these disadvantages, considerable research data using MEG have been accumulated in recent years, and MEG is becoming a useful diagnostic test for clinical patients.

Closing Remarks

For close to 90 years since the discovery of brain electrical activity in humans by Berger, EEG and its related fields have provided vast contributions to the advancement of neurological and neurophysiologic sciences as a diagnostic as well as research tool. However, introduction of neuroimaging studies (CT and MRI) and the development of functional imaging studies (fMRI, SPECT, and PET) have weakened the role of EEG as a neurological diagnostic study and brain function measurement tool. One has to realize that there is a fundamental difference between electroneurodiagnostic (END) testing and neuroimaging studies; the former reflects brain function while the latter represents anatomical structure. Digital EEG recording with concomitant video recording has allowed continuous EEG recording at bedside, especially in critically ill patients in the ICU setting. Use of this technology has discovered that many acutely ill comatose or stuporous patients have nonconvulsive seizures, which would have been missed without continuous bedside EEG recording. It is well agreed that EEG has

excellent temporal resolution reflecting dynamic brain function in terms of milliseconds. With appropriate quantitative and statistical analyses, the role of EEG will improve further as a brain function diagnostic test. Further, by taking into account the geometry and conductivity of electrical media, spatial and anatomical resolution for localization of an electrical source of a given activity will improve. Finally, collaborating research with MRI, fMRI, PET, and SPECT will further elaborate the relationship between brain function and brain anatomy and will eventually fulfill Berger's dream: "EEG is the window of the human mind."

References

1. Brazier MAB. *A History of the Electrical Activity of the Brain: The First Half-century.* London: Pitman Medical Publishing Co., 1961.
2. Caton R. The electric currents of the brain. *Br Med J* 1875;2:278.
3. Beck A. Die Bestimmung der Gehirn-und Rucken—markfunctionen vermittelst der elektrischen Ersheimungen. *Cbl Physiol* 1890;4:473–476.
4. Berger H. Uber das Elekrenkephalogram des Menschen. *Arch of Psychiat* 1929;87:527–570.
5. Adrian ED, Matthew BHC. The Berger rhythm: Potential changes from occipital lobes in man. *Brain* 1934;57:355–385.
6. Gibbs FA, Davis H, Lennox WG. The electroencephalogram in epilepsy and in condition of impaired consciousness. *Arch Neurol Psychiatry (Chicago)* 1935;34:1133–1148.
7. Jasper HH. Localized analyses of the function of human brain by the electroencephalogram. *Arch Neurol Psychiatry* 1936;36:1131–1134.
8. Walter WG. The location of cerebral tumors by electroencephalography. *Proc R Soc Med* 1936;30:579–598.
9. Dawson GD. A summation technique for detecting small signals in a large irregular background. *J Physiol (London)* 1951;115:2.
10. Jewett DL, Williston JS. Auditory-evoked far fields averaged from scalp of human. *Brain* 1971;94:681–696.
11. Stockard JJ, Stockard JE, Sharbrough FW. Detection and localization of occult lesions with brainstem auditory responses. *Mayo Clin Proc* 1977;52:761–769.
12. Cracco RQ, Cracco JB. Somatosensory evoked potentials in man: Far-field potentials. *Electroencephalogr Clin Neurophysiol* 1976;41:460–466.
13. Sherg M. Fundamentals of dipole source analysis. In: Grandori F, Hoki M, Rommani GL, eds. *Auditory Evoked Magnetic Fields and Electronic Potentials. Advances in Audiology.* Vol. 6. Basel: Karger, 1990:40–69.
14. Cohen D. Magnetoencephalography: Evidence of magnetic fields produced by alpha-rhythm currents. *Science* 1968;161:784–786.

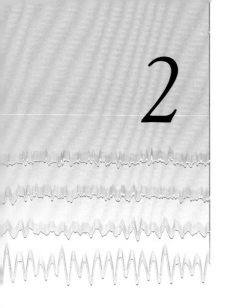

2

Basic EEG Technology

THORU YAMADA and ELIZABETH MENG

Personnel in the EEG Laboratory

All EEG laboratories have, at minimum, two members of the staff: an EEG technologist and an electroencephalographer. An EEG technologist or NDT (neurodiagnostic technologist) is an allied health care employee who specializes in the recording of EEG and other neurodiagnostic procedures. An electroencephalographer (or so-called EEGer) is a physician (usually a neurologist) who has expertise in clinical neurophysiology. The role of the technologist is to explain the testing procedure to the patient, prepare the patient, and perform the EEG recording. The technologist is skilled in obtaining technically satisfactory recordings by modifying recording parameters and noting patient behaviors and other factors that may affect the recording, allowing for appropriate and accurate EEG interpretation by the EEGer. The EEGer should also have a technical background and be able to recognize various artifacts, technical modification, or technical errors in order to avoid misdiagnosis (see Chapter 15).

Most laboratories will find it invaluable to employ a secretary to register patients, schedule procedures, and type and file reports. It is also very helpful to have a biomedical technician or an electrical engineer to take care of equipment maintenance, troubleshoot problems, and do periodic electrical safety checks on the instruments.

Electrodes

CONVENTIONAL ELECTRODES

An EEG is recorded from electrodes attached to the scalp. These electrodes are made of metal, most commonly platinum, gold, or silver–silver chloride. They are 4- to 10-mm discs attached to a wire that is plugged into an electrode board and, eventually, the EEG instrument (Fig. 2-1). The choice of electrode metals is based on cost, convenience, and quality. Platinum electrodes are very expensive and used for special recording purposes. Gold electrodes are actually silver with a gold overlay. The silver–silver chloride electrode is the most commonly used electrode consisting of silver that is treated with a salt solution that changes the surface of the electrode. This electrode requires some maintenance to keep the electrode chlorided. All three of these metals have good recording qualities with minimal drift of electrical potentials and a long time constant (TC; see "Filter Settings" in this chapter), allowing better reproduction of many recording frequencies. Whichever metal is chosen, it is preferable to use the same metal for all electrodes since a pair of electrodes of different metals has different TCs, resulting in an alteration of the waveform.

An electrode placed on the scalp will have an electrolyte (conductive jelly) placed between the scalp and the electrode.

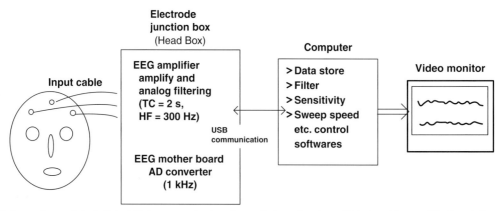

FIGURE 2-1 | Schematic model of digital EEG system. In the electrode junction box, EEG signal is amplified and filtered (analog filter) commonly with high frequency of 300 Hz and TC of 2 s. Restricting the bandpass of the amplified signal eliminates external interference. The filtered signal is then sent to the A/D converter, with a sampling rate of 1,000 Hz. The digitized data are then sent to the computer for data storage (data from each channel are stored with a single reference format) and also for reformatting to appropriate parameters (montage, sensitivity, filter bandpass, etc.) to be displayed on the video monitor screen.

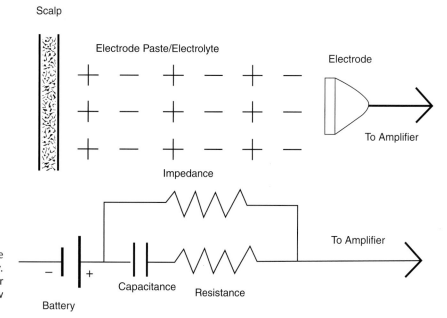

FIGURE 2-2 | Schematic model of electrode attached to the scalp with conductive jelly. (Modified from Tyner FS, Knott JR, Mayer WB Jr. *Fundamentals of EEG Technology*. New York: Raven Press, 1983, with permission.)

This interface has properties of capacitors and resistors (Fig. 2-2) and forms an *impedance* that is "resistance" against alternating current (AC) flow. After the electrodes are placed on the scalp, it is important to lower the electrode impedance. It is preferred that electrode impedance be less than 5 kΩ, but at minimum, less than 10 kΩ.[1,2] Because of the properties of the amplifiers used in EEG, unequal impedance between two electrodes in a pair creates an imbalance that can hinder the recording quality (see next paragraph). Impedance of less than 5 kΩ on all electrodes is best, but if that is not possible, impedances of 9 to 10 kΩ on all electrodes would be preferable to having impedance difference at 1 kΩ for one and at 10 kΩ for the other. It is best to have no more than 5 kΩ difference between the highest and the lowest impedance readings. Most EEG equipment has some method of checking impedance built into the instrument. High-electrode impedance tends to produce artifacts by slight movements of the head, body, or even the electrode wires.

A common artifact, "electrode pop," may mimic abnormal EEG activity (see Fig. 15-26A and B). This electrically unstable electrode pop can be caused by an electrolyte that has become dry or by an unstable electrode surface contact with the skin. The electrode pop is not related to electrode impedance; therefore, it may occur even when impedances are low. The pop may occur when silver–silver chloride electrodes are not well chlorided. If using silver–silver chloride electrodes, chloriding should be done periodically.[3] This can be done by placing silver electrodes into 1% to 5% sodium chloride (NaCl) solution in a nonmetallic container and sending a weak current (<1 mA) to the electrodes to be chlorided. Bright, unchlorided silver electrodes will darken slowly to a uniform gray color as chloriding progresses.

SPECIAL ELECTRODES

Subdermal Needle Electrodes

These electrodes are inserted just beneath the skin. Because of infection control issues, these electrodes should be of a disposable type. There are many problems associated with the use of needle electrodes[4]; therefore, the American Clinical Neurophysiology Society[5] (ACNS) (formerly the American EEG Society) does not recommend their use for routine EEG recording. However, subdermal needle electrodes have been commonly used for intraoperative monitoring because they are quickly and easily placed without discomfort to the patient under anesthesia. Special care must be taken when placing needle electrodes in order to (i) maintain sterility of the puncture site and (ii) dispose of the used needles in a proper "sharps" container.

Nasopharyngeal Electrodes

Nasopharyngeal (NP) electrodes are usually referred to as PG1 and PG2 and are used to noninvasively record activity from the *inferior* and *mesial temporal lobe* as well as *orbitofrontal* activity (Fig. 2-3B). They are inserted via the nostril and are carefully rotated so that the tip will be in contact with the roof of nasopharynx. They are usually made of insulated semiflexible Z-shaped wire of about 12.5 cm in length with a silver ball exposed at the tip.

The use of NP electrodes results in a higher yield of epileptiform activity when compared to recording with only scalp electrodes.[6,7] Because of unstable contact with the pharyngeal mucosa, NP recordings are often contaminated by respiration, eye movement, or other artifacts, especially when used on patients who are awake. Generally, an NP electrode study without a sleep recording is unyielding. If NP electrodes are to be used, it is recommended that the patient is sedated or sleep deprived prior to the study to increase the probability of gaining a sleep recording. NP electrodes are not suitable for long-term EEG monitoring. Other special electrodes have been developed for this specialized use.

Some studies have indicated that surface electrodes over the cheeks, T1 and T2 (see "Electrode Nomenclature"), or the use of long interelectrode distances are equally as effective for detecting mesial temporal lobe abnormalities.[8,9]

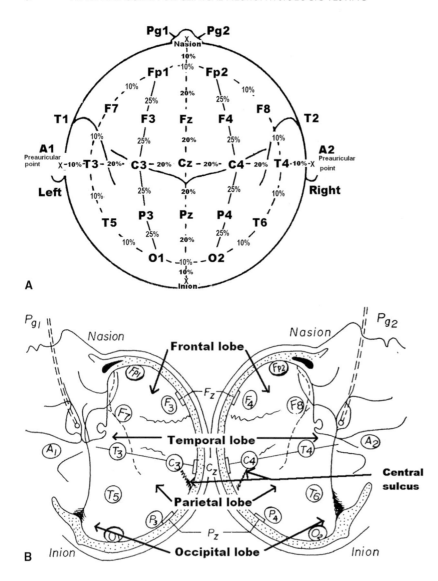

FIGURE 2-3 | **A:** Top view of the International 10–20 system for electrode placement. **B:** Lateral view of the International 10–20 system in relation to the surface of the brain. (From Jasper HH. Report of the committee on methods of clinical examination in electroencephalography. *Electroencephalogr Clin Neurophysiol* 1958;10:370–375, with permission.)

OTHER SPECIAL ELECTRODES

Electrodes have been developed to monitor specific body functions. There are electrodes to record air flow from the nose or mouth, movement of the chest with respirations, tremors of the extremities, etc. Use of these special electrodes can make the interpretation of EEG more accurate and should be used when necessary.

For long-term EEG monitoring, especially for the evaluation of a seizure focus in patients with intractable epilepsy who are candidates for surgical treatment, special electrodes have been developed. These include sphenoidal electrodes,[10] foramen ovale electrodes,[11] tympanic electrodes,[12] ethmoidal electrodes,[13] depth electrodes,[14] and subdural electrodes.[15] These will be discussed in more detail in Volume II.

Electrode Placement

Standard electrode placement uses 21 electrodes in accordance with the *10–20 International System of Electrode Placement* recommended by the International Federation of Societies for EEG and Clinical Neurophysiology in 1958[16] (Fig. 2-3A). This system was developed to gain consistency between laboratories. It also ensures consistency for each patient as follow-up EEG recordings

are done. The system is based on percentages (10% or 20%) of the total size of the head. Anatomical landmarks are identified that can be found on most people. These landmarks are the *nasion* and the *inion* (for the anterior–posterior plane) and the left and right *preauricular points* (for the transverse plane) (Fig. 2-3A and B). The nasion is located at the bridge of the nose. The inion is the bump midline on the back of the skull above the hairline. It can be felt more easily if the patient is directed to move his head forward and back while the tech feels the back of the head. The preauricular points are on each side of the head. The actual point is at the notch that can be felt just anterior to the tragus of the ear. It can be more readily palpated if the patient is directed to slightly open and close the jaw. For practical purposes, the notch just above the tragus may be used as a preauricular point. Accurate measurement with equal interelectrode distances for homologous electrode pairs is essential; unequal distances will cause a spurious amplitude asymmetry (the shorter the interelectrode distance, the lower the amplitude) (see Fig. 15-48A and B). The only changes in this system should occur when the skull does not allow adherence. It might be necessary to misplace the electrodes, if, for example, there is a bandage on a portion of the skull that cannot be removed. Symmetry between homologous electrode pairs should still be attempted by also misplacing electrodes on the other side. When these changes are necessary, a diagram of the alteration must be documented by technologist. In addition to these electrodes, a ground electrode must be placed, which can be anywhere on the scalp, but often, Fpz (between Fp1 and Fp2) is used.

ELECTRODE NOMENCLATURE

The electrode positions are named according to the relationship with the underlying brain anatomy or lobe (Fig. 2-3B). "F" is designated for electrodes over the frontal lobe, "P" for parietal, "O" for occipital, and "T" for temporal lobe. "C" refers to central electrodes, which closely overlie the *central sulcus* or *Rolandic fissure* of the brain (see Fig. 2-3B). "FP" refers to the frontopolar electrodes, which are placed just above the eyes and located over the frontal poles of the frontal lobes.

Each electrode, besides a letter name, also has a number in it's name. Even numbers represent the right side of the head; odd numbers refer to left side. The middle (or midline) is called "Z". The numbering system starts at the midline (Z) and progresses laterally; thus, F3 is closer to the midline than F7 but both are on the left side. If a technologist chose to add an electrode between F3 and F7, it would be called F5 (according to a new modified nomenclature) (Fig. 2-4).

Generally, 19 electrodes are placed on the scalp and one electrode is placed on each ear lobe (occasionally, it is necessary to use the *mastoid* instead of the ear lobe). The ear electrodes are called A1 and A2 standing for *Auricular 1* and *Auricular 2*. They are commonly used as the reference electrodes (see "Montages" in this chapter).

Instead of using F7 and F8, some prefer to use T1 and T2, which are located 1 cm above and one third the distance from the *external auditory meatus* to the *outer cantus* of the eye. T1 and T2 are closer to the anterior temporal lobe than F7 and F8,[17] but this placement does not follow the rules of the 10–20 system and, therefore, should be labeled as a variance from the International 10–20 system.

In recent years, the application of computer technology has made it possible to analyze spatial potential fields in more detail for EEG and evoked potential studies. The ACNS published a modification of the International 10–20 system with additional electrodes located by further dividing the distances between standard placements (Modified Combinatorial Nomenclature).[18] With this new system, T3 and T4 became T7 and T8, respectively. T5 and T6 became P7 and P8, respectively (Fig. 2-4). This nomenclature has not been widely used for routine clinical EEG but has been proven useful in research fields.

MEASURING FOR ELECTRODE PLACEMENT

An essential role of the EEG technologist is to accurately and securely place electrodes. It can take several months of practice to perfect the technique, but once learned, the procedure can be accomplished in less than 30 minutes.

A grease pencil (china marker) is usually used to place measurement marks on the head. A millimeter tape measurer is important. The retractable measurers are good but must be wiped clean between uses. There are also disposable, paper tapes available. Each technologist develops his or her own preferences and techniques that work for measuring the head. But to have a starting point, step-by-step directions are included from which to practice. You will note that a spot is not ready for electrode placement until it has two marks making a +. Refer to Figure 2-3A when practicing measuring the head. You will also find a video about measuring and marking electrodes on your on-line reference. (The code is under a scratch off inside the front cover of this text.)

1. Measure the distance from the nasion to the inion down the middle of the head (the sagittal plane). Calculate 50% of that number and place a mark perpendicular to the tape at that spot (Cz). Then, starting at the nasion, put another mark at 10% of the total measurement (Fpz). At this time, place a crossing mark at Fpz that is in line with the nose, therefore being on the midline. You can then move the tape to measure between Fpz and Cz. Place a mark halfway between them. (This also turns out to be 20% of the total.) Move the tape again to Cz and measure the same 20% distance back to Pz and again to Oz. (Usually, there is no electrode placed at Fpz and Oz. They are used for measurement of other electrodes only.) There should now be 10% of the total remaining to reach the inion.

2. Measure the total distance from the left preauricular point to the right, going through the partial mark at Cz (the coronal plane). Calculate 50% of that number and place a mark perpendicular to the tape at that spot. The mark should intersect with the original Cz mark to make a +. Then, starting at the left preauricular point, put another perpendicular mark at 10% of the total measurement (T3). You can then move the tape to measure between T3 and Cz. Place a mark halfway between them (C3). (This also turns out to be 20% of the total.) Move the tape again to Cz and measure the same 20% distance down toward the right preauricular (C4) and again to T4. There should now be 10% of the total remaining to reach the right preauricular point.

3. The next measurement is the total circumference of the head. Start at Fpz, part off the hair as much as possible, and continue running the tape all the way around the head, making sure to pass through T3, Oz, and T4. This measurement is then divided into 10 segments, each 10% of the total. The first 10% is between Fp1 and Fp2

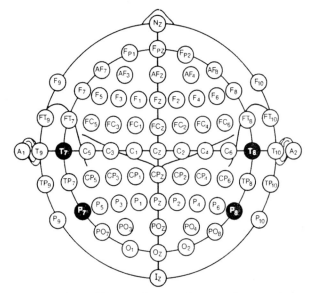

FIGURE 2-4 | Modified combinatorial nomenclature to be used for detailed topographic mapping of EEG activity. (From American Clinical Neurophysiology Society. Guideline 5: Guidelines for standard electrode position nomenclature. *J Clin Neurophysiol* 2006;23(2):107–110, with permission.)

(5% on each side of Fpz). Then, move the tape to Fp1 and measure back toward T3. Put a mark at the 10% number (F7) and another mark at twice that number, which should cross with the previous T3 mark. Move the tape to T3 and measure toward Oz, marking at 10% for T5 and another 10% for O1. O1 can be cross marked by visually lining it up with the original mark placed at Oz. Then, start at Fp2 and move to the right using the same procedure to measure for F8, T4, T6, and O2. O2 can also be cross marked if it is in line with Oz. You will note that F7, F8, T5, and T6 do not have cross marks yet. These can be added at this time. Use the tape measurer as a straight edge. Lay it between Fp1 and T3. Make sure that it is placed above the mark on both ends. Then, find the original mark at F7 and cross that mark by running a mark along the bottom of the tape measure. The same procedure can be used to cross mark the remaining three electrode locations. It is important that if your tape is lined up above two electrodes, the mark you make should be below the tape. You could instead line the tape up below two electrodes, but then the mark would be made above the tape to end up on the same plane.

4. Now, measure from F7, through Fz, to F8. Half that distance should mark the midline at Fz. Measure from F7 to Fz. Place a mark at the halfway spot for the first F3 mark. Move the tape and measure from Fz to F8. Again, half that distance will be the first mark for F4. Do the same in the back of the head by measuring from T5, through Pz, to T6. At half that distance, a mark should intersect the original Pz mark that identifies the midline. Next, measure from T5 to Pz where the first P3 mark will be in the middle. Then, measure from Pz to T6 to place the first P4 mark in the middle. These measurements are somewhat difficult as the tape must follow the curve of the head.

5. The last remaining measurements will cross mark F3, F4, C3, C4, P3, and P4.

6. Start by measuring from Fp1, through the original mark at C3, to O1 (the parasagittal plane). Cross mark C3 at half this distance. Then, move the tape back to Fp1 and measure to C3. Cross F3 at half this distance. Move the tape again to C3 and measure to O1. Cross P3 at half this distance. Do the same on the right to cross F4, C4, and P4. These measurements must also follow the curve of the head.

Electrode Application

SKIN PREPARATION

To ensure low impedance between the electrode and the scalp, the skin should be thoroughly cleaned. Many products are available that serve this purpose. Put a little cleansing gel onto a paper towel and dip a cotton-tipped applicator into it. Gently scrub the area just in the middle of the cross that was made while marking the head. Be aware that these gels are abrasive. Excessive scrubbing can irritate the skin. It will take a little practice to decide how aggressive to be without undue discomfort to the patient. Also, be careful not to clean off the entire mark. The mark is there to guide electrode placement. If it is completely rubbed off, placement will not be accurate. When placing electrodes to be used in a long-term EEG, the gel should be wiped from the scalp before placing the electrode to help in avoiding skin breakdown.

APPLICATION METHODS

The most common adhesives used in routine EEG recording are paste and collodion (ether-based glue). Paste is relatively quick, has no unappealing odors, and cleans off fairly easily. But paste is not a stable application method. Head movement or sweating can cause electrodes to shift or fall off. Therefore, paste is not suitable for difficult patients, children, long-term recordings, or surgical monitoring. Collodion-applied electrodes are very stable and can stay on the head for days to weeks with only minimal maintenance. But collodion is flammable; has a strong, sometimes unpleasant, odor; and must be removed with acetone (another strong-smelling chemical). It also takes longer to apply a set of electrodes with collodion than with paste.

In some institutions, the technologist will be able to choose which method to use. But some practice settings might not allow the use of collodion because of its flammability and odor while others might not allow paste, preferring a more stable application.

Paste Application

Put a small amount of paste on a paper towel. Each technologist tends to develop a system to determine the order of application. If the patient is sitting, starting with the front of the head works well. If the patient is lying down, starting with the back of the head on one side might be preferable. Scoop a small amount of paste from the paper towel into the cup of the electrode. To avoid possible cross contamination, do not dip the electrode into the paste jar. There should be enough paste so that when applied, a very small amount leaks out around the electrode. Excessive amounts of paste must be avoided as the recording area encompasses the entire paste/electrode junction. Once applied, a piece of gauze, cotton, or even paper towel applied over the electrode will secure the stability of the electrodes. It is helpful to run the electrode wire away from the face and in a direction that does not fight gravity.

When the EEG is completed, paste electrodes can be gently pulled off the head and the residue cleaned away with a warm, wet washrag. Electrodes should be cleaned with soap and water using a soft brush and then disinfected with an appropriate solution.

Collodion Application

For collodion application, a supply of pressurized air is necessary to dry the glue. This can be accomplished by tapping into the medical air line (if available) in the wall, by a portable air pump, or by "canned" air sold most typically for dusting electronic parts. Place the electrode on the scalp. While holding it in place, cover it with a 1-inch square piece of gauze that has been dipped into collodion. Then, dry the collodion with air. Care must be taken so that the electrode does not move from the desired location while drying the glue. Protecting the patient's eyes and clothing is also a concern when using collodion and precautions should be observed. Collodion tends to splatter a little when the air is turned on. Once the electrodes are in place, an electrolyte must be added to fill the space between the scalp and the electrode. These products are readily available. The electrolyte can be injected under the electrode (through a small hole in the cup) using a syringe with a blunted needle (or stub adaptor). The electrolyte should just fill the cup, not overfill it. When finished, the blunted needle or stub adaptor should be disposed of in a hospital grade sharps container.

Some technologists use a combination of paste and collodion. A scoop of paste helps to hold the electrode in place while a gauze square soaked in collodion is applied. In this method, additional electrolyte is unnecessary (the paste has electrolyte qualities).

If collodion has been used, acetone (or acetone-free collodion remover) is the only suitable method of removal. It can be applied liberally using a cotton ball, gently rubbing until the electrode falls off. Care must be taken to ensure that acetone does not get into the eyes or on the clothing. Once the electrodes are removed, additional scrubbing with acetone will be necessary to remove residue in the hair and on the scalp. Electrodes should be cleaned with a soft brush and warm, soapy water. It is also helpful to soak them for a few minutes in acetone to remove collodion residue from the electrodes. Once rinsed clean, an appropriate disinfectant should be used.

The Differential Amplifier

A pair of inputs (electrodes) is required to appropriately amplify the EEG signal. These two inputs used to be called "G1" and "G2," corresponding to a "grid" of the "old-fashioned" vacuum tube amplifiers. But in a solid-state amplifier, the differential amplifier is, in effect, made up of two separate amplifiers such that each (input 1 and input 2) records with respect to a third one (usually the ground electrode) (Fig. 2-5). The output of a differential amplifier reflects the voltage difference between the two inputs (input 1 and input 2); if the difference is a negative value, or the activity of input 1 is relatively more negative as compared to input 2, the deflection of the EEG activity goes up. Conversely, if the difference between input 1 and input 2 is a positive value, the deflection goes down. If there is no difference in voltage between input 1 and input 2, there will be no deflection (*equipotential*). This is an important concept in localizing EEG abnormalities and should be clearly understood for appropriate and accurate interpretation.

If the differential amplifier is perfectly matched and balanced, signals of the same phase, polarity, and amplitude entering both inputs should result in total cancellation, that is, zero voltage. For example, external interference such as 60 Hz common to both inputs should be cancelled out if the amplifier is balanced. In reality, the amplifier is never perfectly balanced and the degree of "imperfection" is expressed by the *common mode rejection ratio (CMRR)*, which is the ratio of the amplification gain for the differential signal to that for the common mode noise. The CMRR is commonly at least 10,000:1. Even if the amplifier is balanced with a high CMRR, the balance can be externally disturbed simply by using unbalanced electrode impedances between the two inputs (e.g., one electrode has much higher impedance than the other), which commonly results in the introduction of 60-Hz artifact (see Fig. 15-25A).

The Amplifier Controls

EEG amplifiers have several controls that aid in the proper display of EEG activity. It has traditionally been the role of the EEG technologist to be expert in the use of these controls to best display the abnormalities in the recording. With the advent of digital EEG, however, it is imperative that EEGers also understand these controls as they will frequently review the EEG, making their own control choices rather than using those provided by the technologist.

AMPLITUDE (VERTICAL) SCALE

The amplitude scale is usually expressed by a voltage value per millimeter of deflection. This is based on the traditional analog EEG, which utilized pens writing on paper and a "sensitivity" control that dictated how much voltage was represented by each millimeter of pen movement. A simple calculation can be an aid in sensitivity problems:

$$S = V/H$$

where S = sensitivity (μV/mm), V = voltage (μV), and H = height of pen deflection (mm).

This formula can be used to find any value if the other two are known. If the voltage is unknown, use $V = S \times H$. If the amplitude is unknown, use $H = V/S$.

The most commonly used sensitivity setting is 7 μV/mm. This means that each millimeter represents 7 μV of activity. In a digital system, however, a sensitivity setting may be less accurate because the amplitude scale (or height) may be different or can be adjusted depending on the size of the screen or computer program. Also, the scale may be different when the EEG is printed out on paper, depending on the paper size or the printing program. Nonetheless, adjusting vertical scaling close to a sensitivity of 7 μV/mm would be appropriate for conventional EEG interpretation. Though 7 μV/mm is a good starting point for visual inspection and interpretation of most routine EEGs, the setting should be adjusted according to the activity being recorded. If the activity is very high amplitude, a decrease in sensitivity is in order. Note that a decreased sensitivity will actually have a larger number on the setting. Therefore, S = 10 μV/mm is *less* sensitive than S = 7 μV/mm. Remember, when making this particular adjustment, 1 mm of deflection will now represent 10 μV rather than 7 μV. If, instead, the recorded activity at S = 7 μV/mm is very low amplitude and difficult to see, a more sensitive setting of S = 5 μV/mm will increase the size of EEG activity. Now, each millimeter of deflection represents 5 μV.

Differential amplifier

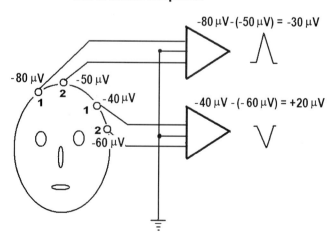

FIGURE 2-5 | Schematic model of a differential amplifier. The output is the result of the difference between input 1 and input 2. If subtracting input 2 from input 1 results in a negative value, the signal deflection is upward. If the difference is a positive value, the signal deflection is downward.

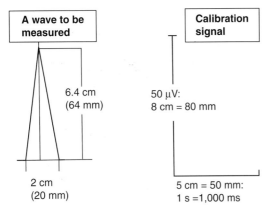

Duration = {calibration scale (ms) x a wave width (mm)}/calibration width (mm)
In this case, the duration of this wave is (1,000 ms x 20 mm)/50 mm = 400 ms

Amplitude = {calibration scale (µV) x a wave height (mm)}/calibration height (mm)
In this case, the amplitude of this wave is (50 µV x 64 mm)/80 mm = 40 µV

FIGURE 2-6 | Amplitude (µV) and duration (ms) based on the calibration scale.

When calibrating the EEG system, a 50 µV signal should measure 5 mm of height on the screen at S = 10 µV/mm. When the EEG is printed on a paper (usually 8 ½ × 11 inch), the scale may be slightly different. For accurate amplitude (µV) measurement of a wave, the following formula is used (Fig. 2-6):

$$\text{Amplitude (µV)} = \frac{\text{Calibration scale (µV)} \times \text{Wave height (mm)}}{\text{Calibration height (mm)}}$$

TIME (HORIZONTAL) SCALE

The time scale in EEG is expressed in one of two ways: (i) the number of millimeters the sweep moves in 1 second (i.e., 30 mm/s) or (ii) the number of seconds visualized on a full video screen (i.e., 10 to 15 s/page). The first option is based on the traditional, paper written (analog) EEG. The instrument was designed to have the paper move at a rate of 30 mm every second. The paper speed control would allow an adjustment to double or half the speed. In some cases, the control would allow for speeds as slow as 6 mm/s. Since digital EEG has no moving paper, it is now more common to describe paper speed in terms of seconds per page. The most common setting is a 10 to 15 s/page. Similar to vertical scale (amplitude scale), horizontal scale (time scale) can be different depending on the monitor size and program. Again, it is reasonable to use a similar scale as was established in analog EEG, that is, a monitor screen should be set as close as possible to 30 mm/s and 10 to 15 s for full screen. Whichever setting is used, it is important to use a standard time scale for ease of visual inspection and interpretation. EEG frequencies appear to be slower when viewed with a faster time scale (i.e., 5 s/page) (see Fig. 15-36A and B) or faster when viewed with a slower time scale (i.e., 30 s/page) (see Fig. 15-37A and B). There are good uses of both the faster and the slower speeds. Faster speeds allow better visual inspection and more accurate measurement of the timing or frequency of a given activity of interest. Slower speeds can sometimes help visualize a subtle slow-wave abnormality or periodicity in case of slow periodic activity (Fig. 10-31). Slower speeds are also commonly used in sleep studies (*polysomnography*): 10 mm/s or 30 s full screen. When a digital EEG is printed on paper, the time scale will change depending on the print program that is used and on the size of the paper. The following formula can be used to calculate the duration (frequency) of a given wave on the paper measured with a ruler (Fig. 2-6):

$$\text{Duration of a wave (ms)} = \frac{\text{Wave width (mm)} \times \text{Calibration time scale (ms)}}{\text{Calibration width (mm)}}$$

The duration of a wave can be converted to frequency (Hz) by using the following formula:

$$\text{Frequency (Hz)} = \frac{1,000 \text{ (ms)}}{\text{Duration of wave (ms)}}$$

Figure 2-7 shows an example of measurement for amplitude, duration, and frequency values of an actual EEG sharp discharge.

FILTER SETTINGS

EEG activity consists of a composite of various frequencies. The bandwidth for routine EEG is conventionally from 1 to 70 Hz. Activity outside of this range is attenuated or totally eliminated. This attenuation or elimination is the result of the function of filters. Filters are used to minimize or eliminate activity that is not of value and to enhance activity of interest. The two filters that are of most use in EEG are (i) the *low-frequency filter* (*LFF*) and (ii) the *high-frequency filter* (*HFF*). The LFF can enhance or eliminate slower (lower) frequency activity without affecting faster (higher) frequency activity. Therefore, it is also called a *high-pass filter*. The HFF, conversely, can enhance or eliminate faster (higher) frequency activity without affecting slower (lower-) frequency activity. Therefore, it is also called a *low-pass filter*. Knowledge of the filtering effects is essential because their use can completely alter the ability to see particular frequencies that might be of value. A frequency response curve for the filters being used can aid in understanding the effect of the filter on various frequencies. Figure 2-8 shows a frequency response curve for four common LFF settings and three HFF settings. Note that the frequency scale on the x-axis is a logarithmic scale. The y-axis shows a percent of the total amplitude that is displayed using each filter.

Wave duration and amplitude measurement

Duration (ms) = calibration (ms) × measured duration (mm)/calibration width (mm)
(In this case, duration of this wave is 400 ms × 6 mm/20 mm = 120 ms)
(By definition, this wave is "sharp" wave and the frequency is 1,000 ms/120 ms = 8.33 Hz)

Amplitude (μV) = calibration (μV) × measured height (mm)/calibration height (mm)
(In this case, amplitude of this wave is 30 μv × 15 mm/8 mm = 56.25 μv)

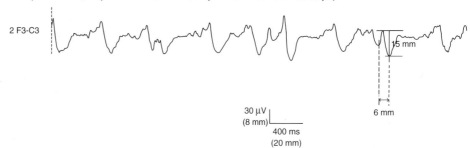

FIGURE 2-7 | The amplitude (μV) and duration (ms) of a given wave from an EEG tracing.

Each filter is named with a number called the "cutoff" frequency. This number designates the frequency at which there will be a 30% reduction in amplitude (3-dB attenuation) as compared to 100% amplitude at 10 Hz. With an HFF of 15 Hz, the amplitude of 15-Hz activity will be reduced by 30%. Recording activity faster than 15 Hz will show more reduction or total elimination. When recording slower frequencies, there will be less or no reduction. The LFF filters are demonstrated on the left side of the diagram. If an LFF of 0.5 Hz is being used, there will be a 30% amplitude reduction of 0.5-Hz activity (0.5 is the cutoff frequency). Slower frequencies will have more amplitude reduction and faster frequencies will have less reduction. Notice that neither set of filters affects the frequency of 10 Hz. The available "cutoff" frequencies for the HFF (low-pass filter) are usually 15, 35, and 70 Hz and for the LFF (high-pass filter) are 0.3, 0.5, 1.6, and 5 Hz, and they are determined by the manufacturer. Adjustment of the filters (HFF or LFF) will *not* change the frequency of the recorded activity. It will change the amplitude only.

Filter settings are sometimes expressed in terms of "time constant" (TC). TC, as it relates to the LFF, is defined as the time it takes for a calibration signal to decay by 63% from full scale (Fig. 2-9). Relating to an HFF, TC refers to the time it takes for the calibration to rise to 63% of its total amplitude. Both high- and low-filter settings relate to the functions of resistance (Ohm) and capacitance (Farad). In a low-filter circuit as shown in Figure 2-10A, low-frequency activity is blocked because the impedance of the capacitor increases as the frequency decreases. In an HFF, the position of the resistor and the capacitor is reversed (Fig. 2-10B). This attenuates the high-frequency activity because the impedance of the capacitor decreases as the frequency increases. TC relates resistance and capacitance mathematically by the equation $TC = R \times C$ [e.g., resistance of 1 mega ohm ($10^6 \, \Omega$) and capacitance of 1 μF (10^{-6} F) gives $TC = 1$ s]. The values of TC and filter (F) setting are inversely related by the equation of $TC = 1/(2\pi F)$ (see Chapter 3, Frequency response of high and low filters, for further detail). Although the "time constant" applies to both HFFs (rise TC) and LFFs (decay TC), it is conventionally used for the LFF control. TCs of 0.03, 0.1, 0.3, and 1.0 s, for example, are equivalent to LFF of 5.3, 1.6, 0.53, and 0.16

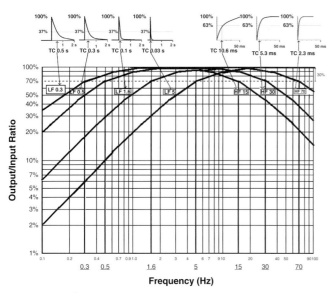

FIGURE 2-8 | Frequency response curves. Note 30% amplitude reduction at each low or high "cutoff" frequency.

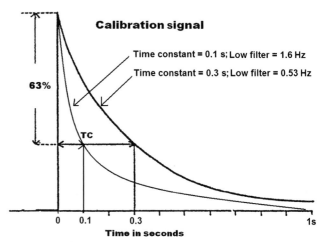

FIGURE 2-9 | Calibration signal with examples of TC. The shorter the TC, the higher the low-filter setting.

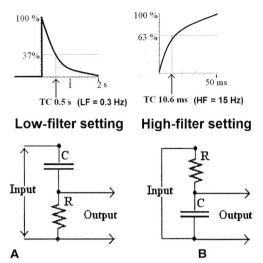

Low-filter setting   **High-filter setting**

A   **B**

FIGURE 2-10 | Resistance and capacitance circuit for low **(A)** and high **(B)** filters. In a calibration signal, 63% delay time and 63% rise time are defined as TC. TC is equal to *R* (resistance in Ohm) × *C* (capacitance in Farad).

Hz, respectively (Fig. 2-8). It should be noted that the longer (greater number) the TC, the lower (smaller number) the low-filter setting.

In a calibration signal, a sharp and pointed rise corresponds to HFF 70 Hz and the top becomes more rounded with a decrease of the HFF setting (Fig. 2-11A). Lowering the HFF (e.g., from 70 to 35 Hz) attenuates the amplitude of fast activity

and raising the HFF (e.g., from 35 to 70 Hz) enhances the fast activity (Fig. 2-11A). Raising the LFF setting from 1.6 to 5.3 Hz (shortening of TC) will attenuate slow waves and the reverse will enhance the slow waves (Fig. 2-11B).

NOTCH FILTER

There is an additional filter called a "notch filter," which specifically eliminates a particular frequency. This is 60-Hz AC (alternating current) activity, which exists abundantly surrounding our environment. Sixty-Hertz activity is well within the bandwidth of EEG and contaminates EEG tracing as artifacts. Fortunately, most of 60-Hz contamination is eliminated (cancelled out) by effective grounding and low and matched electrodes impedances. A notch filter is designed to eliminate 60-Hz activity only without affecting other frequency activity (see Fig. 15-25A and B). Because AC line could be 50 Hz depending on locations (some areas in Japan or Europe), some EEG instrument may offer the choice to set either 50 or 60 Hz as a notch filter. Sixty-Hertz interference can be from other equipment in the vicinity of the EEG, from improper grounding, or from a host of inadequate techniques relating to electrodes, electrode wires, and cables. It is important to eliminate the technical issues as the cause of 60 Hz before resorting to the use of notch filter as these issues can also cause other interpretive dilemmas. Remember, the bandwidth for EEG activity is 1 to 70 Hz. By using a notch filter at 60 Hz, any EEG activity at that frequency will be virtually eliminated but not affecting other frequency activities.

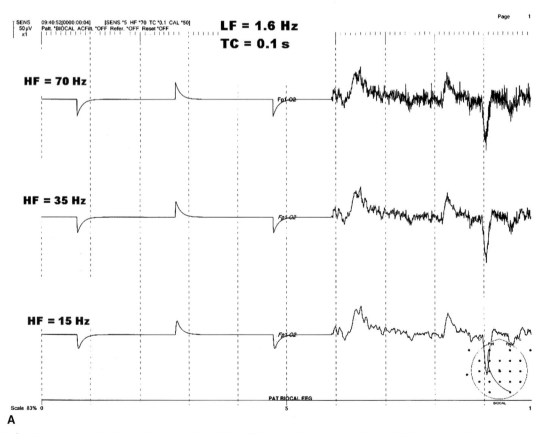

FIGURE 2-11 | Different combinations of high and low filters (TC) in calibration signals and EEG tracings. Changing high-filter setting from 70 to 15 Hz shows blunted peak in calibration signal and decrease of fast activity in EEG tracing **(A)**. Changing from a short to a long TC shows a slower delay time in calibration signal and increases slow wave in EEG **(B)**. (**A** and **B** are reformatted from same EEG sample.)

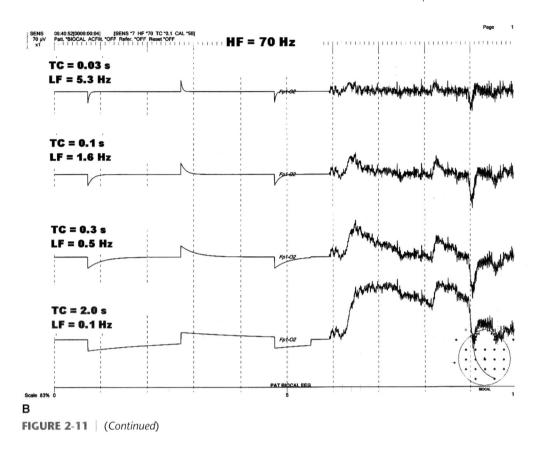

B

FIGURE 2-11 | (Continued)

APPROPRIATE USE OF FILTER SETTINGS

For routine EEG interpretation, an LFF of 1.6 Hz (*TC* = 0.1 s) and HFF of 70 Hz are common. When excessive muscle artifact obscures the underlying EEG activity, the HFF may be reduced to 35 or 15 Hz (Fig. 2-12A and B). However, one should be aware that lowering the HFF may reduce the amplitude of spike or sharp discharges that could be significant in the interpretation. Additionally, it could make muscle artifact appear like a spike, sharp wave, or beta, again hindering

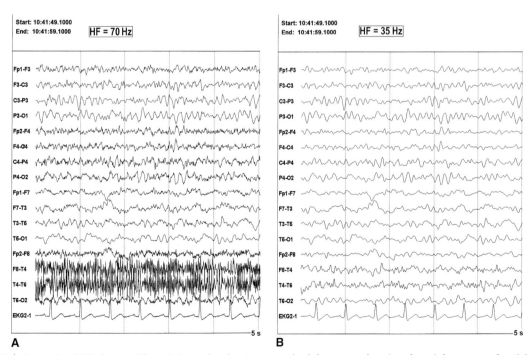

FIGURE 2-12 | Example of HF change. There is irregular slowing over the left temporal region, but right temporal activity is obscured by muscle artifact **(A)**, and it is not certain if there is any slowing in the right temporal region. High-filter (HF) change from 70 to 15 Hz reduces the muscle artifact and verifies that there is no slowing in the right temporal region **(B)**. (**A** and **B** are the same EEG sample.)

interpretation (Fig. 2-13A and B; see also Figs. 15-38A and B, and 15-39A and B). It is preferable to take the steps necessary to make the patient relaxed and comfortable so that the muscle artifact is eliminated at the source. If the recording shows excessive slow-wave activity such as "sweat" artifact (sweat gland potential) (Fig. 2-14A and B) or respiratory movement artifact, the LFF may be changed from 1.6 Hz (*TC* = 0.1 s) to LFF 5 Hz (*TC* = 0.03 s), but one must be aware that this will reduce the amplitude of abnormal delta activity as well (Fig. 2-15A–C; see also Fig. 15-40A and B). Again, it is preferable to eliminate these artifacts at the source.

The higher LFF setting can be used to better visualize "spikes" hidden by large slow waves (Fig. 2-16A and B). By reducing the amplitude of the slow waves, the lower voltage spikes can be seen. Reducing the amplitude of the slow activity will also sometimes allow for an overall increase in sensitivity (amplitude scale). Lowering the LFF (lengthening the TC) can be used to enhance subtle slow waves (Fig. 2-15A and B). Conversely, raising the LFF (shortening the TC) minimizes the slow waves (Fig. 2-15C).

Indiscriminate changing of the filter settings is "dangerous" and could lead to erroneous interpretation. When the HFF is reduced, "trust only slow activity"; and when the LFF is increased, "trust only fast activity." Changing filter setting affects not only the amplitude of filtered activity but also the phase of the waves. It is a common misconception that phase shift does not occur in digital EEG. Most commercially available digital EEG programs mimic analog EEG systems and phase shift does occur. With a shorter TC (higher LFF setting), slow waves shift earlier in time (Fig. 2-17A). Conversely, lowering the HFF setting results in phase delay (i.e., the peak of the wave occurs later) (Fig. 2-17B). This becomes critical if not all channels are recorded using the same filtering. Phase shift does not occur if the filtering is done by using a "zero" phase shift program.

Montages

Montages are systematic and logical combinations of multiple pairs of electrodes using available channels (amplifiers), usually 16 to 21, which allow for the simultaneous recording of EEG activity over the entire scalp. The montages are created primarily to compare activity from homologous electrodes between the two hemispheres. In the United States, most laboratories prefer to display electrodes from the left hemisphere first (higher on the page) followed by electrodes from the right hemisphere (The International Federation recommends the opposite).[19] There are two basic montage design methods, *referential and bipolar montages*.

REFERENTIAL MONTAGES

The referential montage was originally called "monopolar" because it utilized one scalp electrode and one reference electrode in each channel. But this term is misnamed since none of the electrophysiologic recordings are truly "mono"polar. Two inputs are always needed. In a referential montage, multiple scalp electrodes (input 1) are connected to a common reference (input 2). The most commonly used reference is the ear (A1 or A2). Left hemisphere electrodes are usually referred to the left ear (A1) and right hemisphere electrodes are referred to the right ear (A2). The display is usually such that the frontopolar electrodes (Fp1 and Fp2) are at the top of the page followed by the more posterior electrodes with the occipital electrodes at the bottom of the page (Fig. 2-18).

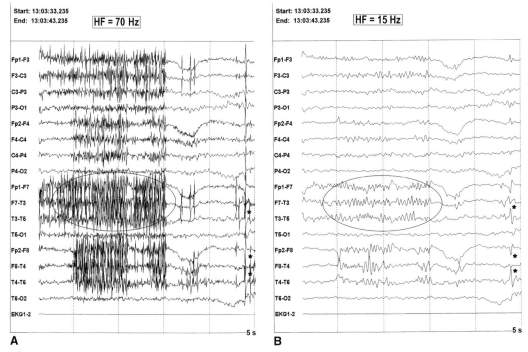

FIGURE 2-13 | **A and B:** Example of HF change. There is increased tonic muscle artifact and twitches (with use of HF at 70 Hz). Decreasing the HF from 70 to 15 Hz changes tonic muscle artifact to look like beta activity (*in circle*) and muscle twitch artifact to look like spike activity (indicated by *). (**A** and **B** are the same EEG samples.)

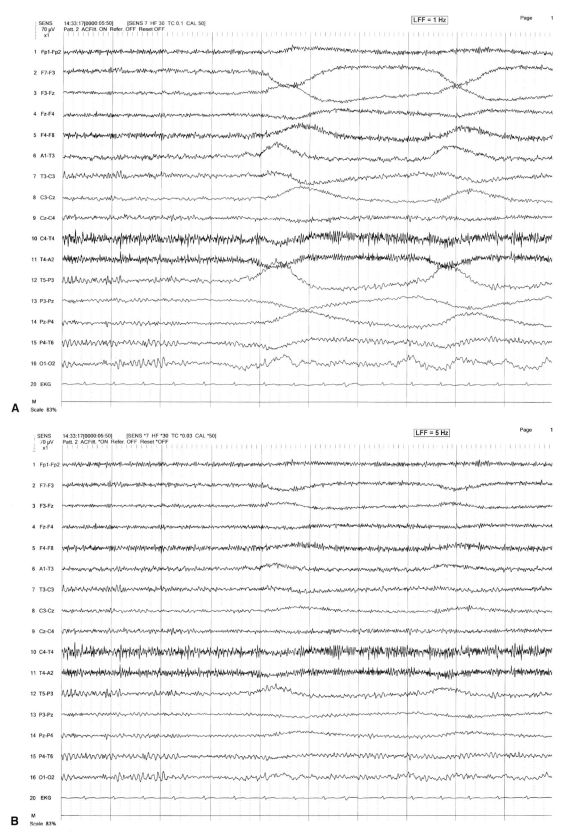

FIGURE 2-14 | Example of LF change. Slow drifting waves caused by sweat gland potential (sweat artifact) recorded with LF 1 Hz **(A)** is reduced by raising low-filter setting to 5 Hz **(B)**. (**A** and **B** are the same EEG samples.)

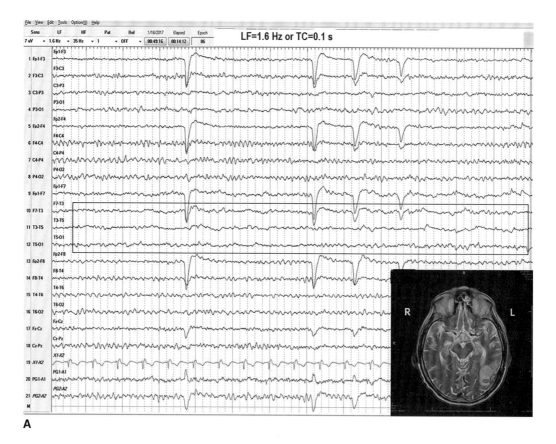

A

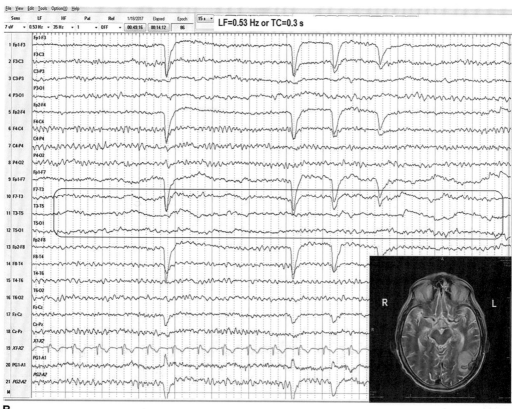

B

FIGURE 2-15 | Example of low-filter changes in a patient with a brain tumor in the left parietal region (shown by MRI). Focal delta activity at temporal electrodes (shown by *rectangular box*) is minimally recognized with LF setting of 1.6 Hz (TC = 0.1 s) **(A)** but more clearly visible with lowering the low-filter setting to 0.53 Hz (TC = 0.3 s) **(B)**. Conversely, using excessive LF setting of 5.3 Hz (TC = 0.03 s) essentially obliterates the delta slow waves **(C)**.

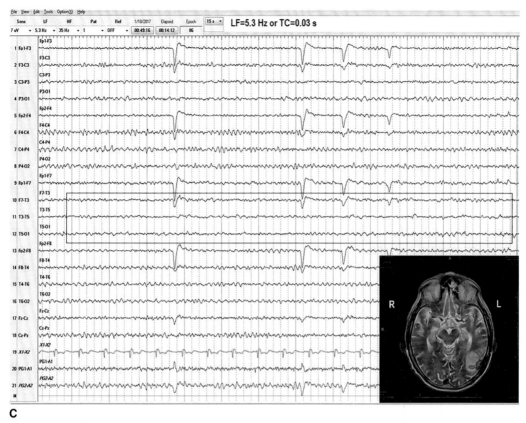

C

FIGURE 2-15 | *(Continued)*

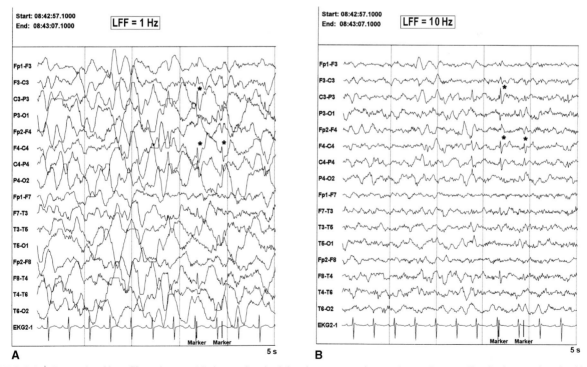

A

B

FIGURE 2-16 | Example of low-filter change. High-amplitude delta slow waves obscure intermittent spike discharges (marked by *) with LF 1 Hz **(A)**. Spikes are better visualized by reducing slow waves with LF 10 Hz **(B)**. (**A** and **B** are the same EEG samples.)

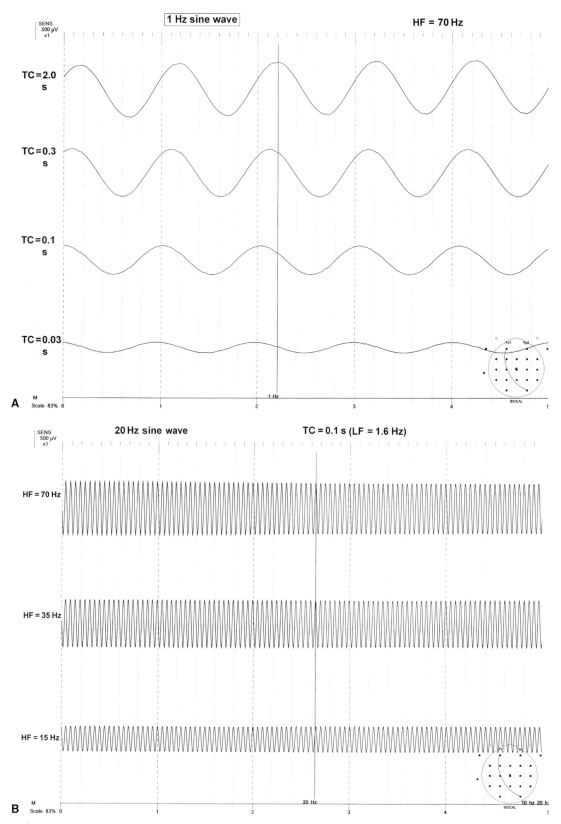

FIGURE 2-17 | **A:** Change in LFF causing a sine wave phase shift. Note that the peak of the 1-Hz sine wave becomes progressively shorter as the TC is shortened. **B:** Change in HFF causing sine wave phase shift. Note the peak of the 20-Hz sine wave becomes slightly later with the lower HFF.

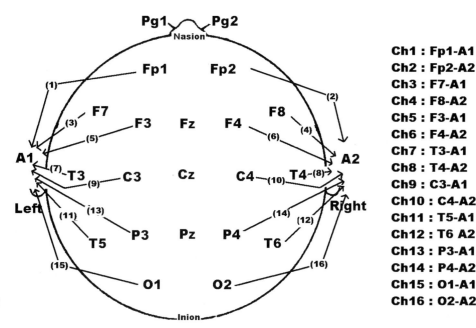

Ch1 : Fp1-A1
Ch2 : Fp2-A2
Ch3 : F7-A1
Ch4 : F8-A2
Ch5 : F3-A1
Ch6 : F4-A2
Ch7 : T3-A1
Ch8 : T4-A2
Ch9 : C3-A1
Ch10 : C4-A2
Ch11 : T5-A1
Ch12 : T6 A2
Ch13 : P3-A1
Ch14 : P4-A2
Ch15 : O1-A1
Ch16 : O2-A2

FIGURE 2-18 | Typical example of referential recording montage.

Some referential montages clump all of the left-sided channels on the top of the page with the right-sided channels toward the bottom. The referential montage in the diagram displays homologous electrode pairs (first left, then right) while moving from the front to the back of the head. With this arrangement, the first two channels show eye movement artifacts and last two channels show alpha rhythm. This allows an easy comparison between activity from the left and the right (Fig. 2-19).

The premise of the referential montage is that the reference electrode is assumed to be electrically "inactive." If this is the case, each channel shows true amplitude, frequency, and phase of the EEG activity at each electrode. This is the ideal situation, but it is never the case. The ear electrodes, indeed, are

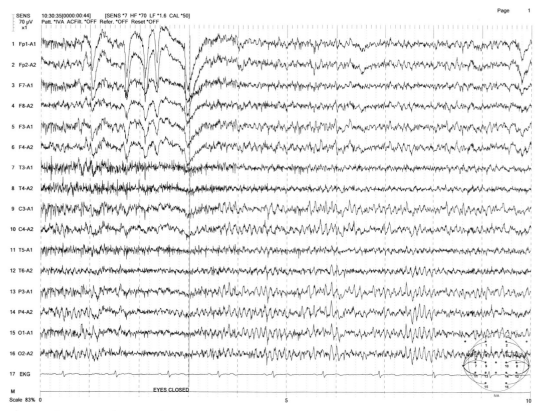

FIGURE 2-19 | Typical example of a normal awake EEG with referential (ear reference) recording. Note the alpha rhythm is focused at occipital electrodes and eye movement artifacts associated with eyes opening and closing are maximal at the frontopolar electrodes. EEG activity from a pair of left and right homologous electrodes is symmetric.

"active" with EEG activity because of their close proximity to the temporal lobes. When there is focal activity close to T3 or T4, A1 or A2, respectively, becomes active by the spread of EEG activity from T3 or T4. This is called "ear contamination." When there is a focal activity at T3 as shown in Figure 2-20, A1 reference becomes "active" or "contaminated" and all scalp electrodes connected to A1 are contaminated by A1 activity (Fig. 2-21A and B; see also Fig. 14-4A and B). In this case, the A1 electrode becomes "active" by spread of negative (upward swing) sharp discharge arising from T3. The T3 to A1 derivation then registers negative potential, smaller than the true amplitude at T3 because of a cancellation effect.

Conversely, electrodes that have no sharp discharge on their own can record large sharp waves that actually originated from A1. These discharges are downgoing or "positive polarity" (see next section for further explanation) because of greater negativity in the reference electrode, A1. To an untrained eye, this discharge might look like a diffusely distributed activity from all electrodes except T3. It could lead to misinterpretation of the field distribution of a wave of interest. Once identified, a montage with a contaminated ear reference can be clarified by choosing an alternate reference. Frequently, the opposite ear is chosen; for example, if A1 is active, all electrodes may be referred to A2 (see Fig. 2-21B). In this case, however, it should be noted that the amplitude between homologous electrodes is no longer comparable because of the unmatched interelectrode distances. But this is a good method to more accurately reflect the amplitude and distribution of the activity within the hemisphere.

Another solution when the focal activity is close to T3 or T4 is to use a Cz reference. This is an excellent way to maintain reliable amplitude comparisons between homologous electrode pairs (Fig. 2-21C). However, a Cz reference is not suitable if the patient becomes drowsy or asleep because Cz becomes highly "active" with vertex sharp waves, sleep spindles, or other physiologic sleep potentials contaminating all electrodes with these sleep activities (Fig. 2-22A and B). Figure 2-21D demonstrates another referential montage, that is, an average reference recording (see "Average Reference Montages").

Ear reference recording tends to pick up EKG artifacts more often than scalp-to-scalp bipolar recording (Fig. 2-23A). Because the polarity of EKG is opposite from A1 and A2 (because the QRS complex of the EKG vector is directed from right to left, EKG deflection is usually upgoing with A1 and downgoing with A2 reference recording), a linked ear reference (A1 + A2) can minimize EKG artifacts by the additive effect of positive and negative polarities (between A1 and A2) of the QRS complex (Fig. 2-23B).

Finding the perfectly "neutral" reference relative to the EEG activity is virtually impossible; chin, nose, or cheek may be used as a reference, but there is no guarantee that these references are "inactive" in reference to EEG activity. In fact, volume-conducted spikes originating from the temporal lobe may be detected from the face or even from the jaw. Chin, nose, or cheek references may also enhance artifacts from eye movement or glossokinetic potentials associated with tongue movement or talking (see Figs. 15-11 to 15-13).

When a distant reference away from the head (noncephalic reference) is used, EKG contamination onto the EEG recording becomes problematic. In order to minimize EKG contamination, a balanced reference offers some solution.[20] This requires an introduction of a potentiometer into the circuit that connects a cervical electrode and chest electrode. By adjusting the potentiometer, EKG artifact can be balanced and cancelled out.

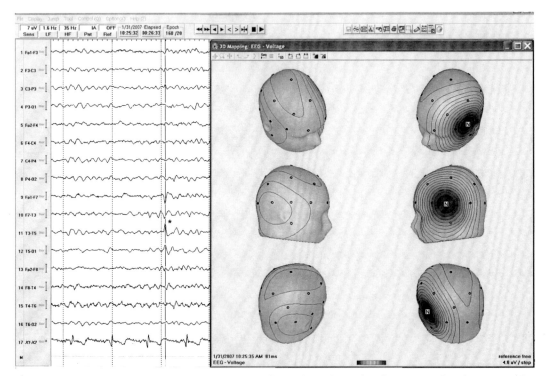

FIGURE 2-20 │ An example of sharp discharge, maximum at T3 electrode, is shown by phase reversal and topographic mapping. "N" in topographic map indicates peak field of negative polarity. Ear (A1) becomes "active" because A1 electrode is within the maximum field of the sharp discharge (see Fig. 2-21A).

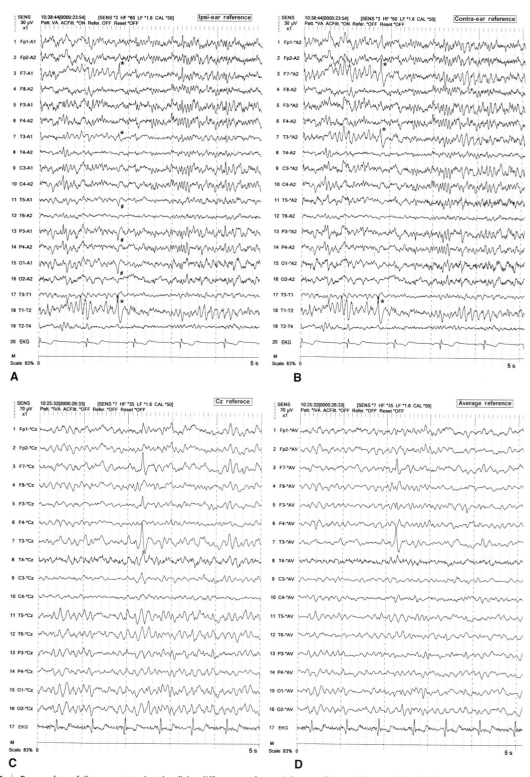

FIGURE 2-21 | Examples of "ear contamination" in different referential recordings. When spike discharge is maximally present at T3, the left ear (A1) is charged with activity similar to T3. This contaminates all electrodes connected to the A1 reference; because A1 is negatively charged, the electrodes where no spike discharges are present show "positive" or downward deflection reflecting the negative potential from A1 electrode **(A)** (shown by # mark in **A**). In order to avoid ear contamination from A1 electrode, contralateral ear (A2) can be used **(B)**. This yields a relatively "true" amplitude and distribution of this spike discharge (shown by * mark in **B**). However, this derivation shows smaller amplitude of EEG activity at F8, T4, and T6 as compared to the activity of homologous electrodes because of cancellation effect due to closer interelectrode distances. Another alternative reference is Cz reference recording to avoid ear contamination **(C)**. Cz is a good reference choice to show a relatively "true" amplitude and distribution of a temporal sharp discharge. Unlike contralateral ear reference (Fig. 2-21B), homologous derivations can be compared for amplitude symmetry. Note the smaller amplitude activity at P3, P4, C3, and C4 because of their shorter electrode distance to Cz. Another referential recording using average reference is shown in **(D)**. (**A** and **B**, **C** and **D** are the same EEG samples.)

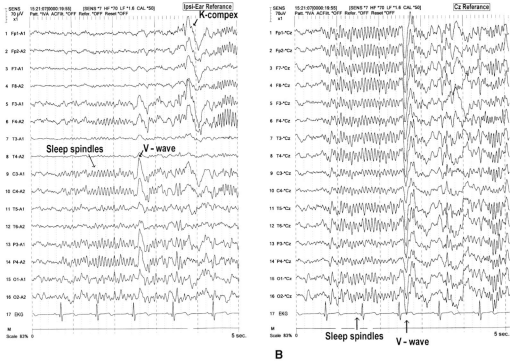

FIGURE 2-22 | A sleep EEG with sleep spindles and V waves in referential montage with ear reference **(A)**. Changing to a Cz reference **(B)** shows contamination of sleep spindles and V waves through all the channels. (**A** and **B** are the same samples.)

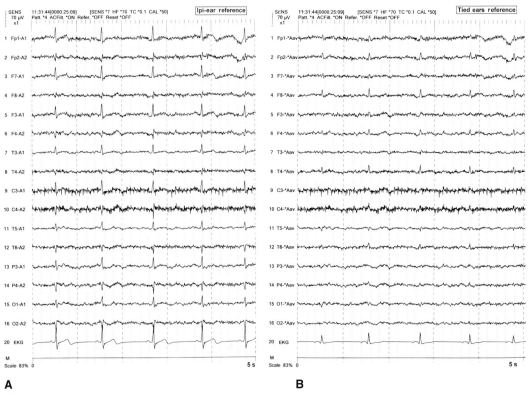

FIGURE 2-23 | Large EKG artifact with ipsilateral ear reference. Note the QRS complex of EKG shows an upward swing on the A1 channels and a downward swing on the A2 channels **(A)**. Combining A1 and A2 (tied or linked ear reference) electronically attenuates the EKG artifact **(B)**. In this example, A1 and A2 are considered as "average" reference. (**A** and **B** are the same EEG samples.)

AVERAGE REFERENCE MONTAGES

Another reference is called "average reference."[21,22] This reference is created by electronically combining the activity from all electrodes, and the mean activity from all electrodes serves as a reference (Fig. 2-24). In a digital system, this is achieved simply by the instantaneous calculation of the average value of all electrodes in use. Because there will be negative and positive polarities at different electrodes, the sum of all values derived from averaged reference recording nears zero. This is based on the theoretical assumption that the sum of all electrical events in the brain is balanced with zero potential.

This principle is true only if the averaging is derived from all the electrodes in use. As a practice, however, most commercially available EEG instruments allow the user to exclude channels that have large amplitude activity in order to minimize contamination. For example, Fp1 and Fp2 channels are often excluded to avoid large eye movement artifacts, which will show an inverted deflection in all channels if these electrodes are included in average. The same is true if an electrode of disproportionately high-amplitude focal activity is included in the average. The average reference recording is useful to delineate focal activity. As shown in Figure 2-25A, ear reference recording shows diffuse and bifrontal dominant spike discharges, although close scrutiny of the discharges shows a slight right-sided dominance at the frontal electrode. The average reference recording delineates a maximum negative spike at the right frontal electrode (F4) and positive polarity at distant electrodes (Fig. 2-25B). The average reference recording is often used for topographic brain mapping and quantitative EEG analyses.

BIPOLAR MONTAGE

In a bipolar montage, serial pairs of electrode are connected in longitudinal, transverse, or circumferential lines. Each pair of electrodes enters input 1 and input 2. When these pairs of electrodes are arranged in a chain, the input 2 electrode shares input 1 of the next channel. Bipolar montages are useful in defining the location of maximum potential. The electrode with the maximum voltage within a series of electrode linkage is expressed by a "phase reversal." If a given activity shows phase reversal between the two channels in a chain, the activity is maximum at the electrode common to both channels.

This is better understood with knowledge of the relationship of deflection to relative polarity. In any one channel, if input 1 is relatively more negative than input 2, the resulting deflection will be upward (i.e., simple subtraction of the values of input 2 from input 1; if the result is negative, this will result in upward defection). If input 2 is relatively more negative than input 1 (subtracted result of input 2 from input 1 is positive), then the deflection will be downward. Conversely, if input 1 is relatively more positive than input 2, the deflection will also be down. (Remember, if an input is more positive, it is also less negative.) And if input 2 is relatively more positive than input 1, the deflection will be upward.

As shown in Figure 2-26A, when input 2 has greater negativity than input 1, subtracting input 2 from input 1 will result in a positive value. Therefore, the deflection is down. Look, now, at the second channel and compare electrode 2 (now in input 1) to electrode 3 (in input 2). Since electrode 2 is more negative than electrode 3, the deflection is up. This results in a negative phase reversal (shown as the two deflections pointing to each other), indicating that this potential is negative in polarity and maximum at the electrode common to both channels, that is, electrode 2. A positive phase reversal (shown as deflections pointing away from each other) is shown in Figure 2-26B. In channel 1, electrode 1, though a positive voltage, is less positive (or more negative) than electrode 2. Therefore, the deflection is up. In channel 2, electrode 2 is more positive (and also less negative) than electrode 3, causing a downward deflection. This indicates that the potential at the electrode common to both channels (electrode 2) is maximally positive. If two electrodes of a pair have equal polarity, there is cancellation (equipotential) between the two and no potential is recorded (Fig. 2-26C and D). Figure 2-27A and B show an example of negative spike shown by peak meeting each other and an example of positive spike shown by peak away from each other, respectively.

The above "positive and negative phase reversal rules" work in most situations because a given activity usually has a single maximum negativity and/or a single maximum positivity at a certain electrode, with progressive potential decline further away from that electrode. If, however, the potential gradient is not progressive or two peaks of the same polarity exist simultaneously as shown in Figure 2-28, two phase reversals can occur. This is often called a "double phase reversal." The double (or triple) phase reversal occurs most frequently in artifactual conditions. If there is a double or triple phase reversal in a bipolar chain, the first choice is artifact unless proven otherwise. An example is shown in Figure 2-29, which shows artifactual delta activity caused by head movement: double phase reversals are occurring between T5 to O1 and O1 to O2 and O1 to O2 and O2 to T6 (see also Figs. 15-23 and 15-24). However, the double or triple phase reversal can be seen in a *rare* case of genuine cerebral activity. For example, when spike discharges are simultaneously distributed at T3 and T4 with both electrodes having greater amplitude than in-between (Cz in this case), a so-called butterfly distribution as shown in Figure 2-30 can occur. The spike shows a negative phase reversal at T3 and T4 with positive phase reversal at Cz simultaneously.

When there is a maximum voltage at input 1 of the first channel or input 2 of the last channel of a bipolar chain (Fig. 2-31A–D), this will result in no phase reversal (i.e., all potentials move in the same direction). This phenomenon is called an *"end of chain"* effect. In this case, the electrode of

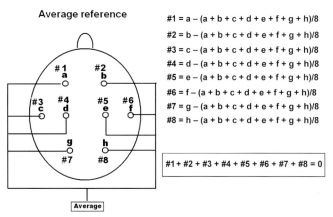

Average reference

#1 = a – (a + b + c + d + e + f + g + h)/8
#2 = b – (a + b + c + d + e + f + g + h)/8
#3 = c – (a + b + c + d + e + f + g + h)/8
#4 = d – (a + b + c + d + e + f + g + h)/8
#5 = e – (a + b + c + d + e + f + g + h)/8
#6 = f – (a + b + c + d + e + f + g + h)/8
#7 = g – (a + b + c + d + e + f + g + h)/8
#8 = h – (a + b + c + d + e + f + g + h)/8

#1 + #2 + #3 + #4 + #5 + #6 + #7 + #8 = 0

FIGURE 2-24 | Schematic model for average reference.

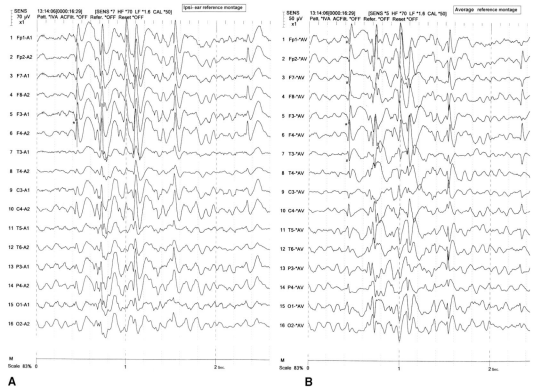

FIGURE 2-25 | Comparison of spike discharges recorded with ipsilateral ear reference **(A)** and with average reference **(B)**. Spike discharges are distributed diffusely with frontal dominance with ipsilateral ear reference recording **(A)**. Only with close scrutiny can one realize that the spike has slightly greater prominence on the right than on the left. All spikes are negative in polarity. In average reference recording **(B)**, negative spike is focused at frontal electrodes (F8, F4, and C4) with surrounding positive spikes. Adding all negative and positive spikes will result in "0." (**A** and **B** are the same EEG samples.)

maximum amplitude could be input 1 of the first channel or input 2 of the last channel, but it might lie even further out from these electrodes. To complete the phase reversal, additional electrodes may be added in the chain until a phase reversal can be found or changing the montage may show a phase reversal and clarify the site of highest activity (Fig. 2-32A and B).

SOURCE REFERENCE DERIVATION OR LAPLACIAN METHOD

In this method, each electrode is referred to its own unique reference, which is created by a weighted average derived from adjacent electrodes (Fig. 2-33). The theory behind this is that the activity measured at the scalp electrode is the sum of

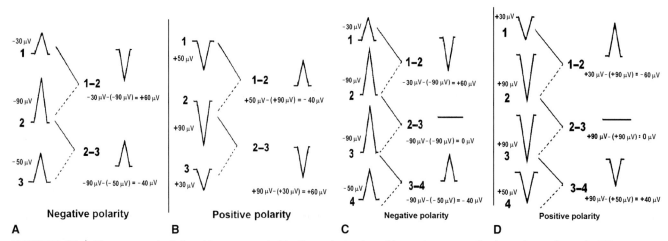

FIGURE 2-26 | Phase reversal relationships represented by three electrodes with maximum amplitude at electrode no. 2. **(A)** represents a negative phase reversal when the focus has a negative polarity and **(B)** represents a positive phase reversal for the positive polarity focus. Phase reversal relationship with the same amplitude at no. 2 and no. 3 electrodes. With either negative **(C)** or positive **(D)** polarity, a pair of two electrodes with the same amplitude results in "0" potential (cancellation effect).

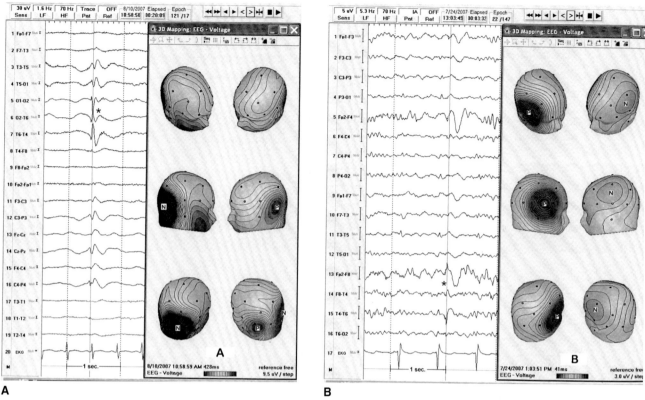

FIGURE 2-27 | Negative spike with phase reversal at O_2, corresponding with negative (*N*) field in topographic map **(A)** and positive spike with phase reversal at F8 and T4 (near equipotential at F8 and T4), corresponding positive (*P*) field in topographic map **(B)**.

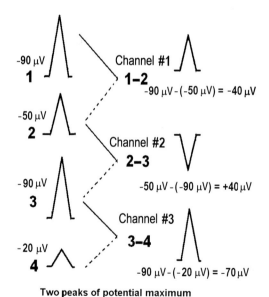

Two peaks of potential maximum at electrodes #1 and #3

FIGURE 2-28 | Phase reversal relationship when the potential gradient is not linear, that is, maximum negativity at no. 1 and at no. 3 electrodes with smaller negativity in-between these two electrodes. Note the phase reversal between channels 1 and 2 and also between channels 2 and 3, creating a "double phase reversal." Although the potential at each electrode is negative in polarity, the no. 2 electrode is "relatively" less negative as compared to no. 1 and no. 3, resulting in a positive phase reversal between channels 1 and 2. At the same time, no. 3 electrode is "relatively" more negative when compared to no. 2 and no. 4 electrodes, causing a negative phase reversal between channels 2 and 3.

numerous current sources in the underlying and adjacent cortex, resulting in a much wider potential field than the actual field distribution over the cortex. The source reference derivation attempts to mimic a "true" potential field of the activity over the cortex. This method involves the application of Laplacian's equation.[23,24] The mathematical calculation is as follows: the activity of each electrode is derived by subtraction of the reference created by the average value of four surrounding electrodes.

Practically, the Laplacian method has characteristics intermediate between bipolar and average reference montages. As in the averaged reference recording, this also creates steeper potential gradients and causes focal features to stand out from neighboring electrodes (Fig. 2-34A and B). This method is also used commonly for topographic brain mapping for detection of source localization of a given wave by dipole field distribution (Fig. 2-34C). Accuracy improves when a larger number of electrodes are used.

CREATION AND SELECTION OF MONTAGES

The most commonly used referential montage arranges electrodes from left and right homologous areas and refers those electrodes to the ipsilateral (same side) ear. The montage starts from the frontopolar electrodes (Fp1 and Fp2) in the first two channels and progresses to more posterior electrodes, and finally to the occipital electrodes (O1 and O2) in the last two channels (Fig. 2-18). Figure 2-35A shows a typical awake EEG showing alpha rhythm maximally at occipital electrodes and eye movement artifacts maximally at frontopolar electrodes.

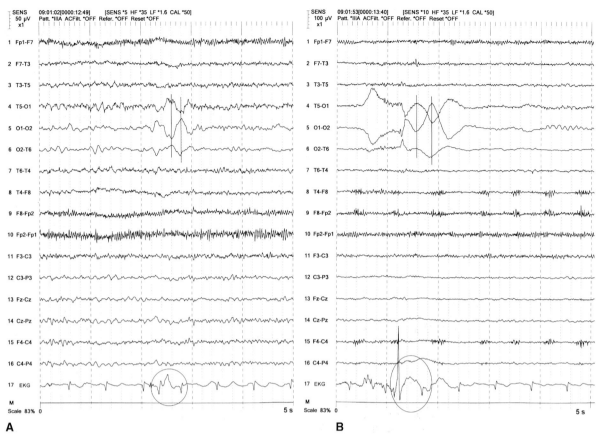

FIGURE 2-29 | A and B: Double phase reversal relationship caused by head movement. Note the double phase relationship of delta activity between T5 to O1 and O1 to O2 and between O1 to O2 and O2 to T6 (see Figs. 15-23 and 15-24, see also Video 15-10).

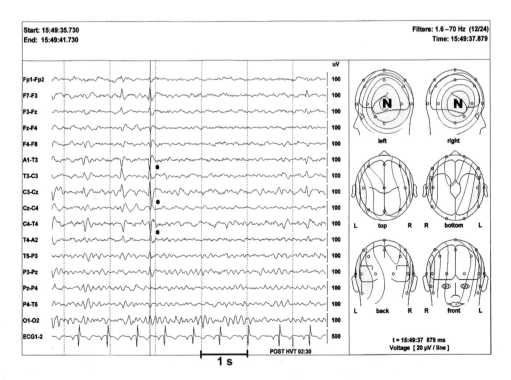

FIGURE 2-30 | Double phase reversal relationship in synchronous bitemporal spikes. This is an unusual spike distribution arising from temporal electrodes. As shown in topographic mapping, spike discharges of negative polarity appear on both temporal lobes simultaneously (indicated by "N"). Because the potential gradient is not linear from the left to right temporal transverse line (there are two peaks of spike discharges simultaneously), transverse derivation shows a "triple" phase reversal as indicated by *dot*.

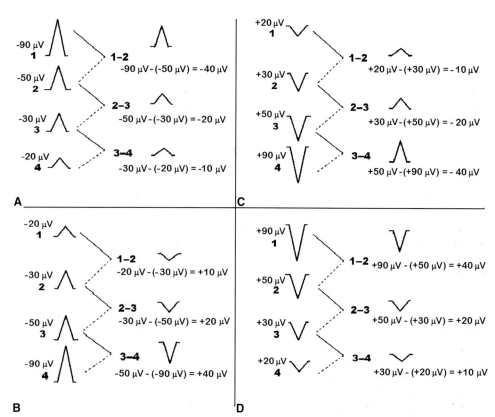

FIGURE 2-31 | A–D: "End of chain" relationship in a series of bipolar linkages. In this case, either input 1 of the first channel or input 2 of the last channel has maximum amplitude.

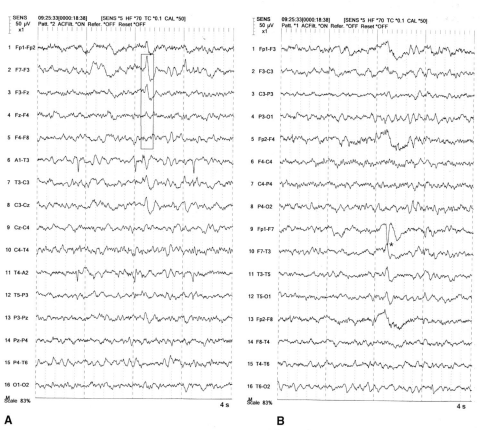

FIGURE 2-32 | An example of an "end of chain" effect with no phase reversal showing all upward deflection of the sharp discharge shown by rectangular box in **(A)**. This indicates this discharge has higher amplitude at F7 than at F3. **(B)** shows the same sample on a different montage that now reveal phase reversal between channels 9 and 10 (shown by * mark in **B**) indicating F7 has highest amplitude activity as compared to Fp1 or T3 activity, though the true focus could lie outside the electrodes currently being used and may require additional electrode (e.g., T1) to localize maximum amplitude of this sharp discharge.

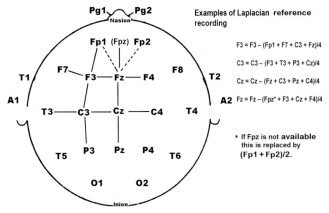

Examples of Laplacian reference recording

F3 = F3 – (Fp1 + F7 + C3 + Fz)/4

C3 = C3 – (F3 + T3 + P3 + Cz)/4

Cz = Cz – (Fz + C3 + Pz + C4)/4

Fz = Fz – (Fpz* + F3 + Cz + F4)/4

* If Fpz is not available this is replaced by (Fp1 + Fp2)/2.

FIGURE 2-33 | Schematic model of Laplacian method. Each electrode is referenced to the average of four surrounding electrodes. If there is no electrode at an equidistant site, the value is estimated by the neighboring electrodes.

Figure 2-35B shows a typical sleep EEG showing sleep spindles and vertex sharp waves at fronto-central-parietal regions and frontal dominant K complex (see "Normal Sleep EEG," Chapter 7; see also Figs. 7-37 to 7-40, and 7-42 for normal sleep patterns). Because the ear is relatively inactive, the amplitude of a given electrode fairly closely represents the true amplitude at each electrode, with the exception of T3 and T4, which shows spuriously low amplitude because of the short interelectrode difference between those electrodes and their respective reference electrodes. Instead of a single electrode alternating

from the left and right homologous areas, some laboratories prefer to arrange a group of electrodes from the left and right hemispheres, for example, left and right parasagittal electrodes, followed by left and right temporal electrodes. Neither option is necessarily better than the other. Physicians, like technologists, develop a preference usually based on experience.

In bipolar montages, there are two basic arrangements, longitudinal (anterior–posterior direction) and transverse (left-to-right direction). The most commonly used longitudinal montage is often called the "double banana" montage, which, when diagrammed, looks like two bananas, one on each hemisphere facing each other (Fig. 2-36). This montage is useful to view the symmetry of EEG activity between left and right hemispheres by comparing channels 1 to 4 and 5 to 8 from the parasagittal chains and 9 to 12 and 13 to 16 from the temporal chains. This shows eye movement artifacts at channels 1, 5, 9, and 13 and alpha rhythm at channels 4, 8, 12, and 16 (Fig. 2-37A). Figure 2-38A shows normal sleep pattern in "banana" montage, compared with referential montage (Fig. 2-38B). Some prefer to arrange the first eight channels from the left hemisphere and the last eight channels from the right hemisphere with the left temporal chain at channels 1 to 4 and the right temporal chain at channels 12 to 16.

With a longitudinal montage like these, it is not possible to accurately determine if the activity of interest is dominant in the parasagittal or the temporal region within the hemisphere. A transverse montage is used for this purpose.

Since a transverse montage runs sequentially from the left temporal, left parasagittal, midline, right parasagittal, and right temporal (Fig. 2-39), it is useful to determine if a given activity

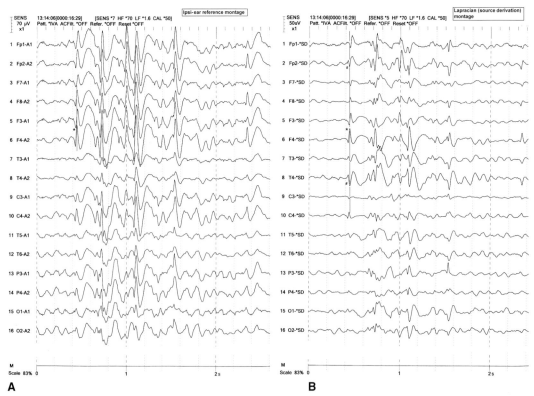

FIGURE 2-34 | **A and B:** An example of EEG reformatted by Laplacian method. This is the same EEG sample as in Figure 2-25A and B. The potential distribution is similar to that of the average reference recording (Fig. 2-25B) showing maximum negativity at F4 with positivity at Fp1, Fp2, and F3 electrodes. (**A** and **B** are the same EEG samples.) **C:** Example of a topographic map that uses Laplacian montage. Note positive and negative dipole distribution of potential fields.

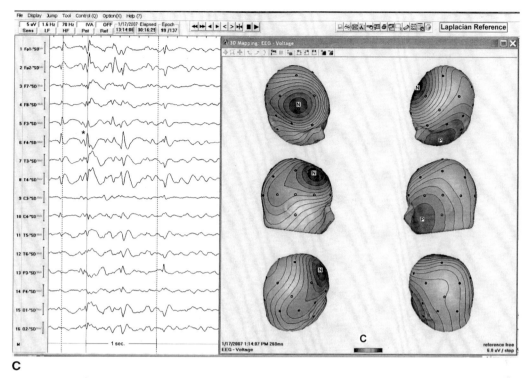

C

FIGURE 2-34 | (Continued)

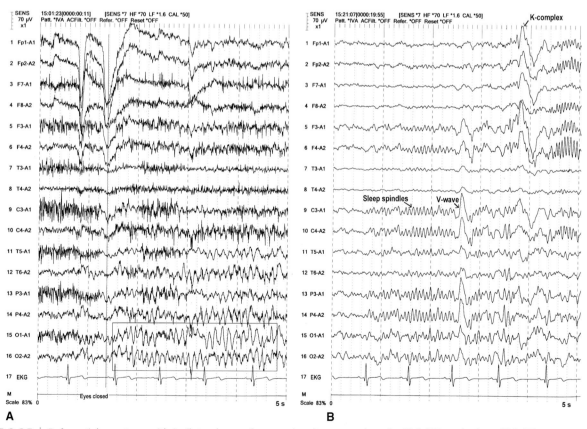

A

B

FIGURE 2-35 | Referential montage with ipsilateral ear reference showing normal awake EEG **(A)** and asleep EEG **(B)**.

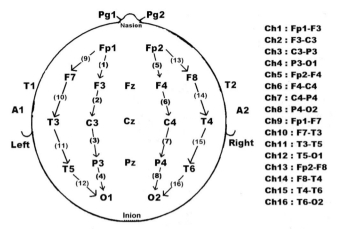

Ch1 : Fp1-F3
Ch2 : F3-C3
Ch3 : C3-P3
Ch4 : P3-O1
Ch5 : Fp2-F4
Ch6 : F4-C4
Ch7 : C4-P4
Ch8 : P4-O2
Ch9 : Fp1-F7
Ch10 : F7-T3
Ch11 : T3-T5
Ch12 : T5-O1
Ch13 : Fp2-F8
Ch14 : F8-T4
Ch15 : T4-T6
Ch16 : T6-O2

FIGURE 2-36 | Schematic model of longitudinal ("double banana") montage.

has temporal or parasagittal dominance, but it is less useful to determine the potential gradient in the anterior–posterior direction. Although the Fp1 to Fp2 derivation on a transverse montage does not have a homologous pair for comparison, this channel is useful to determine the symmetry of Fp1 and Fp2 activity (Fig. 2-40B). If Fp1 and Fp2 activities are symmetric, a relatively low-amplitude tracing is expected (in this derivation, vertical eye movement artifacts noted in other montages are cancelled out because of equipotentiality between Fp1 and Fp2). If the alpha rhythm between O1 and O2 has the same phase and amplitude, the O1 to O2 derivation should also

show a low-amplitude alpha or flat tracing. But O1 to O2 derivation usually shows alpha rhythm, at times even higher amplitude than O1 or O2 with referential recording, indicating that alpha rhythms are neither symmetric nor having same phase activities between O1 and O2 (Fig. 2-40B). This montage is especially useful in sleep recordings as it reveals better defined vertex sharp-wave phase reversals at the midline electrodes (Fig. 2-41B; see also Figs. 7-40, 7-42, and 7-45B and C). The K complex also shows a phase reversal at the midline, but with more frontal dominance (see Figs. 7-42 and 7-45B and C; see also Video 7-2).

The transverse and longitudinal montages are mutually complementary. With a longitudinal montage, it is not possible to accurately determine if the activity of interest is dominant in the parasagittal or the temporal region within the hemisphere. A transverse montage is used for this purpose. As shown in Figure 2-42A, a spike discharge in a longitudinal montage shows phase reversal between F4 to C4 and C4 to P4 and also at F8 to T4 and T4 to T6 derivations, but this does not clarify which of the two electrodes has higher amplitude of the spike. The transverse montage then gives the answer by the phase reversal between C4 to T4 and T4 to A2 derivations, indicating that T4 has higher-amplitude spike than C4 (Fig. 2-42B).

Because the transverse montage runs sequentially from the left temporal, left parasagittal, midline, right parasagittal, and right temporal, it is useful to determine if a given activity has temporal or parasagittal dominance, but it is less useful to determine the potential gradient in the anterior–posterior direction. An example for this is shown in Figure 2-43A and B; the spike

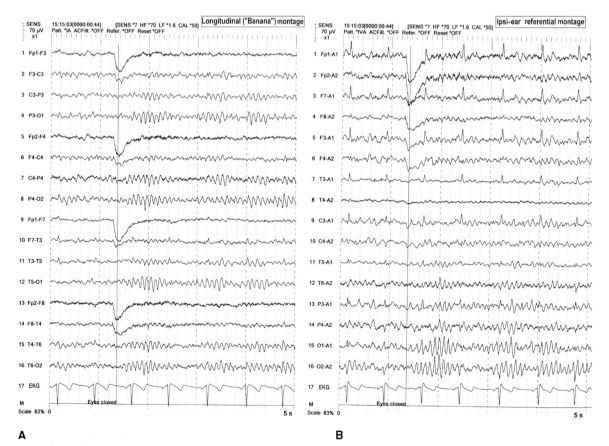

FIGURE 2-37 | Normal awake EEG with longitudinal bipolar montage **(A)** and referential montage **(B)** (**A** and **B** are from the same EEG samples).

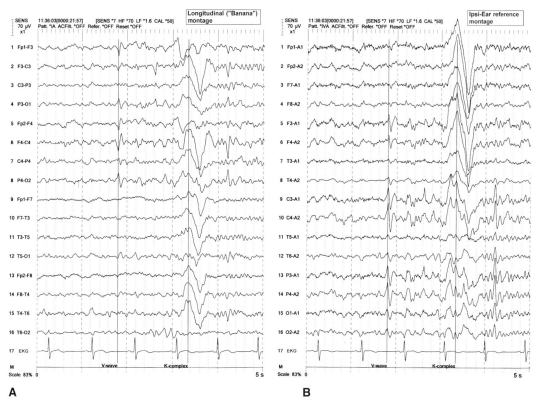

FIGURE 2-38 | Normal asleep montage with longitudinal bipolar montage on the left **(A)** and referential montage on the right **(B)**. (**A** and **B** are the same EEG samples.)

discharges show phase reversal between T3 to C3 and C3 to Cz and T5 to P3 and P3 to Pz, indicating the spike focus at C3 or P3, respectively, but this derivation is unable to determine which electrode of the two has larger amplitude when C3 and P3 electrodes are compared (Fig. 2-43A). The "double banana" montage reveals the phase reversal between C3 to P3 and P3 to O1 derivations, deciding that the P3 electrode has higher-amplitude spike than the C3 electrode (Fig. 2-43B).

Another commonly used montage is primarily longitudinal but arranged in a circumferential manner. It is called a "hat band" montage (Fig. 2-44). This montage is useful to visualize occipital activity (Fig. 2-45A). With this montage, posterior–temporal and occipital activities are conveniently arranged in channels 3 through 7, which makes it easy to evaluate the posterior activity, but not ideal for frontopolar and anterior–tem-

poral activity. Channels 4 to 6 show alpha rhythm in an awake EEG and *positive occipital sharp transients of sleep (POSTs)* in an asleep EEG (Fig. 2-46A; see Figs. 7-39A and B, 7-40B, and 7-45C; see Video 7-1B). Also in sleep, this derivation shows vertex sharp waves as a phase reversal at Cz in channels 13 and 14. Reversing this montage (i.e., posterior–anterior circumferential derivation) (Fig. 2-47), frontopolar and anterior–temporal activities are focused in channels 4 through 6, which makes for easier evaluation of these regions, but it is not convenient for examination of posterior activities. Focal activity at either frontopolar or anterior–temporal electrode is better localized by this *"reversed hat band"* montage when localization is not clear in other montages (Fig. 2-48A and B).

In some cases, long interelectrode distances are useful to delineate small potentials, which may not be well visualized with either transverse or longitudinal montages because of cancellation between two neighboring electrodes. Figure 2-49 shows such a montage, commonly called a "triangular montage." In a conventional longitudinal montage, only a small sharp transient is visible (Fig. 2-50A), but this becomes a distinct sharp discharge if using long interelectrode distances as in the triangular montage (Fig. 2-50B).

Each montage has advantages and disadvantages. It is also possible that the abnormality noted in one derivation may be obscured in another derivation. For example, if a spike discharge has equal amplitude at the anterior and midtemporal electrodes, this will be cancelled out in a longitudinal montage because of equipotentiality between the two electrodes (see Fig. 15-45B) but could be clearly visible using a transverse montage (see Fig. 15-45A). Conversely, in some cases, the asymmetry between two hemispheres is clearly visible in longitudinal montage but not in trans-

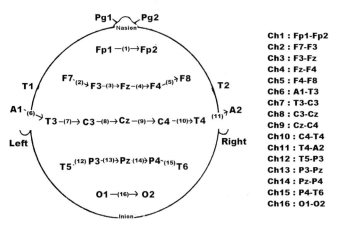

Ch1 : Fp1-Fp2
Ch2 : F7-F3
Ch3 : F3-Fz
Ch4 : Fz-F4
Ch5 : F4-F8
Ch6 : A1-T3
Ch7 : T3-C3
Ch8 : C3-Cz
Ch9 : Cz-C4
Ch10 : C4-T4
Ch11 : T4-A2
Ch12 : T5-P3
Ch13 : P3-Pz
Ch14 : Pz-P4
Ch15 : P4-T6
Ch16 : O1-O2

FIGURE 2-39 | Schematic model of transverse montage.

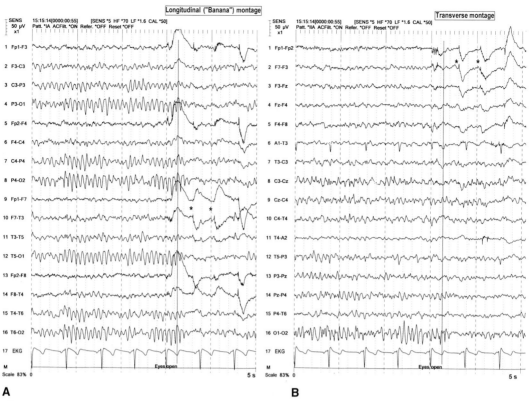

FIGURE 2-40 | Normal awake EEG with longitudinal bipolar montage on the left **(A)** and transverse montage on the right **(B)**. Note vertical eye movement associated with eyes opening (*vertical lines*) in "banana" montage **(A)** is cancelled out in transverse montage **(B)** but horizontal eye movements (shown by * mark) are visible in both montages. (**A** and **B** are the same EEG samples.)

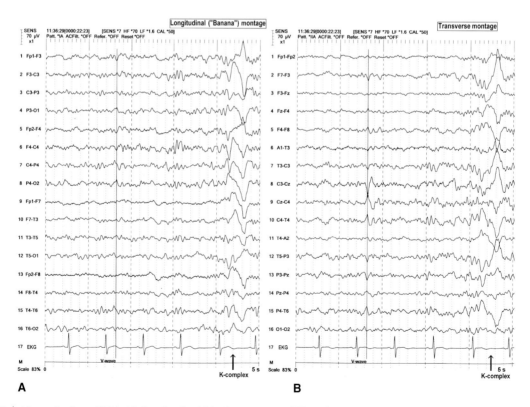

FIGURE 2-41 | Normal asleep EEG with longitudinal bipolar montage **(A)** and transverse montage **(B)**. Vertical lines indicate vertex sharp wave. (**A** and **B** are the same EEG samples.)

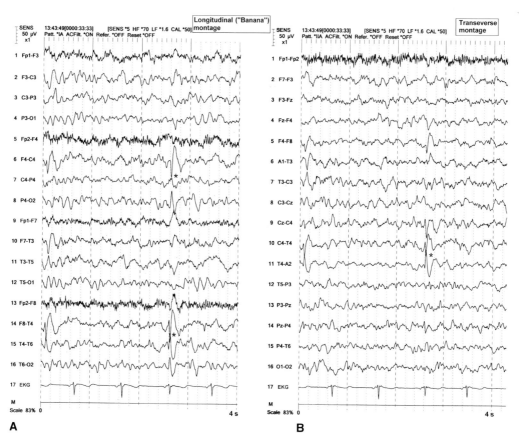

FIGURE 2-42 | Spike discharges recorded with "double banana" **(A)** and transverse montage **(B)**. In "double banana" montage, phase reversal of spike occurred at C4 and T4 electrodes (marked by * marks), but this does not clarify which of the two electrodes has higher amplitude of spike **(A)**. The transverse montage gives the answer by showing phase reversal at T4 (shown by * mark), indicating higher amplitude at T4 than at C4 **(B)**. (**A** and **B** are reformatted from the same EEG sample.)

verse montage (see Fig. 15-46A and B). It is vital that EEGs should not be interpreted after viewing solely on one montage.

Additional channels', including T1 and T2, electrodes often aid to delineate anterior–temporal activity, especially if longer interelectrode distances are used. The montage in Figure 2-50B includes three channels with such derivations. Channels 17 to 19 are Fz to T1, T1 to T2, and T2 to Fz. Viewing different montages is sometimes helpful to differentiate significant versus insignificant patterns or true EEG activity versus artifacts (see "Technical Pitfalls and Errors," Chapter 15). Digital EEG allows us to change the montage after the recording is completed. This can lead to more accurate and appropriate interpretation. This was not possible before the advent of digital EEG.

Calibration Signal

In analog EEG systems that involved mechanical movement of a pen by means of an oscillograph on moving paper, it was customary and essential to check the *square-wave calibration* signal [a direct current (DC) electrical source] and *"bio-calibration"* (an AC electrical source) in which all channels are connected to the same input, for example, Fp1 to O2. Most EEG labs chose Fp1 and O2 for this purpose because of the long interelectrode distance yielding large amplitudes and a variety of frequencies, including slow waves, generated by eye movements (from Fp1)

and alpha rhythm (from O2). These two calibrations were done before the start of the EEG recording to verify that all the channels were functioning equally. The square-wave calibration checked both mechanical and electrical properties resultant from a DC signal (calibration battery). And the biological calibration was an added component to verify the integrity of the EEG instrument in response to an AC signal (the brain activity). For digital EEG recording, some claim that the calibration signal and bio-calibration recording are not needed and meaningless. However, checking calibration routinely helps to avoid unforeseen mistakes and to recognize quickly if one or more channels are not programmed properly (i.e., filter or sensitivity programming errors). For example, Figure 2-51A shows how one is able to quickly recognize that channels 2, 4, 7, and 10 are different from the others: channel 2 shows a rounded peak in the calibration signal and smoother EEG (decreased fast activity), channel 4 shows quicker decay in calibration and decreased slow waves in EEG, channel 7 shows slower decay in calibration and increased slow EEG waves, and channel 10 shows decreased amplitude of both calibration and EEG without changes in waveforms. These are due to the HFF setting of 15 Hz instead of 70 Hz at channel 2, LFF setting of 5 Hz (*TC* = 0.03 s) at channel 4, and LFF setting of 0.5 Hz (*TC* = 0.3 s) at channel 7 instead of 1 Hz. At channel 10, the sensitivity is 15 μV/mm instead of 7 μV/mm. All square-wave calibrations and biological calibrations become identical after correcting these errors (Fig. 2-51B).

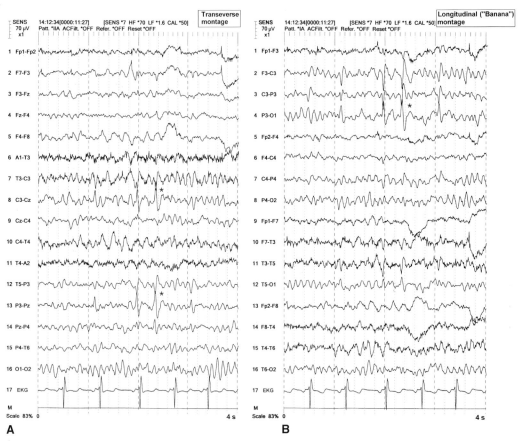

FIGURE 2-43 | Spike discharges recorded with transverse **(A)** and "banana" montage **(B)**. In transverse montage, phase reversal of spike occurred at C3 and P3 (marked by * marks), but this does not clarify which of the two electrodes has higher amplitude of spike **(A)**. The "banana" montage gives the answer, showing phase reversal at P3 (shown by * mark), indicating higher amplitude at P3 than C3 electrode. (**A** and **B** are reformatted from the same EEG sample.)

Administrative Issues in the EEG Lab

There is a variety of administrative chores that are a part of every EEG Lab. Paper work associated with the EEG process usually includes an EEG request (prescription), a technologist's worksheet, and a final report or interpretation of the EEG. The request and the final report become a part of the patient's permanent file. In modern EEG labs, these pieces of paper work might be stored in digital media, but the information should be available in one form or another. The technologist's worksheet can be kept in the EEG lab, but it is not a part of a patient's chart. Its purpose is to provide the electroencephalographer with the information necessary for proper interpretation. It should include:

1. Patient information such as name, age (date of birth), and identification number
2. Referring physician and referring service
3. Reason for EEG request
4. Patient's current and past history that is relevant to the EEG and relevant family history
5. Medications that the patient is taking, especially neuroleptic, psychiatric, sedative, and anticonvulsant drugs
6. Time of the last meal
7. If there is a seizure history or a history of episodes of altered consciousness, the date of the last event and description of the event, including aura and postictal state, etc.
8. The patient's mental and cognitive state
9. Presence of skull defects, edema, or unusual skull shape

An EEG lab should also have a Policy and Procedure manual. General hospital-wide policies are usually kept in a separate binding and cover items of interest to all employees in the hospital, such as general work rules and the rights and privileges of employment. A Policy and Procedure manual specific to the EEG lab outlines proper techniques involved in providing each service offered by the lab. This manual includes

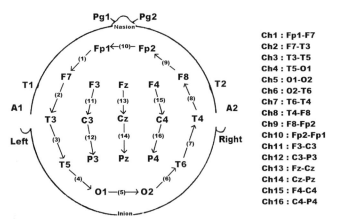

FIGURE 2-44 | Schematic model of anterior to posterior circumferential ("hat band") montage.

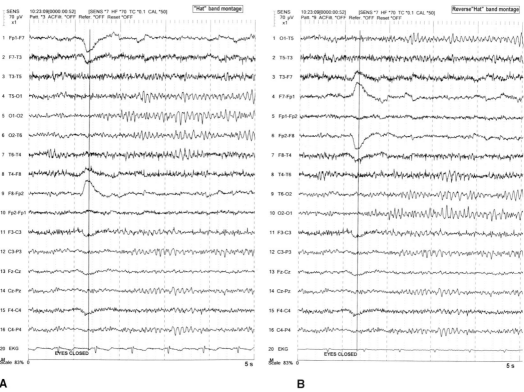

FIGURE 2-45 | Normal awake EEG with circumferential montage on the left **(A)** and reversed circumferential montage on the right **(B)**. Vertical lines indicate horizontal eye movement artifact. (**A** and **B** are the same EEG samples.)

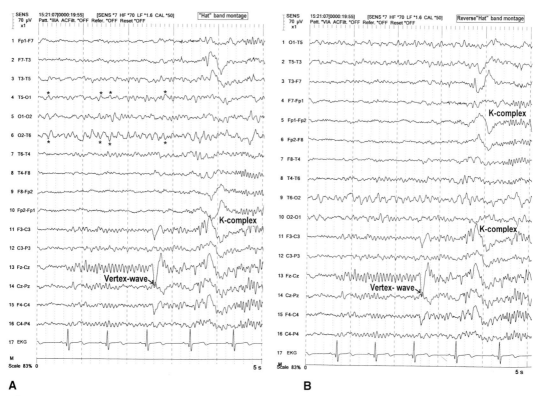

FIGURE 2-46 | Normal asleep EEG with circumferential montage on the left **(A)** and reversed circumferential montage on the right **(B)**. "POSTs" are indicated by * marks in **A**. (**A** and **B** are the same EEG samples.)

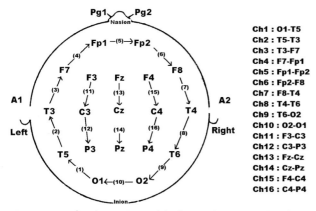

Ch1 : O1-T5
Ch2 : T5-T3
Ch3 : T3-F7
Ch4 : F7-Fp1
Ch5 : Fp1-Fp2
Ch6 : Fp2-F8
Ch7 : F8-T4
Ch8 : T4-T6
Ch9 : T6-O2
Ch10 : O2-O1
Ch11 : F3-C3
Ch12 : C3-P3
Ch13 : Fz-Cz
Ch14 : Cz-Pz
Ch15 : F4-C4
Ch16 : C4-P4

FIGURE 2-47 | Schematic model of posterior to anterior circumferential montage (reversed hat band montage).

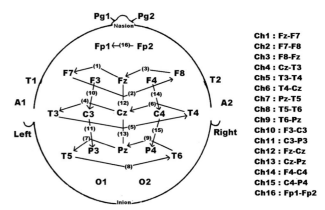

Ch1 : Fz-F7
Ch2 : F7-F8
Ch3 : F8-Fz
Ch4 : Cz-T3
Ch5 : T3-T4
Ch6 : T4-Cz
Ch7 : Pz-T5
Ch8 : T5-T6
Ch9 : T6-Pz
Ch10 : F3-C3
Ch11 : C3-P3
Ch12 : Fz-Cz
Ch13 : Cz-Pz
Ch14 : F4-C4
Ch15 : C4-P4
Ch16 : Fp1-Fp2

FIGURE 2-49 | Schematic model of long interelectrode distance "triangle" montage.

itemized procedures as well as general policies. With proper EEG training and a good Policy and Procedure manual, a new EEG technologist should be able to handle any problem that comes up in the lab if the supervisor is unavailable. The EEG specific Policy and Procedure manual is generally a large volume that includes items like:

1. Treatment of hazardous materials (acetone, collodion, sharp objects, etc.). This section should also include material safety data sheets (MSDS) for all chemicals found in the lab. The MSDS gives important information regarding chemical properties, safe storage, proper handling of a spill, etc., and needs to be readily available.

2. Infection control. This section discusses how to handle infective patients. It should outline proper techniques for entering and exiting an isolated patient room. It should also include information regarding specific illness and how the EEG procedure is affected. Additionally, it

should include specific guidelines for cleaning or disposal of contaminated equipment.

3. Sedation policy. Many EEG labs will give a mild sedative (with an order from and under the direction of a physician). Policy regarding the procurement of this permission, safe dosing, and proper monitoring is *a must* if sedation is to be used in the EEG laboratory.

4. Equipment maintenance. Policy should be written to dictate the frequency of routine testing of equipment in the EEG lab. Additionally, there should be a section outlining a procedure for repair of malfunctioning equipment.

5. Maintaining credentials. Policy and Procedure should be written to outline the process of maintaining EEG credentials. This section can also house a statement of Scope of Practice for the EEG technologist.

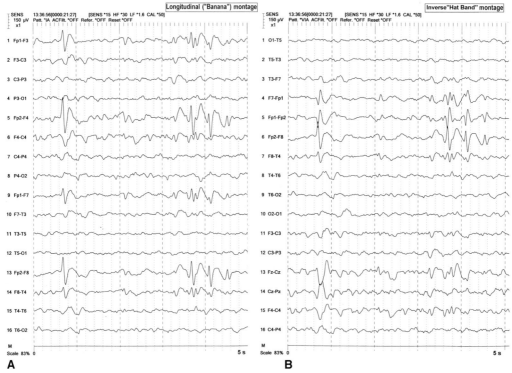

FIGURE 2-48 | An "end of chain" effect on a longitudinal bipolar montage (**A**) becomes a phase reversal when viewed on a reversed circumferential montage (**B**). (**A** and **B** are reformatted from the same EEG sample.)

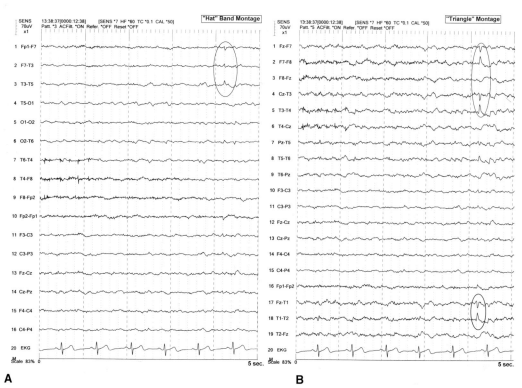

FIGURE 2-50 | Circumferential montage shows small spike at channels 1 to 3 **(A)** while triangle montage shows more distinct spikes in F7 and T3 **(B)**. Small spikes are shown by elongated *circles*. (**A** and **B** are reformatted from the same EEG sample.)

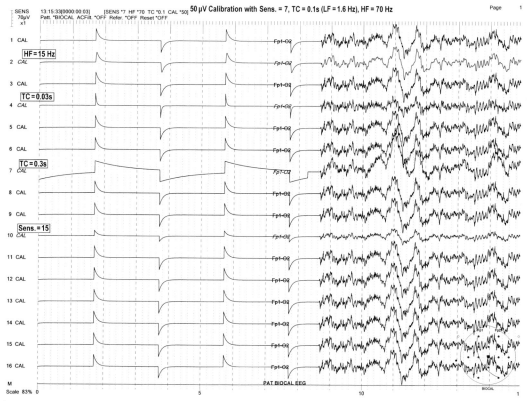

FIGURE 2-51 | **A:** Errors in square-wave calibration and bio-calibration. Note that square-wave calibration and bio-calibration are different at channels 2, 4, 7, and 10, resulting in dissimilar calibration signals and EEG patterns. **B:** Corrected calibration signals showing identical calibration signals and EEG patterns throughout all channels.

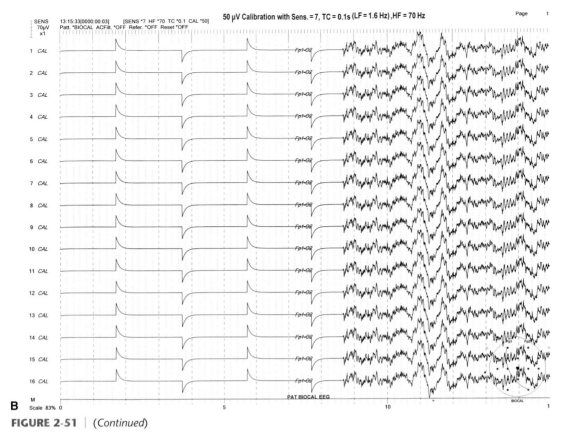

FIGURE 2-51 | (Continued)

References

1. Geddes LA. Bioelectrodes. Part II: The nature of electrode impedance. *Am J EEG Technol* 1974;14:205–210.
2. Geddes LA. Bioelectrodes. Part III: The importance of amplifier input impedance. *Am J EEG Technol* 1975;15:99–106.
3. Tyner FS, Knott JR, Mayer WB Jr. *Fundamentals of EEG Technology.* New York: Raven Press, 1983.
4. Tyner FS, Knott JR. Amplitude asymmetries when using subdermal electrodes: Is accurate head marking sufficient? *Am J EEG Technol* 1976;15:179–187.
5. American Clinical Neurophysiology Society. Guideline 1: Minimal technical requirement for performing clinical electroencephalography. *J Clin Neurophysiol* 2006;23(2):86–91.
6. de Jesus PV, Masland WS. The role of nasopharyngeal electrodes in clinical electroencephalography. *Neurology (Minneap)* 1970;20:869–878.
7. Kashing DM, Celesia GG. Nasopharyngeal electrodes in the diagnosis of partial seizures with complex symptoms. *Arch Neurol (Chicago)* 1976;35:519–529.
8. Morris HH, Lueders H, Lesser RP, et al. The value of closely spaced scalp electrodes in the localization of epileptiform foci: A study of 26 patients with complex partial seizures. *Electroencephalogr Clin Neurophysiol* 1986;63:107–111.
9. Sperling MR, Engel J Jr. Electroencephalographic recording from the temporal lobes: A comparison of ear, anterior temporal and nasopharyngeal electrodes. *Ann Neurol* 1985;17(5):510–513.
10. Ives JR, Gloor P. New sphenoidal electrode assembly to permit long-term monitoring of the patients' ictal or interictal EEG. *Electroencephalogr Clin Neurophysiol* 1977;42:575–580.
11. Wieser HG, Hajek M. Foramen ovale and peg electrodes. *Acta Neurol Scand Suppl* 1994;152:33–35.
12. Arellano AP. A tympanic lead. *Electroencephalogr Clin Neurophysiol* 1949;1:112–113.
13. Lethinen OJ, Bergsrom L. Clinical and laboratory notes. Naso-ethmoidal electrode for recording the electrical activity of the inferior surface of the frontal lobe. *Electroencephalogr Clin Neurophysiol* 1970;29:303–305.
14. Lueders H, Lesser RP, Dinner DS, et al. Commentary: Chronic intracranial recording and stimulation with subdural electrodes. In: Engel J Jr, ed. *Surgical Treatment of the Epilepsies.* New York: Raven Press, 1987:297–321.
15. Engel J Jr, Rausch R, Lieb JP, et al. Correlation of criteria used for localizing epileptic foci in patients considered for surgical treatment of epilepsy. *Ann Neurol* 1981;9:215–224.
16. Jasper HH. Report of the committee on methods of clinical examination in electroencephalography. *Electroencephalogr Clin Neurophysiol* 1958;10:370–375.
17. Silverman D. The anterior temporal electrode and the ten-twenty system. *Electroencephalogr Clin Neurophysiol* 1960;12:735–737.
18. American Clinical Neurophysiology Society. Guideline 5: Guidelines for standard electrode position nomenclature. *J Clin Neurophysiol* 2006;23(2):107–110.
19. IFSECN Proceedings. EEG instrumentation standards. *Electroencephalogr Clin Neurophysiol* 1978;45:144.
20. Stephenson WA, Gibbs FA. A balanced noncephalic reference electrode. *Electroencephalogr Clin Neurophysiol* 1951;3:139–143.
21. Offner FF. The EEG as potential mapping: The value of the average monopolar reference. *Electroencephalogr Clin Neurophysiol* 1950;2:215–216.
22. Goldman D. The clinical case of "average" reference electrode in monopolar recording. *Electroencephalogr Clin Neurophysiol* 1950;2:211–214.
23. Hjorth B. An on-line transformation of EEG scalp potentials into orthogonal source derivation. *Electroencephalogr Clin Neurophysiol* 1975;39:526–530.
24. Nunez PL, Pilgreen KL. The Spline-Laplacian in clinical neurophysiology: A method to improve EEG spatial resolution. *J Clin Neurophysiol* 1991;8:397–413.

3

Basic Electronics and Electrical Safety

PETER SEABA and THORU YAMADA

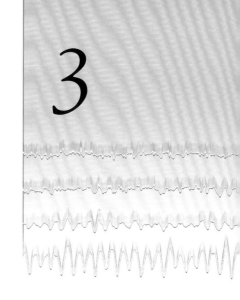

Basic Electricity and Electronics

The following is a synopsis of the "basic electricity" concepts that are important for one to know when studying EEG instrumentation. This chapter should be read while studying the figures to understand the concepts being described.

Basic electricity consists of units (volts, amperes, ohms, watts), components (*resistors, capacitors, inductors*), and formulas (*Ohm's law, power,* components in series/parallel). In addition, there are special topics unique to EEG instrumentation. Understanding these basic concepts will ensure the understanding of EEG-related concepts found later in this chapter.

BASIC ELECTRONIC UNITS

Table 3-1 lists the basic electronic units.

OHM'S LAW

Ohm's law is a formula which is used in many EEG applications. It describes how current, resistance, and voltage are interrelated in a circuit. To understand Ohm's law, one should know that voltage (*E*) is the electrical force that moves electrons through wires and electrical devices. Current (*I*) is the rate of electron flow. Resistance (*R*) is a property that limits current.

$$Flow \sim Pressure \quad \& \quad Flow \sim \frac{1}{Resistance}$$

$$\Rightarrow \quad Flow \sim \frac{Pressure}{Resistance}$$

FIGURE 3-1 | Hydraulic analogy of Ohm's law.

It might also be helpful to use an analogy between hydraulics and electricity. In a hydraulic system, the flow of water will depend on the water pressure and the dimension of the pipe or hose (resistance). The flow of water is proportional to the water pressure. If someone squeezes the hose, increasing its resistance, the flow decreases. Flow is inversely proportional to resistance. We can combine the two relationships as shown in Figure 3-1.

In a similar manner, electromotive force (EMF) will cause current to flow through a wire. The electrical analogy is that electrical current (*I*) is proportional to voltage (*E*) but inversely proportional to resistance (*R*). This can be stated in the following formula, where "*I*" is current, "*E*" is voltage, and "*R*" is resistance.

$$I = E \times 1/R \quad or \quad I = E/R$$

This is one form of *Ohm's law.* By algebraic manipulation (multiply both sides of the equation by *R*), we have the more familiar form: $E = I \times R$.

The unit of power is watt. Power can be calculated by the following formulas:

1. Power = $E \times I$
2. Power = I^2R (since $E = I \times R$)
3. Power = E^2/R (since $I = E/R$)

RESISTORS

Resistors are electronic components in a circuit which are meant to impede current flow. They can be arranged in a series or in parallel, and the total resistance depends on this arrangement.

Resistors in Series

Resistors can be placed in a circuit one after another in a series. When a string of resistors is connected in a series, the

TABLE 3-1 BASIC ELECTRONIC UNITS		
Name	Symbol	Units
Charge	*Q*	Coulomb (6.25 × 10^18 e⁻)
Voltage	*E*	Volt [Requires 0.799 V to remove outer electron from silver (ionization potential). Also listed as EMF]
Current	*I*	Ampere (or amp) [flow of 6.25 × 10^18 e⁻ per second (1 C/s)]
Resistance	*R*	Ohm
Impedance	*Z*	Ohm
Power	*P*	Watt

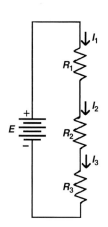

1. The voltage across the three resistors equals the battery voltage E.

2. Using Ohm's Law, the voltage across the resistors are: $R_1 \times I_1$, $R_2 \times I_2$, $R_3 \times I_3$.

$$E = I_1R_1 + I_2R_2 + I_3R_3$$

3. Since it is the same current going through all three resistors, $I_1 = I_2 = I_3 = "I."$

$$E = IR_1 + IR_2 + IR_3$$

$$E = I(R_1 + R_2 + R_3)$$

4. We now have a equivalent resistance, one that fits the equation: $E = IR_{eq}$.

$$R_{series} = R_1 + R_2 + R_3 + \dots\dots$$

FIGURE 3-2 | Equivalent resistance of resistors in series.

combined resistance is equal to the individual resistances added together. Therefore, an appropriate single resistor can replace several individual resistors in series. The equivalent resistor must equal the sum of all the resistor values. For example, if resistors R_1 and R_2 are connected in series, their combined resistance, R, is given by

Combined resistance in series: $R = R_1 + R_2$.

This will be true for more resistors: $R_{series} = R_1 + R_2 + R_3 + \dots$

One important point to remember is that the combined resistance in series will always be greater than any of the individual resistances. A derivation of the equivalent resistor is shown in Figure 3-2.

Using the hydraulic analogy, if you add another section of hose to the existing hose, the resistance increases.

Resistors in Parallel

Notice that parallel resistors provide several individual routes for the current to complete the circuit and return to the negative side of the battery (Fig. 3-3). Thus, the resistance will be lowered, and it will be lower than that of any single resistor. The total resistance of resistors in parallel will always be less than the resistance of any single resistor.

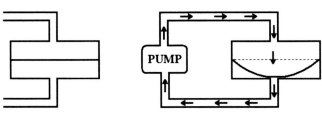

FIGURE 3-4 | Hydraulic analogy of a capacitor.

What is the equivalent resistance of three resistors in parallel? This time, we do not have a single loop of current, but one path for each resistor. The equivalent resistance of three resistors in parallel is

$$R_{parallel} = \frac{1}{1/R_1 + 1/R_2 + 1/R_3}$$

CAPACITORS

Capacitors are electronic components of a circuit that are designed to store a charge between compartments. A pump can store pressure by pumping water from one side to the other. The hydraulic analogy of a capacitor is a pressure vessel with a diaphragm between compartments (Fig. 3-4). A capacitor is a component that can store electrical energy analogous to the hydraulic pressure storage system. It has a similar design as shown in Figure 3-5.

The voltage–current relationship changes with time. The rules for adding capacitors in series and parallel are reversed from those for adding resistors in series and parallel, respectively. The capacitance of this device is defined by how much charge is moved per volt applied. A capacitor that will store 1 C when 1 V is applied is a 1 F capacitor.

Capacitance is proportional to the area of the plates or conductors (the more area, the more electrons that can be stored). However, it is inversely proportional to the distance between the plates. The closer the plates, the more the attraction between + and − and the more electrons you can store per volt. These factors, plate area and distance between the plates, affect how capacitors behave in series and parallel.

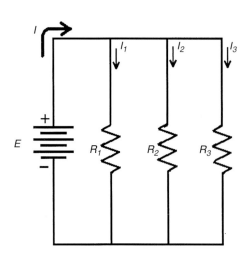

1. The current from the battery is the sum of the individual currents.

$$I = I_1 + I_2 + I_3$$

2. $I = E/R_1 + E/R_2 + E/R_3$

$$I = E(1/R_1 + 1/R_2 + 1/R_3)$$

3. Multiply both sides by $(1/R_1 + 1/R_2 + 1/R_3)$ and the equation becomes:

$$"E = I/(1/[R_1 + R_2 + R_3])"$$

$R_{equivalent}$: $1/(1/R_1 + 1/R_2 + 1/R_3)$

FIGURE 3-3 | Equivalent resistance of resistors in parallel.

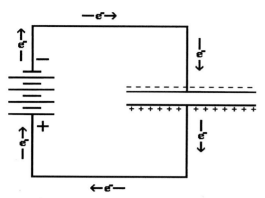

FIGURE 3-5 | Charging the capacitor.

Capacitors in Parallel

When capacitors are in parallel, the plate area increases. Thus, the capacitance increases proportionately (Fig. 3-6):

$$C_{parallel} = C_1 + C_2 + C_3 + \cdots$$

Capacitors in Series

When capacitors are in series, the distance between the plates increases. Capacitance then decreases. The formula is the same as that for resistors in parallel (Fig. 3-7):

$$C_{series} = \frac{1}{1/C_1 + 1/C_2 + 1/C_3 + \cdots}$$

INDUCTANCE

Inductance is the ratio of magnetic flux to the current in a circuit. Inductance opposes any change in current through the conductor.

Capacitors and the effects of capacitance are common in medical instruments. Inductors are seen more often in high-frequency circuits, such as radios. Inductors used for low-frequency applications are physically large.

Current flowing through a wire produces a magnetic field around the wire. Coiling the wire increases the intensity of the magnetic field. As the current flows, a magnetic field expands around the coil of wire. This generates an opposing voltage and opposes the increase in current. If, once the current is flowing, the switch is suddenly opened, the magnetic field will begin to decrease and collapse around the coil. Whenever a magnetic field changes in intensity, the intensity

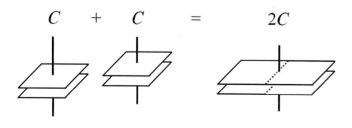

$$C_{parallel} = C_1 + C_2 + C_3 + \cdots$$

FIGURE 3-6 | Equivalent capacitance of capacitors in parallel.

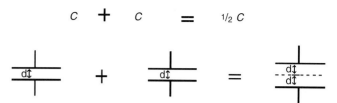

FIGURE 3-7 | Equivalent capacitance of capacitors in series.

change will induce a current in the coil of wire (Fig. 3-8). In this case, the diminishing magnetic field will induce current flow in the same direction. Inductance also opposes a decrease in current.

The hydraulic analogy of inductance is inertia. Fluid at rest tends to remain at rest and fluid in motion tends to remain in motion. Similar to inertia, inductance opposes any change in current through the inductor. The unit of inductance is the henry. Inductors in series and parallel circuits are combined like resistors in series and parallel, respectively.

Power Transformers

Power transformers are devices that transfer electrical energy from one circuit to another. They are used to "step up" or "step down" the voltage.

If you induce current in a wire, the wire will develop a magnetic field around it (Fig. 3-9, left). If this magnetic field cuts through a nearby coil of wire, the wire will develop a voltage since it is experiencing a change in the magnetic field strength (Fig. 3-9, right). The transformer combines these two phenomena. An AC voltage is applied to the input called the primary coil. The primary coil will generate a varying magnetic field. The magnetic field then cuts the second coil (secondary) and then induces electricity within the second coil.

The ratio of the number of windings on each side of the transformer affects the voltages. If you have the same number of windings on each side, the output voltage will be the same as the input voltage (Fig. 3-10). If a transformer has a turns ratio greater than 1, the output voltage is less than the input voltage.

If the ratio is 10:1, 120 V would produce 12 V at the output (Fig. 3-11). Even though the voltage is reduced, the amount of current available increases by the same factor. A load of 0.4 Ω would draw 30 A. The power consumed by the resistor would be 360 W (30 A × 12 V). The same power would have to be flowing into the transformer. Since the input voltage is 120 V, the current flowing into the transformer is only 3 A (120 V × 3 A = 360 W).

ISOLATION TRANSFORMER

The isolation transformer is a simple 1:1 transformer as shown in Figure 3-10. This eliminated the problem of one side of the outlet (neutral) being grounded. When nearly all of the anesthetics were explosive, personnel were required to be grounded to avoid static sparks. Since they are grounded, they need only come in contact with a faulty drill, saw, or some other device that has a fault. To reduce the chance of the staff being electrocuted, isolated power is provided. Neither side is grounded, so that leakage current will not flow through a person to the nearest ground. Even though flammable anesthetics are rare and people are no longer required to be grounded, the isolation transformer is still required.

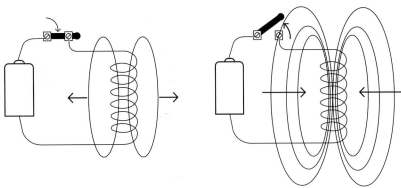

As the switch closes, the current generates an expanding magnetic field.

As the switch opens, the magnetic field collapses around the wire.

FIGURE 3-8 | Expanding magnetic field induces opposing field. Collapsing tries to maintain the field.

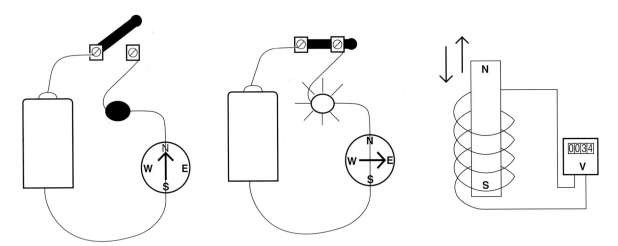

Electrical current generates magnetic field

Moving magnetic field generates electricity

FIGURE 3-9 | Current flowing through wire generates magnetic field. Magnetic field cutting wire induces current.

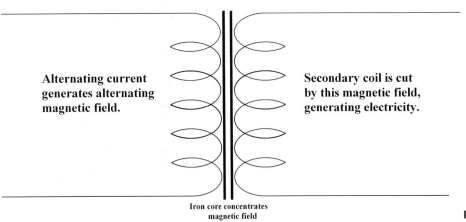

Alternating current generates alternating magnetic field.

Secondary coil is cut by this magnetic field, generating electricity.

Iron core concentrates magnetic field

FIGURE 3-10 | Transformer operation.

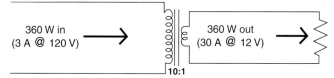

FIGURE 3-11 | Transformer decreases voltage and increases current.

Isolation transformers are also used on portable systems that have excessive leakage current. If an isolation transformer is used, the leakage current is only that of the input of the transformer.

THE GROUND LOOP

The ground loop may be problematic for patient safety or may introduce interference into the recording. The ground loop is a loop of wire around a room. Its path may go from an electrical outlet to the instrument attached, through patient connections, to another instrument, to an outlet at the far side of the room, and, through the ground wire, back to the first outlet. This can be avoided by plugging all of the patient-connected instrumentation into the same group of outlets.

The ground loop gets its power from the transformer effect. Current in the primary windings creates a magnetic field, which in turn creates current in the wire it "cuts" (the secondary). Instead of the primary, we have various instruments generating magnetic fields. The secondary is a single loop of wire around the room. Each of the devices around the room generates a magnetic field, which in turn generates current in the loop. We

are not able to estimate how many "turns" are on the primary, but the single loop ensures that the voltage will be low while the current is high.

In Figure 3-12, the EEG is plugged into an outlet across the room and the chassis touches the grounded bed, completing the loop. The resistance of the ground wires around the room would be low, allowing maximum current to flow through the loop. The current generates noise on the EEG's ground line. It can even flow through the patient.

Voltage Divider

The voltage divider is used in many EEG applications. One of the most commonly used voltage dividers is amplification or gain control. The divider passes a portion of the input signal to the output.

Consider a circuit with three resistors, two 25 Ω and one 50 Ω resistors. If 10 V is applied to the circuit, what is the voltage across one of the 25 Ω resistors (Fig. 3-13)? Since we know the resistance value, we only need the current through the resistor to get the voltage. The three resistors are in series, so the three seem like a single 100 Ω resistor. 10 V applied to 100 Ω yields a current of 10/100 or 0.1 A. 0.1 A × 25 Ω yields 2.5 V (Fig. 3-13, left). If the input voltage were increased to 100 V, the current flowing through the 100 Ω would be 100/100 or 1 A. The output across the 25 Ω resistor is $I \times R$ = 1 A × 25 Ω = 25 V (Fig. 3-13, right).

A long string of resistors could be used to adjust the signal level. With 10 equal resistors, each of 10 steps can be selected to obtain 0% to 100% of the total resistance (Fig. 3-14).

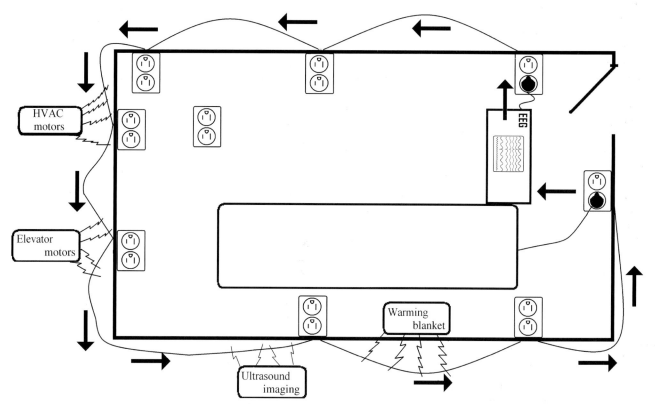

FIGURE 3-12 | Path of a ground loop around a patient room.

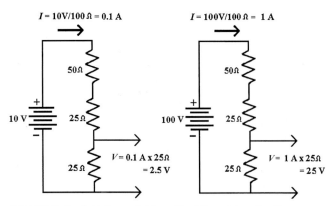

FIGURE 3-13 | Voltage divider with different input voltages.

The voltage divider can be continually variable, as with potentiometers or volume controls.

Frequency Response of High and Low Filters

Both high- and low-frequency filters can cause attenuation of amplitude and phase shift. You can use a frequency response curve (Fig. 3-15) to see if the waveforms are being attenuated and by how much. Knowing the attenuation, you can estimate the waveform's actual amplitude. Actual voltage × X% = apparent voltage. First, look at the waveforms of interest. If the frequency is well within the bandpass (filter settings), X% is 100% and the observed or apparent voltage is equal to the actual voltage. If the waveform of interest is beyond the bandwidth of the filters, the curves can be used to determine the actual voltages.

As an example, assume the frequency of a slow wave is 1 Hz, the low filter setting is 5, and the amplitude measured is 50 μV. First, find the frequency of interest along the bottom of the graph. Then, locate the curve for your filter (LF 5). Where do the vertical line 1 Hz and the curve LF 5 meet? The curve crosses at 20%. Then, go back to the formula. The apparent amplitude was 50 μV (arrow in Fig. 3-15). Actual voltage × 20% = 50 μV. Actual voltage was 50/0.2 or 250 μV.

How are these curves generated? Imagine a voltage divider consisting of a fixed element (resistor) and an element whose resistance varies with frequency (capacitor). The low filter is such a circuit, with the output across the frequency-varying element (the capacitor). At high frequency, the capacitor is near zero impedance, shorting the output. At low frequencies, the capacitor has no effect and the output is near 100% of the input.

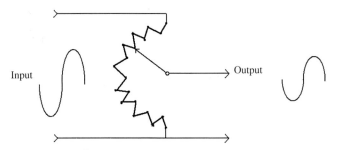

FIGURE 3-14 | A round voltage divider—the volume control.

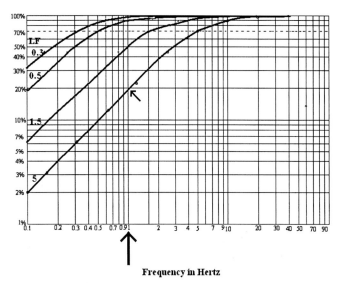

FIGURE 3-15 | Frequency response of four low-frequency filters.

HIGH-FREQUENCY FILTER

The high-frequency filter (HFF) (Fig. 3-16, right) is similar to the two-resistor voltage divider (Fig. 3-16, left). There are two differences between them: (i) the capacitor's impedance (AC resistance) varies with frequency, and (ii) the total impedance is a vector sum.

The impedance of a capacitor (Z_C) is determined by the value of the capacitor, and the frequency of the voltage is used to measure the reactance. The formula for calculating impedance is $Z_C = 1/2 \pi CF$ (Fig. 3-17, left). The reactance/AC resistance gets larger as the frequency (F) gets lower.

Figure 3-17 is a graphical representation of resistance and capacitance. R has a fixed value that does not change with frequency. The impedance of the capacitor changes with frequency and is 90° out of phase (Fig. 3-17, center). The sum of R and C is the vector sum of the two. Pythagoras, around 500 BC, gave us the answer: $A^2 + B^2 = C^2$. (Given a right triangle, the square of the hypotenuse is equal to the sum of the squares of the other two sides.) The resistance and capacitance are squared and added together, and then the square root is taken to get the vector sum as seen in Figure 3-17 (right) and Figure 3-18.

The HFFs are characterized by the cutoff frequency. At this frequency, the output is 70% of the input and the phase shift is 45°. Why is it 70% instead of 50% (which would be easier to use in calculations)?

Resistance (R) and capacitive impedance (Z_C) are graphically represented by two sides of a triangle, with 90° between the two. The vector sum is represented by the third side of the triangle. The Z_C side of the triangle varies in length with frequency (Fig. 3-18, left).

There is a frequency at which the Z_C side will equal the R side of the triangle. What is the vector sum of the two sides when the sides have the same magnitude? If $R = Z_C$, then we have a right triangle with the third side being $2^{1/2}R$. The divider ratio is $Z_C/R + Z_C$. $R + Z_C$ are added as a vector sum, so it is the square root of $R^2 + Z_C^2$. Since the magnitude of $Z_C = R$, the sum is $(2R^2)^{1/2}$. Since the magnitudes are the same, divider ratio is now $R/2^{1/2}R = 70.7\%$ (Fig. 3-18, right). This is why the 70% is associated with the *cutoff frequency*.

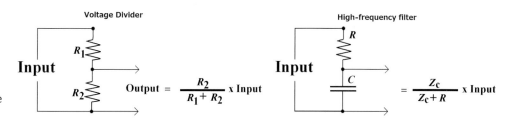

FIGURE 3-16 | The voltage divider and HFF as a divider.

$$Z_c = \frac{1}{2\Pi CF}$$

Capacitive reactance as a function of frequency and Capacitance

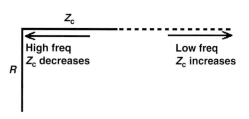

Capacitive reactance changes with frequency. It become small at high frequencies and an open circuit at low frequencies

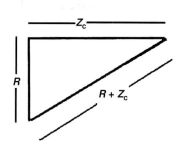

Vector addition of R and Z_c

FIGURE 3-17 | Voltage divider ratio using vector addition.

HFF Response at the Cutoff Frequency (@ $R = Zc$)

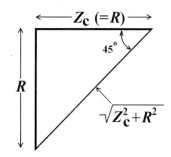

Adding R and Zc (Vector Addition)

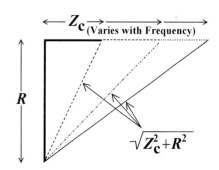

Divider Ratio at Cutoff Frequency =

$$\frac{\text{Capacitive Impedance}}{\text{Capacitive Impedance + Resistance}} = \frac{Z_c}{\sqrt{Z_c^2 + R^2}} \quad \text{(R=Zc)}$$

$$= \frac{Z_c}{\sqrt{Z_c^2 + Z_c^2}}$$

Phase Shift:
Phase shift if equal to the angle between the Z_c side of the triangle and the hypoteneuse. The angle can be found by taking the inverse tangent of R/Zc. Here $R = Zc$ and the tangent is 1. The angle with a tangent of 1 is $45°$.

$$= \frac{Z_c}{\sqrt{2Z_c^2}} = \frac{Z_c}{Z_c\sqrt{2}}$$

$$= \frac{1}{\sqrt{2}}$$

$$\underline{\textbf{Tangent}^{-1}\ \textbf{1} = \textbf{45}°} \qquad = \underline{\textbf{70.7\%}}$$

FIGURE 3-18 | Calculating attenuation (divider ratio) for HFF.

The R-C voltage divider not only attenuates the output based on frequency, it also shifts the phase of the output based on frequency.

High-frequency filter

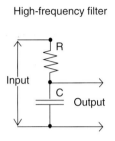

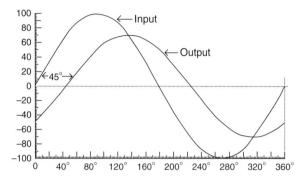

FIGURE 3-19 | Effect of the HFF at the cutoff frequency.

The cutoff frequency from the component (R and C) values can be calculated by the following formula. The capacitive impedance is $1/(2\pi FC)$. If $Z_C = R$, then $1/(2\pi FC) = R$. Multiply both sides of the equation by the same amount (F/R), and we have $1/(2\pi RC)$ = frequency.

In addition to the amplitude reduction, there will be a phase shift of waveform as shown in Figure 3-19.

In summary, the HFF setting (15, 30, or 70 Hz) is related to the rise time constant, $R \times C$. An HFF will attenuate signals 70% at the frequency (F) where $F = 1/(2\pi RC)$. There is also a 45° delayed phase shift as shown in Figure 3-19.

The longest rise time constant is seen in the lowest HFF, usually HF = 15 Hz. The rise time is calculated to be about 10 ms (0.01 s). Using an analog EEG, this would be 30 mm/s × 0.01 s = 0.3 mm at normal chart speed. Even the longest rise time constant is difficult to see.

What about digital EEG? The common sampling rate for clinical EEG is 200 samples/s or one sample every 5 ms. There would be two samples per time constant, using the longest time constant. If the HF 70 filter was used, the time constant would be $1/(2\pi \times 70) = 0.0023$ s = 2.3 ms. More than two constants would pass before a second sample is taken. With appropriate calculations, the time constant could be derived from two

samples, the beginning and end points. But, observation of the rise time constant remains elusive.

LOW-FREQUENCY FILTER

Similar calculations are used for the low-frequency filter. An LF 5 filter also has $Z_C = R$ at the cutoff frequency. The output of this voltage divider is across the resistor, so the ratio is now $R/(R + Z_C)$ (Fig. 3-20).

In summary, at the cutoff frequency, the divider ratio is the same as the HFF, that is, 70% reduction with time constant measured by $R \times C$. The phase shift is the same, 45°, but the phase shift is ahead in time as shown in Figure 3-21.

Amplifier

The basic theory of an amplifier is also based on a voltage divider across a series of resistors as shown in Figure 3-22. The length of the resistors in the diagram below is exaggerated to make the division of the voltage across the resistors more intuitive.

Instead of a fixed resistor, one of the resistors can be made variable as shown in Figure 3-23 (variable voltage divider).

At the cuttoff frequency

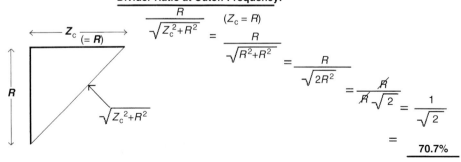

Phase Shift:
Phase shift is equal to the angle between the Z_c side of the triangle and the hypotenuse. This angle can be found by taking the inverse tangent of R/Z_c. Here where $R = Z_c$, the tangent is 1. The angle with a tangent of 1 is 45°.

$$\text{Tan}^{-1} = \underline{45°}$$

FIGURE 3-20 | Calculating attenuation (divider ratio) for low-frequency filter.

The R-C voltage divider not only attenuates the output based on frequency, it also shifts the phase of the output based on frequency.

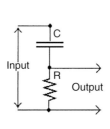

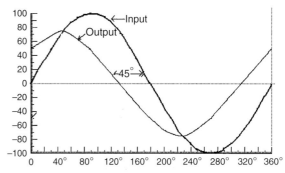

FIGURE 3-21 | Effect of the low-frequency filter at the cutoff frequency.

In summary, at the cutoff frequency, the divider ratio is the same as the high-frequency filter (HFF), that is, 70% reduction with time constant measured by $R \times C$. The phase shift is the same, $45°$, but the phase shift is ahead in time as shown in the figure above.

Instead of turning a knob of a variable resistor, the variable resistor is replaced with a device that changes resistance depending on a small "input" current, that is, the resistance is proportional to the input current. A small amount of current flowing into this device can vary the resistance from zero to infinity (from a short to an open). The device is called "**TRANSISTOR**" (derived from **TRAN**sfer re**SISTOR**). When it is used in the voltage divider circuit, we have a one-transistor amplifier (Fig. 3-24).

With a few modifications, several of the transistor amplifiers can be connected in series: the output of the first transistor goes on to control the second, the output of the second transistor goes on to control the third, and so on. In this way, the input signal is amplified many times.

DIFFERENTIAL AMPLIFICATION

A simple model of the differential amplifier consists of two single-ended amplifiers (Fig. 3-25). The output of the amplifier is gain × input voltage. If a −5 μV signal is connected between input and ground of the +100 gain amplifier, the output voltage is (+100 × −5) = −500 μV. If a −10 μV signal is connected to the second amplifier with a negative gain of −100 (called an inverting amplifier), the output would be (−100 × −10) = +1,000 μV (Fig. 3-25, left).

To create a differential amplifier, all that needs to be added is a summing circuit. The interconnected amplifiers and a summing circuit constitute a *differential amplifier*. The difference between −5 μV and −10 μV is +5 μV. The output of the differential amplifier is the difference between the input voltages × 100 = +500 μV (Fig. 3-25, right).

The purpose of the differential amplifier is to cancel out the external noise (interference) common to both inputs. To simulate common mode noise, a sine wave function generator is connected to both inputs of the amplifier (Fig. 3-26). The upper amplifier acquires and amplifies the 1,000 μV to 100,000 μV. The lower amplifier not only does the same but also inverts it. The sum is zero! In reality, the differential amplifier does not remove all of the noise. The problem lies in the amplifier. The gains are fixed by components, such as precision resistors. Thus, a differential amplifier may have one amplifier with a gain of 100.5 and the other with a gain of 99.5 (Fig. 3-27). A figure of merit for the amplifier is the *common mode rejection ratio* (CMRR). It compares the differential gain to the common mode gain. With perfectly matched amplifier gains, the common mode gain is zero and the CMRR is infinity. However, if the gains were realistic, such as 100.5 and 95.5, some of the common mode signal would be amplified (Fig. 3-27). The ideal CMRR value should be infinite but this is not realistically

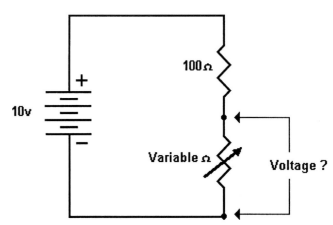

FIGURE 3-22 | Basic voltage divider.

FIGURE 3-23 | Output of divider varies with variable resistor.

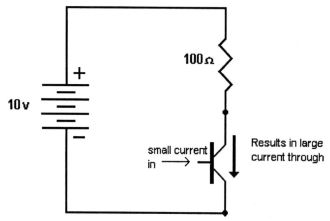

FIGURE 3-24 | A device that changes resistance with input voltage changes (transistor).

possible. The guideline suggests that the acceptable CMRR is 10,000.

The CMRR is a function of design, construction, and tuning of the amplifier. It is not something over which the user has control. However, there are factors that we do control. The prime factor is electrode impedance. There is a practical limit set by the electrode impedance imbalance and input impedance of the amplifier. If the two input electrodes had a large impedance difference, for example, one is 6,000 Ω and the other is 1,000 Ω and the amplifier had an input impedance of 1,000,000 Ω, the limit would be 1,000,000/(6,000 − 1,000) or 200:1! If the amplifier had an input impedance of 10,000,000, the ratio would be 10,000,000/5,000 = 2,000:1. If the electrodes' impedances were closer, such as 3,000 and 2,000 Ω, the limit imposed by the electrodes would be 10,000,000/1,000 or 10,000:1. Therefore, it is important to keep the electrodes impedance balanced.

Electrical Safety

GENERAL PROBLEMS

The electrical safety problem affects all of us. It is not just in hospitals or other health care facilities. The general public is at risk of being electrocuted.

The problem starts with the generation of electricity at a distant site. It is much more economical to send power through power lines at high voltages. The losses along the power line are equal to I^2R. Figure 3-28 is an example of sending power

at 120 V compared to stepping up the voltage to 12,000 V for transmission. The first loses 200 W of power in the two power lines, while the second loses only 0.02 W. With the power being sent at high voltages, there is little loss from current through the transmission cables. At the remote site, the high voltage must be again stepped down to standard line voltages of 120 and 240. With the high voltages on the input/primary side of the transformer, some current will leak through to the secondary side. To keep the secondary from "floating," one side of the secondary is grounded. This will keep the secondary from rising to greater than the line voltage.

The standard outlet has three connectors: (i) long slot connected to neutral, (ii) short slot connected to the hot line, and (iii) U shaped connected to ground (Fig. 3-29). The second tap is also 120 V from ground. However, this second tap is out of phase with the upper tap and voltage between them is 240 V. The U-shaped connector is for the ground. Normally, it does not carry current. It is meant to conduct stray currents from the case of the instrument.

Grounding one side of the power line solves one problem but creates another. To be shocked, a person needs to come into contact with two points. No one would intentionally touch both sides of an outlet at once. However, you are often in contact with one side of the power line: the ground! This is why certain areas will have special electrical requirements. Wet areas such as bathrooms, kitchen sinks, outdoor construction, etc., require ground fault current interrupters (GFCIs). The requirements for these areas are found in the National Fire Protection Association's (NFPA) national electrical code.[1] The current flows into and out of the instrument, but some "leaks" to the metal chassis. The ground line then carries this leakage, through ground, to the neutral (Fig. 3-29).

HOSPITAL SETTING

The health care facility has its own set of codes to follow: NFPA-99.[1]

Patients are more at risk because of the following:
1. The patient is grounded.
2. Patients are often connected to multiple, 120 volts alternating current (VAC)-powered instruments, with multiple chances for leakage current.
3. The dry, outer layer of skin is compromised by well-applied electrodes.
4. The patient may be weakened or comatose and not be able to withdraw from the painful shock.
5. The patient's heart may be weakened and susceptible to lower levels of current than normal.

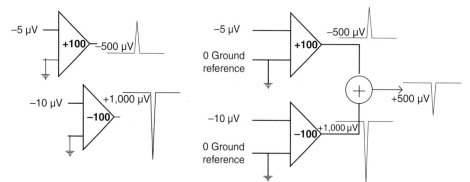

FIGURE 3-25 | Using two amplifiers to measure the difference.

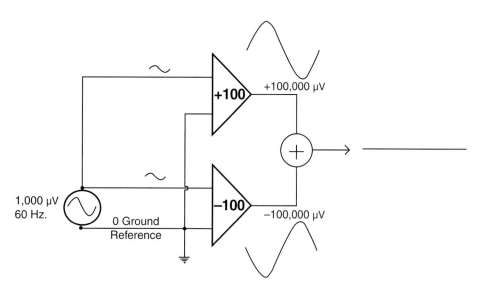

FIGURE 3-26 | When a common signal is amplified.

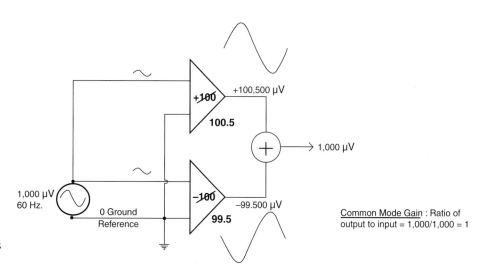

FIGURE 3-27 | Mismatched inputs and common mode gain.

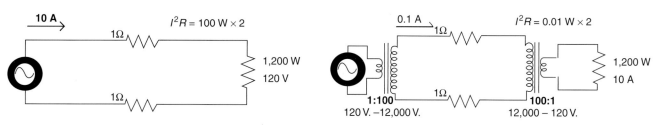

FIGURE 3-28 | Why high-voltage transmission is needed.

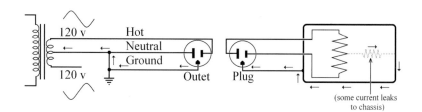

FIGURE 3-29 | One side of the line is grounded.

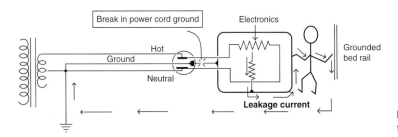

FIGURE 3-30 | If the ground fails, leakage current flows through the patient.

As seen in Figure 3-29, some current finds its way from the electronics to the chassis. This is called leakage current. If instruments are designed with low leakage current and are grounded, why should we be concerned? The reason is that if the leakage current were to increase and the ground connection fails, large currents could flow through the patient (or you) (Fig. 3-30). Neither fault is readily evident. Leakage currents should be well under 1/1,000 A. However, it would require currents 10,000 times this value (or more) before the circuit breaker would trip. Because EEG is sensitive in the microvolts range, it is one of the fields where loss of the ground connection might be noticed by the appearance of the 60-Hz artifacts on EEG recording. But, use of the 60 Hz filter would hide the symptom. The ground wire does not carry current under normal circumstances, so loss of ground is usually not noticed. Consider how many plugs you have encountered with the ground pin missing!

Grounding and Chassis Leakage

Safety inspections are intended to detect increasing leakage current and failing ground connections before they become a problem. If the ground were to break, we would want to know what current would flow through a grounded patient (or operator); leakage current is measured by interrupting the ground line, diverting the leakage current through the meter as shown in Figure 3-31.

The ground integrity of your instrument can be tested with an ohmmeter. With the instrument unplugged, measure the resistance from the U-shaped terminal (ground connection) on the instrument's plug to a metal point on the chassis. The reading should be less than 0.15 Ω (Fig. 3-32).

The leakage current limit has changed in the past several years.[1] NFPA lists the limit as 300 μA, and up to 500 μA in some cases. It had been 100 μA for many years.[1,2] This increase was to bring the US limits in line with international standards. Individual hospitals may choose to retain the more stringent *patient lead leakage* limits.

Even with the ground connection intact, we have to consider current that leaks to the electrode jacks as shown in Figure 3-33. The leakage current meter is placed between a patient input and ground. Current is measured with the ground–chassis connection open and closed. The test is repeated for each input. Another test measures current flowing between patient inputs. The leakage current limit for all leads/inputs connected together and ground is 100 μA.[1] This is measured with or without the chassis connected to ground.

Isolated Inputs

Isolated inputs are intended for conductors with direct pathways to the heart. This may be a direct wire connection (such as that used for pacing) or a nonconductive catheter filled with conductive liquid.[1,2] The electrical isolation test applies 120 VAC and measures the current flowing into the inputs.

Figure 3-34 is a simplified diagram of one of the isolation tests. Safety precautions must be exercised when performing this test since line voltages are involved. The current flowing into the inputs shall not exceed 20 μA.

The actual tests are more complex than the figures indicate. The impedance of the meter in the above diagram is designed to simulate well-applied electrodes and the response to various frequencies. The "hot" and "neutral" connections are reversed during the test, simulating an improperly wired outlet. The ohmmeter used must be capable of measuring resistance in the 0.05 Ω range.

Circuits that meet the isolation test above are readily available. However, for medical equipment to be recognized by Underwriter's Laboratories (UL), the input must withstand 2,500 V for 1 minute without failing. With nonisolated inputs,

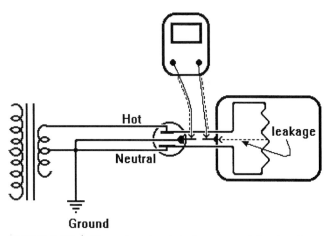

FIGURE 3-31 | Measuring chassis leakage current flowing down ground wire.

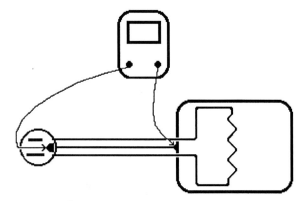

FIGURE 3-32 | Checking ground integrity.

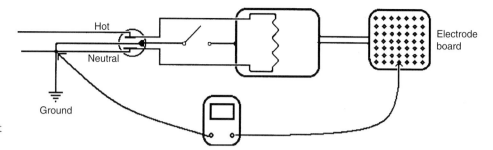

FIGURE 3-33 | Measuring patient lead leakage.

the 2,500 V appears across the power transformer, which is designed to withstand the voltage. In the case of isolated inputs, most of the 2,500 V appears across the isolation circuitry. Isolation circuitry that will pass microvolt level signals and not be destroyed by kilovolt level signals is difficult to design.

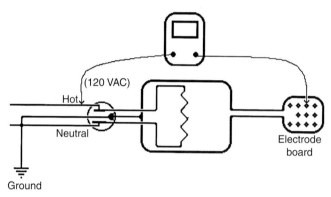

FIGURE 3-34 | Isolation tests at 120 VAC.

WHAT YOU SHOULD DO TO PROTECT PATIENT'S SAFETY

General Precautions

Most of the recommendations are common sense. Inspect power cords for damage. There should be no ungrounded (two-wire) devices within the patient's reach. Use an outlet in the same area used by other patient-related devices. No extension cords. Turn on and calibrate before using the instrument. Have the biomedical department inspect the "ground" patient input. Report abnormal interference (noting equipment in the area) to the biomedical department. Ensure that the patient is not connected to the instrument when powering on or off.

References

1. NFPA 99. *Health Care Facilities.* Quincy, MA: National Fire Protection Association, 2002:2169–7471.
2. Federal Register. Electrode lead wires and patient cables: Performance standard. *Fed Reg* 1997;62(90):25477–25498.

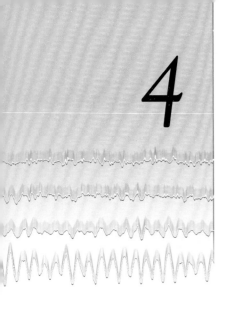

4

Digital EEG

MALCOLM YEH

Introduction

Traditional electroencephalogram (EEG) recordings are typically used for medical diagnosis and neurobiological research. One EEG channel, commonly recorded from a surface electrode attached to the scalp, is a graphical representation of the voltage as it varies with time. When multiple electrodes are used, more than one location on the scalp can be monitored simultaneously to produce a multiple channel EEG recording. In essence, the EEG record is a picture of the electrical activity of the brain. The amplitude of the wave represents the amount of voltage and can be displayed on a paper recorder using a galvanometer-driven pen-writing system or a digital video screen driven by a computer.

Since the invention of the EEG machine in 1929 by Hans Berger, the basic components of an EEG system have remained the same. That includes electrodes (the actual voltage sensors), amplifiers, and output devices. Over the years, there has been continual improvement of each component with the latest improvement being on the output device.

The classical paper-recorded EEG for clinical diagnostic purposes remained in common clinical use for about 45 years before advances in computer technology made it more economical to store EEG recordings digitally. Digital recording technology was first applied commercially in the music industry in the 1960s as a means of reproducing musical data without loss of quality in the recording during the duplication. In the 1970s, clinical neurophysiology began recording digital data in evoked potential recordings. Because evoked potentials are short in duration and resolved with averaging techniques, storage of small static data files was not a problem. However, storage for a continuous stream of data from an EEG recording only became possible when two advancements occurred. The first occurred when computer processors became fast enough to capture the large amount of streaming data from a multichannel EEG system. The second advancement occurred in about 1990, when long-term computer storage media dropped low enough in price to allow economical storage of large amounts of data. At that time, digital EEG systems quickly came on the market to compete with the analog (paper) recording systems. Digital EEG proved to have many advantages including (i) filing and storage of the recording in a much smaller space (i.e., tape, CD, DVD, flash drives, and remote servers), (ii) the ability to reformat the data postrecording with regard to the viewing montages, filter

adjustments, adjustments in sensitivity (vertical scaling), and time base settings (horizontal scaling), (iii) more accurate measurements of frequency and timing in regard to phase relationships between channels, and (iv) the ability to quantify EEG characteristics numerically with statistical tools such as power spectrum analysis and topographic voltage maps.[1,2] Digitized EEG data certainly provided many more advantages and were a major advancement over the analog recordings.[3]

However, there were a few pitfalls for the early commercial EEG systems. When the first generation of commercial digital EEG systems appeared in the early 1990s, the recordings were merely analog EEG systems with a low-resolution display attached to magnetic storage media. This first generation of digital EEG recorders offered digital storage as the main advantage. However, reading the EEG could not be done instantaneously as a paper recording could.[4] In addition, the technologist's job of monitoring and making adjustments to optimize the recording was a slower and more complicated process because adjustments were made through tedious keyboard commands. As a result, many technologists at that time found it easier to perform a paper recording. Because of the ease in storing large amounts of data, there is created the problem of accurately analyzing large amounts of continuous EEG data in a timely manner making EEG bedside interpretation impossible. As a result, quantitative EEG (qEEG) analysis has seen the invention of numerous tools to improve the efficiency and reduce the burden of analyzing massive amounts of data. Since the data can be processed mathematically by any number of algorithms, a large array of techniques have come into being to help visualized continuous EEG in a more compact form. Some examples of these techniques include (i) comparing for asymmetries in various amplitudes and frequencies over analogous areas of brain, (ii) assessing for changes in frequencies in the time domain to identify state changes or seizure activity, and (iii) recognizing patterns of potentially epileptiform discharges. Many of these techniques have been included in the EEG reading software, though validation is still needed when more subtle findings are being sought.[5]

ANALOG EEG (PAPER) RECORDERS

The classic analog pen-writing EEG recorders required dividing the technologist's attention between the patient and to the many parts of the EEG equipment. This would include intermittently

Comparison of analog EEG and digitized EEG recordings

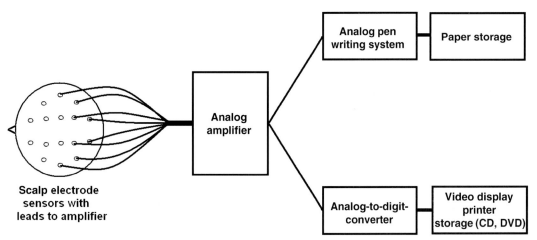

FIGURE 4-1 | Analog EEG and digitized EEG recordings have common features using scalp electrode sensors and analog amplifiers. However, they differ in the third component where the analog EEG typically has the amplifier send the signals to an analog pen-writing system, but the digital system has the amplifier send the signals to an ADC circuit. This allows much more flexibility with the display and storage of the data.

monitoring the amplitude of the waveforms for pen blocking or extremely low amplitudes that would require adjustments of the sensitivity setting of the amplifiers. Messy mechanical ink pens would occasionally malfunction and require maintenance while the recording was in progress. Maintaining accurate pen alignment was tedious but was required to maintain the time phase relationships between channels. From time to time, there would be noise in the recording that would obscure the EEG, and optimizing the recording of a desired signal would require further adjustments of filters or paper-speed. Finally, observation and notation of the patient's behavior during the recording were performed by writing directly on the moving paper as it was rolling past the moving EEG pens.

DIGITAL EEG RECORDERS

Second-generation digital EEG machines came into the market in the late 1990s, with the main improvement being better display monitors while streamlining the technical aspects of the recording process. From the technologist's point of view, there were fewer steps and fewer factors that had to be addressed in order to complete an EEG recording. With the digitally recorded EEG, the ink pens have been replaced with a computer display that requires no maintenance. The amplitude range of digital EEG is much larger in comparison to paper-generated records. In effect, this eliminates the need to periodically adjust the gain of the amplifiers. Monitoring and adjusting the amplitude of the signal has become an option for the technologist rather than a necessity. Because digital frequency filters can be applied when the recording is reviewed, applying frequency filters in real time is used to monitor the quality of the recording and to aid the technologist in viewing abnormalities. Timing in regard to phase relationships between channels is now automatic and no longer requires alignment in comparison to the pen-writing system. As a result of these conveniences, more time can be spent monitoring and documenting the patient's behavior and symptoms.

A schematic of a digital EEG recording system in comparison to the classic pen-writing system is shown in Figure 4-1.

Components of the Digital EEG System

SENSORS

The first component in the recording of biological signals is the sensor, which in the case of EEG would be the scalp electrodes. The electrode is an extremely important element in determining the quality of the recorded signal. It is the technologist's responsibility to be sure that the recorded signal at the sensor level is adequate; otherwise, junk signals into the system will only generate junk signals out. This means being sure that the electrode is applied in the correct location and that the electrical contact is adequate (impedance <5 kΩ) in addition to keeping external electrical noise to a minimum.

The recorded voltage from the scalp electrode is a continuously varying signal. A signal that is continuous without breaks or discontinuities is, by definition, an analog signal. Nature surrounds us with analog signals. Examples include sound wave amplitudes, intensities of light, and magnitudes of weights to name just a few of the measurable analog properties that can be measured as a continuous analog signal. To recapitulate, the voltage recorded from a scalp electrode is an example of a continuous analog signal that will be compared to a digitized signal later in our discussion.

AMPLIFIERS

The analog amplifier is the second component in the recording pathway. The continuous analog signal is fed into the amplifier that typically boosts the signal so that it can be further processed in the recording system. For a pen-writing system, the signal voltage would be converted to pen displacement that would produce a paper recording.

DATA STORAGE AND PROCESSING

The third component in a digital EEG system has the amplifier sending the amplified signal to a special electrical circuit known as an *ADC* (*analog-to-digital converter*) circuit. This is to be contrasted to the analog EEG system, where the third component would be the pen-writing system. The ADC circuit is also called a digitizer because its function is to transform an analog measurement into a number. This circuit is a specialized digital voltmeter with a rapid response time that can make a voltage measurement almost instantaneously. It measures the amplified signal voltage and converts it into a number that is then sent to a computer to process. It is this step that changes the analog signal to a digital signal and allows the signal to be represented as a number that machines can easily process and store on a variety of mediums (i.e., storage tape, CD, DVD).

Analog signals, being continuous by nature, have a continuously changing value over time. However, digitized signals are only a sampling of the original analog signal since only a finite number of values can be stored and processed (Fig. 4-2). When digital EEG recordings were in their infancy, the slower computer processors could not match the quality of the analog recordings because sampling rates were too low. However, second-generation digital EEG systems allow much faster sampling rates and have easily matched the resolution of analog EEG. Typically, computer processors in current digital EEG systems are fast enough that digital data can be stored as well as providing a simultaneous data display to monitor the quality of the recording. One nice aspect of storing data in digitized form is that there is no degradation of the quality of the data no matter how many times the data are copied. This is certainly an advantage over analog recordings, where the information degrades each time it is duplicated.

Factors and Limitations of Digitized Data

Digital recordings have certainly made EEG recording more efficient both in the use of the technologist's time and in archiving

Amplitude resolution with different amplitude ranges

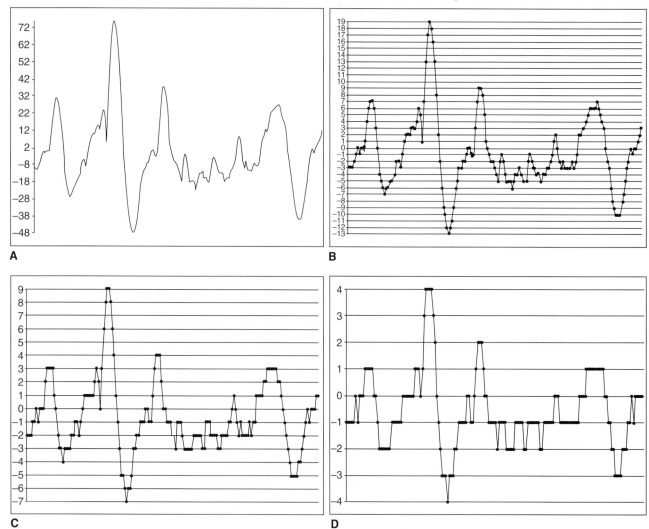

FIGURE 4-2 | The original analog signal is shown in **panel A**. In **panel B**, a 5-bit ADC processor has an amplitude range of 32 steps. In **panel C**, a 4-bit processor has an amplitude range of 16 steps. In **panel D**, a 3-bit processor has an amplitude range of eight steps. The fewer the number of steps in the amplitude range, the more blocky the appearance of the waveforms.

records. However, because the analog data are digitized, there are additional factors and limitations that ultimately affect the quality and interpretation of the recording. The technologist will need to be aware of the frequency and amplitude of the signal of interest in comparison to the resolution of the digital record in terms of amplitude resolution and time resolution. Amplitude and time factors will determine the types of EEG signals that could be recorded. Some of the pitfalls in recording and interpreting digitized data would include the introduction of virtual signals that occur in the reconstruction process of the original analog signal. These virtual signals are called *alias* signals (or aliasing), which are easily seen in cyclical recorded signals. An example of this is in the recording of a regular sine wave signal.

Two main factors that determine resolution of the digitized data are the amplitude range and the sampling rate of the ADC circuit. Raw digital EEG data are still displayed in the traditional paper format due to familiarity of presenting data in graph form. The EEG is a graph of the voltage of the scalp over time.

AMPLITUDE RESOLUTION (*Y*-AXIS)

The amplitude of a signal is the magnitude or vertical height of the signal and is displayed along the vertical axis (*Y*-axis) of the display. The ADC circuit translates the measured voltage into a binary numerical value of amplitude. The range of the numerical value will depend on the largest binary number that the ADC circuit can hold in its memory banks for one sample measurement in time.

Let us take, as an example, an ADC circuit that can capture a voltage measurement and store it as a number between 0 and 7 (which is a three-digit binary number "3-bit number" in computer terms using base 2. In base 2, the number seven will be represented as the binary digit 111. Each digit is a placeholder for powers of 2 so that the number $111 = 1 \times 2^2 + 1 \times 2^1 + 1 \times 2^0 = 7$). There will be eight possible amplitude steps that can be generated from such a range. As a result, the figure will come out looking quite blocky (Fig. 4-2D). If we upgrade our ADC circuit to store a four-digit binary number from 0 to 15, the resolution increases to 16 possible amplitude steps in the range. The upgraded ADC certainly improves the resolution, but some blocky appearance still exists (Fig. 4-2C).

If we continue to upgrade to ADC circuits that store larger numbers at a time, the amplitude resolution continues to improve (Fig. 4-2B). First-generation EEG systems used 8-bit ADC processors (256 steps in the amplitude range). Even at this resolution, displays appeared blocky for low-amplitude signals.[6] Currently, many digital systems will store an amplitude range of 65,536 steps, which, in "base 2," is a 16-bit number (2 to the 16th power turns out to be the binary number 1 with 16 trailing zeros: 10000000000000000). This is a resolution that is beyond the video display. One may ask, "Why would one want to have such a large range in amplitude?" A main advantage is the ability to record both high- and low-amplitude signals at the same time with reasonable resolution, without having to manually adjust the gain of the amplifier. In regard to the display, the video display may not be able to show all resolutions of amplitude since the recorded amplitude range may be well beyond the resolution of the video screen. An example would be a very low-amplitude signal that cannot be displayed well

due to pixel size or extremely large amplitudes that go beyond the limits of the screen.

To get around this limitation of the video screen resolution, the amplitude axis of the video screen can be adjusted by software to make it appear as if the sensitivity of the analog amplifiers had been changed. This gives the appearance of zooming in or out on various portions of the waveform. The effects of having a very large amplitude range to work with allows one to avoid the blocky appearance of very small waveforms when zooming in and allows the display of large amplitude waveforms by zooming out.

To describe this advantage conversely, there is a disadvantage to having an ADC circuit with a small range in amplitude as was the case for earlier computers that worked with 8-bit numbers or less since one would have to maintain constant attention to the amplitude of the signal from the amplifiers to be sure that the signal being recorded was in the range of the processor. With a small range of amplitudes to work with, the technologist has to continually monitor the amplitude during the recording so that adjustments in the amplifier gain can be made to allow the ADC circuit to record the signal within its full amplitude range. (See Fig. 4-3, which illustrates this problem.) If one has a large amplitude range to work with, continuous monitoring of the signal is not necessary since adjustments of the virtual gain (sensitivity) of the screen allows one to use the amplitude range of the screen more conveniently. As a result, we now have the convenience of adjusting the amplitude when the recording is being acquired or after the recording has been completed.

Another advantage of having the data in numerical form is the ability to continue to process the information after the recording is complete. Examples of further processing include

Examples of amplifier gains that do not use the full extent of the amplitude range

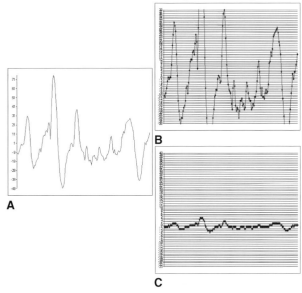

FIGURE 4-3 | The original analog signal is shown in **panel A**. In **panel B**, the amplifier gain is too high, resulting in clipping the signal outside the range of the digitizer. In **panel C**, the amplifier gain is well within the range of the digitizer; however, the gain is so low that it does not use the full range of the digitizer optimally, and as a result, the recorded waveform has a coarse, blocky appearance.

viewing the data with a different montage that allows one to change the references of the channels being viewed. This can be done algebraically to allow one to take the waveform in one channel and add or subtract it from the waveform in another channel. An example of this can be seen in Figure 4-4. This figure shows the raw data sampled at electrodes P4 and O2 being compared to a common reference denoted as "−rfr" (raw data in the first two columns and sample in the first two frames). Since this waveform contains the value differences between electrodes P4 and −rfr as well as O2 and −rfr, one can now view this as a mathematical sentence of subtraction:

$$P4 - rfr = (Signal\ waveform\ 1)$$
$$O2 - rfr = (Signal\ waveform\ 2)$$

One can now manipulate this data to create the new channel P4 − O2, where electrode P4 is being referenced (or compared) to electrode O2. This channel (raw values in the third column and sample in the bottom frame) is a virtual channel that is derived by subtracting waveform 2 from waveform 1.

$$(signal\ waveform\ 1) - (signal\ waveform\ 2) = (P4 - rfr) - (O2 - rfr)$$

Since the "−rfr" term is present in both waveforms, it just drops out to zero and the result is

$$(signal\ waveform\ 1) - (signal\ waveform\ 2) = P4 - O2$$

This is now a new derived channel P4 − O2, which shows a posterior sharp transient of sleep.

Graphical representation of numerical EEG data

P4 − rfr	O2 − rfr	P4 − O2
−8.0665	−10.535	2.4685
−4.6193	−5.0635	0.4442
1.38759	−5.3857	6.77329
1.36788	−7.0365	8.40438
−1.1545	−7.1771	6.0226
0.30436	−5.8879	6.19226
0.65954	−6.7057	7.36524
0.97933	−5.718	6.69733
3.95065	−1.9697	5.92035
1.48987	−7.494	8.98387
−4.4415	−17.05	12.6085
−5.3844	−17.558	12.1736
−1.1804	−15.326	14.1456
2.79212	−18.704	21.49612
1.06906	−24.225	25.29406
−0.2977	−25.502	25.2043
3.8417	−25.235	29.0767
6.3786	−27.901	34.2796
5.56817	−31.183	36.75117
5.34218	−34.301	39.64318
5.10301	−36.252	41.35501
4.8511	−35.841	40.6921
6.34388	−33.892	40.23588
7.22221	−29.582	36.80421
5.3011	−25.48	30.7811
3.97848	−21.405	25.38348
5.11631	−12.713	17.82931
4.68929	−3.6789	8.36819
0.83283	1.43918	−0.60635
−2.4313	6.87862	−9.30992
−3.9412	12.6206	−16.5618
−6.1202	15.8249	−21.9451
−4.6038	19.9073	−24.5111
3.14731	26.149	−23.0017
7.95767	30.6776	−22.7199
5.53576	32.5003	−26.9645
1.34654	32.211	−30.8645
−1.5065	29.3427	−30.8492
−1.3185	28.536	−29.8545
1.51475	33.7087	−32.194
1.747	−35.8405	−34.0935

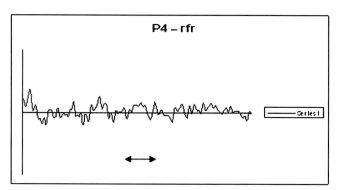

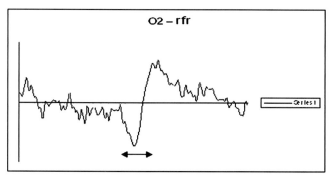

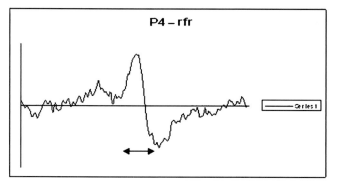

FIGURE 4-4 | The numerical EEG data denoted between the short horizontal *arrows* under each of the waveforms for three channels (P4 − rfr, O2 − rfr, and P4 − O2) are shown in a three-column table on the left with the waveforms for each channel shown to the right. If the second channel (second column of numbers) is subtracted from the first channel (first column of numbers), the results are seen as a third channel (third column of numbers). In effect, the waveform for channel O2 − rfr has been subtracted from the waveform for channel P4–rfr to give a new waveform in a derived channel P4 − O2.

TIME RESOLUTION (X-AXIS)

In EEG recordings, the ADC circuit uses time along the horizontal axis (X-axis) of the recording. As a result, the time setting will depend on how it records and displays increments of time along the horizontal axis. The smallest unit of time recorded by the ADC circuit is called the *dwell* time. Dwell time is the amount of time between two sampling points. It is within this dwell time that the voltage amplitude of the signal is captured and recorded. The mathematical inverse of the dwell time is the sampling frequency, which is the number of samples per second that the ADC circuit is able to record. When dwell times are long, the number of samples per second (sampling rate) is low, making the resolution low along the time axis. When the sampling rate is increased, the time axis resolution increases and more details about the signal in time are recorded. For example, when the dwell time is 0.005 second, the sampling rate is 200 samples/s. If the dwell time is increased to 0.05 second, the sampling rate is 20 samples/s. This is demonstrated in Figure 4-5, where a spike is being recorded at different sampling rates. Note that more fine details of the wave drop out when the sampling rate decreases. This, in effect, is like applying a high-frequency (HF) filter to the data so that higher frequencies in the signal drop out. This is seen in Figure 4-5, which demonstrates loss of higher frequencies in an EEG signal.

In some instances, high frequency loss can be much more obvious, such as when recording the regular repetitive signal of an EKG signal. The sampling frequency could cause the appearance of missing or abnormally conducted heartbeats when, in fact, it was an artifact of the digital recording

Signal resolution with various digitizer sampling rates

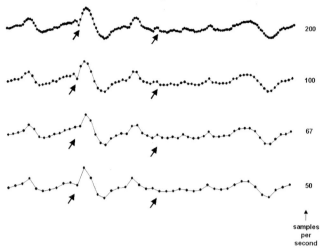

FIGURE 4-5 | An EEG spike-and-slow wave complex recording is displayed using various digitizer sampling rates. Note that the spike portion of the spike-and-slow wave complex is lost at lower sampling rates. As a result, an epileptiform discharge would not be detected at low sampling rates. The *arrows* indicate small notched waves visible in 200 sampling rate, which become unclear with decreasing sampling rates.

process or reconstruction that resulted in losing the details of the time resolution as it was being digitized. This can certainly lead to misinterpretations of the data clinically (Figs. 4-6).

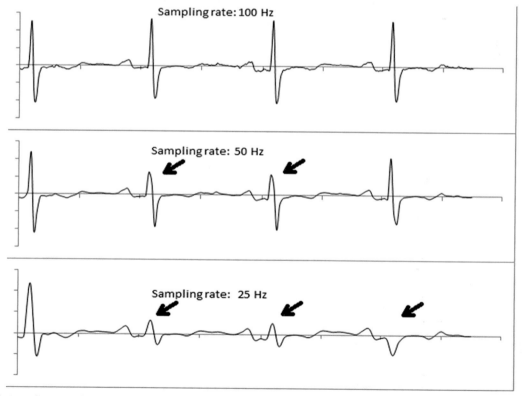

FIGURE 4-6 | A cardiac EKG channel recording is displayed using various digitizer sampling rates. Note the dropout of the QRS complex at the position of the *arrows*. This would result in an erroneous diagnosis of cardiac dysrhythmias.

Nyquist Frequency

So why pay attention to the ADC circuit (digitizer) sampling rate? It turns out that the sampling rate will determine the highest frequency recordable by the system. The Nyquist theorem states that for digitized data, the fastest signal that can be recorded is a frequency that is half the sampling rate of the digitizer. Half the sampling rate of the digitizer is defined as the Nyquist frequency and is the highest frequency the system can record at that specific sampling rate. For example, if the sampling rate was 50 samples/s, then the Nyquist frequency would be 25 samples/s, which means the highest frequency that the system can record is 25 Hz. In most digital EEG recording systems, the sampling rate is 200 samples/s or higher, which means one would be able to record frequencies up to 100 Hz (since the Nyquist frequency is 100). This is slightly faster than paper recordings that have a limit of about 70 Hz.

Alias Signals

With digitized recordings, an interesting problem occurs as signals of various frequencies are recorded. Phantom signals appear as a part of the digitization process.[7] The first problem one notices is that the maximum amplitude of the original analog signal is not always faithfully represented as one approaches the Nyquist frequency. As a result, the superimposition of amplitude modulations of lower frequencies appears on top of the signal. The low-frequency signals are amplitude artifacts generated from the digitizing process (which limits the time resolution) and that apparent signal can be quite different from the original signal. In addition, if the analog input signal has a higher frequency than the Nyquist frequency of the digitizer, then the recorded frequency is slower than the original signal. In the sine wave example, this recorded frequency will be quite low if the signal frequency is close to the digitizer's sampling rate (Fig. 4-7).

One can easily detect alias signals by playing with a sine wave signal made from a signal generator that is recorded on a digital EEG system. If one slowly increases the signal frequency to approach the Nyquist frequency, bizarre low-frequency low-amplitude modulations are intermixed with the original signal. This is due to sampling of points on the wave that are not at the peaks, and as a result, our eye try to fit the incomplete data into a different frequency. As one continues to increase the sine wave frequency beyond the Nyquist frequency to approach

Digitized alias signal from original analog signal

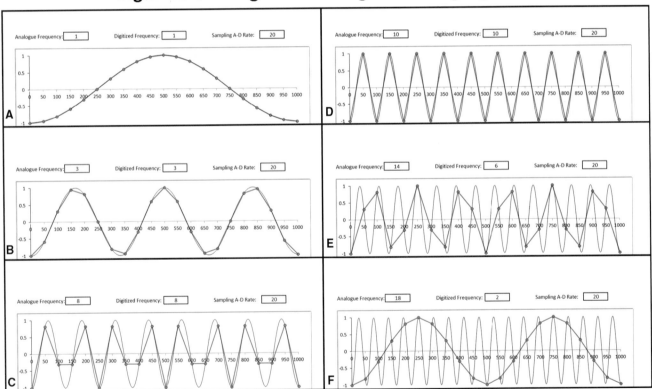

FIGURE 4-7 | This illustration shows how an analog signal is converted to a digitized recording. In all these examples, the digitizer has a sampling rate of 20 Hz or 20 samples/s. The Nyquist frequency is half the sampling rate or 10 Hz, which is the highest frequency the digitizer can record and display. In these examples, we see the digitized reconstructed wave superimposed on the original analog wave. Increasing frequency of the analog signal is noted sequentially from display **A–F**. Note that at low frequencies, the digitized wave closely approximates the original analog wave. However, apparent angular or "blocky" distortion of the original waveform becomes noticeable at about 1/3rd of the Nyquist frequency (or 1/6th of the digitizer's sampling rate) and worsens with higher frequencies. This is due to increasing loss of the details of the original analog wave due to the sampling process. Also notice that the frequency for the digitized waveform is accurate up to the Nyquist frequency (which for this digitizer is 10 Hz). When the digitizer tries to record frequencies above the Nyquist frequency (as seen in figures **E** and **F**), there is noted a slower frequency since the sampling interval is greater than half the analog waveform. We start seeing slower and slower digitized waveforms when trying to record analog frequencies between the Nyquist frequency (in this case 10 Hz) and the sampling rate (in this case 20 Hz).

values near the sampling rate of the digitizer, then very slow alias frequencies are recorded, even though it is known that the original signal frequency is much higher.

Figure 4-7 shows a system that samples at 20 Hz. You can see that the frequency and the details of the waveform are well preserved at 1 Hz, which is well below the sampling rate of 20 Hz. At this frequency, you can see 1 peak. The number of peaks in signals of faster frequency is preserved until you go beyond 10 Hz. At 10 Hz, the number of peaks matches the frequency. Since the sampling rate is 20 Hz, half the frequency of the sampling rate would be 10 Hz, which is the defined Nyquist frequency for this digitizer. When one tries to record frequencies faster than the Nyquist frequency, it results in a recorded signal that has fewer peaks. As Figure 4-7 shows, a 12-Hz signal is recorded as 8 Hz (8 peaks), and a 16-Hz signal is recorded as 4 Hz (4 peaks). These are signals that are perceived as slower frequencies, even though a higher frequency was in the original analog signal. (Refer to the video illustration that describes the process of recording an analog signal in digital format.) For a more dynamic view of alias signals, view Video 4-1 that demonstrates how analog signals are recorded and represented in digitized form.

To reduce aliasing, one should condition the analog signal by filtering out the unwanted frequencies before they are digitized.[8] To do this, one would place an HF filter (low bandpass filter) on the analog amplifier that is low enough to filter out frequencies below the Nyquist frequency. One may ask, "How low should the HF filter be?" A good rule of thumb is to use an HF filter that is about one sixth the sampling frequency or one third the Nyquist frequency since amplitude aliasing starts to be noticed at about half the Nyquist frequency. As an example, if the sampling rate were 200 samples/s or 200 Hz (as is the case for most commercial digital EEG systems), the Nyquist frequency will be 100 Hz. Therefore, an optimal HF filter would be about one third the Nyquist frequency or about 33 Hz. Finally, the display of the digital data can cause additional problems if the equipment used to display the data is also digital, such as printers or video monitors. Commonly, a digital video display that displays the digitized data can add more alias signals to the waveform by the very fact that the video display is now adding an additional sampling rate (in this case, a spatial sampling rate) to the data on the display.[9] One can experiment with the screen resolution by viewing a sine wave in a graphic program. If one were to resize the sine wave display to smaller displays on the same screen, bizarre amplitude variations occur, which produce slower alias signals that are, in fact, are there as a result of the digitization process and can be misleading. Alias signals may be appreciated when viewing actual EEG data when the time base of the waveform is varied on the digital display. These alias signals from the display can be minimized by looking at the data in a "zoomed-in" mode in which the highest time resolution is viewed.

Required Technical EEG Parameters for Digital Recordings: Guidelines for the Technical Parameters of Digital EEG Recordings in Clinical Practice Have Been Published by the American Clinical Neurophysiology Society and Include:

1. Use of a sampling rate of at least 256 samples per second to ensure at least capturing the frequency of 70 Hz (which has been the traditional high-frequency bandpass filter on the traditional paper recording systems). However, if morphology of the waveform is to be reasonably pre-

served, then a sampling rate of 512 is recommended. At this rate, one can safely say that both frequency and at least 90% of the amplitude from the original analog signal are faithfully recorded.

2. Amplitude resolution should allow resolution to below 2 µV since this would be a requirement for recordings to support the confirmation of cortical brain death. The digitizer should be able to store at least 16-bit numbers with a range that allows resolution to go down to 0.05 µV to allow adequate morphology resolution of a 2-µV wave. Using 16-bit numbers per sample permits a maximum excursion of ±1.638 mV (±1638 µV). With this dynamic range being this wide, it will easily allow high signals such as cardiac EKG to be recorded along side channels recording at 2 µV or less.[10]

SUMMARY

Digital EEG recording systems have evolved over the past 20 years, with the major advances being improved amplitude and time resolution of the recordings. The main advantage over pen-writing systems is the ability to store large volumes of data in a smaller space with no loss of information in the data when copied. In addition, digitized EEG data have a higher-amplitude range and more accurate timing with regard to phase relationships between channels. Digital EEG has been a major improvement in the recording of the data, reducing the overall amount of work compared to pen-writing systems where amplitude and pen alignment had to be constantly monitored. A major advantage of digital EEG over analog is the ability to further manipulate the raw data after the recording is complete. Common digital processing techniques that were not available on paper recorders include the ability to view the same recording in different montages or with different filter and sensitivity settings, which is done after the recording is complete in the early systems and is now done in real time on current EEG recording systems. Further processing can compress the data so that the data can be viewed at different time frames to uncover possible trends in the data.

There are new factors and limitations to be aware of with digital EEG data. The first is the amplitude range of the recording. Early EEG systems would have a smaller amplitude range, which would require continual monitoring of the signal to be sure that the sensitivity of the amplifier was adjusted appropriately to optimize recording the signal.[6] Current EEG systems now store data in 16 bits or more, which is a large enough amplitude range to record the amplitudes of all signals of interest without having to adjust the gain of the amplifier. The technologist will need to be aware of the sampling rates of the digitizer because this will determine the frequency limitations that the system can record. Finally, the technologist will also need to pay attention to alias signals that can be minimized by preconditioning the analog signal with analog filters before it reaches the ADC digitizer circuit. In this way, only the signals of interest will be recorded.

References

1. Gotman J. Computer analysis during intensive monitoring of epileptic patients. *Adv Neurol* 1987;46:249–269.
2. Scherg M, Ebersole JS. Brain source imaging of focal and multifocal epileptiform EEG activity. *Neurophysiol Clin* 1994;24:51–60.

3. Swartz BE. The advantages of digital over analog recording techniques. *Electroencephalogr Clin Neurophysiol* 1998;106(2):113–117.

4. Epstein CM. Digital EEG: Trouble in paradise? *J Clin Neurophysiol* 2006;23(3):190–193.

5. Sinha SR. Quantitative EEG analysis: Basics. In: Husain AM, Sinha SR, eds. *Continuous EEG Monitoring: Principles and Practice*. Switzerland: Springer International Publishing, 2017:173–191.

6. Risk WS. Viewing speed and frequency resolution in digital EEG. *Electroencephalogr Clin Neurophysiol* 1993;87(6):347–353.

7. Krauss GL, Weber WRS. Digital EEG. In: Niedermeyer E, Fernando Lopes Da Silva M, eds. *Electroencephalography Basic Principles, Clinical Applications, and Related Fields*. Philadelphia, PA: Lippincott Williams & Wilkins, 2005:707–813.

8. Blum DE. Computer-based electroencephalography: Technical basics, basis for new applications, and potential pitfalls. *Electroencephalogr Clin Neurophysiol* 1998;106(2):118–126.

9. Schevon CA, Thompson T, Hirsch LJ, et al. Inadequacy of standard screen resolution for localization of seizures recorded from intracranial electrodes. *Epilepsia* 2004;45(11):1453–1458.

10. Halford JJ, Sabau D, Drislane FW, et al. American clinical neurophysiology society guideline 4: Recording clinical EEG on digital media. *J Clin Neurophysiol* 2016;33:317–319.

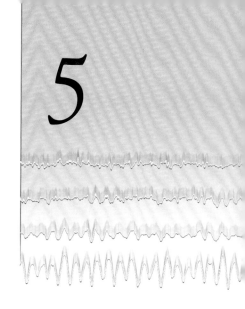

Neuroanatomical and Neurophysiologic Basis of EEG

THORU YAMADA and ELIZABETH MENG

To understand the electroencephalogram (EEG) and its related field of clinical neurophysiology, it is important to know basic neuroanatomy and neurophysiology. In this chapter, neuroanatomical and neurophysiologic aspects of the nervous system are presented.

Basic Anatomical Structures of the Nervous System

The nervous system is divided into two basic parts, the *central nervous system* (CNS) and the *peripheral nervous system* (PNS). The CNS consists of the brain (cerebrum), brainstem, cerebellum, and spinal cord. The brainstem is divided into three parts, midbrain, pons, and medulla oblongata. The spinal cord is divided into cervical, thoracic, lumbar, and sacral cord (Fig. 5-1).

BRAIN (CEREBRUM)

The brain lies in the cranial cavity and is protected by the scalp and skull. Both the brain and the spinal cord are covered by three membranes: *dura mater*, *arachnoid mater*, and *pia mater* (Fig. 5-2). The dura mater is a thick membrane that lies just beneath the skull (cf: *subdural hematoma* is the collection of blood underneath the dura, and *epidural hematoma* is the collection of blood outside the dura, i.e., between the dura and the skull). The pia mater directly covers the entire brain surface including the cortical convolutions. Between the dura mater and pia mater, there is the arachnoid mater (cf: *subarachnoid hemorrhage* is bleeding underneath the arachnoid) and the *cerebrospinal fluid* (CSF), which is a clear and colorless fluid filling the space between the arachnoid and pia mater (the *subarachnoid space*).

The CNS is composed of *gray matter* and *white matter*. The gray matter, which appears grayish in color, consists of billions of nerve cells called *neurons*. The white matter consists of bundles of nerve fibers arising from neurons. The cerebral cortex that covers the brain surface, *thalamus*, and *basal ganglia* (such as the caudate nucleus, putamen, and globus pallidus occupying the deeper portion of the brain) is the gray matter (Fig. 5-3). The white matter of the brain is located underneath the cerebral cortex and outside the thalamus and basal ganglia.

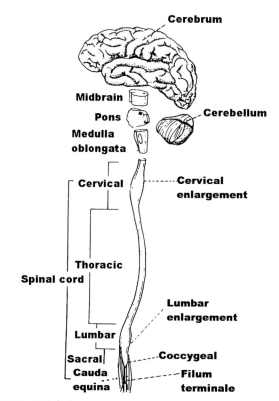

FIGURE 5-1 | Gross anatomy of the cerebrum, brainstem, cerebellum, and spinal cord. (Modified from Snell RS. *Clinical Neurophysiology for Medical Students.* 5th Ed. Baltimore, MD: Lippincott Williams & Wilkins, 2001, with permission.)

The *cerebrum* is the largest part of the brain. It consists of two cerebral hemispheres, which are connected by a mass of white matter called the *corpus callosum* (Fig. 5-3). The cerebral cortex has multiple folds separating multiple *gyri* (gyrus in the singular term). The major folds are called *sulci* (sulcus in the singular term) or *fissures*. Several large fissures or sulci separate the lateral surface of the cortex into four major lobes: *frontal lobe*, *parietal lobe*, *temporal lobe*, and *occipital lobe* (Fig. 5-4). The frontal and parietal lobes are separated by the *central sulcus* or *Rolandic fissure*. The temporal lobe is separated from the frontal and parietal lobes by the *lateral sulcus* or *sylvian fissure*. Parietal and occipital lobes are separated by the *parieto-occipital fissure*.

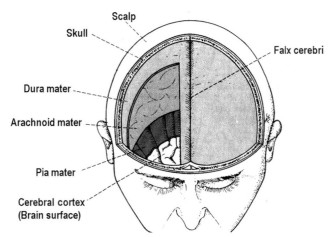

FIGURE 5-2 | Protective coverings of the brain. (Modified from Snell RS. *Clinical Neurophysiology for Medical Students.* 5th Ed. Baltimore, MD: Lippincott Williams & Wilkins, 2001, with permission.)

Each lobe has specific, elaborate, and extremely complicated brain functions. Details of those functions are beyond the scope of this chapter. Very basic and primary functions are described here. The *precentral gyrus* in the frontal lobe, situated just anterior to the central sulcus, controls motor functions (*primary motor cortex*). The superior–medial part of the precentral gyrus represents motor function for the lower extremities, and more lateral and inferior portions of the gyrus represent

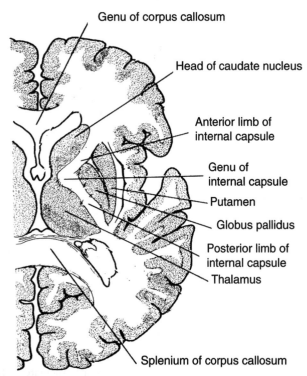

FIGURE 5-3 | Axial section of a brain hemisphere. Shaded areas are the gray matter, which includes the cortex and basal ganglia. White area consists of the nerve fibers, that is, white matter. (Modified from Gatz AJ. *Manter's Essential of Clinical Neuroanatomy and Neurophysiology.* 4th Ed. Philadelphia, PA: FA Davis Co., 1970, with permission.)

motor functions for the trunk and upper extremities. The lowest portion of the *precentral gyrus*, that is, closest portion to the temporal lobe, controls face and tongue movements (Fig. 5-5). Since movements of the face, tongue, mouth, and fingers require much more delicate and elaborate motions than the trunk or lower extremity, these occupy much larger areas of cortex than that for the trunk or lower extremity. Damage, such as a stroke or brain tumor, or excitation, such as a seizure, in the *motor cortex* area would result in motor paralysis or muscle movement/twitches, respectively, in the body part corresponding to the damaged or excited area of motor cortex (see motor evoked potential section in Volume II for further detail; see also Video 14-8).

The postcentral gyrus in the parietal lobe is situated just posterior to the central sulcus (*Rolandic fissure*) and receives sensory input (*primary sensory cortex*) from the entire body (Fig. 5-4). The area corresponding to each body part is arranged in the same way as that for the motor cortex, that is, an upside-down representation with the lower extremities at the top of the gyrus and the face at the bottom of the gyrus (Fig. 5-5). Damage or excitation of an area of sensory cortex would result in sensory loss or sensory hallucination, such as numbness or tingling (see somatosensory evoked potential section of Volume II for further detail). *Primary visual cortex* is situated in the tip and mesial aspect of the occipital cortex (Fig. 5-4). Damage causes a visual field defect, and excitation causes visual hallucinations (see visual evoked potentials in Volume II for further detail; see Video 10-5A). In the superior gyrus of the temporal lobe, there is the *primary auditory cortex*, which receives auditory information. Due to extensive bilateral representation (hearing input from one ear reaches the temporal lobe in both hemispheres), damage to the auditory cortex of one side does not cause deafness in either ear, unlike other sensory or motor functions (see brainstem auditory evoked potential section in Volume II for further detail).

Most brain functions are in a mirror-imaged arrangement between the left and right hemispheres; left hemisphere receives information from or controls the right side of the body and vice versa. Some functions, especially language, have dominance in only one hemisphere. In most individuals and especially in right-handed people, the language or speech center resides in the left hemisphere, often referred to as the *dominant hemisphere.* Speech may be divided into separate motor and sensory functions. In the motor function, elaborate and coordinated movements of the mouth, tongue, larynx, soft palate, and respiratory muscles are required to articulate words and to speak. The motor cortex of speech is called *Broca's area* and is strategically located in the inferior part of the frontal gyrus, just anterior to the primary motor cortex controlling muscles for speech, that is, mouth, lips, tongue, etc. (Figs. 5-4 and 5-5). When Broca's area is damaged, a person can understand the spoken language but is unable to articulate words or sentences. This is called *motor aphasia.* In the sensory function of speech, information received through the ears reaches the primary auditory cortex located in the superior gyrus of the temporal lobe. This information needs to be interpreted to understand what is spoken. Just posterior to the primary auditory cortex, there is an area for interpretation of spoken words called *Wernicke's area* (Fig. 5-4). When the Wernicke's area is damaged, a person can speak but is unable to understand spoken language. This is called *sensory or receptive aphasia.*

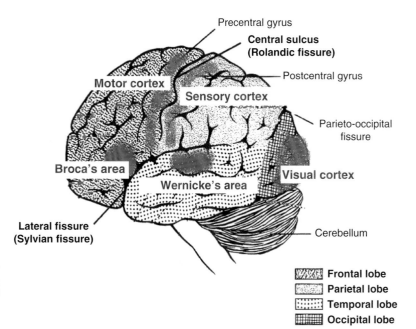

FIGURE 5-4 | Lateral view of the brain (left hemisphere). Note the motor speech area (Broca's area) is located just anterior to the motor cortex (precentral gyrus), which controls the face, tongue, and oropharyngeal muscles necessary for speech. Note that the sensory speech area (Wernicke's area) is situated in the superior temporal gyrus, just posterior to the primary hearing center. (Modified from Gatz AJ. *Manter's Essential of Clinical Neuroanatomy and Neurophysiology.* 4th Ed. Philadelphia, PA: FA Davis Co., 1970, with permission.)

Other elaborate cortical functional areas are also conveniently located near the primary sensory areas; just posterior to the primary sensory cortex in the postcentral gyrus, there is an area which interprets the information received in the primary sensory cortex. If this area is damaged, a person can feel an object with the hand but is unable to interpret or identify that object. This is called *sensory agnosia*. Similarly, there is an interpretation center for visual information just anterior to the visual cortex in the occipital lobe. Damaging this area causes *visual agnosia*. This is when an object can be seen but not recognized.

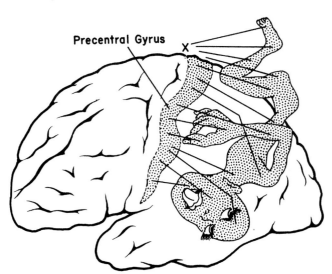

FIGURE 5-5 | Topographic representation of motor cortical functions at precentral gyrus (primary motor cortex). Motor system from the brain to the spinal cord. Note that the area of cortical representation for the face, tongue, and hand in the lower portion of the precentral gyrus is much larger than the area of the trunk or lower extremity. The cortical representation for the leg and foot are situated in the mesial aspect of the hemisphere (not shown here). (Modified from Gatz AJ. *Manter's Essential of Clinical Neuroanatomy and Neurophysiology.* 4th Ed. Philadelphia, PA: FA Davis Co., 1970, with permission.)

Other cortical dysfunctions include (i) *alexia* (unable to read) and *agraphia* (unable to write) due to a lesion at the angular gyrus in the posterior parietal lobe, (ii) *astereognosis* (unable to appreciate texture, size, and form by touching objects) due to a lesion at superior parietal lobe, (iii) *apraxia* (unable to perform purposeful and learned act such as driving a car, playing a piano, etc.) due to a lesion of various association cortex, especially in the dominant hemisphere, and (iv) *amnesia* (loss of memory) due to a lesion in the hippocampus.

BRAINSTEM

The *brainstem* lies between the brain and spinal cord and consists of *the midbrain, pons,* and *medulla oblongata* (Figs. 5-1 and 5-6). The brainstem has three major functions: (i) it functions as a conduit gathering and transmitting multiple ascending and descending tracts between the spinal cord and brain; (ii) it controls elementary life-sustaining functions such as respiration, the cardiovascular system, and level of consciousness; and (iii) it contains multiple nuclei of the *cranial nerves* (CN) (CN III to XII).

The details of brainstem anatomy and functions are beyond the scope of this chapter, and only basic anatomy and function will be described here.

The midbrain has four colliculi (*corpora quadrigemina*), which are rounded eminences that are divided into superior and inferior parts. The *superior colliculi* (colliculus in the singular term) are gray matter with collections of various nuclei. They relate to a part of the visual reflex system and have multiple motor and sensory traits. They connect to the *lateral geniculate body* (see visual evoked potential section of Volume II for further details). *Inferior colliculi* also have multiple nuclei and relate to the auditory pathway, having multiple sensory and motor pathways. They connect to the medial geniculate body (see brainstem auditory evoked potential section in Volume II for further details). The *oculomotor nerve* (CN III) and *trochlear nerve* (CN IV) exit from the midbrain. Both of these cranial nerves control eye movement. CN III also functions in the *pupillary reflex.*

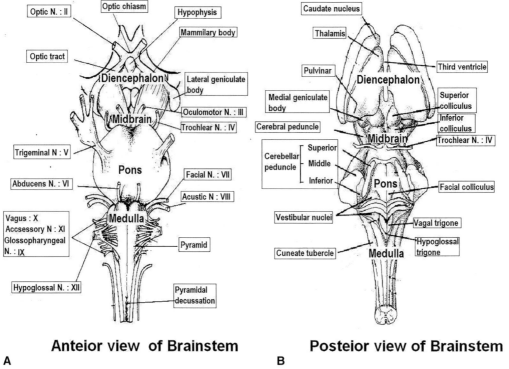

Anteior view of Brainstem

A

Posteior view of Brainstem

B

FIGURE 5-6 | Anterior **(A)** and posterior **(B)** views of the brainstem. Note that multiple cranial nerves originate from the brainstem. (Modified from Gatz AJ. *Manter's Essential of Clinical Neuroanatomy and Neurophysiology*. 4th Ed. Philadelphia, PA: FA Davis Co., 1970, with permission.)

The pons connects the medulla oblongata to the midbrain. The posterior portion of the pons, called the tegmentum, extends from the midbrain. The pons contains numerous nuclei and fiber tracts including the *medial lemniscus,* which carries the ascending sensory fibers for proprioceptive (position sense) and vibratory sensation. The pons also functions as a bridge connecting the left and right cerebellar hemispheres. The *trigeminal nerve* (CN V), which receives facial sensation and controls masticatory muscles, enters and exits from midpons. The medulla connects the pons superiorly and spinal cord inferiorly. On each side of the median fissure, there is an elongated eminence called the *pyramid.* The pyramids are composed of bundles of nerve fibers originating from the motor cortex (precentral gyrus) descending as the *corticospinal tract.* The majority of descending fibers cross over to the opposite side, forming the *pyramidal decussation. The abducens nerve* (CN VI, controls eye movements), *facial nerve* (CN VII, controls facial muscles), and *acoustic* or *vestibulocochlear nerve* (CN VIII, receives hearing input) emerge from the border of the pons and medulla. The remaining cranial nerves (CN IX, *glossopharyngeal nerve* controls oropharyngeal muscles; CN X, *vagus nerve* controls autonomic function; CN XI, accessory nerve controls sternocleidomastoid and trapezius muscles; and CN XII, *hypoglossal nerve* controls tongue movement) exit from the medulla oblongata (cf: CN I is the *olfactory nerve* and arises from the base of the brain. CN II is the *optic nerve* and passes between the base of the brain and brainstem).

CEREBELLUM

The *cerebellum* is located in the posterior cranial fossa and lies posterior to the fourth ventricle, pons, and the *medulla oblongata.* It consists of two cerebellar hemispheres joined by a narrow *median vermis.* The cerebellum receives afferent information concerning voluntary movement from the cerebral cortex and also from muscles, tendons, and joints. Cerebellar output is conducted to the sites that influence motor activity at the segmental spinal level. The cerebellum functions as a coordinator for precise voluntary movement, which requires a continuous balance between output from the cerebral motor cortex and feedback of proprioceptive information from the muscles. This then allows the degree of muscle contraction necessary for a precise voluntary movement to be adjusted.

Damage to one cerebellar hemisphere causes a disturbance of voluntary movement called *ataxia* on the same side of the body; the muscle group fails to work harmoniously, and the patient may have difficulty in picking up an object, writing, or shaving (*dysmetria*). The patient may have difficulty walking and may tend to fall to the same side as the lesion (*ataxia*). The patient may have difficulty articulating words, called *dysarthria,* due to a failure of coordinated movements of the tongue, mouth, and larynx (cf: this is different from motor aphasia resulting from damage to the cerebral cortex or Broca's area). Damage in the midline of the cerebellum (vermis) causes a disturbance in the midline body parts, such as the head and trunk; the patient may have difficulty in holding the trunk straight (*truncal ataxia*).

Despite the important and fundamental functions of the cerebellum for daily living activities, there is no specific neurophysiologic test that directly measures cerebellar function.

SPINAL CORD

The spinal cord begins at the *foramen magnum* in the skull base where it connects to the medulla oblongata rostrally.

It is protected by multiple vertebrae that allow for flexible movement. The spinal cord terminates inferiorly at the level of the lower border of the first lumbar vertebra in an adult. The spinal cord in children ends at the upper border of the third lumbar vertebra. Like the brain, the spinal cord is also surrounded by pia mater, arachnoid mater, and dura mater, and there is CSF in the subarachnoid space.

The spinal cord is enlarged (see Fig. 5-1) at the cervical level (cervical enlargement) to allow abundant nerves to exit and enter the brachial plexus, connecting peripheral nerves of the upper limbs (Fig. 5-7). Similarly, at the lumbar level, there is a lumbar enlargement (see Fig. 5-1) allowing abundant nerves to exit and enter the sacral plexus, connecting the nerves of the lower limb. The spinal cord tapers into the conus medullaris and progresses to the filum terminale, which ends at the coccyx (see Fig. 5-1). There are abundant peripheral nerves descending from the first lumbar vertebrae to the coccyx, which are called the cauda equina (because it looks like a horse's tail).

Along the entire length of the spinal cord, 31 pairs of spinal nerves (8 cervical, 12 thoracic, 5 lumbar, 5 sacral, and 1 coccygeal) are attached. The spinal nerves consist of two nerve roots, one posterior and another anterior. The posterior root carries sensory information and enters the posterior part of spinal cord. Each posterior root has a posterior (or dorsal) root ganglion containing the cell body that gives rise to the peripheral and central portions of the nerve fiber. The anterior root carries motor information and exits from the anterior part of the spinal cord. The peripheral nerves may contain sensory and motor fibers (*mixed nerve*) or either sensory or motor fibers alone. The *median and ulnar nerves* are mixed nerves at the wrist but contain sensory fibers only in the fingers. The *posterior tibial nerve* is a mixed nerve, and the sural nerve is a sensory nerve (see somatosensory evoked potential in Volume II for further details of peripheral nerve innervations).

THE AFFERENT AND EFFERENT SYSTEMS

Both the CNS and the PNS comprise afferent and efferent pathways. The typical example of an afferent pathway is the *sensory system* in which sensory signals originate from the peripheral receptors (such as muscle spindles in the muscle tissue, joint receptors from the joint, etc.) and travel to the CNS via the PNS.

The peripheral nerve fibers from pain, temperature, and touch receptors traveling through small *myelinated or unmyelinated fibers* (Fig. 5-8A) enter the posterior portion of the spinal cord. The fibers then cross over to the opposite side of the spinal cord after synaptic connection at the *substantia gelatinosa* and ascend as the *spinothalamic (lateral or anterior) tract* (Fig. 5-8A). The fibers then ascend as *spinal lemniscus* at the brainstem and proceed to the *ventroposterolateral (VPL) nucleus* of the *thalamus*, finally reaching the postcentral gyrus.

The peripheral nerve fibers from muscle spindles and joint receptors carrying proprioceptive sense and discriminative touch sense consist of large *myelinated fibers*. They enter the posterior part of the spinal cord, the same way as the fibers of pain/temperature senses. But unlike pain/temperature pathways crossing to the opposite side of spinal cord, these ascend to the brainstem via the *dorsal column* on the same side as they entered the *fasciculus cuneatus* (from upper extremity) and the *fasciculus gracilis* (from lower extremity) (Fig. 5-8B). At the brainstem, synaptic connections occur in the *cuneate nucleus* (for nerve fibers from the upper extremity) and in the *gracile nucleus* (for nerve fibers from the lower extremity). After *synaptic connections* in the cuneate or gracile nucleus, the fibers then cross to the opposite side and ascend the brainstem as the *medial lemniscus* to the *VPL nucleus* of the thalamus. After the thalamus, the sensory fibers reach the sensory cortex (postcentral gyrus) via the internal capsule.

A typical efferent pathway is the motor system in which signals originating from the motor cortex (precentral gyrus) travel through the *internal capsule* down to the brainstem where the majority of fibers cross to the opposite side (*pyramidal decussation*) at the level of the medulla (Fig. 5-9; see also Fig. 5-6A). The fibers then descend to the anterior horn cells of the spinal cord and exit from the anterior portion of the spinal cord. They finally reach their designated muscles via the PNS.

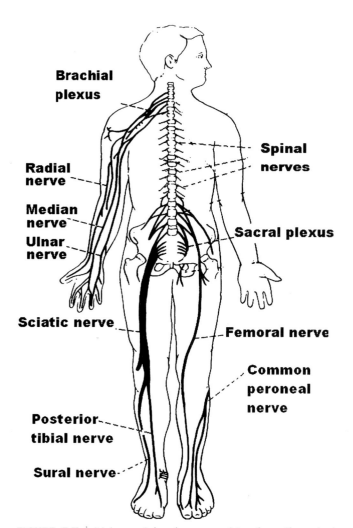

Brachial plexus

Radial nerve

Median nerve

Ulnar nerve

Spinal nerves

Sacral plexus

Sciatic nerve

Femoral nerve

Common peroneal nerve

Posterior tibial nerve

Sural nerve

FIGURE 5-7 | Major peripheral nerves arising from the spinal cord (commonly used for studies of somatosensory evoked potentials). (Modified from Snell RS. *Clinical Neurophysiology for Medical Students.* 5th Ed. Baltimore, MD: Lippincott Williams & Wilkins, 2001, with permission.)

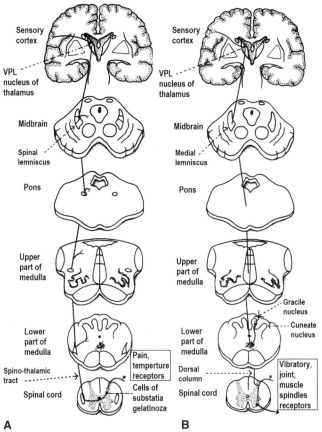

FIGURE 5-8 | Sensory system from the peripheral nerve through the spinal cord and the brain. Small myelinated fibers carrying touch, pressure, and nonmyelinated fibers carrying pain/temperature senses enter the spinal cord through the posterior spinal root **(A)**. After entering the spinal cord, the fibers cross to the opposite side and ascend the anterior and lateral portion of the spinal cord through the spinothalamic tract. The fibers then pass through the spinal lemniscus at the brainstem and reach the VPL nucleus of the thalamus. They finally reach the primary sensory cortex. Large myelinated fibers carrying the information from the joint and muscle spindles receptors and vibratory sensation enter the posterior portion of the spinal cord through posterior spinal root, the same way as for the pain/touch sensory pathway **(B)**. Unlike the pain/temperature pathway, which cross to the opposite side of spinal cord, however, these fibers ascend in the dorsal column (fasciculus gracilis from the lower and fasciculus cuneatus from upper extremities) on the same side of entrance and reach the cuneatus and gracilis nuclei for the upper and lower extremities, respectively, where synaptic changes occur. The fibers then cross to the opposite side and ascend as the medial lemniscus in the brainstem, connect to the VPL nucleus of the thalamus, and finally reach the primary sensory cortex at the postcentral gyrus. (Modified from Snell RS. *Clinical Neurophysiology for Medical Students.* 5th Ed. Baltimore, MD: Lippincott Williams & Wilkins, 2001, with permission.)

Vascular System of the Brain and Spinal Cord

ARTERIES OF THE BRAIN

The brain is supplied by the two *internal carotid arteries* and two *vertebral arteries*.

Internal Carotid Artery

The internal carotid artery starts at the bifurcation of the common carotid artery, where the external carotid artery also gives rise. The right common carotid artery arises from the *brachiocephalic artery* branching from the aortic arch, which directly connects to the heart (Fig. 5-10). The left common carotid artery directly arises from aortic arch. The internal carotid artery divides into the anterior and *middle cerebral arteries* after entering the cranium (Figs. 5-10 and 5-11). The *anterior cerebral artery* runs forward and medially and supplies a large portion of medial surface of the brain including the frontal and parietal lobes. Left and right *anterior cerebral arteries* are connected via the *anterior communicating artery* (as a part of Circle of Willis). The *middle cerebral artery* runs laterally and supplies a large portion of the lateral hemisphere including the frontal, parietal lobes, and superior and middle temporal gyri. The *corpus striatum* and the *internal capsule* are also supplied by the middle cerebral artery.

Vertebral Artery

The *vertebral artery* arises from the *subclavian artery* (a part of the aortic arch) and ascends the neck by passing through the foramina of the transverse process of the cervical vertebra. It enters the skull through the *foramen magnum*. The vertebral artery gives rise to the posterior inferior cerebellar artery, supplying a large portion of the cerebellum. Left and right vertebral arteries then join at the lower border of the pons and form the basilar artery. The basilar artery splits into left and right posterior cerebral arteries at the midbrain level. The *posterior cerebral artery* supplies the posterior portion of medial hemisphere and inferior and medial temporal gyri. The posterior cerebral artery also sends a branch to the *posterior communicating artery*, which connects to the internal carotid artery (Figs. 5-10 and 5-11).

Circle of Willis

The anterior communicating, anterior cerebral, internal carotid, posterior communicating, posterior cerebral, and basilar arteries form the Circle of Willis by multiple anastomoses. This allows blood to be distributed to any part of the cerebral hemisphere by either the internal carotid or the vertebral/basilar arteries should either artery fail (Fig. 5-11).

VENOUS DRAINAGE OF THE BRAIN

There are six major sinuses that collect venous drainage from various veins. They are the superior sagittal sinus, inferior sagittal sinus, straight sinus, occipital sinus, transverse sinus, and sigmoid sinus. All sinuses join together at the sigmoid sinus, which connects to the internal jugular vein, returning venous blood to the heart (Fig. 5-12).

ARTERIES OF THE SPINAL CORD

The spinal cord receives arterial supply from two (left and right) *posterior spinal arteries* and one *anterior spinal artery*. All spinal arteries arise from the left and right vertebral arteries (Fig. 5-13). At each intervertebral foramen, the posterior spinal artery sends a segmental spinal artery. The lower two thirds of the spinal cord is mainly supplied by one large, important

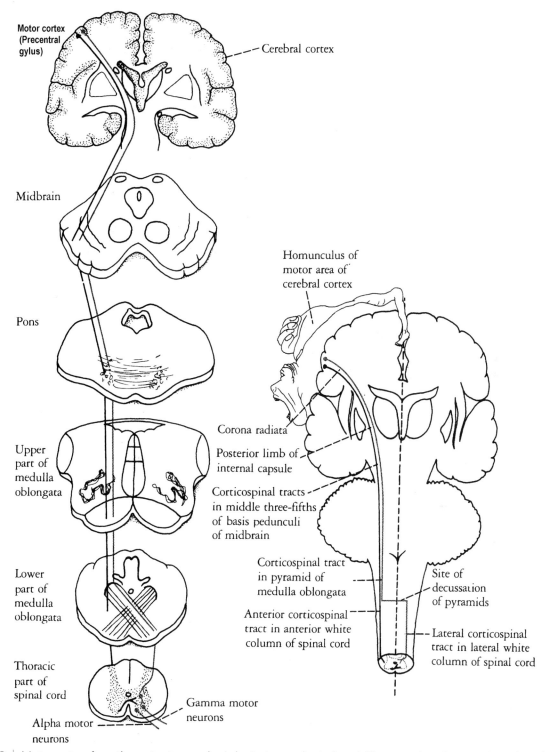

FIGURE 5-9 | Motor system from the cortex to muscle via brainstem and spinal cord. The motor impulse starts from the primary motor cortex (precentral gyrus) and descends through posterior limb of internal capsule as the corticospinal tract. At the medulla, most of the fibers cross to the opposite side at the pyramidal decussation. The fibers then descend through the lateral portion of the spinal cord as the corticospinal tract and reach the anterior horn cells where synaptic connection occurs. The motor fibers then exit the spinal cord via anterior spinal root and finally reach the designated muscles. (From Snell RS. *Clinical Neurophysiology for Medical Students*. 5th Ed. Baltimore, MD: Lippincott Williams & Wilkins, 2001, with permission.)

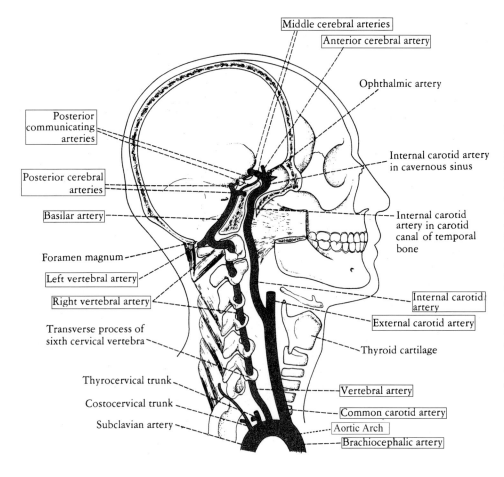

FIGURE 5-10 | Vascular supply to the brain. The right common carotid artery arises from brachiocephalic artery and splits into internal and external carotid arteries. The left common carotid artery arises directory from aortic arch (not shown in this figure). The internal carotid artery gives rise to the middle and anterior cerebral arteries. The vertebral artery arises from subclavian artery and ascends through transverse process of the cervical vertebra. Left and right vertebral arteries join and form basilar artery, which gives rise to posterior cerebral artery. Left and right posterior cerebral arteries are connected (anastomoses) with internal carotid arteries via posterior communicating arteries (Fig. 5-11). (From Snell RS. *Clinical Neurophysiology for Medical Students.* 5th Ed. Baltimore, MD: Lippincott Williams & Wilkins, 2001, with permission.)

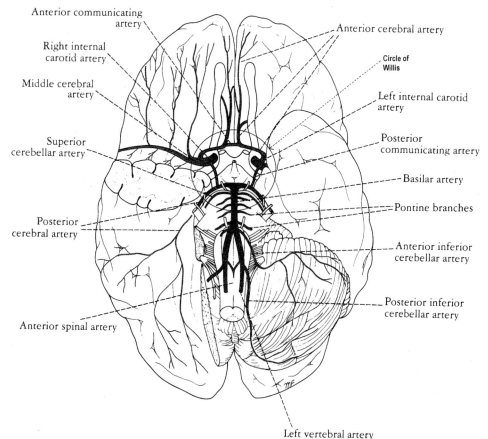

FIGURE 5-11 | The inferior view of vascular supply to the brain. Left and right posterior cerebral arteries are connected with left and right internal carotid arteries via left and right posterior communicating arteries, respectively. Left and right anterior cerebral arteries are connected by anterior communicating artery. These anastomoses form the Circle of Willis (shown by *circle*). Also note that the two vertebral arteries and anterior spinal artery branched from left and right vertebral arteries, which supply blood to the spinal cord (Fig. 5-13). (From Snell RS. *Clinical Neurophysiology for Medical Students.* 5th Ed. Baltimore, MD: Lippincott Williams & Wilkins, 2001, with permission.)

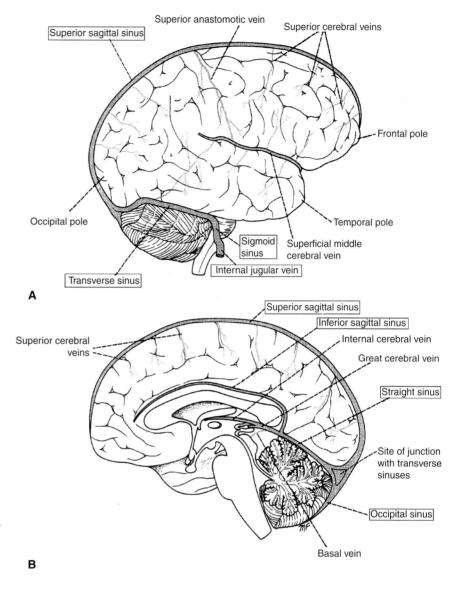

FIGURE 5-12 | Venous drainage of brain [lateral view, **(A)**; medial view, **(B)**]. Major sinuses are shown in rectangular boxes. (From Snell RS. *Clinical Neurophysiology for Medical Students.* 5th Ed. Baltimore, MD: Lippincott Williams & Wilkins, 2001, with permission.)

FIGURE 5-13 | Arterial supply of the spinal cord. Three major arteries (left and right posterior spinal arteries and anterior spinal artery), which arise from the vertebral arteries **(A)**. The posterior spinal artery gives rise to segmental artery, which splits into anterior and posterior radicular arteries at each spinal segment **(B)**. The segmental and posterior spinal arteries supply blood to most of posterior and lateral spinal cord and anterior spinal artery covers anterior and central portion of spinal cord. (From Snell RS. *Clinical Neurophysiology for Medical Students.* 5th Ed. Baltimore, MD: Lippincott Williams & Wilkins, 2001, with permission.)

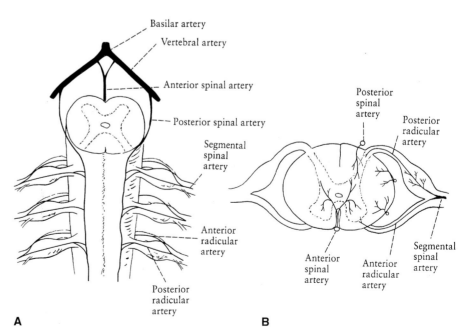

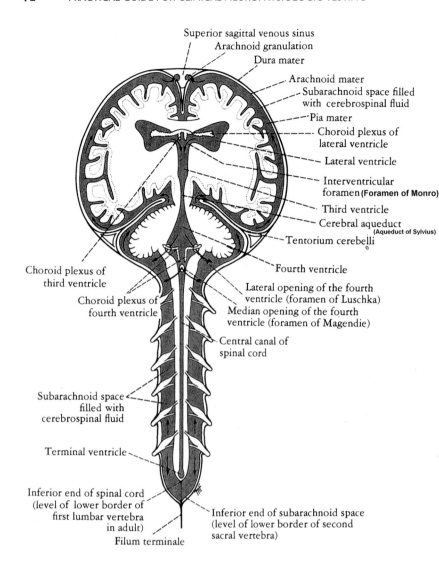

Superior sagittal venous sinus
Arachnoid granulation
Dura mater
Arachnoid mater
Subarachnoid space filled
with cerebrospinal fluid
Pia mater
Choroid plexus of
lateral ventricle
Lateral ventricle
Interventricular
foramen (Foramen of Monro)
Third ventricle
Cerebral aqueduct
(Aqueduct of Sylvius)
Tentorium cerebelli
Fourth ventricle
Choroid plexus of
third ventricle
Lateral opening of the fourth
ventricle (foramen of Luschka)
Choroid plexus of
fourth ventricle
Median opening of the fourth
ventricle (foramen of Magendie)
Central canal of
spinal cord
Subarachnoid space
filled with
cerebrospinal fluid
Terminal ventricle
Inferior end of spinal cord
(level of lower border of
first lumbar vertebra
in adult)
Inferior end of subarachnoid space
(level of lower border of second
sacral vertebra)
Filum terminale

FIGURE 5-14 | Ventricular system and CSF. Three ventricles consisting of lateral, third, and fourth ventricles located at the center of the brain and the brainstem. The lateral and third ventricles are connected via interventricular foramen (foramen of Monro), and the third and fourth ventricles are connected via cerebral aqueduct (aqueduct of Sylvius). The fourth ventricle and central canal of spinal cord are connected via median opening of the fourth ventricle (foramen of Magendie). There is also an opening to the subarachnoid space of the spinal cord via lateral opening of the fourth ventricle (foramen of Luschka). CSF circulates through these ventricles and the subarachnoid space.

feeder artery called the great anterior medullary *artery of Adamkiewicz*, which arises from the abdominal aorta at the lower thoracic or upper lumbar vertebral levels. (See section of intraoperative monitoring in volume II for further details.)

Ventricular System

There are three major cavities in the brain called ventricles, which communicate with the central canal of the spinal cord. They are the lateral ventricles, the third ventricle, and the fourth ventricle (Fig. 5-14). The left and right lateral ventricles communicate via the *interventricular foramina* (*foramen of Monro*) with the third ventricle. The third ventricle is connected to the fourth ventricle by the *cerebral aqueduct* (*aqueduct of Sylvius*). The fourth ventricle continues to the central canal of spinal cord via the two *foramina, the foramen of Luschka,* and the *foramen of Magendie.* CSF is manufactured in these ventricles and circulates thru the ventricles, central canal of spinal cord, and the subarachnoid space.

Cellular Anatomy and Physiology

To understand how the working nervous system can be recorded by electrodes placed on the scalp, we must start

with an understanding of what lies below the scalp. The different structures in the nervous system are all interconnected. Understanding the manner in which each works and how they work together gives us insight into the working of the whole.

PERIPHERAL NERVE

A peripheral nerve is a nerve outside of the CNS. The peripheral nerve consists of bundles of nerve fibers, each of which is covered by a fine connective tissue called the *endoneurium* (Fig. 5-15). A group of nerve fibers is then surrounded by another connective tissue called the *perineurium*. Several groups of nerve fibers covered by perineurium are further covered by the *epineurium*.

The individual nerve fibers have different diameters related to different functions. Each nerve fiber arises from the *soma* (cell body) of the *neuron* (nerve cell) through a long extended process called the "*axon.*"

There are two types of axons: one is a large diameter axon, which is wrapped by multiple layers of highly lipid material called *myelin*. The myelin is derived from the extended membrane of a *Schwann cell* (Fig. 5-16) and covers most of the length of an axon. There is a small space in between two myelin sheaths where the axon is not covered by myelin, exposing the nerve. This space is the "*node of Ranvier*" (Fig. 5-17; see

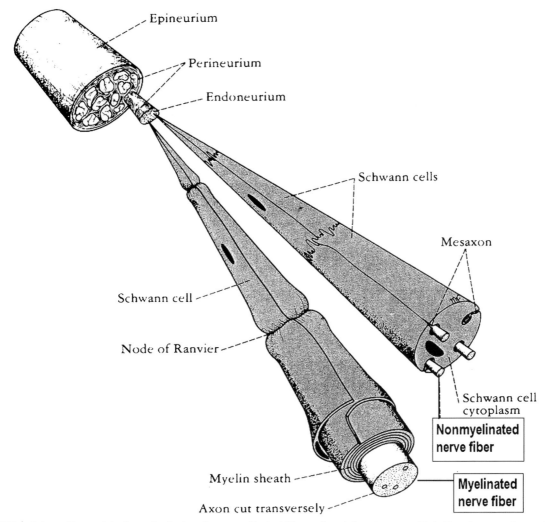

FIGURE 5-15 | Schematic model of myelinated and nonmyelinated fibers of peripheral nerves. Note the absence of a node of Ranvier and the small diameter of a nonmyelinated nerve fiber. (From Snell RS. *Clinical Neurophysiology for Medical Students.* 5th Ed. Baltimore, MD: Lippincott Williams & Wilkins, 2001, with permission.)

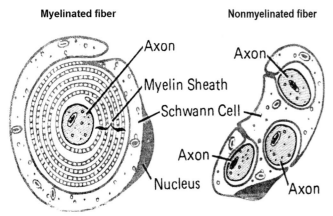

FIGURE 5-16 | Schematic model of a cross section of non-myelinated and myelinated fibers. Although both fibers (axons) are wrapped by a Schwann cell, only the myelinated fiber is covered by multiple layers of myelin sheaths derived from a Schwann cell. (From Schmidt RF, ed. *Fundamentals of Neurophysiology.* New York: Springer-Verlag New York, 1975, with permission.)

also Fig. 5-15). This unique anatomical arrangement of myelin sheaths wrapping the axon interrupted by the node of Ranvier allows the electrical current to jump from one node to the next instead of traveling steadily within the axon. This facilitates the speed of impulse conduction along the nerve fibers and is called "*saltatory conduction*" (Fig. 5-17).

The second type of axon is the nerve fiber, which is not wrapped by the myelin sheath, called "*nonmyelinated fiber*" (Figs. 5-15 to 5-17). The nonmyelinated fiber has a much smaller diameter than the myelinated fiber and is imbedded in the Schwann cell. Due to its small diameter, conduction velocity of a nonmyelinated fiber is much slower than myelinated fiber. In addition, the impulse of the nonmyelinated fiber travels within the axon (instead of jumping from one node of Ranvier to the next node as in a myelinated fiber), which further slows the conduction (Fig. 5-17).

Impulse transmission along the nerve is mostly controlled by chemical properties of sodium (Na^+) and potassium (K^+) ions. When the nerve is at a resting state, the inside of the nerve is negatively charged, typically at around -70 mV. This is called the *resting membrane potential* (Fig. 5-18; see "Resting

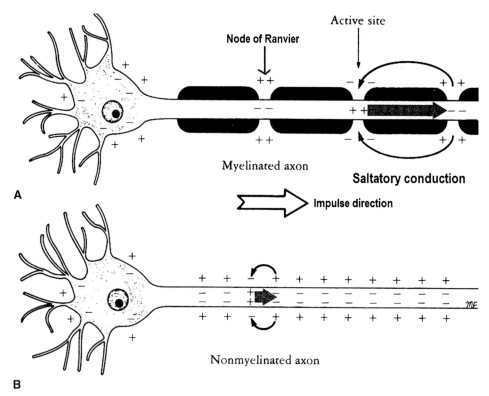

FIGURE 5-17 | The impulse propagation of myelinated **(A)** and nonmyelinated **(B)** axons. The traveling impulse originating from the nerve cell (soma) successively changes the membrane potential inside the axon from negative to positive, which results in current flow from the positive to the negative site; current flows toward the direction of impulse transmission inside the axon and toward the opposite direction outside the axon. In the myelinated fiber, the current jumps from one node of Ranvier to the next (saltatory conduction) resulting in faster conduction than in nonmyelinated fibers in which the current flows in a step-by-step process within the axon. (Modified from Snell RS. *Clinical Neurophysiology for Medical Students.* 5th Ed. Baltimore, MD: Lippincott Williams & Wilkins, 2001, with permission.)

Membrane Potentials and Postsynaptic Potentials," for further details). Stimulating the nerve alters the permeability of Na+ (sodium) ions at the point of stimulation. This causes diffusion of Na+ from outside the axon to inside, changing the membrane potential from more negative to less negative (toward the positive side) called *depolarization*. When the membrane potential reaches a certain level of depolarization (−50 to −60 mV), a sudden influx of Na+ occurs producing the *action potential*, and the membrane potential changes to a positive polarity at about 30 to 40 mV inside the axon. At this point, the outside of the axon becomes negatively charged and acts as a new stimulus to the adjacent point, changing its membrane potential to the positive polarity. As the action potential propagates, the site action potential becomes sequentially positive inside the axon, and the tail end of propagation then becomes negative, restoring the resting membrane potential.

There are three major types of peripheral fibers having different functions, diameters, and conduction velocities, that is, A, B, and C fibers. The fastest conducting fibers [*Group A alpha,* diameter 12 to 20 µm (1 mm = 1,000 µm)] have a conduction velocity of 70 to 120 m/s. These fibers carry efferent impulses to skeletal muscles. The slowest conducting fibers (*Group C fibers,* diameter 0.4 to 1.2 µm) have a conduction velocity of 0.5 to 2.0 m/s. The *C fibers* carry afferent impulses from pain and temperature receptors (often referred to as superficial sensation). In between these fastest and slowest fibers, there are Group A beta, gamma, and delta fibers. *Group A beta fibers* (diameter 5 to 12 µm) have a conduction velocity of 40 to 70 m/s and

involve touch, pressure, and vibration senses. *Group A gamma fibers* (diameter 3 to 6 µm) with a conduction velocity of 10 to 50 ms carry afferent impulses from muscle spindles. *Group A delta fibers* (diameter 2 to 5 µm) move at 6 to 30 m/s and carry localized pain, temperature, and touch sensations. B fibers (diameter of <3 µm) with conduction velocity of 3 to 15 m/s carry impulse related to autonomic functions. With the exception of C fibers, all fibers are myelinated.

NEURONS

A *neuron* is a nerve cell. It is estimated that the human brain possesses about 25 billion neurons. The cell body, called "soma," has one or two long nerve fibers called "*axons*" and several branches of short nerve fibers called "*dendrites*" (Fig. 5-19). Neurons transmit electrical signals or impulses to other neurons or to the effector organs such as muscle fibers. The outgoing signal is transmitted by the axon, which can be as short as 1 mm (millimeter) or as long as 1 m (meter) in length.

There are three types of neurons: (i) the *afferent neuron,* which receives signals from other cells; (ii) the *efferent neuron,* which transmits signals to other cells; and (iii) the *interneuron,* which lies exclusively within the CNS and integrates activity between afferent and efferent neurons. The final communication between the two neurons occurs at a specialized anatomical structure called the "*synapse.*" This communication may occur from axon to dendrite, axon to soma, or axon to axon (Fig. 5-20).

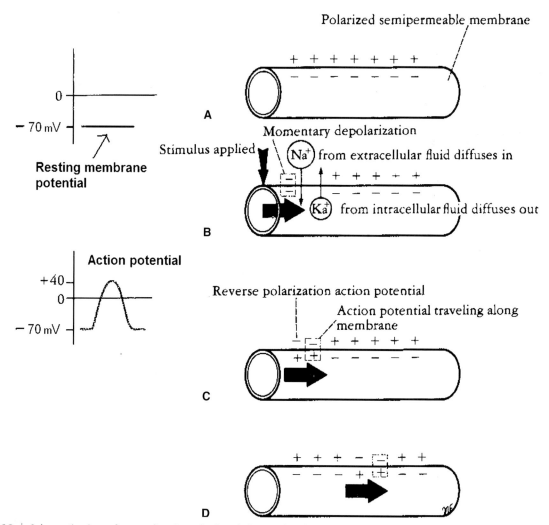

FIGURE 5-18 | Schematic view of a traveling impulse in relation to the change of membrane potentials. At the resting state, the inside of the cell (axon) is negatively charged at −70 mV called the "polarized state" **(A)**. When the stimulus is applied, sodium ions (Na⁺) from the extracellular fluid enter the axon, and potassium ions (K⁺) from the intracellular fluid exit the axon, changing the intracellular membrane potential toward the positive side called "depolarization" **(B)**. When the depolarization reaches a certain level (threshold), an action potential arises changing the intracellular membrane potential to a positive value at around +40 mV **(C)**. Once the action potential is generated, it spreads to the next site, changing the membrane potential to the positive value bringing about another action potential. This sequence continues, and action potentials self-propagate along the axon **(D)**. (From Snell RS. *Clinical Neurophysiology for Medical Students*. 5th Ed. Baltimore, MD: Lippincott Williams & Wilkins, 2001, with permission.)

SYNAPSES

The synapse is the anatomical structure where the signal (electrical impulse) from one cell is transmitted to another cell; the action potential traveling through the axon (Figs. 5-17 and 5-18) reaches the axon terminal as a *presynaptic potential* (Fig. 5-21). The axon terminal is separated from the surface of the soma or dendrites of another cell (*postsynaptic neuron*) by a narrow surface (about 2 nm) called the "*synaptic cleft*." The electrical signal reaching the presynaptic terminal is transmitted to the postsynaptic neurons as a "postsynaptic potential (PSP)" by chemical transmission at the synaptic cleft. The PSP is generated as follows: the axon terminal contains vesicles of a neurotransmitter. The arrival of the action potential at the presynaptic terminal promotes the inflow of Ca²⁺ ions, which triggers the release of the *neurotransmitter* from the synaptic vesicle to the cleft. The released neurotransmitter diffuses across the cleft and acts on the *postsynaptic membrane* to open

a specific ion channel allowing the specific ion to enter the postsynaptic membrane. This results in changes of the membrane potential at the postsynaptic site. There are two types of *PSP*, one is *excitatory PSP (EPSP)* and the other is *inhibitory PSP (IPSP)*.

RESTING MEMBRANE POTENTIALS AND POSTSYNAPTIC POTENTIALS

The cell membrane has channels that may open or close allowing particular ions to enter or exit the membrane, selectively. At the resting state, the concentration of potassium (K⁺) is 20 times greater inside the cell than outside (20 mM outside vs. 400 mM inside), and the concentration gradient is reversed for sodium (Na⁺), which is about 10 times greater outside than inside the cell (440 mM outside vs. 50 mM inside). The difference in concentration is established and

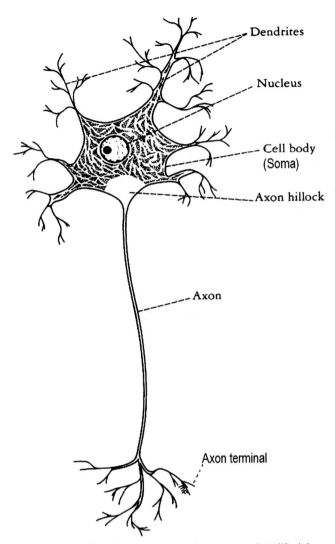

FIGURE 5-19 | Cellular structure of a neuron. (Modified from Snell RS. *Clinical Neurophysiology for Medical Students.* 5th Ed. Baltimore, MD: Lippincott Williams & Wilkins, 2001, with permission.)

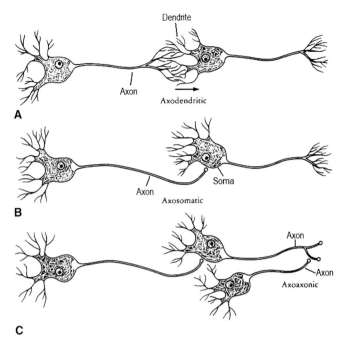

FIGURE 5-20 | Three types of synaptic connections between two neurons. (Modified from Snell RS. *Clinical Neurophysiology for Medical Students.* 5th Ed. Baltimore, MD: Lippincott Williams & Wilkins, 2001, with permission.)

The resting membrane potential is close to the Cl⁻ equilibrium potential, and for mammalian nerve and muscle cells, it lies between −70 and −100 mV, generally at around −70 to −80 mV. This is referred to as the membrane being "polarized."

Various conditions and mechanisms can alter the membrane resting potential. The stimulation of peripheral nerves or sensory receptors by electrical stimulation either naturally or artificially affects the sodium and potassium balance between inside and outside the cell, resulting in a change of the membrane potential.

SYNAPTIC POTENTIALS AND ACTION POTENTIALS

Whether a postsynaptic membrane potential is EPSP or IPSP is dependent on the type of *neurotransmitter*. If the neurotransmitter, for example *acetylcholine*, increases sodium (Na^+) permeability of the postsynaptic membrane, it is an EPSP. The greater the sodium influx, the greater the degree of *depolarization* shift occurs; that is, the membrane potential moves toward a more positive side. When the depolarization shift reaches a certain level (−50 to −60 mV), which is the threshold, the ionic permeability to Na^+ increases dramatically, and this sudden influx of Na^+ creates the "action potential" (Fig. 5-23). The action potential is an all or none phenomenon and is unable to stop once it starts. This is in contrast to the graded property of the PSP, which allows an increase in parallel to the degree and time course of Na^+ influx. When the membrane potential reaches around +30 mV, there is an abrupt decrease in permeability to Na^+ followed by a quick increase of K^+ permeability, which brings the membrane potential back to negative polarity. This event lasts only 1 to 1.5 ms (milliseconds) and is followed by some residual increase of K^+ permeability leading to an overshift of the membrane potential and resulting in greater negativity

maintained by an active mechanism called the "*sodium–potassium pump*" (Fig. 5-22). The differences of K^+ from inside to outside and that of Na^+ from outside to inside are counterbalanced by the sodium–potassium pump. The energy for this sodium–potassium pump is derived from hydrolysis of adenosine triphosphate.

The concentration of *chloride* (Cl⁻) is also different inside and outside the cell (100 vs. 580 mM). The membrane permeability for negatively charged Cl⁻ is high, and there is no active transport for Cl⁻ across the cell membrane. The high concentration of extracellular Na^+ is primarily balanced by a high extracellular concentration of Cl⁻. The Cl⁻ equilibrium potential is about −70 mV. The membrane potential based on ionic influx and efflux is then calculated by the equilibrium potential using the "*Nernst equation.*" Nernst equation of potassium equilibrium potential, for example, is calculated by

$$EqK^+ = +61\log\frac{\left[K^{\pm}\text{outside}\right]}{\left[K^+\text{inside}\right]} = +61\log\frac{20}{400} = \sim -90\text{mV}$$

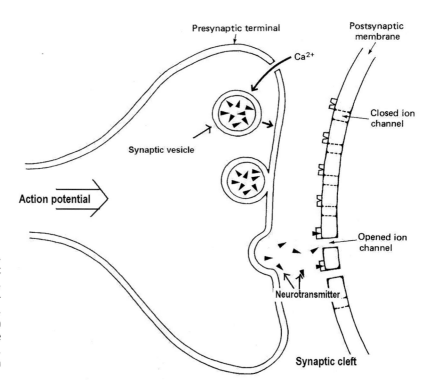

FIGURE 5-21 | Schematic view of a synapse. The action potential reached at the presynaptic terminal triggers the entrance of the calcium ion, which triggers the release of a neurotransmitter from synaptic vesicles into the synaptic cleft. The neurotransmitter in the synaptic cleft then opens the ion channel's postsynaptic membrane to allow the Na$^+$ ion to enter into the next cell. A sufficient sodium influx then creates the action potential.

than the original resting membrane potential. This is called the "*hyperpolarized state*," which lasts about 2 to 3 ms. During the hyperpolarized state, the cell is more difficult to excite than during the resting state, that is, refractory state.

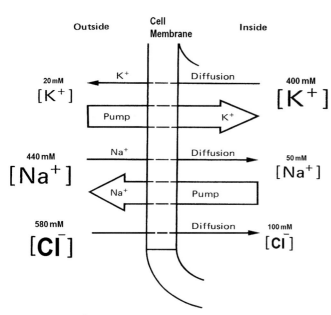

FIGURE 5-22 | Potassium (K$^+$), sodium (Na$^+$), and chloride (Cl$^-$) concentrations at the resting state. The concentration of sodium and chloride is much higher outside the cell than inside, and the concentration of potassium is much higher inside the cell than outside, which maintains a polarized resting membrane potential. The differences of K$^+$ from inside to outside and those of Na$^+$ from outside to inside are counterbalanced by the sodium–potassium pump. (Modified from Stratton DB. *Neurophysiology.* New York: McGraw-Hill, 1981, with permission.)

Some synapses have a property of specifically inducing *hyperpolarization* when excited. This is called IPSP. Instead of an excitatory transmitter such as acetylcholine, inhibitory synapses release an inhibitory transmitter, for example, *gamma-aminobutyric acid (GABA)*, which increases the permeabilities of K$^+$ and Cl$^-$ pushing K$^+$ out and pulling Cl$^-$ inside the cell. The IPSP is reflected by a hyperpolarized membrane potential with greater negative polarity (−90 mV) than the resting membrane potential (Fig. 5-24).

Relationship between Cellular Activity and Cortical Waves

Nerve cell membranes exhibit several types of activity: propagating dendritic potential, somatic and dendritic PSPs, and action potentials from the axon, axon hillock, and soma. The question is then "Which activity contributes to the oscillation of cortical waves?" It is unlikely that the activity from axons or fine dendrites contributes to the surface cortical waves since the narrow diameter of the structure imposes considerable internal resistance to the flow of ionic current. In contrast, the action potential developed in the soma is relatively large. However, the duration of the action potential is too brief (<1 to 2 ms) to be compatible with the much longer duration of a cortical wave (50 to 200 ms). Also, elimination of an action potential by deep anesthesia does not abolish cortical rhythms.[1] It is thus unlikely that the soma action potential is a primary contributor to the cortical rhythm.

Unlike the all or none characteristic of the action potential, PSPs have a graded property as described in the previous section. Since many synapses converge on the dendrite and soma of a single neuron, PSP from many synapses can be summated simultaneously. This integrated process is called

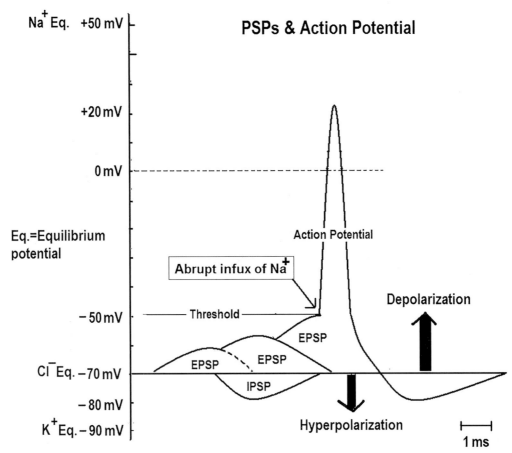

FIGURE 5-23 | The characteristics of EPSP, IPSP, and action potential in relation to the resting membrane potential. When the EPSP reaches a certain level (threshold) by membrane depolarization, sudden and massive influx of sodium ions triggers the action potential. After the action potential, the membrane potential becomes more negative than the resting state, which is called hyperpolarization. The EPSP and IPSP have "graded" functions, while the action potential is characterized by "all or none" property.

"spatial summation." PSPs that do not occur simultaneously but overlap in time can also be additive or "temporal summation" (Fig. 5-23). In addition, overlapping EPSPs and IPSPs are capable of producing waves with varieties of duration, amplitude, and waveform, which is compatible with the cortical (EEG) rhythm. Indeed, simultaneous recordings of EEG (cortical activity) and the intracellular recording show a close correlation between cortical rhythm and PSPs (Fig. 5-25).[2]

Polarity of Surface Potential in Relation to Cortical Cellular Activity

There are six cortical layers (molecular layer I, external granular layer II, external pyramidal layer III, internal granular layer IV, internal pyramidal layer V, and multiform layer VI).

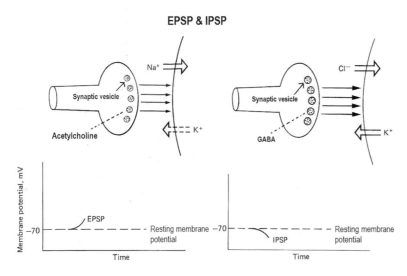

FIGURE 5-24 | EPSP and IPSP triggered by an excitatory neurotransmitter (e.g., acetylcholine) and an inhibitory neurotransmitter (e.g., GABA) causing depolarization and hyperpolarization, respectively, of the membrane potential. (Modified from Stratton DB. *Neurophysiology*. New York: McGraw-Hill, 1981, with permission.)

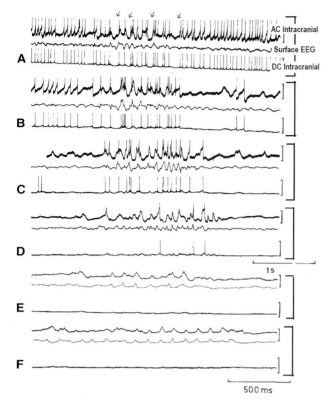

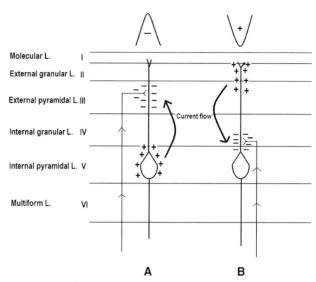

FIGURE 5-26 | Schematic model of cortical activity (polarity) in relation to cellular activity. Note the polarity of surface cortical activity is dependent upon the depth of the source and sink of the current flow. In **(A)**, thalamocortical inputs enter superficial layer of the cortex, while in **(B)**, it enters into deeper layer of the cortex.

The Controlling Mechanisms of Cortical Rhythm

There are two major subcortical structures that control and influence the cortical EEG activity. They are brainstem and thalamus.

BRAINSTEM CONTROL ON CORTICAL RHYTHM

Isolated cortical neurons from a cortical slab are capable of producing autonomous rhythmic activity at a frequency of 1 to 20 Hz.[4] However, abundant evidence indicates that the cortical rhythm is controlled by other brain structures. A classical and pioneering experiment by Bremer[5] showed that a waking pattern prevailed in the nonanesthetized cat following bulbospinal transection (*encéphale isolé prep*aration) but that the cortex fell into a type of sleep pattern after mesencephalic midcollicular transection (*cerveau isolé preparation*). These preparations led him to believe that sleep is the result of deafferentation of sensory input to the cerebral cortex. Later, Lindsley et al.[6] showed more specific brainstem areas, which altered cortical activity. Transection of successively more rostral levels of the brainstem resulted in progressive alteration in the EEG (Fig. 5-27). There was no significant EEG change observed after transection between the spinal cord and the medulla (Fig. 5-27A). After transection between the pons and the medulla, some increase in slow waves was noted (Fig. 5-27B). Further rostral transection at the pons and the midbrain junction resulted in a dramatic increase in slow waves (Fig. 5-27C). A more selective experimental lesion in the midbrain found a clearer relationship between brainstem structure and cortical rhythm (Fig. 5-28). A lesion of periaqueductal gray matter did not alter the EEG pattern (Fig. 5-28A). A mesencephalic lesion placed laterally showed only minimal changes with slightly more synchronized activity (Fig. 5-28B). By contrast, a mesencephalic lesion, which destroyed a large area of the tegmentum, abolished the

FIGURE 5-25 | Intracellular records (*first line,* AC amplification; *third line,* DC amplification) and surface EEG (*middle line*) during and after barbiturate anesthesia. **(A)** is the control, and **(B–F)** are progressively deepening anesthesia. The action potentials (shown by needle-like spikes) are progressively decreased with deepening anesthesia (from **B** to **F**). The action potentials can no longer be elicited at **(E)**. Close relationship between PSPs (EPSP and IPSP) and the cortical rhythm becomes progressively more evident with deepening anesthesia. (From Creutzfeldt OD, Watanabe S, Lux HD. Relations between EEG phenomena and potentials of single cortical cells. I: Evoked response after thalamic and epicortical stimulation. *Electroencephalogr Clin Neurophysiol* 1966;201:1–18, with permission.)

An EEG recording from either the scalp or cortex is viewed from the perspective of the extracellular space. The polarity of the extracellular recording depends on whether the potential generated is EPSP or IPSP or whether the electrode position is close to the current source or sink. The axons of the pyramidal cells are oriented perpendicular to the cortical surface. Since the main source of EEG activity arises from pyramidal cells from layer III or V, the current flows perpendicular to the cortical surface creating a vertically oriented dipole. In case of an EPSP, the site where the synapse terminates holds negative charge extracellularly and acts as a sink of current flow.[3] If a synapse terminates in a superficial layer of cortex (layer II or III), the current flows from a deeper layer to a superficial layer, causing negativity on the cortical surface (Fig. 5-26A). If a synapse terminates in a deeper layer (layer IV or V) of cortex at the soma, the current flows from a superficial to deeper layer, resulting in a positive deflection on the cortical surface (Fig. 5-26B). This relationship is reversed when the IPSP is generated. The above is an extremely simplified model. In reality, EEG reflects a complex summation and integration of IPSP and EPSP arising from thousands of neighboring cortical neurons.

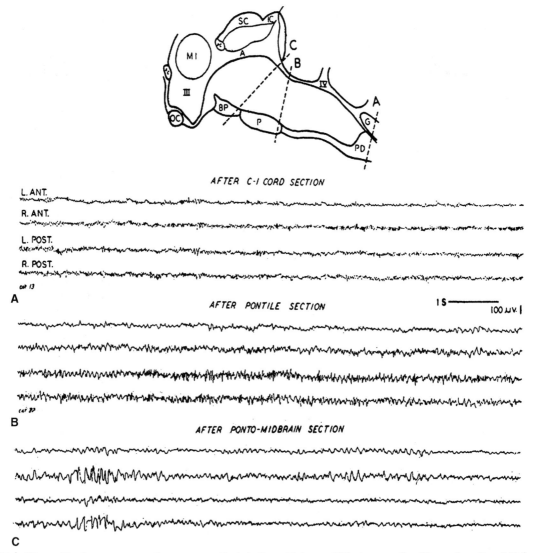

FIGURE 5-27 | Effect of brainstem transection upon cortical rhythm. Note no EEG change after C1 cord section **(A)** but increase of alpha-like synchrony after pontobulbar transection **(B)** and further increase of slow waves after pontomidbrain transection **(C)**. (From Lindsley DB, Bowden JW, Magoun HW. Effect upon the EEG of acute injury to the brain stem activating system. *Electroencephalogr Clin Neurophysiol* 1949;1:475–486, with permission.)

electrocortical pattern of activation (desynchronized pattern) and was replaced by recurring bursts of spindles and slow waves (synchronized pattern) (Fig. 5-28C and D). The lesions producing these changes (synchronous EEG resembling sleep pattern) were distributed in the tegmentum of the midbrain and subthalamus and hypothalamus of the diencephalon. This corresponded to the area of the "*ascending reticular activating system* (RAS)." These changes can be attributed to the specific destruction of the brainstem RAS, and in this view, this system at the midbrain and diencephalic levels contribute an indispensable control for the preservation of EEG activation and wakefulness. Conversely, a stimulation experiment of the brainstem RAS performed by Moruzzi and Magoun[7] further supported the same concept. The reticular stimulation resulted in cessation of the synchronized slow discharges produced by anesthesia and changed to a low-voltage desynchronized pattern, similar to the waking EEG (Fig. 5-29A–C). The activation effect was limited to the hemisphere ipsilateral to the side of stimulation when the stimulus frequency was reduced (Fig. 5-29D).

Simply put, the ascending RAS is responsible for the awake state recorded in the EEG.

SYNCHRONIZING MECHANISM IN LOWER BRAINSTEM

Thus far, the evidence suggested that EEG synchronization, such as the sleep state, is a passive phenomenon or a release from the RAS. Contrary to this assumption, Batini et al.[8] showed that a midpontine pretegmental transection of the brainstem altered the cat's electrocortical activity to a nearly permanent state of desynchronization, that is, awake state. This suggested that a high degree of EEG activation by a midpontine transection in the cat is due to withdrawal of some synchronizing or sleep-inducing mechanism from the caudal parts of the brainstem. To further support experiments by Batini et al.[8], Cordeau and Mancia[9] carried out an experiment of midpontine pretegmental hemisection. After the midpontine hemisection, synchronized activity was confined to the contralateral side of the section, and

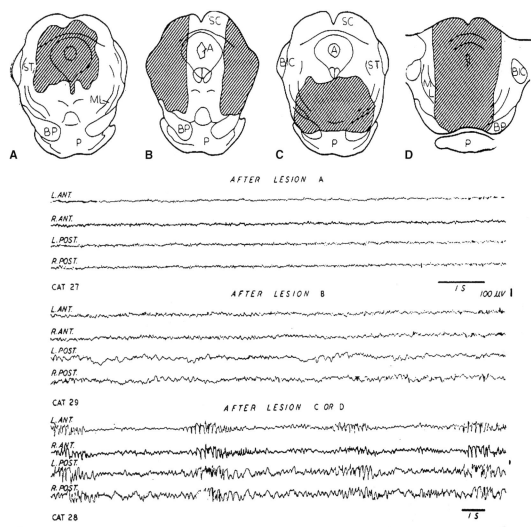

FIGURE 5-28 | Transverse sections through the midbrain with lesions at periaqueductal gray **(A)**, lateral sensory paths **(B)**, and tegmentum **(C and D)**. Note greater slowing and synchronization with spindle bursts after ventral tegmental lesions **(C and D)**. (From Lindsley DB, Bowden JW, Magoun HW. Effect upon the EEG of acute injury to the brain stem activating system. *Electroencephalogr Clin Neurophysiol* 1949;1:475–486, with permission.)

an awake pattern prevailed on the ipsilateral side (Fig. 5-30). This preparation produced an asymmetry in the electrocortical activity between the two hemispheres. The asymmetry is characterized by the greater tendency to synchronize in the contralateral hemisphere to hemisection, or expressed differently and perhaps more accurately, by the greater tendency of the ipsilateral cortex to remain permanently activated. In their second experiment, after a midpontine hemisection, a second hemisection was carried out at the level of the midbrain on the same side of the pontine hemisection. After the midpontine hemisection, desynchronized and synchronized patterns prevailed on the ipsilateral and contralateral sides of hemisection, respectively, as found in the first experiment. Arousal stimulation changed the synchronized pattern to desynchronized EEG on the contralateral hemisphere (Fig. 5-31A). Following the second intervention, a dramatic shift in the EEG asymmetry occurred. On the side of both the mesencephalic and pontine hemisections, the cerebral hemisphere was now deeply and permanently synchronized (Fig. 5-31B). Arousal stimuli, while producing *desynchronization* on the contralateral side to the hemisection, were no longer effective in activating the ipsilateral hemisphere to the hemisection.

The results of the first experiment (midpontine hemisection alone) can be attributed to the view that the unilateral synchronization in the contralateral hemisphere to the hemisection occurred through the intact afferent flow from the synchronizing mechanism of the lower brainstem, whereas the synchronizing mechanism was interrupted on the side of hemisection (Fig. 5-32A), resulting in permanent desynchronized (awake) state. Ipsilateral synchronization in the second experiment is due to the permanent interruption of afferent flow from the desynchronizing mechanism, that is, RAS (Fig. 5-32B), resulting in coma/sleep state. The results indicated the existence of a synchronizing mechanism originating from the caudal part of the brainstem. This, in turn, supports that sleep is not a passive state secondary to inactivity of the awake state but rather is an active state regulated by a sleep-promoting mechanism originating from the lower brainstem.

In summary, the sleep state recorded in EEG is not merely deactivating state or passive state of wakefulness. Instead, it is an actively promoted state originating from the lower brainstem. Therefore, awake and sleep patterns are actively controlled by respective brainstem structures.

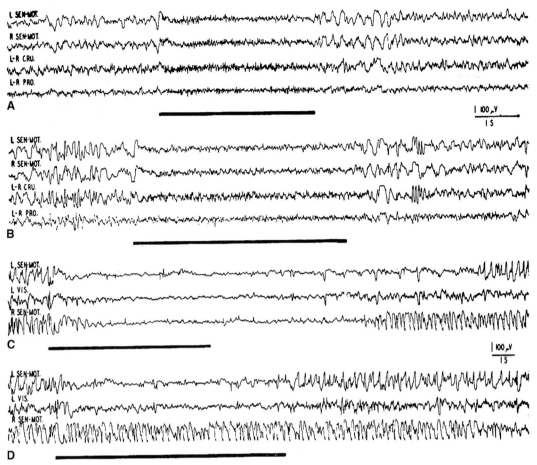

FIGURE 5-29 | Effect of stimulating the brainstem reticular formation upon electrocortical activity in chloralose-anesthetized cats. **A** and **B** were "encephalo-isolé" preparations, and **C** and **D** were intact cat. Note replacement of high-voltage slow waves by low-voltage fast activity (desynchronized pattern) with left bulboreticular stimulation (1.5 V, 300 Hz) in **A** and **B** and greater and more prolonged change on the ipsilateral cortex by greater amplitude of stimulation (3 V, 300 Hz) with left bulboreticular stimulation **(C)**. When the frequency of the stimulus is reduced to 100 Hz, the effect is limited to the ipsilateral cortex **(D)**. (From Moruzzi G, Magoun HW. Brainstem reticular formation and activation of the EEG. *Electroencephalogr Clin Neurophysiol* 1949;1:455–473, with permission.)

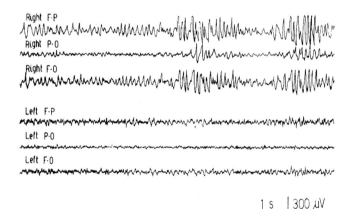

FIGURE 5-30 | EEG changes after left midpontine hemisection in a cat experiment. Note persistent low-voltage fast EEG activity (desynchronized or awake pattern) in the hemisphere ipsilateral (*left*) to the side of hemisection, contrasting with synchronized bursts of slow waves (sleep pattern) in the hemisphere contralateral (*right*) to the hemisection. (From Cordeau JP, Mancia M. Evidence for the existence of an electroencephalographic synchronization mechanism originating in the lower brain stem. *Electroencephalogr Clin Neurophysiol* 1959;11:551–564, with permission.)

THALAMIC CONTROL ON THE CORTICAL RHYTHM

The pioneering work by Morison and Dempsey[10] found that the *thalamus* has powerful influence over the cortical rhythm. They reported that rhythmic waves similar to the cortical rhythm were predominantly found among the midline thalamic nuclei and that the stimulation of these nuclei induced a widespread cortical activity similar to the spontaneous EEG waves. A single pulse stimulation in the midline thalamus, massa intermedia (nucleus centralis lateralis), induced rhythmic bursts (recruiting response) over wide cortical areas (Fig. 5-33). Repetitive stimulation at close frequency to the cortical rhythm produced EEG activity similar to the spontaneous rhythm, having waxing and waning characteristics (augmenting response) (Fig. 5-34). This effect was strikingly similar to the spindle waves occurring in a barbiturate-anesthetized animal. The experiment of Morison and Dempsey leads to the "*midline thalamic pacemaker theory*," implying the existence of a pacemaker in the midline thalamus controlling the cortical rhythm.

Jasper[11] further extended the original concept of Morison and Dempsey and introduced the diffuse projection system of the *thalamus*. The thalamus is the rostral end of the RAS of

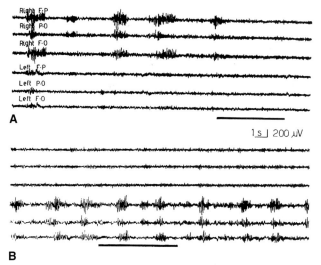

A

1 s ⌋ 200 μV

B

FIGURE 5-31 | EEG changes after left midpontine hemisection **(A)** and after second hemisection at the left midbrain level **(B)**. Similar to Figure 5-30, synchronized EEG pattern dominated in the contralateral hemisphere (*right*) but changed to the low-voltage desynchronized pattern by the auditory stimulation (*indicated by horizontal line*) shown in **(A)**. After the second midbrain hemisection, dominant desynchronized pattern in the hemisphere ipsilateral (*left*) to the hemisection changed to a synchronized slow-wave pattern. The external stimulation (indicated by *horizontal line*) was no longer effective in altering the synchronized pattern to a desynchronized EEG. (From Cordeau JP, Mancia M. Evidence for the existence of an electroencephalographic synchronization mechanism originating in the lower brain stem. *Electroencephalogr Clin Neurophysiol* 1959;11:551–564, with permission.)

the brainstem and functions as an important relay and integrative station receiving information from various sensory organs as well as from the basal ganglia and cerebellum and passing information to the cortex.

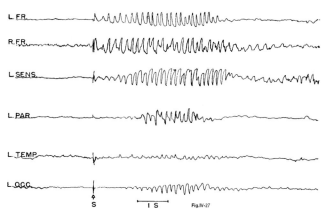

FIGURE 5-33 | Cortical response to a single pulse (1-ms duration, 3 V) in the massa intermedia (nucleus centralis lateralis) in unanesthetized cat. Note the diffuse rhythmic bursts at 7- to 8-Hz activity. (From Jasper HH. Diffuse projection systems: The integrative action of the thalamic reticular system. *Electroencephalogr Clin Neurophysiol* 1949;1:405–420, with permission.)

The thalamus has two types of projection systems. One is specific and the other is a nonspecific projection system. The *specific projection system* receives input from specific organs and reaches a specific area of the cortex. The specific projection system has two types of nuclei, relay and association nuclei. The relay nuclei are the VPL and VPM (ventroposteromedial), which receive sensory information from the extremities and from the face, respectively, and project to the primary sensory cortex at the postcentral gyrus (Fig. 5-4). Other relay nuclei are the *medial geniculate nucleus* for auditory and *lateral geniculate nucleus* for the visual system. The association nuclei receive afferent information from structures outside the thalamus, for example, the mamillothalamic tract from the mammillary bodies, the dentatorubrothalamic tract from the cerebellum, etc.

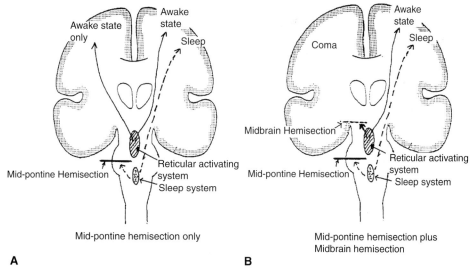

A   **B**

FIGURE 5-32 | Schematic illustration of experiments by Cordeau and Mancia[9] (**A:** first experiment, Fig. 5-30; second experiment, Fig. 5-31). Awake pattern (desynchronized EEG) prevailed in the hemisphere ipsilateral to the midpontine hemisection because of the intact awake structure of the RAS and deprived sleep-inducing structure situated below the hemisection **(A)**. Additional hemisection at the midbrain now deprived the awake-promoting mechanism (RAS), resulting in permanent coma with a synchronized EEG pattern **(B)**. In both experiments, the hemisphere contralateral to the hemisection was capable of producing both awake and asleep patterns.

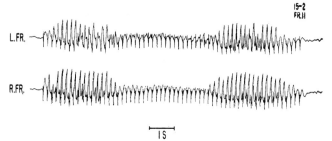

FIGURE 5-34 | Cortical responses from the left and right frontal regions in the cat under Nembutal anesthesia. Repetitive stimulation at 7 Hz (pulse duration 1 ms, 2.5 V) at nucleus centralis medialis brought out the same frequency activity over the cortex bilaterally with gradual augmentation and subsequent decline and augmentation again, that is, waxing and waning characteristics, similar to the spontaneous cortical alpha rhythm. (From Jasper HH. Diffuse projection systems: The integrative action of the thalamic reticular system. *Electroencephalogr Clin Neurophysiol* 1949;1:405–420, with permission.)

The *nonspecific projection system* consists of the midline (M) nuclei, intralaminar nuclei, ventralis anterior (VA) nuclei, and reticular (R) nuclei. In contrast to the specific projection system, the nonspecific projection system projects diffusely to the entire cortex. Jasper[11] and Hambery and Jasper[12] found that widespread rhythmic activity following midline thalamic stimulation discovered by Morison and Dempsy[10] required VA nuclei and reticular nuclei and proposed a modified midline pacemaker theory (Fig. 5-35). They regarded the intrathalamic system, consisting of midline nuclei, intralaminar nuclei, nucleus VA, and reticular nuclei, as the rostral end of the RAS discovered by Moruzzi and Magoun.[7]

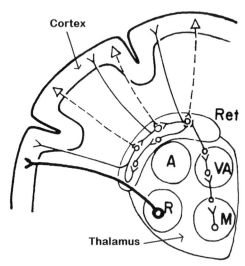

FIGURE 5-35 | Diagrammatic representation of the modified midline pacemaker theory proposed by Hambery and Jasper.[12] The rhythmic activity is imposed upon widespread cortical areas via a multineuronal system, including midline nuclei, VA nucleus, and the reticular (Ret) nucleus. The cortical projection from the relay (R) nuclei is separate from the diffuse rhythm-inducing system. (From Andersen P, Andersson SA. Development of ideas on the rhythmicity of the brain waves. In: Andersen P, Andersson SA, eds. *Physiological Basis of the Alpha Rhythm*. New York: Appleton-Century-Crofts, 1968, with permission.)

In summary, in addition to the brainstem, the thalamus possesses strong influencing and regulating functions upon the cortical rhythm.

The Relationship of EEG Activity Recorded from Cortex and Scalp

As discussed in earlier sections, EEG activity arises from ionic current generated by PSP caused by a change in the ionic permeability of dendrites and soma. In principle, the amplitude of the scalp EEG is dependent on four factors: (i) the attenuation factor (square of the distance between the generator source and recording electrodes), (ii) spatial spread, (iii) orientation of the generators, and (iv) frequency of activity.

1. *The attenuation factor.* The amplitude of an intracellular recording is much larger, in the range of millivolt as compared with amplitude of cortical rhythm, which is in the range of microvolt. Cortical activity is further attenuated at the scalp by intervening tissues, that is, CSF, dura, skull, and scalp. For example, the amplitude of alpha rhythm over the scalp is usually less than 100 µV, but this can be 300 µV or greater when EEG is recorded directly over the cortex.

2. *Spatial spread.* There are striking differences in the EEG activity recorded from intracerebral electrodes and from scalp electrodes. For example, it is not uncommon that intracerebral electrodes, placed for presurgical evaluation in patients with intractable epilepsy, register frequent spike discharges arising from closely spaced (<5 mm) multiple electrodes independently, but most of these localized spikes are not detected by the scalp electrodes (Fig. 5-36). This indicates that these activities have very limited and "close" electrical fields. Only widespread and synchronous cortical activity is detected from the scalp electrode. Generally speaking, it requires approximately 6 cm² cortical spread of a given activity to be recorded at the scalp electrode.[13]

3. *Orientation of the generators.* EEG primarily reflects activities of the pyramidal cell because perpendicularly oriented cell structures (axons run vertically toward cortex) yield a radially oriented dipole field, which is easily detected at the cortex or scalp. On the other hand, a tangentially (horizontally) oriented dipole that is parallel to the cortex is a relatively weak signal for cortical recording. This characteristic is contrasted with *magnetoencephalography* (MEG), which is weak in detecting radially oriented current flow but sensitive to the tangentially oriented current flow.

4. *Frequency of activity.* Scalp-recorded EEG loses much of the information generated at the cortical surface. The amplitude attenuation can be as high as 5,000:1 for the localized activity, but for the coherent widespread activity, it may be only 2:1. Also, the faster frequency activity is attenuated more than the slower frequency activity by intervening tissues between the cortex and the scalp. For this reason, the activity recorded at or nearby a burr hole (skull defect after brain surgery) shows increased amplitude of all frequencies but a greater degree of fast (beta) activity, often forming a mu-shaped wave (*breach rhythm*) (see Figs. 7-20 and 12-13).

If all EEG could be recorded directly from the cortex, more accurate interpretation, revealing more detailed cortical

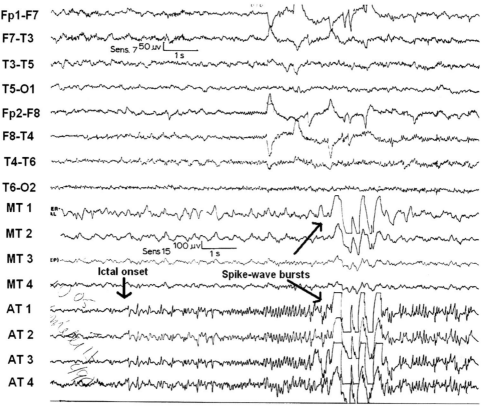

FIGURE 5-36 | Simultaneous recording from surface cortical electrodes (bottom eight channels from midtemporal MT and anterior–temporal AT regions and scalp electrodes. This is the onset of an ictal (seizure) event. Note the recurrent spikes and fast activity at the AT electrodes, and the large spike-wave burst did not appear on the scalp-recorded EEG.

functions, could be expected. But, without that ability, clinical EEG recordings are limited. It is the technologists' and EEGers' role to bring out as much information as possible by technical modification and adaptation of recording parameters from limited data of scalp-recorded EEG.

References

1. Li CH, McLennan H, Jasper H. Brain waves and unit discharge in cerebral cortex. *Science* 1952;116:656–657.
2. Creutzfeldt OD, Watanabe S, Lux HD. Relations between EEG phenomena and potentials of single cortical cells. I: Evoked response after thalamic and epicortical stimulation. *Electroencephalogr Clin Neurophysiol* 1966;201:1–18.
3. Spencer WA, Brookhart JM. Electrical patterns of augmenting and recruiting waves in depths of sensorimotor cortex of cat. *J Neurophysiol* 1961;24:26–49.
4. Burns BO. Some properties of the isolated cortex. *J Physiol (London)* 1950;111:50–68.
5. Bremer F. L'activite cerebrale au cours du sommeil et de la narcose: Contribution a l'etude du mecanisme du sommeil. *Bull Acad Roy Med Belg* 1937;2:68–86.
6. Lindsley DB, Bowden JW, Magoun HW. Effect upon the EEG of acute injury to the brain stem activating system. *Electroencephalogr Clin Neurophysiol* 1949;1:475–486.
7. Moruzzi G, Magoun HW. Brainstem reticular formation and activation of the EEG. *Electroencephalogr Clin Neurophysiol* 1949;1:455–473.
8. Batini C, Moruzzi G, Palestini M, et al. Persistent patterns of wakefulness in the pretrigeminal midpontine preparation. *Science* 1958;128:30–32.
9. Cordeau JP, Mancia M. Evidence for the existence of an electroencephalographic synchronization mechanism originating in the lower brain stem. *Electroencephalogr Clin Neurophysiol* 1959;11:551–564.
10. Morison RS, Dempsey EW. A study of thalamo-cortical relations. *Am J Physiol* 1942;135:281–292.
11. Jasper HH. Diffuse projection systems: The integrative action of the thalamic reticular system. *Electroencephalogr Clin Neurophysiol* 1949;1:405–420.
12. Hambery JC, Jasper H. Independence of diffuse thalamo-cortical projection system shown by specific nuclear destructions. *J Neurophysiol* 1953;16:252–271.
13. Cooper R, Winter AL, Crow HJ, et al. Comparison of subcortical, cortical and scalp activity using chronically indwelling electrodes. *Electroencephalogr Clin Neurophysiol* 1965;18:217–228.

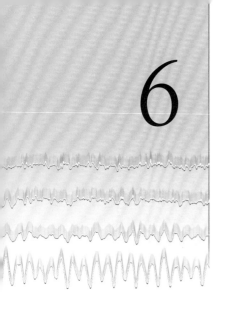

6

Principles of Visual Analysis of EEG

THORU YAMADA and ELIZABETH MENG

The most characteristic features that distinguish EEG from other neurodiagnostic studies are (i) the dynamic nature by which it expresses various physiological and pathological brain functions and (ii) the manner in which it instantaneously reflects the level of consciousness. EEG is dependent upon one's age and has considerable interindividual variabilities. For accurate assessment of an EEG and to determine its normality, it is essential to understand these complex variables. The following are the main features to be examined when recording and evaluating an EEG.

Amplitude

The amplitude may vary over a wide range, from a few microvolts to several hundred microvolts. Generally, *alpha rhythm* (8 to 13 Hz posterior dominant rhythm) in adults is usually less than 100 µV. Most of the alpha amplitude in adults falls within the 40 to 100 µV range and is higher (100 to 200 µV) in children. Abnormal activity could reach as high as 1,000 µV. An example of this is *hypsarrhythmia*, which is characterized by extremely high-amplitude slow waves, seen in children with *infantile spasms* or *West syndrome* (see "Infantile Spasms, Salaam Spasms, West Syndrome," Chapter 10; see also Figs. 10-25A and B, 10-26, and 10-27A and B). Generally speaking, faster frequency activity has lower amplitude, and slower frequency activity has higher amplitude.

It should be noted that the amplitude measured in a bipolar recording does not reflect the true (absolute) amplitude of activity from either electrode; one should always keep in mind that the EEG records the amplitude difference between the two electrodes. A more accurate amplitude measurement may be made by using a referential derivation, assuming that the reference electrode is relatively "inactive." The amplitude of the alpha rhythm from the occipital electrode is thus measured more accurately, for example, from O1 to A1 than from O1 to T5 or O1 to P3 (see Fig. 7-1A and B). With an ipsilateral ear reference recording, however, T3 and T4 amplitudes are erroneously low because of a cancelation effect due to the short interelectrode distances between T3 and T4 and their respective ipsilateral ear electrodes (see Fig. 7-1A). Conversely, frontocentral alpha activity will show lower amplitude on a bipolar than a referential recording (see Fig. 7-1A and B). This occurs because of the cancelation effect from electrodes having similar activities, such as between Fp1 and F3.

An amplitude asymmetry between homologous electrodes in a bipolar montage may be due to technical problems rather than a true amplitude asymmetry. These technical problems may include an erroneously short interelectrode distance (see Fig. 15-48A and B), a salt bridge (shorting of two electrodes by excessive electrode paste), or mistakenly recorded parameters, such as sensitivity or filter settings (see Figs. 15-32A and B and 15-33A and B). Depression of amplitude noted in a bipolar derivation, especially if only in one channel, must be confirmed by a referential recording (see "Technical Pitfalls and Errors," Chapter 15; see also Fig. 15-47A and B).

Frequency

The frequency of EEG activity is conventionally classified as follows:

delta waves < 4 Hz, theta waves 4 to 7.5 Hz, alpha waves 8 to 13 Hz, beta waves 14 to 30 Hz, and gamma waves 30 to 80 Hz.

The *alpha rhythm* is specifically designated as the posterior background rhythm and is attenuated by eye opening (see Fig. 7-1A and B). Most normal adults have an alpha rhythm faster than 9 Hz during the awake state. An alpha rhythm consistently at or less than 8 Hz during the awake state is abnormally slow at any age except in children less than 3 or 4 years old. The frequency may be measured or estimated by counting the number of waves occurring within 1 second, as long as waves with the same frequency appear repeatedly. If the appearance of waves is sporadic or a series of waves is irregular, the frequency must be determined by measuring the duration, which can be converted to the frequency (see Figs. 2-6 and 2-7).

Waveform (Morphology) and Rhythmicity

Many EEG patterns have characteristic waveforms. Alpha rhythm usually appears as a repetition of similar waveforms or rhythmically recurring waves, with waxing and waning amplitude changes, but not exactly sinusoidal. Alpha activity in the central electrodes usually has a different waveform than the posterior alpha rhythm. This has a pointed negative peak followed by a rounded positive phase forming a wicket-shaped

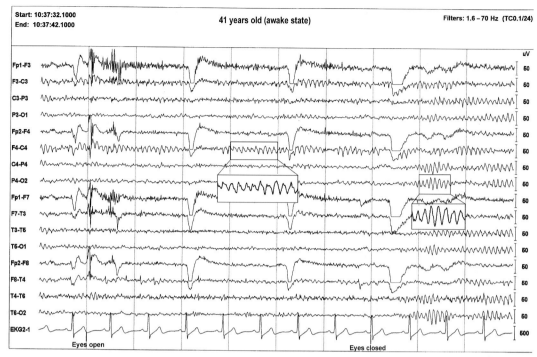

FIGURE 6-1 | An example of mu rhythm. Note the persistence of mu rhythm during the eye-opening period when the alpha rhythm is attenuated (a part of the mu rhythm is enlarged and shown in the *box*).

appearance often referred to as "*mu rhythm*" (synonyms: *wicket rhythm, comb rhythm, and rythme en arceau*) (Fig. 6-1; see also Figs. 7-18 and 7-19A and B). Sometimes, posterior alpha rhythm may also appear as mu-shaped form when associated with beta activity (Fig. 6-2). This occurs because mu waveform is a mixture of alpha and beta activities.

Slow waves, usually consisting of delta activity, are categorized into two forms. One is *serial rhythmic* (or *monomorphic*) or *intermittent rhythmic delta activity* (IRDA), which consists of a series of slow waves having similar wave form, amplitude, and frequency. An example of this is *FIRDA* (*frontal intermittent rhythmic delta activity*) or *frontally predominant RDA** often seen in patients with diffuse encephalopathy (Fig. 6-3; see also Fig. 8-14). Another example of IRDA is *OIRDA* (*occipital intermittent rhythmic delta activity*) or *occipitally predominant RDA**, which is commonly seen in children, especially in patients with absence seizure (see "Intermittent rhythmic delta activity," Chapter 8; see also Fig. 8-15; see also Video 10-6).

The other form of slow waves is serial irregular (or *polymorphic*), which consists of a series of slow waves having different amplitude, frequency, or waveform (Fig. 6-4). This pattern is often seen as a localized (focal) slow wave in patients with a focal brain lesion or pathology (see "Focal Delta Activity," Chapter 12).

Transients and Bursts

Transients and bursts are paroxysmal activities that appear and disappear suddenly and are clearly distinguishable from the ongoing and sustained EEG activities. A *transient* is a single wave consisting of a brief mono-, bi-, or triphasic waveform. A *burst* is a group of mixed waves that could be either a stereotyped sequence of waves (*monomorphic, monorhythmic, or serial rhythmic*) or a mixture of various waveforms (*polymorphic or serial irregular*). Examples of transients are *spike* or *sharp* discharges, which are defined as sharply contoured waves (distinguishable from the background activity) with waveform duration of less than 70 ms for spike (Fig. 6-5A) and 70 to 200 ms for sharp waves (Fig. 6-5B). The spike discharge has higher correlation with seizure diagnosis than the sharp discharge. Some sharp discharges show a waveform having a steep declining phase, which are considered to be "spike-equivalent" potentials, and have equal clinical significance as spike discharge (Fig. 6-5C).

An example of a monomorphic paroxysmal burst is represented by the *3-Hz spike-wave discharge* (*GSW** = *generalized spike-wave*), which is a diagnostic pattern for absence seizures and consists of a stereotyped rhythmic spike and wave complex lasting a few to several seconds (Fig. 6-6A; see also Figs. 10-15 and 10-16; see also Videos 9-2 and 10-6). Bursts may also consist of various irregularly mixed waves called polymorphic bursts (Fig. 6-6B; see also Figs. 10-17B and 10-18A; see also Videos 10-7 and 10-10).

Not all bursts or transients are abnormal. There are many physiological bursts or transients, especially in sleep. Whether these are normal or abnormal is dependent on when and where a given discharge appears, which is discussed in the next section. The abnormal paroxysmal activity of any waveform raises suspicion for an epileptogenic discharge, but the presence of a spike or a spike-wave discharge is more specifically correlated with seizure diagnosis than other types of paroxysmal discharges.

---

*According to the new (2012) ACNS Standardized Critical Care EEG Terminology, FIRDA is named as frontally predominant *RDA* (*Rhythmic Delta Activity*) and OIRDA is named *occipitally predominant RDA*[1] (see Table 13-1).

---

*In this and subsequent chapters, new nomenclatures recommended by ACNS (2013) are labeled with * mark (see Table 13-1).[1]

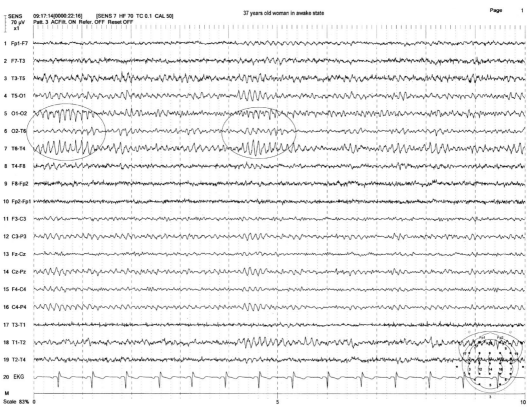

FIGURE 6-2 | An example of "mu"-shaped alpha rhythm (shown by *oval circles*). The mu-shaped wave forms are resulted from the amalgam of alpha and beta frequency activities.

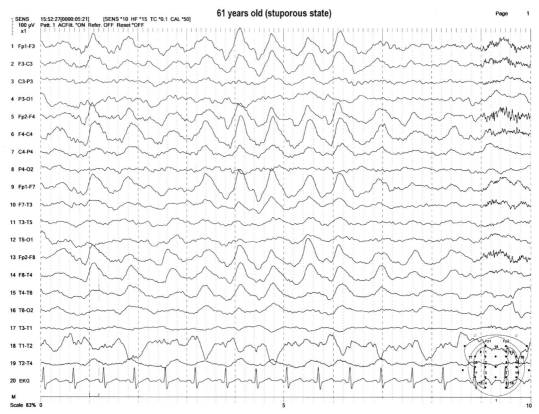

FIGURE 6-3 | An example of FIRDA secondary to metabolic encephalopathy. Note frontal dominant 1.5- to 2-Hz monomorphic (monorhythmic) delta activity.

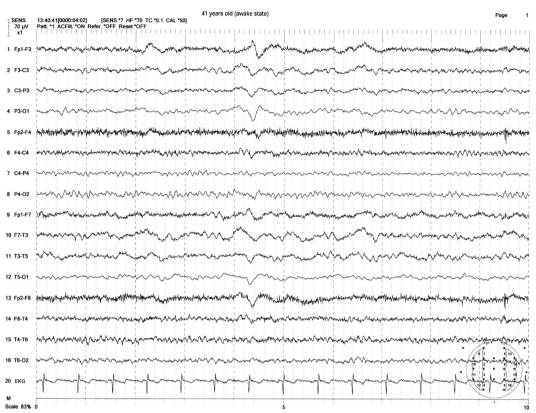

FIGURE 6-4 | An example of polymorphic (irregular) delta activity secondary to a left hemisphere stroke. Note 1- to 2-Hz delta slow waves in the left hemisphere, associated with slower and decreased background activity.

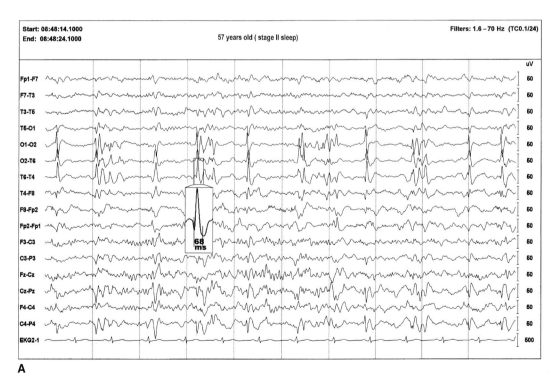

A

FIGURE 6-5 | Examples of focal spike **(A)** and sharp discharges **(B)**. Note the repetitive spikes **(A)** (duration <70 ms) and sharp discharges **(B)** (duration of 70 to 200 ms). (An example of a spike discharge and a sharp discharge is enlarged and shown in *boxes in* **A** *and* **B**, respectively.) **C:** An example of "spike-equivalent" potential. Although this discharge with duration of 155 ms is "sharp wave" by definition, steep descending phase of the wave form is considered to be equivalent to "spike" discharge (an example of "spike-equivalent" potential is enlarged and shown in *boxes* in **C**).

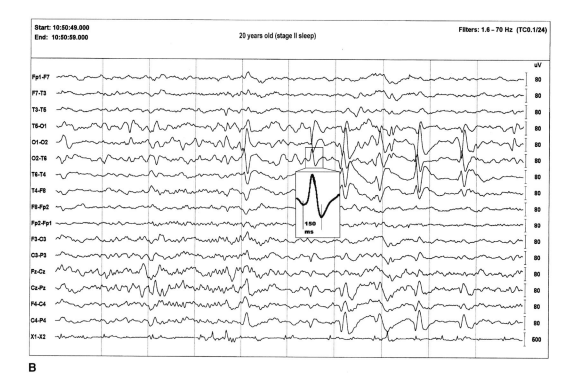

B

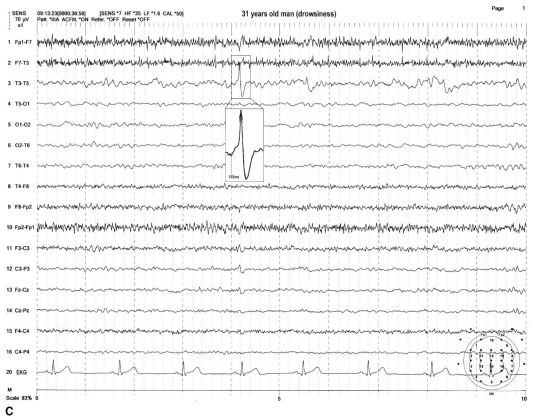

C

FIGURE 6-5 | (*Continued*)

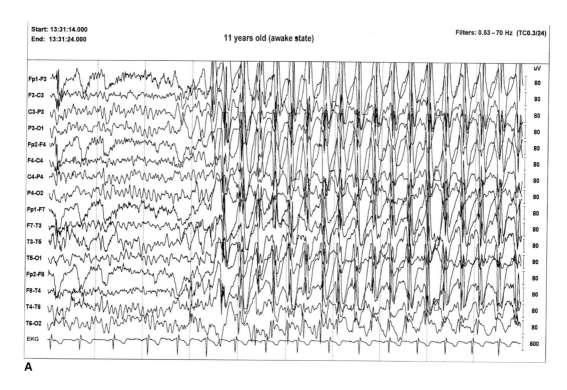

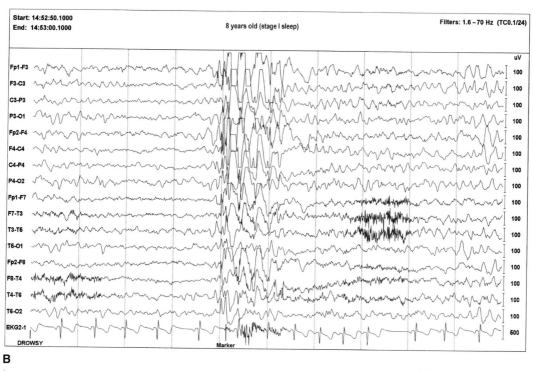

FIGURE 6-6 | An example of a rhythmic (monomorphic) paroxysmal discharge shown as 3-Hz spike–wave burst in an absence seizure **(A)**. An example of an irregular (polymorphic) paroxysmal discharge shown as irregular spike–wave bursts in a myoclonic seizure **(B)**.

Temporal and Spatial Factors

In addition to examining the amplitude, frequency, and wave-form of a given activity, it is important to assess the timing (temporal factor) and location (spatial factor) of the activity. The following is an example of a spatial factor: a vertex sharp wave is a sharply contoured transient spatially maximum at the

midline (vertex) with symmetrical spread to the parasagittal regions in normal sleep (Fig. 6-7A). But if similar discharges appear in only one hemisphere or consistently asymmetric, they would represent an abnormal pattern (Fig. 6-7B).

Temporal factors are also important in distinguishing normal from abnormal activity. For example, paroxysmal bursts are a physiological pattern in sleep or during an arousal period

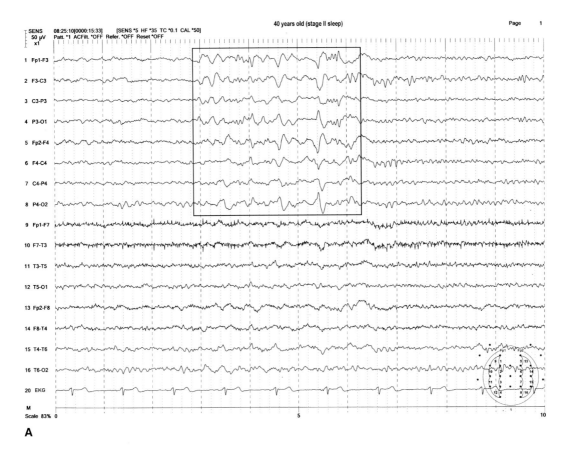

A

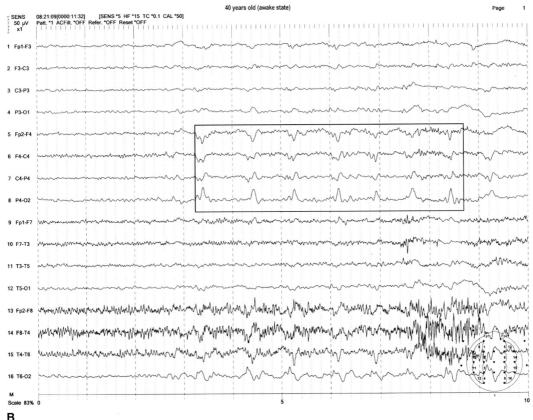

B

FIGURE 6-7 | Physiological V wave in stage II sleep **(A)** and focal epileptiform discharges **(B)** during awake state in a 40-year-old patient with history of epilepsy. Note the similarity of the sharp waveform but with a different distribution; bilaterally symmetric for the physiological V waves (shown in *box*) **(A)** and lateralized to the right hemisphere for the epileptiform discharges (shown in *box*) **(B)**.

(see Figs. 7-32B and 7-33A and B), but if a similar paroxysmal burst appears in the awake state, it would be abnormal (Fig. 6-8). These spatial or temporal factors in determining normal versus abnormal or artifact versus cerebral origin will be described in more detail in Chapters 10 through 13.

Symmetry and Synchrony

The basic principle of normal EEG activity is the symmetry between homologous electrode pairs during both awake and asleep states. The amplitude, frequency, waveform, and amount or incidence of activities should be symmetric overall between two homologous derivations. However, exact symmetry is not expected; for example, amplitude of the alpha rhythm is often higher in the right than in the left occipital region. Also, the timing of the alpha phase is not exactly the same, that is, not synchronous. If the alpha rhythm is symmetric and synchronous between the left and right occipital electrodes, an EEG recording between O1 and O2 would be "flat." In reality, the O1–O2 derivation often shows prominent alpha, even larger in amplitude than that from either O1 or O2 alone, indicating that the alpha rhythm from O1 and O2 is asymmetric and asynchronous (see Fig. 2-40; see also Fig. 7-13A and B).

If there is an amplitude asymmetry of the basic background activity, the side of the lower amplitude is usually abnormal (Fig. 6-9). However, the amplitude asymmetry of alpha rhythm less than 50% is still considered to be normal. If there is a frequency difference in the basic background activity, the side with slower frequency is abnormal (Fig. 6-10). If there is a difference in the amount, abundance, or incidence of basic background activity, the side with decreased background activity is usually abnormal (Fig. 6-11). When there is an asymmetry in slow waves, the side with slower frequency is more abnormal irrespective of the amplitude difference (Fig. 6-12). Focal slowing often becomes more distinct in awake (Fig. 6-13A) than in sleep (Fig. 6-13B). In fact, it is not uncommon that focal EEG reflecting focal pathology in awake state totally disappears in sleep. In some cases, however, a focal feature is not evident in the awake EEG (Fig. 6-14A) but becomes apparent in sleep expressed by depressed sleep spindles (Fig. 6-14B).

Occasionally, a seemingly bilaterally synchronous spike/wave discharge may indeed have an onset on one hemisphere, which is more readily visible when viewing at a faster sweep speed (60 mm/s or 5 s/page instead of the standard 30 mm/s or 10 s/page) (see Fig. 10-31A and B).

Many EEG patterns are asynchronous in premature babies (see Chapter 16). Sleep spindles are normally asynchronous until the age of 1 year (see Fig. 7-42). Persistent and totally asynchronous activities including sleep spindles have been noted in patients with *Aicardi's syndrome* (Fig. 6-15).[2] Clinically, the Aicardi's syndrome is characterized by *flexion spasms* (*infantile spasm*), chorioretinal abnormalities, and agenesis of corpus callosum, seen solely in girls. Another example of asynchronous sleep patterns (spindle, vertex sharp waves, and K complex) may be seen in patients with *obstructive hydrocephalus* (Fig. 6-16).[3]

Reactivity

The commonly known reactive EEG change is "*alpha blocking*" or "*alpha attenuation*" in which the alpha rhythm best developed during the eyes-closed, awake, and relaxed state decreases or disappears when the eyes are opened (see Fig. 7-1A and B). Asking the patient to open and close his/her eyes a few times at the beginning of the EEG recording is a routine procedure.

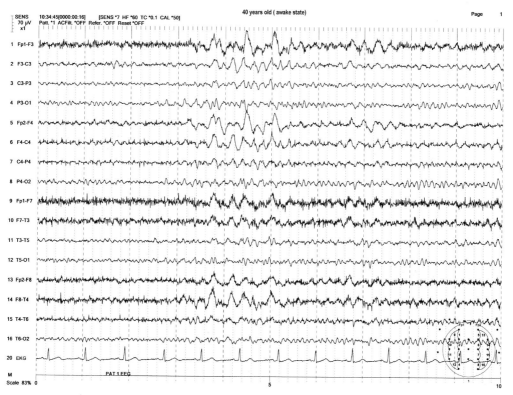

FIGURE 6-8 | An abnormal burst consisting of sharply contoured theta activity during awake state.

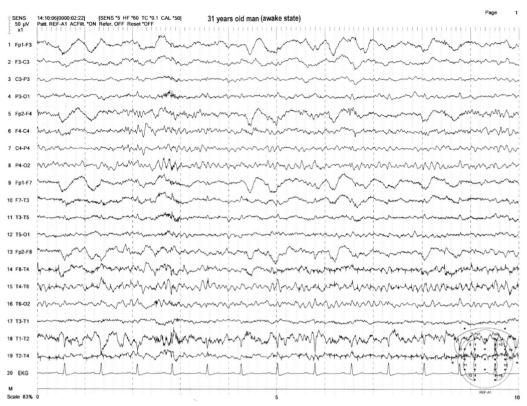

FIGURE 6-9 | Consistent depression of the alpha rhythm on the left (secondary to a subdural hematoma) in a 21-year-old man shown in a longitudinal bipolar montage.

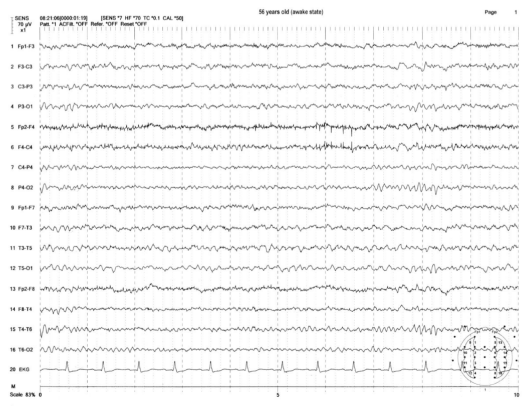

FIGURE 6-10 | An asymmetric background activity with slower frequency in the left hemisphere in a patient with remote history of a left hemisphere stroke. Note 8.5- to 9-Hz alpha rhythm on the right versus 6- to 7-Hz theta rhythm on the left.

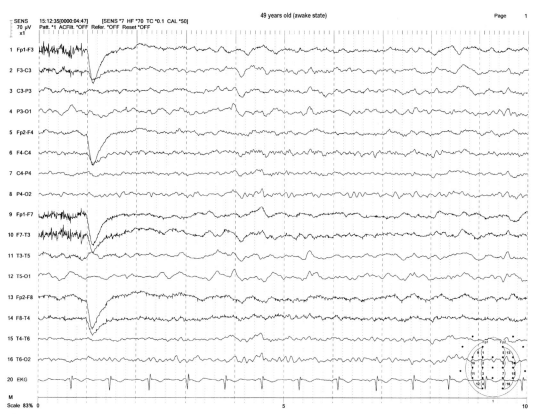

FIGURE 6-11 | Bilateral delta–theta slow waves but with left greater than right prominence in a patient with a recent stroke in the left hemisphere. Note the decreased alpha rhythm on the left indicating worse function in the left hemisphere.

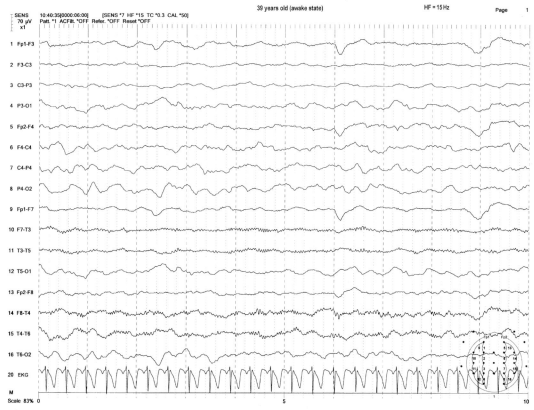

FIGURE 6-12 | Bilaterally diffuse delta–theta slow waves but with decreased theta in the left hemisphere in a patient with recent intra-cerebral hemorrhage. Note the slower frequency and decreased amplitude of delta on the left than on the right indicating worse function in the left hemisphere.

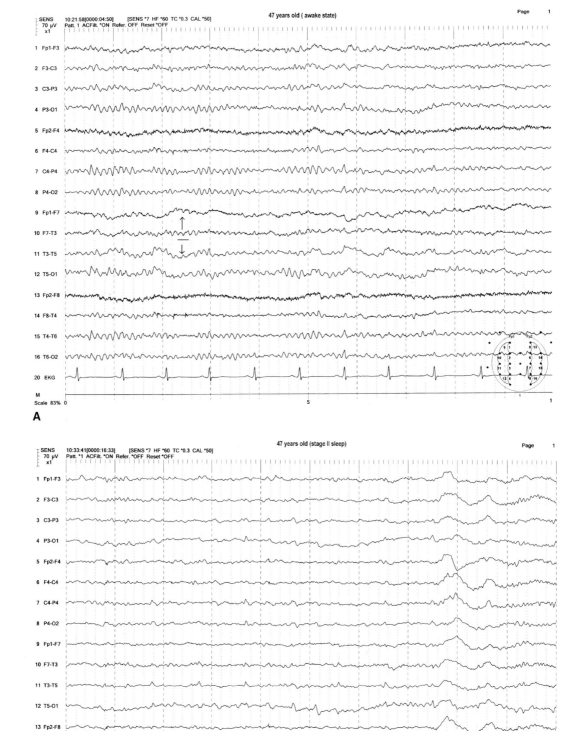

FIGURE 6-13 | Irregular delta slow waves in the left hemisphere, more prominent in the temporal than parasagittal region in a patient with stroke in the left hemisphere. Note that the delta activity is maximum in the F7 and T3 electrodes with phase reversal between Fp1–F7 and T3–T5 (indicated by *arrows*) with equipotential activity between F7 and T3 electrodes (indicated by the *line*) **(A)**. However, background alpha rhythm is well preserved bilaterally. The above distinct focal slow waves become unrecognizable in sleep **(B)**.

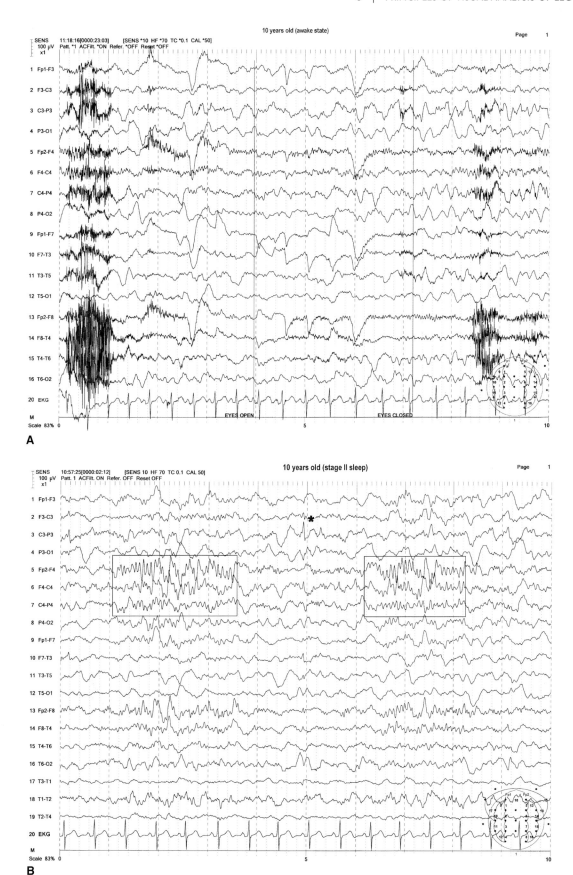

FIGURE 6-14 | EEG of a 10-year-old girl with a history of epilepsy, showing slow background activity consisting of irregularly mixed theta–delta activity but without focal finding in the awake state **(A)**. In sleep, the focal feature becomes evident by consistent depression of sleep spindles on the left (the spindles in the right hemisphere are indicated in the *box*) indicating focal pathology **(B)** (in addition to bilateral cerebral dysfunction). Note the isolated spike discharges from the left hemisphere, maximum in the frontocentral region (indicated by the *asterisk*).

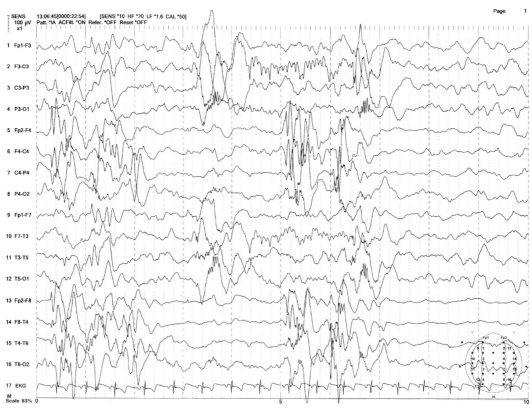

FIGURE 6-15 | EEG of Aicardi's syndrome in a 15-month-old girl with infantile spasms and hypsarrhythmic EEG. Note gross asynchrony of EEG patterns between the two hemispheres.

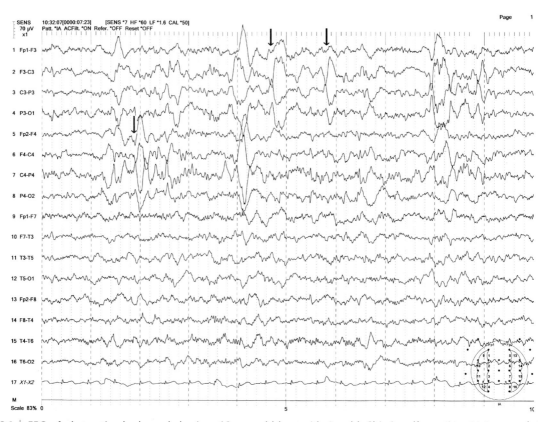

FIGURE 6-16 | EEG of obstructive hydrocephalus in a 13-year-old boy with Arnold–Chiari malformation. Note asynchronous vertex sharp waves of sleep (examples are shown by *arrows*).

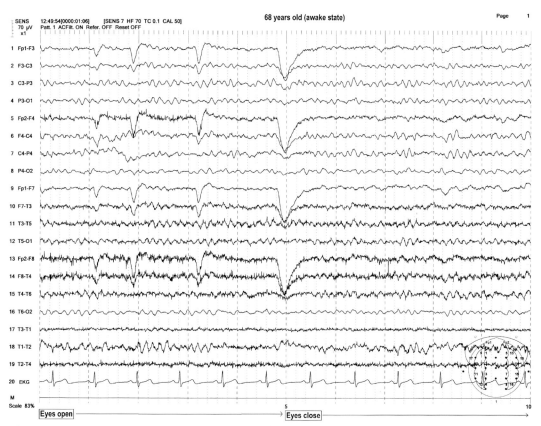

FIGURE 6-17 | Nonreactive background rhythm to eye opening in a 68-year-old patient with dementia. Note the unchanged background activity, which is slightly slow at 6.5 to 7 Hz, when the eyes are opened and closed. The alpha rhythm may be slightly decreased on the right.

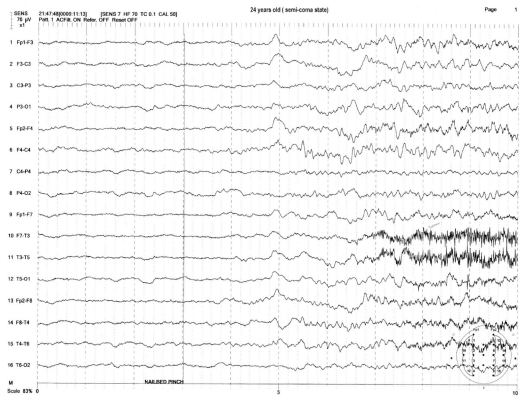

FIGURE 6-18 | Arousal response in a semicomatose patient. Note changes in the EEG pattern from diffuse low-voltage delta activity with minimal theta components to higher amplitude and faster frequency activities along with increased muscle artifact after external (noxious) stimulation.

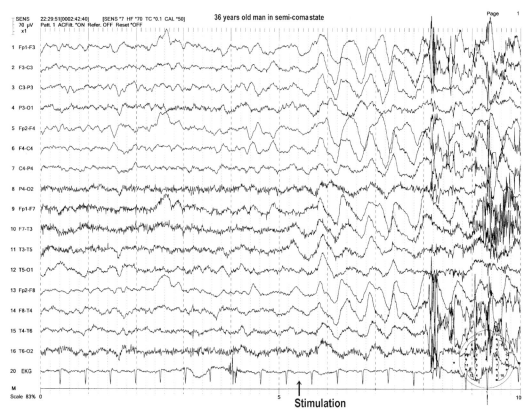

FIGURE 6-19 | Paradoxical arousal response in a patient in a stuporous state secondary to anoxic cerebral injury. Note reactive EEG change with the greater and more prominent delta slow waves after noxious stimulation as compared to the prestimulus state.

In the rare case when alpha blocking occurs in only one hemisphere, the abnormal side is the one in which the alpha does not attenuate. This is referred to as the "*Bancaud's phenomenon.*"[4] The slow waking background activity often seen in patients with dementia may not show reactive changes when the eyes are open (Fig. 6-17).

If the patient is sleepy or stuporous, it is important to record at least part of the EEG during a time when the patient is at the highest level of consciousness. To test this, the EEG technologist should ask the patient several simple questions such as the date, names of the presidents or states, counting backwards, etc., during the recording. When the patient is comatose or unresponsive, it is also important to obtain a part of the EEG during a period when the patient is alerted with external or noxious stimuli such as calling the patient's name or pinching the toes or fingernail. This examines any reactive EEG changes to external stimulation. Generally, a reactive EEG suggests a better prognosis than a nonreactive EEG (Fig. 6-18).[5] If there is a reactive EEG change, it usually consists of faster frequency activity than that before stimulated. Occasionally, an unresponsive patient, when stimulated, will have the opposite reaction and the EEG pattern changes to an even slower frequency activity. This is called a "*paradoxical arousal response*" (Fig. 6-19).[6]

It is not uncommon that diffuse delta/theta slow EEG in obtunded or stuporous patients reveals rhythmic paroxysmal discharges consisting of spike–wave or triphasic waves resembling electrographic ictal (seizure)-like events by external stimulus or spontaneous self-arousal. This has been termed *SIRPIDs* (stimulus-induced rhythmic periodic or ictal discharges).[7] Whether this should be treated as ictal or seizure event has been in dispute and may be treated on a case by case scenario (see Chapter for more detail; also see Figs. 10-38A and B and 13-1A–C, Video 13-3A and B).

References

1. Hirsch LJ, Roche SM, Gaspard N, et al. American Clinical Neurophysiology Society's standardized critical care EEG terminology: 2012 version. *J Clin Neurophysiol* 2013;30:1–27.
2. Farriello RG, Chun RWM, Doro JM, et al. EEG recognition of Aicardi's syndrome. *Arch Neurol (Chicago)* 1977;34:563–566.
3. Fois A, Gibbs EL, Gibbs FA. Bilaterally independent sleep patterns in hydrocephalus. *Arch Neurol Psychiatry* 1957;79:264.
4. Bancaud J, Hecaen H, Lairy GC. Modifications de la reactivite EEG, troubles de fonctions symboliques et troubles confusionnels dans les lesions hemispheriques localisees. *Electroencephalogr Clin Neurophysiol* 1955;7:179–192.
5. Arfel G. Introduction to clinical and EEG studies in coma. In: Remond AE, ed. *Handbook of Electroencephalography and Clinical Neurophysiology.* Vol. 12. Amsterdam: Elsevier Science, 1975:5–23.
6. Evans BM, Bartelett JR. Prediction of outcome in severe head injury based on recognition of sleep related activity in polygraphic electroencephalogram. *J Neurol Neurosurg Psychiatry* 1995;59:17–25.
7. Hirsch LJ, Claassen J, Mayer SA, et al. Stimulus-induced rhythmic, periodic, or ictal discharges (SIRPIDs): A common EEG phenomenon in the critically ill. *Epilepsia* 2004;45:109–123.

7

Characteristics of Normal EEG

THORU YAMADA and ELIZABETH MENG

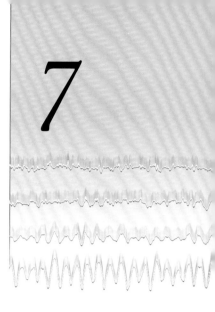

Normal Awake EEG

EEG shows considerable interindividual variability and also changes significantly depending on the level of consciousness. Further, there are progressive maturational changes from infancy, childhood, adolescence, young adulthood, and to the elderly. Despite a great deal of variability, there are general characteristics of EEG patterns according to age, level of consciousness, and state of brain function, which enable us to determine normality and abnormality.

ALPHA RHYTHM

Definition of Alpha Rhythm

The majority of normal adult subjects, during the awake state with the eyes closed, have a dominant rhythm of about 10 Hz. The *alpha rhythm*, defined as 8- to 13-Hz activity, occurs predominantly in the posterior half of the brain, especially in the occipital region. The International Federation of Societies of Electrophysiology and Clinical Neurophysiology[1] (IFSECN) defines alpha rhythm as follows: *Rhythm is at 8 to 13 Hz occurring during wakefulness over the posterior regions of the head, generally maximum amplitude over the occipital areas. Amplitude varies but is mostly below 50 μV in the adult. It is best seen with eyes closed during physical relaxation and relative mental inactivity and blocked or attenuated by attention, especially visual, and mental effort.*

The IFSECN emphasizes that the term "alpha rhythm" should be used specifically for those rhythms that fulfill the above criteria. Activity in the alpha frequency band (which differs from the alpha rhythm in respect to topography and/or reactivity) should be referred to as *rhythm of alpha frequency* or simply *alpha activity.*

Alpha rhythm is most prominent when the subject is awake but relaxed with eyes closed. As Hans Berger discovered, the alpha rhythm is diminished or abolished by eye opening, described as *alpha blocking* or *desynchronization* (Fig. 7-1A and B). Mental concentration or external stimulation also reduces the alpha rhythm. Opening the eyes in total darkness attenuates the alpha rhythm only transiently, and the rhythm soon reappears, although it is again reduced by conscious effort to see in the darkness.

Frequency of Alpha Rhythm

In the normal adult population, the mean frequency of the alpha rhythm is 10.2 Hz, and in less than 5%, it is faster than

11.5 Hz or slower than 8.5 Hz.[2] Under stable conditions, the frequency generally varies only about ±0.5 Hz in one recording. There are progressive maturational changes in the basic waking background activity from infancy, young childhood, adolescence, and to young adulthood. It is, therefore, important to know the evolution of EEG changes with age. Before the age of 3 months, the occipital rhythm is not well defined and may not react to eyes opening (Fig. 7-2). By 6 months of age, a measurable background activity appears (Fig. 7-3), and by 1 year of age, a more sustained 5- to 6-Hz theta rhythm can be recognized[3,4] (Fig. 7-4). The activity becomes close to 8 Hz (7.5- to 9.5-Hz range) by the age of 3 years[3,4] (Fig. 7-5). The frequency of the alpha rhythm progressively increases to 10 Hz until age 15 to 16 years and then plateaus[5] (Figs. 7-6 to 7-8). As age increases, there is a progressive reduction of the theta–delta slow waves (posterior slow of youth; see "Morphology, Amplitude, and Frequency Variation of Background Activity" in this chapter) intervening in the alpha rhythm.

Later in life, the frequency of the occipital alpha rhythm tends to decrease slightly, but the mean frequency is generally maintained at or above 9 Hz[6,7] (Figs. 7-9 and 7-10). An alpha rhythm occurring consistently at or slower than 8 Hz should be considered abnormal even in elderly individuals.[8,9] The frequency of the alpha rhythm has been shown to be closely related to cerebral blood flow. Significant slowing of the alpha rhythm frequency occurs with a decrease of cerebral blood flow, and a faster frequency occurs with an increase of blood flow.[10] A frequency faster than 11 Hz is more often found in women, and there may be a slight increase in the mean frequency during the luteinized phase prior to menstruation.[11]

For a reliable measurement of the basic waking background activity, it is important to record the EEG during the fully awake state, but relaxed with the eyes closed. Occasionally, the first few seconds after closing the eyes might produce an alpha rhythm that is slightly faster than in other resting and eyes-closed state ("*squeak effect*"). Alpha rhythm should be measured after this faster rhythm disappears. In the eyes-open state, especially in children, the EEG appears to be slower. In the young child age group, spontaneous eye closure is a sign of drowsiness; therefore, the background activity measured during this state may be slower than that during the fully awake state. It is necessary to record at least a portion (10 to 30 seconds) of the EEG during a passive eyes-closed state when the child is fully awake. This may require the eyes to be held closed by a technologist (Fig. 7-11).

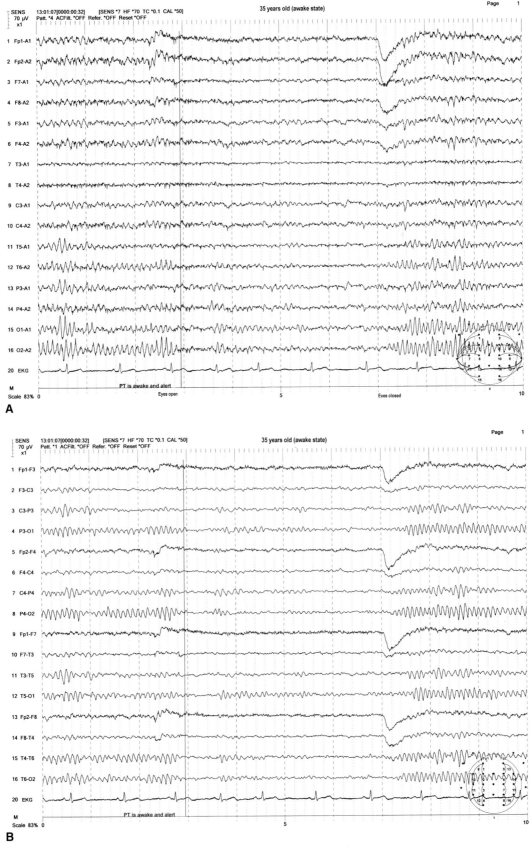

FIGURE 7-1 │ Typical normal alpha rhythm during the eyes-closed awake state in a 35-year-old man. Note attenuation of alpha rhythm by eyes opening. **(A)** is a referential montage and **(B)** is a longitudinal bipolar montage. (**A** and **B** are the same EEG samples.)

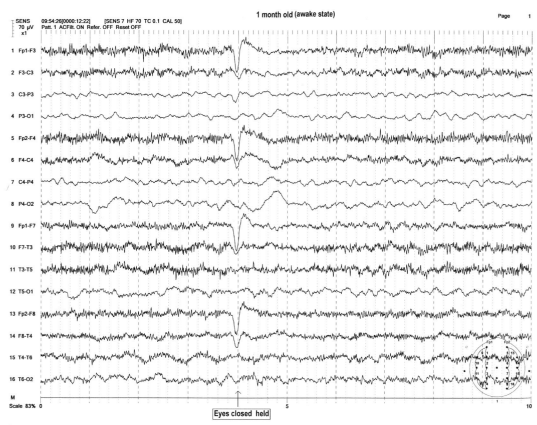

FIGURE 7-2 | EEG of a 1-month-old baby in the awake state. The basic background activity consists of a various mixture of 2- to 3-Hz delta and 4- to 5-Hz theta waves. There is little difference between eyes-open and eyes-closed states.

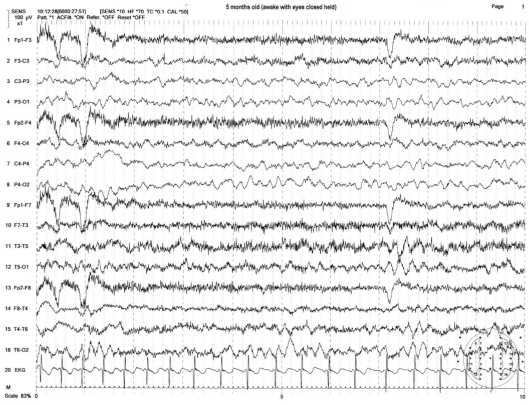

FIGURE 7-3 | EEG of a 5-month-old baby in the awake state. Note the more sustained theta rhythm (4 to 5 Hz) as the basic background activity, as compared to the EEG of a 1-month-old baby.

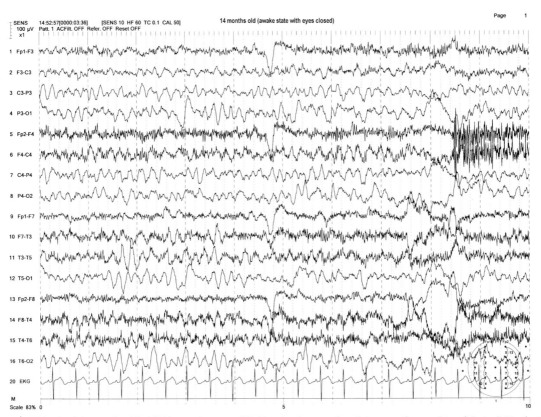

FIGURE 7-4 | EEG of a 14-month-old child in awake state. Waking background activity mostly consists of 5- to 7-Hz theta rhythm.

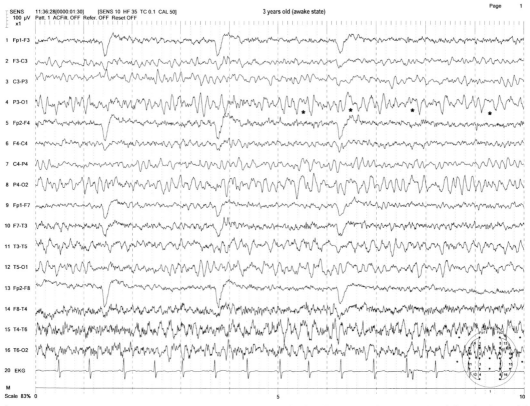

FIGURE 7-5 | EEG of a 3-year-old child in the awake state. Dominant rhythm becomes close to 8-Hz alpha rhythm with interspersed delta slow waves, that is, posterior slow waves of youth (a few examples are indicated by *asterisk marks*).

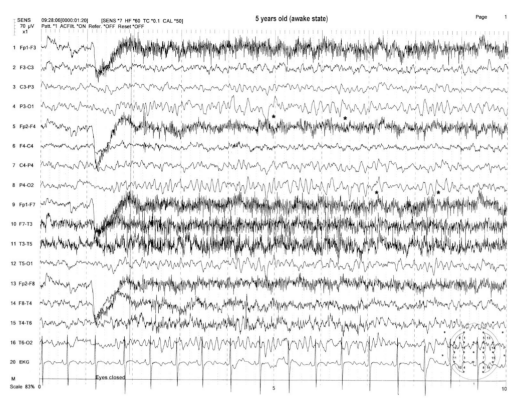

FIGURE 7-6 | EEG of a 5-year-old child in the awake state. Background activity consists of 9- to 10-Hz alpha rhythm with interspersed delta waves, that is, posterior slow waves of youth (a few examples are indicated by *asterisk mark*).

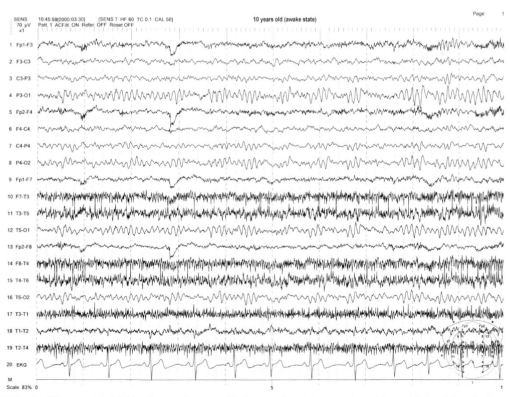

FIGURE 7-7 | EEG of a 10-year-old child in the awake state. Background activity consists of 9- to 10-Hz alpha rhythm with fewer posterior slow waves of youth.

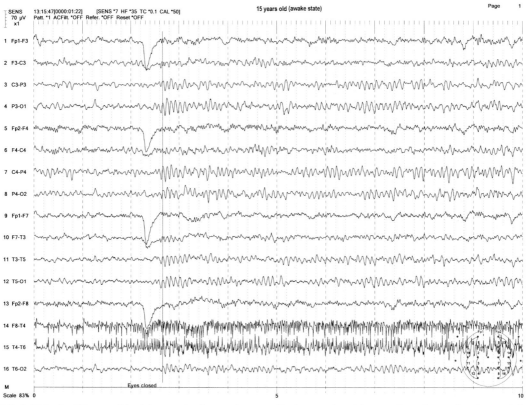

FIGURE 7-8 | EEG of a 15-year-old adolescent in the awake state. Background activity consists of a predominant alpha rhythm.

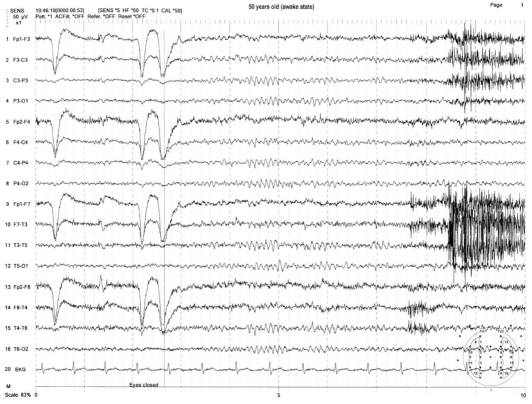

FIGURE 7-9 | EEG of a 50-year-old in the awake state. The amplitude is generally lower than the EEG of youth.

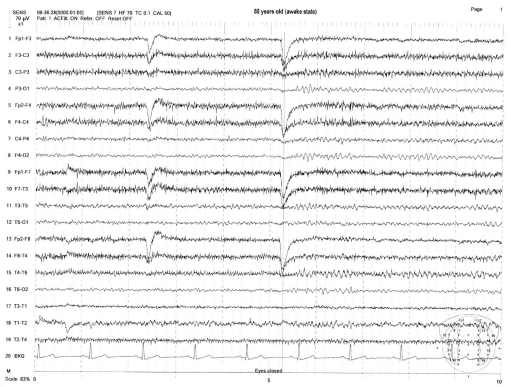

FIGURE 7-10 | EEG of an 80-year-old in the awake state. In general, there may be slight reduction of alpha rhythm frequency in an elderly individual, but the frequency should not be at or slower than 8 Hz.

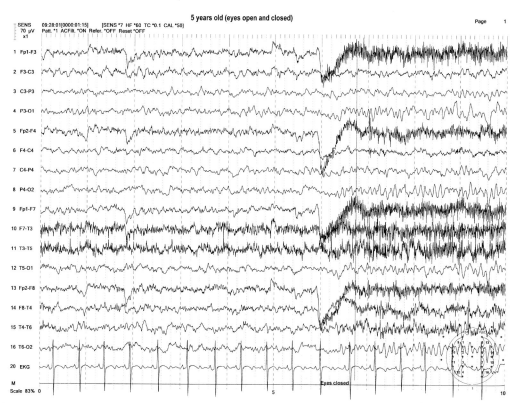

FIGURE 7-11 | EEG of a 5-year-old child during the eyes-open state. This is the same individual as that in Figure 7-6 (eyes-closed state). Note irregular theta–delta slow waves as background with eyes-open and well-modulated 9- to 10-Hz alpha rhythm after eyes closed.

Amplitude of Alpha Rhythm

The amplitude of the alpha rhythm in an adult measured by the referential (ear reference) montage is generally 40 to 50 µV. The amplitude measurement differs depending on the electrode derivation; a derivation of short interelectrode distance, such as T6–O2 or P4–O2, shows smaller amplitude than a long interelectrode derivation, such as O2–A2. Using the P4–O2 derivation, 75% of normal adults have alpha rhythm amplitude of 15 to 45 µV.[2] In about 10% of the normal population, the background activity is very low voltage without a measurable alpha rhythm.[12] In some recordings, the alpha rhythm is hardly recognized shortly after the recording starts, but may soon appear as the subject relaxes as the recording proceeds. In some individuals with low-voltage background activity without appreciable alpha rhythm, hyperventilation may bring out a better defined alpha rhythm. The alpha rhythm in children usually has a larger amplitude than in adults; the average amplitude of an alpha rhythm in the T5–O1 derivation is 50 to 60 µV (age 3 to 15 years), and about 10% of children (age 6 to 9 years) show greater than 100 µV.[4] Very low-voltage alpha rhythm, less than 30 µV, is extremely rare, especially in children less than 10 years old, and may be considered abnormal.

The amplitude of alpha rhythm generally diminishes with increasing age. This may be due to changes in the attenuation factors by intervening structures between the brain and scalp, such as density of the bone, increased electrical impedance or increased space due to brain atrophy, rather than a decrease in the electrical activity of the brain itself.

Symmetry of Alpha Rhythm

Amplitude asymmetry of the occipital alpha rhythm is seen in 60% of adults and in general, the right side shows higher amplitude and wider distribution than the left side (Fig. 7-12). The right being greater than left amplitude asymmetry is especially true in children; 95% of all children show the asymmetric amplitude, but the difference is generally less than 20%.[5] This asymmetry has been attributed to the difference in skull thickness,[13,14] rather than to handedness or speech dominance. Consistent amplitude asymmetry with depression greater than 50% either in an adult or a child is generally considered clinically significant, and this is especially true if the amplitude of the right-sided alpha rhythm is depressed. If, however, the amplitude asymmetry is the only finding, without slowing or other accompanied abnormality, interpretation for determining an abnormality should be rather conservative and cautious; it is always good practice to look for possible technical reasons such as electrode impedance, placement, interelectrode distance (see Fig. 15-48), burr hole (skull defect) effect causing *Breach rhythm* (see Fig. 7-20; see also Fig. 12-12), scalp edema, etc. (see "Technical Pitfalls and Errors," Chapter 15). It is the technologist's role to find, document, and correct possible technical reasons for the asymmetric amplitude.

In determining an abnormality, asymmetric frequency is more reliable than asymmetric amplitude. The difference in alpha frequency between the two sides is small, and a consistent difference of 0.5 Hz or more should be considered abnormal on the side of the slower frequency (see Fig. 6-10). The phase of alpha rhythm varies from ±2.5 ms to ±20 ms.[15] If the alpha rhythms at the O1 and O2 electrodes have the same amplitude and same morphology, and appear with exact synchrony, the O1–O2 derivation should show a "flat" tracing. In reality, the O1–O2 derivation usually shows abundant alpha rhythm with waxing and waning modulation. This indicates that the O1 and O2 alpha rhythms are neither exactly symmetric nor synchronous. Although a routine sweep speed (10 to 15 s/page) appears to show symmetric alpha activity (Fig. 7-13A), a fast sweep tracing reveals intermittently *asynchrony* of the alpha rhythm between the O1 and O2 electrodes (Fig. 7-13B). Also, the alpha activity is not synchronous between anterior and posterior head regions (Fig. 7-13B).

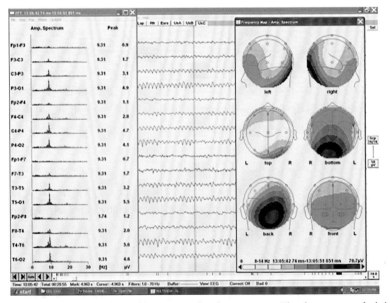

FIGURE 7-12 | Distribution of alpha activity expressed by an amplitude spectrum. The frequency of alpha activity (alpha rhythm) is 10 Hz **(left column)**. The topographic map shows maximum alpha amplitude at the occipital region and asymmetrical spread more to the right side (*darker area* indicates greater amplitude of alpha power shown in the **right column**).

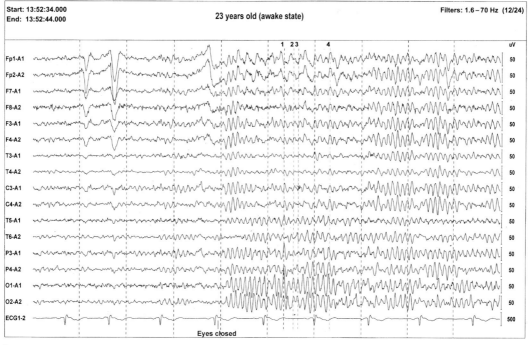

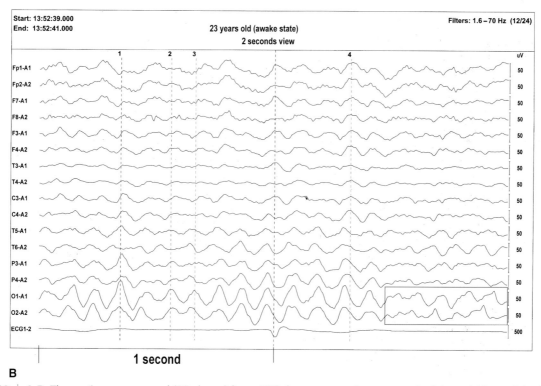

FIGURE 7-13 | **A,B:** The routine sweep speed (10 s/page) for an EEG shows more or less symmetric alpha activities and rhythm between homologous electrodes **(A)**. When a faster sweep speed (2 s/page) is used **(B)**, considerable asymmetry and asynchrony become evident between homologous electrodes (most asynchronous alpha rhythm is shown by *rectangular box*). Also, note the asynchrony of alpha activity from an anterior to poster plane (1, 2, 3, and 4 markers in **A** and **B** correspond to each other).

Distribution of Alpha Activity

The majority of adults and children have a posterior dominant alpha rhythm, but in some individuals, alpha activity is maximal in the central-parietal region. In about one third of adults, alpha activity is widely distributed.[12] In a referential recording, the alpha activity often appears more widely distributed than that in an anterior–posterior bipolar derivation (Fig. 7-14A and B). In fact, the alpha activity is often not visible in the Fp1–F3 or Fp1–F7 bipolar derivation.

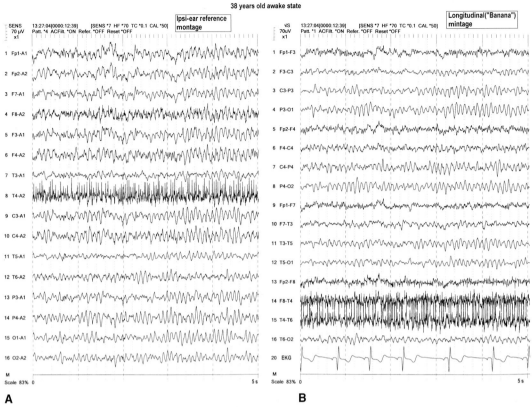

FIGURE 7-14 │ Comparison of alpha distribution between a referential **(A)** and anterior–posterior bipolar derivation **(B)**. **(A** and **B** are the same EEG sample.) Note the relatively widespread alpha activity shown in the referential recording **(A)** becomes posterior dominant with little alpha activity in anterior head region (Fp1–F3, Fp2–F4, Fp1–F7, and Fp2–F8) in longitudinal bipolar derivation **(B)**.

Morphology, Amplitude, and Frequency Variation of Background Activity

The alpha rhythm is rarely a simple sinusoidal waveform. However, the complex EEG waveform can be broken down into a small number of sine waves at different frequencies. A mixture of 9- and 10-Hz sine waves, for example, results in waxing and waning rhythmic waves that resemble a spontaneous alpha rhythm (Fig. 7-15), which in turn implies that the normal alpha rhythm is a composite of at least two different activities of close frequency. From the age of 3 years to the late teen years, the basic waking background activity consists of a mixture of alpha rhythm and theta–delta slow waves (see *posterior slow waves of youth* in "Delta Activity" in this chapter; see also Fig. 7-25). The posterior slow waves of youth progressively decrease toward the end of the teen years. In adults, the frequency of the occipital alpha rhythm is remarkably consistent and shows little variation throughout the day or for long periods of time.[11,15]

Alpha Variants

The alpha rhythm may abruptly assume a frequency, which is half of the ongoing alpha activity, that is, 5-Hz theta rhythm instead of 10-Hz activity (Fig. 7-16A and B). This theta rhythm, called the *alpha variant rhythm*, usually has a bifurcated configuration implying a subharmonic alpha rhythm. Alpha variants may appear sporadically, persistently, or asymmetrically. When persistent, it could mistakenly be regarded as an abnormally slow background activity (Fig. 7-16A). When asymmetric, it

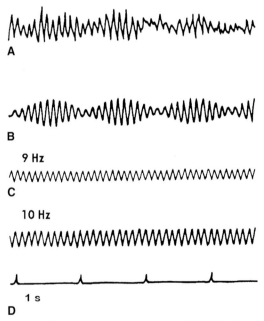

FIGURE 7-15 │ Model for decompression of the background alpha rhythm. Mixture of 9-Hz **(C)** and 10-Hz **(D)** sine waves results in waxing and waning sinusoidal morphology **(B)**, resembling the actual normal alpha rhythm **(A)**. (Modified from Kiloh LG, McComas AJ, Osselton JW, et al. Technology and methodology. In: *Clinical Electroencephalography*. 4th Ed. London: Butterworth & Co., 1981, with permission.)

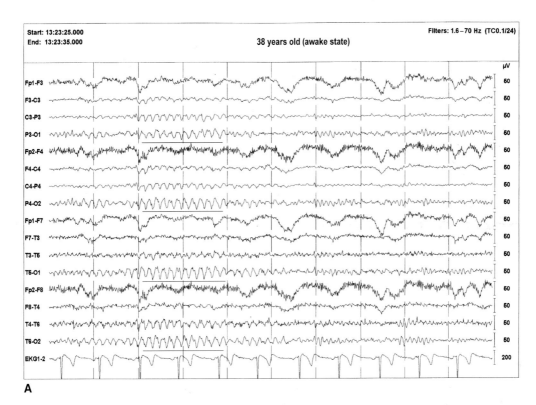

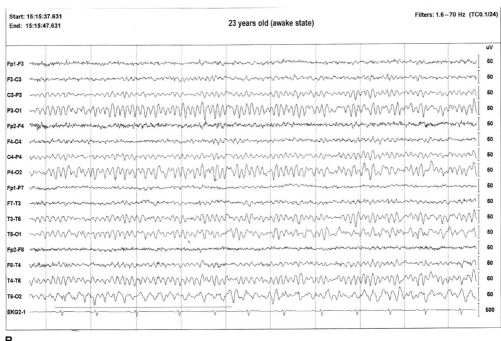

FIGURE 7-16 | Bilateral **(A)** and unilateral dominant *alpha variant rhythm* **(B)** *indicated by underlines*. Note the notched wave configuration in the alpha variant waveform indicating a subcomponent corresponding to the subharmonic alpha rhythm.

may appear as focal slowing (Fig. 7-16B). On some occasions, the frequency becomes "double," appearing as beta activity, which is referred to as *"fast" alpha variants*. The fast alpha variant rhythm can be induced by hypnotic or anxiolytic medications such as barbiturates or benzodiazepines (Fig. 7-17). The incidence of alpha variants is less than 1% of the normal adult population[16]; and there is no known clinical significance or correlate associated with the alpha variant rhythm.

MU RHYTHM

The *mu rhythm* is alpha activity (8 to 10 Hz) in the central region. Some may be slightly slower than alpha frequency. Due to its characteristic arch-shaped waveform, the mu rhythm has been named *"comb"* or *"wicket rhythm,"* or *"rhythme rolandique en arceau"* ("arch" rhythm in French) (Fig. 7-18; see also Fig. 6-1). Mu rhythm is more commonly seen in adoles-

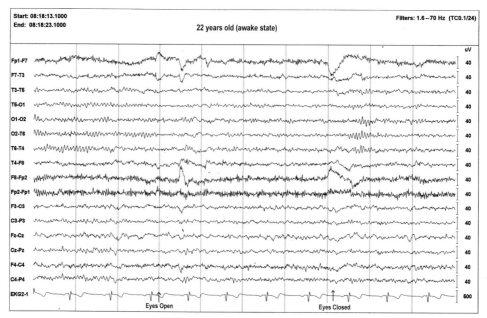

FIGURE 7-17 | Fast alpha variant consisting of beta activity, which is attenuated by eyes opening, acting like an ordinary alpha rhythm.

cents and young adults (17% to 19%) and less commonly in the elderly and in children less than 4 years old.[2,17] The incidence could be as high as 60% in some studies.[18–20] It is twice as common in girls as in boys.[4,5] Before the first description of mu rhythm by Gastaut et al.[20] in 1952, in which the mu rhythm was blocked by contralateral limb movement, Jasper and Penfield[21] found that the central beta rhythm recorded by electrocorticogram was attenuated by contralateral limb movement. In fact, the mu rhythm waveform consists of a mixture of alpha activity and the second harmonic beta rhythm. Indeed, beta rhythm always accompanies mu rhythm. The mu rhythm is also suppressed by intention of movement, sensory stimulation, and, to some extent, mental activity.[22–24]

In contrast to the more or less symmetric appearance of the occipital alpha rhythm, mu rhythm is often asynchronous and asymmetric (see Fig. 7-18). In some normal subjects, it may appear exclusively in only one side throughout the recording. Eye opening affects the occipital alpha rhythm independently from the mu rhythm so that alpha is blocked, but mu rhythm persists (see Fig. 7-18). Although the mu rhythm is primarily a waking pattern, in some individuals, mu may be seen in stage I or even stage II sleep without concomitant appearance of alpha rhythm (Fig. 7-19A and B).[25] This also supports the independent functions of mu and alpha rhythms. Mu rhythm accentuation is common in patients with a history of a craniotomy where there is a burr hole near the C3 or C4 electrode

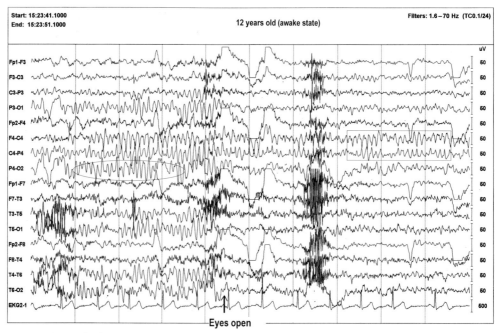

FIGURE 7-18 | Asymmetric mu rhythm. With eyes opening, alpha rhythm (shown by *oval circle*) disappears, while mu rhythm at right central electrodes persists (shown by *a rectangular box*).

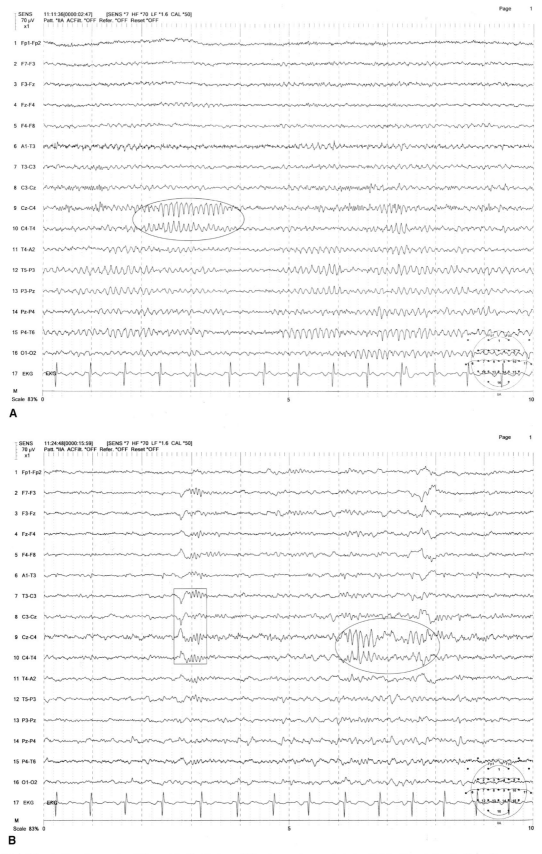

FIGURE 7-19 | Mu rhythm in awake **(A)** and in light sleep **(B)**, shown by *oval circles*. While the alpha rhythm disappears, mu rhythm still appears intermittently in light sleep **(B)** indicating dissociated function between alpha and mu rhythm. Sleep spindles and vertex sharp wave shown by *rectangular box* indicate stage 2 sleep. (**A** and **B** are from the same subject.)

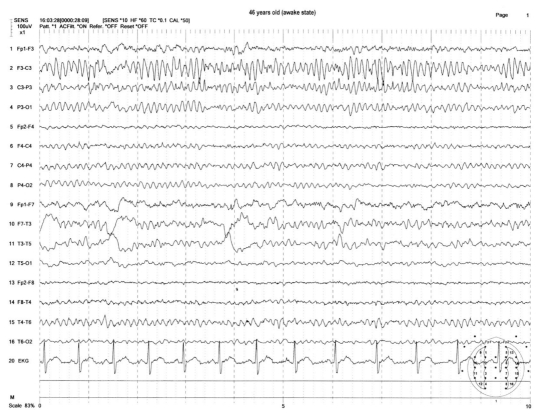

FIGURE 7-20 | Breach rhythm at C3 electrode secondary to the skull defect near C3 electrode from previous craniotomy. Note the large mu rhythm at C3 electrode. Also, irregular delta waves are present at T3 electrode.

(Fig. 7-20). This is due to enhancement of alpha and beta amplitudes with a greater degree of beta rhythm secondary to bone (skull) defect as *Breach rhythm* (see next chapter).

BETA RHYTHM/ACTIVITY

Activity with a frequency higher than 14 Hz but less than 30 Hz is defined as *beta activity*. Beta activity may appear diffusely or more prominently in the frontal regions. The amplitude is usually less than 20 μV. There is considerable interindividual variability and no particular age preference in the incidence of beta activity. Overall, however, beta activity is more common in infants and young children less than 1½ years old and then diminishes in both amplitude and incidence with increasing age.[26] Whenever beta activity is abundant, other EEG activities, namely, alpha or theta waves, assume a "spiky" appearance.

Beta activity is enhanced by sedative, hypnotic, or anxiolytic drugs (barbiturates, benzodiazepines) (Fig. 7-21A; see Fig. 8-2). It usually becomes more prominent and slower in frequency appearing waveform of sleep "spindle-like" activity in sleep (Fig. 7-21B; see also Figs. 8-3 and 8-4; see also "Anxiolytic or Hypnotic Drugs," Chapter 11). Beta enhancement by medication is not dose-dependent but depends more on the individual's sensitivity.

Beta activity is usually symmetrical in amplitude and frequency but could be asynchronous between the two hemispheres. Less than 50% of amplitude asymmetry may be present, possibly secondary to the difference in skull thickness. Greater than 50% amplitude difference suggests an abnormality on the side of decreased beta activity. Consistent depression of beta activity,

either focal or hemispheric, is a sensitive indicator of focal cortical dysfunction (see Fig. 8-5) and may be the first EEG sign of acute cortical injury. This is especially true if the patient is taking a sedative, hypnotic, or anxiolytic drug. Beta depression may be the first sign of an EEG change after cross-clamping the carotid artery during an endarterectomy surgery (see Video 11-1).

Beta activity is usually enhanced in the region of a burr hole or skull defect. This is because beta activity is normally more attenuated than the slower-frequency activities by intervening tissues (dura, CSF, skull, scalp) between the cortex and scalp. The absence of bone, therefore, enhances beta activity more than other slower-frequency activities. This produces a "mu-like" waveform activity referred to as a "breach rhythm"[27] (see Fig. 7-20). The breach rhythm is usually most prominent when a burr hole is near the central electrode. Conversely, beta activity is attenuated by a subgaleal, subdural, or epidural fluid collection. It is important for the technologist to note the presence of such conditions.

Extreme high voltage (>200 μV), generalized but anterior dominant fast activity appearing as continuous sleep spindles, has been referred to as *extreme spindles* and may be a sign of brain damage (see Fig. 8-7).[28]

GAMMA RHYTHM/ACTIVITY

Gamma rhythm is defined as the waves with a frequency faster than 30 Hz and less than 80 to 100 Hz and was largely ignored before the era of digital EEG. With digital EEG, we are now able to investigate much faster frequency activity (ultrafast activity as fast as 400 to 600 Hz), which was not visible in

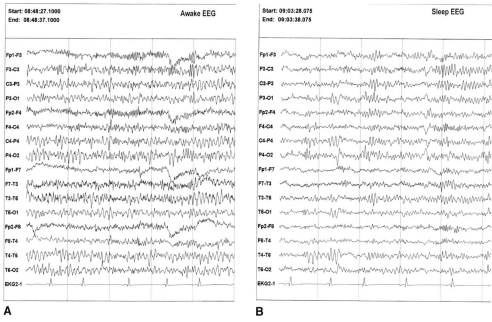

FIGURE 7-21 | Increased beta activity secondary to benzodiazepine in an awake state **(A)** and in sleep **(B)** in a 22-year-old woman. Note increased beta in bianterior head regions in the awake state **(A)**. In stage II sleep, a mixture of abundant sleep spindles and slow beta activity is noted **(B)**.

analog EEG due to the limitation of mechanical oscillation of pen movement. Investigations of gamma rhythm and ultrafast brain activity have brought newer insights to neurophysiological and clinical correlates of EEG activity which have never been explored. Gamma can be easily recorded from cortical as well as subcortical areas,[29,30] although gamma activity is much attenuated when recorded from the scalp. The gamma rhythm

has received a great deal of attention in recent years in relationship with various cognitive functions such as visual awareness,[31] memories,[32] attentiveness,[33] and meditation.[34] Gamma has also been studied in clinical conditions including schizophrenia,[35] Alzheimer's disease,[36] and epilepsy[37] (see Figs. 8-8 to 8-10). The gamma rhythm may be seen in normal sleep EEG (Fig. 7-22). Further investigation of gamma rhythm in relationship with

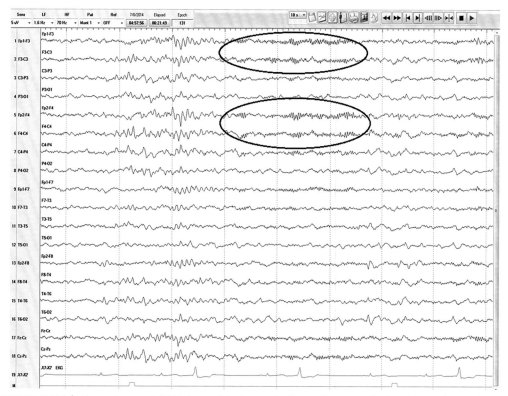

FIGURE 7-22 | Normal stage 2 (N2) sleep with sleep spindles and gamma rhythm (shown by *oval circle*).

neurophysiological and clinical correlates may lead to new discoveries of brain functions (see also "Abnormal gamma rhythm," Chapter 8).

THETA ACTIVITY

Theta activity is defined as frequency less than 8 Hz and faster than 4.0 Hz. The presence of a small amount of intermittently appearing theta activity mixed with alpha rhythm may be seen in a normal awake subject, especially in the younger age group. Six- to seven-Hz theta activity may be the dominant rhythm in the frontal and frontocentral regions in a young adult during the awake state (Fig. 7-23).

Unlike the posterior alpha rhythm, there is considerable individual variation in waveform, frequency, and amplitude of the frontal and frontocentral theta activity. Hence, there is no well-defined point at which frontal theta activity is considered to be abnormal. Increased theta activity in the frontocentral or occipital region replacing the alpha rhythm is a common sign of drowsiness in adults and children. It has been reported that heightened emotional states enhance rhythmic frontal theta activity (6 to 7 Hz) in young adults or in children.[38–42] However, rhythmic frontal theta activity can be recorded during a quiet and ordinary recording session in children. Thus, the differentiation between a heightened emotional state and a "normal" state is difficult, and this should not be considered an "abnormal" pattern. Another rhythmic theta pattern with 4 to 7 Hz monorhythmic waves has been described in children, mostly aged 2 to 6 years. This pattern was thought to be associated with primary as well as secondary epilepsy by some

authors.[43,44] Again, it is not possible to differentiate this pattern with certainty from a normal drowsy pattern or an age-related normal pattern.

Sinusoidal or mu-shaped theta (6 to 7 Hz) activity at the vertex region appearing in drowsiness has been described as the "*midline theta rhythm*" in children and adults (Fig. 7-24). The original description by Ciganek[45] found a high correlation with temporal lobe epilepsy, but later studies have found that the pattern can be seen in one fourth of the nonepileptic population.[46] Another type of midline theta rhythm, not at the central but at the frontal region, called the *Fm theta rhythm*, has been extensively investigated by Japanese researchers in relation to mental tasks, such as reading, mental calculation, etc.[47]

DELTA ACTIVITY

Delta activity is defined as frequency less than 4 Hz. Persistent delta activity without theta or alpha activity is abnormal if seen during wakefulness at any age. In sleep, delta activity increases progressively as the sleep stages (non-REM sleep) deepen. In children, however, delta activity is common especially in the posterior head region. These physiological slow waves usually occur singly and randomly with intermixed alpha rhythm (Fig. 7-25 and also see Figs. 7-5 to 7-8). Since the waveform resembles the "sail" of a sail boat, this has sometimes been referred to as a "*sail wave*."[48] They are more abundant in younger children. The "*posterior slow wave of youth*" becomes progressively less prevalent toward the age of 20 years but could be seen as late as 25 years of age. The posterior slow waves of youth are uncommon in children less

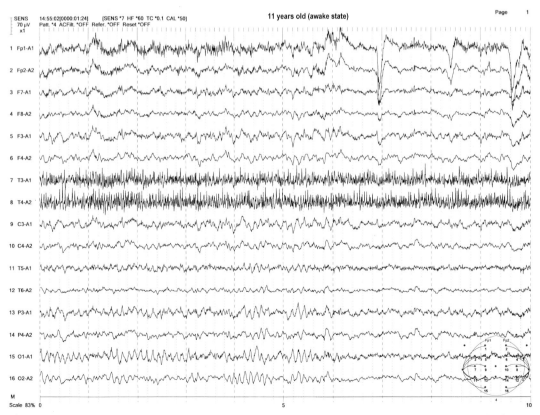

FIGURE 7-23 | EEG of an 11-year-old child in the awake state. Note the abundant theta and delta activities in the frontocentral region contrasting with the well-defined and abundant alpha rhythm posteriorly.

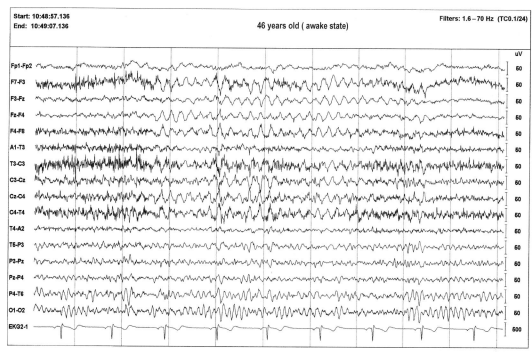

FIGURE 7-24 | Midline theta rhythm in a 46-year-old man. Note rhythmic 4.5- to 5-Hz theta rhythm maximum at Fz and Cz electrodes evidenced by phase reversal.

than 2 years old and become maximum between ages 9 and 14. They are not always symmetric or synchronous between the left and right occipital electrodes and tend to be greater in amplitude and incidence on the right side. They may be more prominent during the early portion of the recording and tend to diminish toward the end of recording. They are attenuated by eye opening and may be accentuated by hyperventi-

lation or possibly by stress. Earlier studies have suggested that posterior slow waves of youth are more commonly seen in children with behavioral problems.[38,49] Although later studies have suggested that these slow waves are more likely an age-related variation, the statistically based evidence appears to support a greater incidence of posterior slow activity in children with behavioral problems than the age-matched

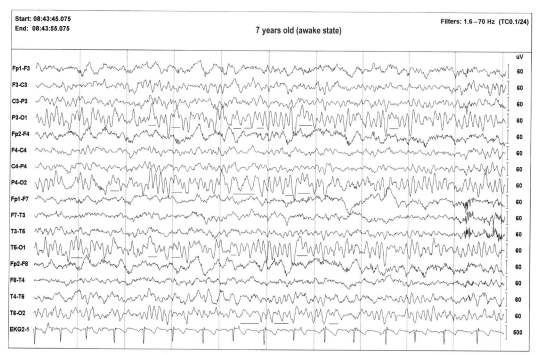

FIGURE 7-25 | Posterior slow waves of youth in 7-year-old child. Note the underlying delta with superimposed alpha rhythm and intermittent 3- to 4-Hz theta–delta waves (some examples are *underlined*) in the occipital regions.

controls.[50–55] However, due to the great variation in amplitude, waveform, and occurrence among normal children, it is difficult to distinguish between normal and abnormal posterior delta in an individual EEG. If occipital slow waves occur with the following appearance, they may be considered abnormal: (a) disproportionately high amplitude as compared to the alpha rhythm (>1.5 times the voltage of the alpha rhythm or >200 µV); (b) serial rhythmic waveform, which constitutes OIRDA (*occipital intermittent rhythmic delta activity or occipitally predominant RDA*[*]; see Fig. 8-15, also see Video 10-6); (c) widespread distribution involving the central or midtemporal electrodes; (d) predominantly unilateral; or (e) persistent after eye opening.

LAMBDA WAVES

Unlike other EEG waveforms, lambda waves originally described by Gastaut[56] are not spontaneously occurring waves, but instead are transient activity associated with eye movements while an individual's eyes are open. They are elicited by saccadic eye movements often seen, for example, while watching TV or reading.[57,58] The waveform consists of a bi- or triphasic configuration with a predominant positive potential at the occipital electrodes (Fig. 7-26A, Video 7-1A). The lambda waves are often asymmetric and tend to have greater amplitude in the right compared to the left occipital electrode. The waveform, distribution, and asymmetry of lambda waves are remarkably similar to POSTS (see "Positive Occipital Sharp Transients of Sleep" in this chapter) (Fig. 7-26B, Video 7-1A and B) and also to photic responses to a slow-frequency rate (Fig. 7-26C).

Lambda waves are more common in children aged between 2 and 15 years than in adults. The amplitude is usually less than 20 to 30 µV but could be greater than 40 µV in children (Fig. 7-27). In some children, a large and predominantly negative wave instead of those with positive polarity at the occipital electrodes may be seen in association with eye movement, especially during scanning of a complex geometric pattern (Fig. 7-28).

It remains puzzling why lambda waves and occipital photic responses, both elicited by visual stimuli, closely resemble the spontaneously appearing POSTS in sleep when the subject's eyes are closed. Also, it is generally true that the subject who has prominent lambda waves also shows prominent POSTs and photic responses by slow-frequency (1 to 3 Hz) photic flashes.

Normal Sleep EEG

DROWSINESS (STAGE I OR N1* SLEEP)

EEG is the most sensitive tool to reflect the level of consciousness instantaneously. During transition from an awake state to drowsiness (stage I or N1* sleep), the occipital alpha rhythm starts to disappear. In some, EEG activity becomes relatively "flat" (Fig. 7-29), while in others, the alpha frequency slows down to a theta rhythm (Fig. 7-30). In the central or frontocentral region, semirhythmic theta rhythm appears. Other than EEG changes, the following physiological parameters assist in determining drowsiness: (a) decreased eye blinking, (b) slow-drifting horizontal eye movements (these are revealed by opposite polarity of the electrooculogram between F7 and

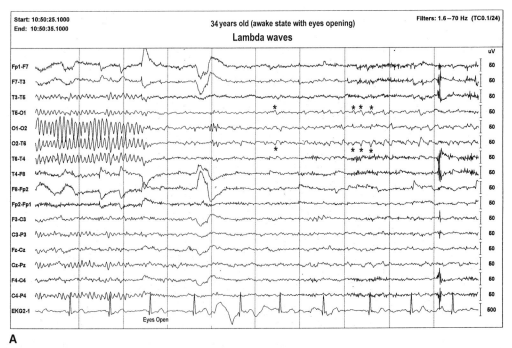

A

FIGURE 7-26 | Lambda waves in relation with POSTS and photic responses in a 34-year-old woman. Note the repetitive small positive sharp waves (examples are shown by *asterisk marks*) at the occipital regions appearing after eyes opening, concomitant with the attenuation of the alpha rhythm **(A)**. Lambda waveform and distribution are similar to POSTS (examples are shown by *asterisk mark*) **(B)** and also photic response (evoked potential) elicited by low-frequency flashes **(C)**. Photic driving responses are indicated by *oval circle* and evoked potentials are shown by *rectangular boxes*. **(A to C** are from the same subject.)

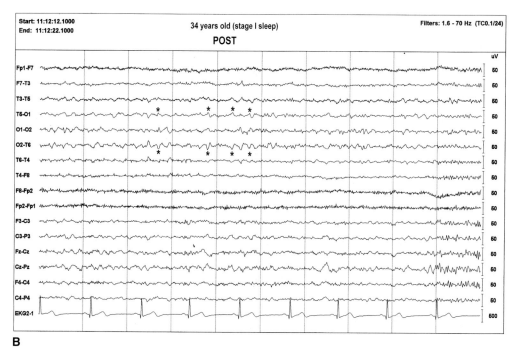

B

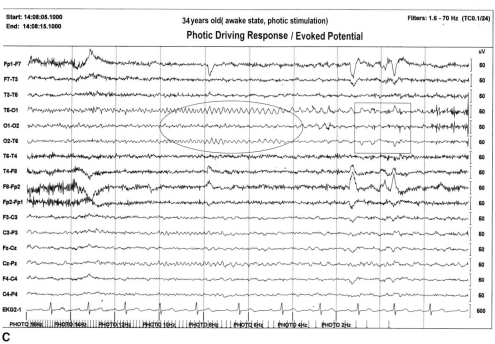

C

FIGURE 7-26 | (Continued)

F8 electrodes) (see Fig. 7-29, also see Fig. 7-31B), and (c) decreased muscle tone or movement artifact. It is important for technologists to recognize these transition signs from wakefulness to drowsiness (Fig. 7-31A and B); the patient should not be disturbed during this transition period so that a sleep recording can be obtained.

Before entering a steady state of sleep, there are usually intermittent arousal episodes during drowsiness. This arousal pattern in adults consists of initial brief delta–theta slow waves, followed by alpha waves, which may be more anterior dominant than the occipital alpha rhythm in the awake state

(Fig. 7-32B; compare with Fig. 7-32A). In children, the arousal patterns show more complex and prominent waveforms, with either diffuse theta or delta bursts with frontocentral prominence (Fig. 7-33A and B).

In children, before the age of 10 years, drowsiness is characterized by the paroxysmal bursts of 3- to 5-Hz theta–delta activity in the frontocentral regions, called *hypnagogic hypersynchrony* (Fig. 7-34). The frequency may be 3 to 4 Hz in infants below the age of 3 months and 4 to 5 Hz in older children. These bursts may become more sustained as drowsiness deepens (Fig. 7-35). The hypnagogic hypersynchrony is most

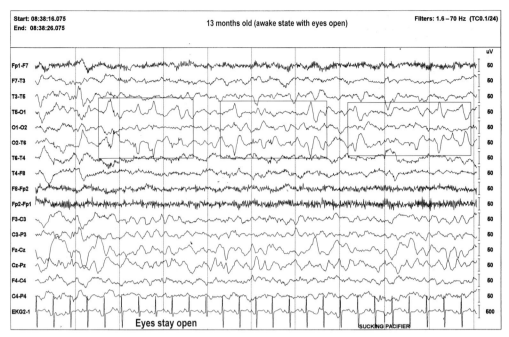

FIGURE 7-27 | Large lambda waves in a 13-month-old baby during eyes-opening state. Lambda waves are shown in *rectangular box*.

prominent at around the age of 1 year and decreases toward the age of 10 years.[5] Similar hypersynchronous theta bursts may occur intermittently associated with brief arousal from light sleep (see Fig. 7-33A and B). The children also show similar but less rhythmic theta–delta bursts upon arousal, called *hypnopompic hypersynchrony* (Fig. 7-36). This lasts from a few seconds to a few minutes, depending on how sleepy the child is upon awakening from sleep.

These hypersynchronous theta–delta bursts sometimes include "spiky" components and could be mistakenly interpreted as abnormal. If similar bursts occur in the fully awake state, however, they should be considered abnormal (see Fig. 6-8).

There are two specific sleep patterns that start to appear in stage I sleep: *positive occipital sharp transient of sleep (POSTS)* and *vertex sharp waves (V waves)*.

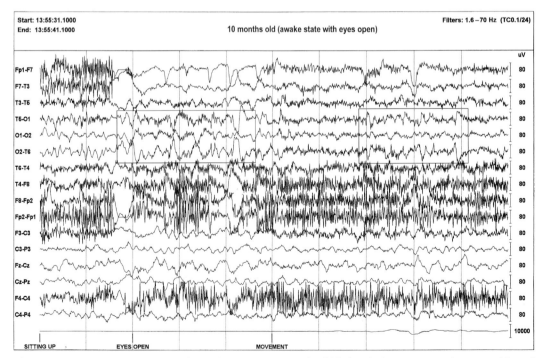

FIGURE 7-28 | The prominent negative occipital transients in a 10-month-old baby during eyes-opening state. Note the large sharp transient predominantly negative in polarity, which appears to be associated with eyes blinking (shown in *rectangular box*).

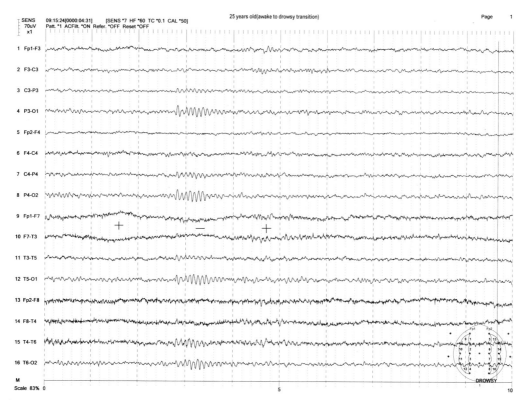

FIGURE 7-29 | Transition from awake to drowsy state in a 25-year-old man. Note loss of persistent alpha rhythm and brief alpha bursts indicating brief arousal during drowsiness. Drifting eye movement is shown by slow positive–negative–positive changes at F7 electrode.

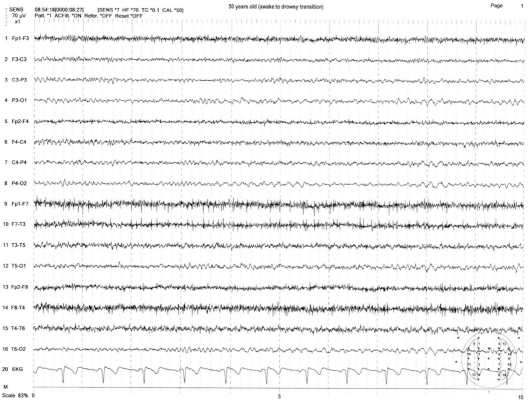

FIGURE 7-30 | Transition from awake to drowsy state in a 50-year-old woman. Note that the alpha rhythm is replaced by 5-Hz theta rhythm at the middle of the page.

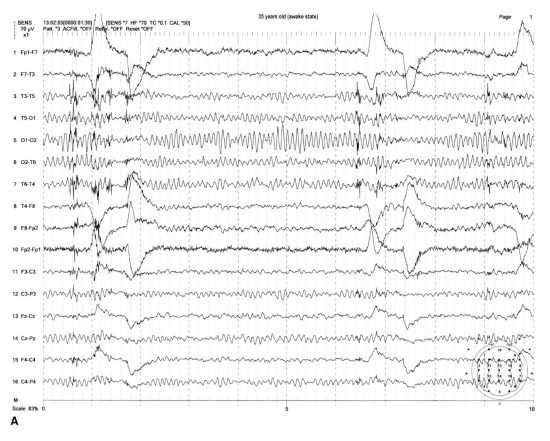

A

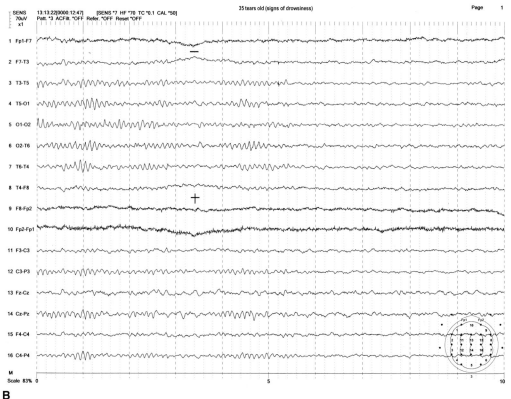

B

FIGURE 7-31 | Waking pattern **(A)** to drowsy pattern **(B)** in a 35-year-old man. Note decrease of tonic muscles, eyes blinking, and movement artifacts in **(B)** as compared to **(A)**. Also note the drifting horizontal slow eye movement's characteristics of approaching to drowsiness (shown by opposite polarities between F7 and F8 electrodes in **B**) (**A** and **B** are from the same subject).

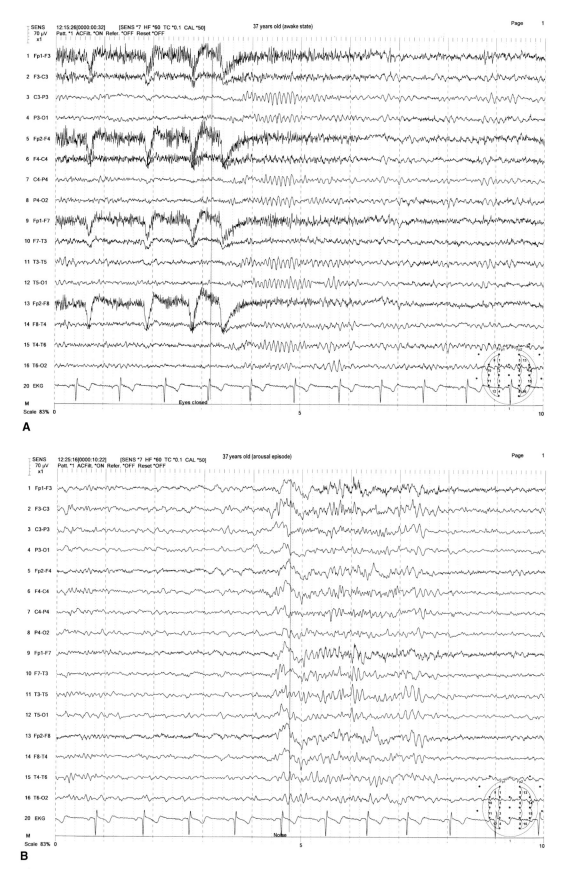

FIGURE 7-32 | EEG in awake **(A)** and in brief arousal episode from drowsiness **(B)** in a 37-year-old woman. Note the paroxysmal bursts of mixture of alpha, theta, and delta activity including some sharp transients lasting about 3 seconds during stage I sleep **(B)**. The alpha activity is more diffusely distributed during arousal period **(B)** compared to the posterior dominant alpha rhythm in the awake state **(A)**.

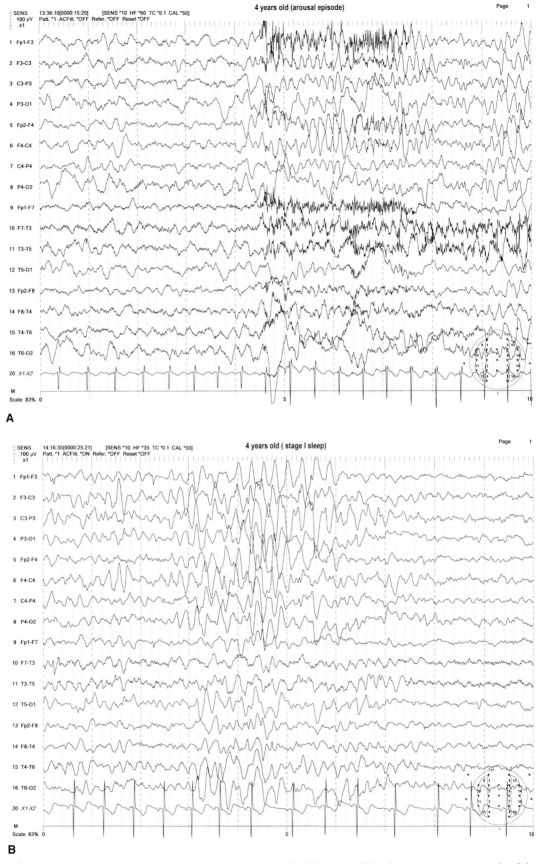

FIGURE 7-33 | **A,B:** An arousal bursts from stage I sleep in a 4-year-old child. Note diffuse bursts consisting mostly of theta with some mixture of delta activities. Degrees of arousal were different between **(A)** and **(B)**, that is, greater arousal in **A** than in **B** evidenced by faster frequency of the burst and lighter sleep stage after the burst in **(A)** than in **(B)**.

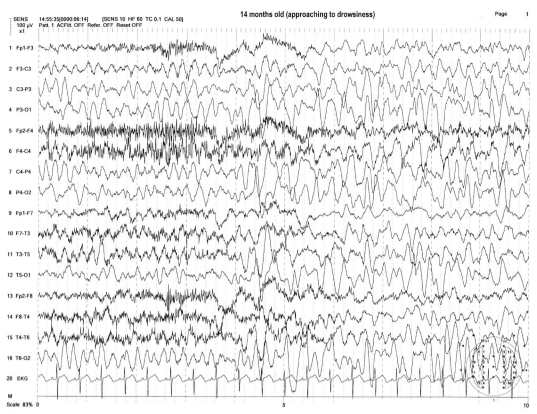

FIGURE 7-34 | Hypnagogic hypersynchronous theta–delta bursts during transition from awake to drowsy state in a 14-month-old baby. Note the dominant delta mixed with theta bursts. Note decreased muscle tone concomitant with the appearance of the bursts.

Positive Occipital Sharp Transients of Sleep

POSTS are surface-positive sharp transients that may have a monophasic or diphasic configuration with the dominant positive potential followed by a small negative phase. It occurs singly or in serial runs of 4 to 5 Hz (Fig. 7-37A and B and Fig. 7-26B; see also Video 7-1B). POSTS are rarely seen before the age of 5 years, presumably because the occipital activity is dominated by high-amplitude delta activity in young children (see Fig. 7-41). It appears that a decrease in occipital delta of

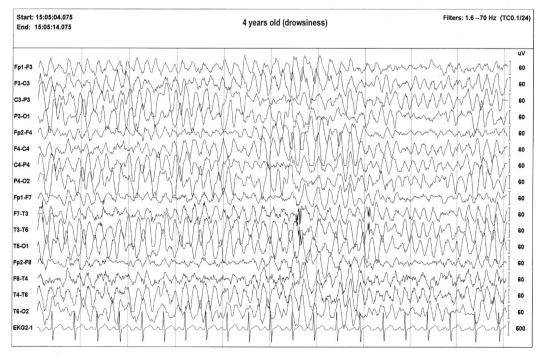

FIGURE 7-35 | Hypnagogic hypersynchronous 5-Hz theta bursts persisting more than 10 seconds in a 4-year-old child.

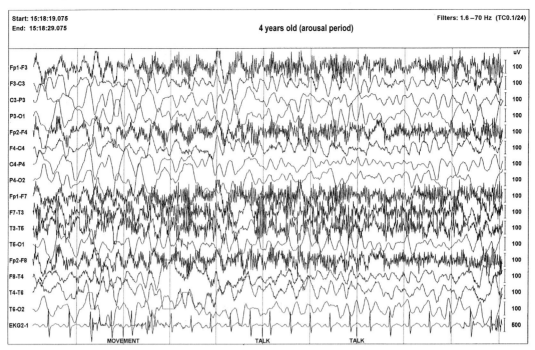

FIGURE 7-36 | An example of hypnopompic theta–delta bursts recording during attempt to wake up from sleep in a 4-year-old child (the same child as in Fig. 7-34). The bursts are less rhythmic and more irregular as compared to hypnagogic bursts (compared with Fig. 7-34).

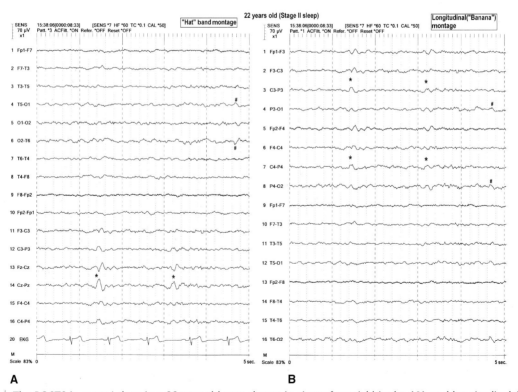

FIGURE 7-37 | The POSTS in stage I sleep in a 22-year-old man shown in circumferential bipolar **(A)** and longitudinal **(B)** montages. (**A** and **B** are the same EEG epoch). Note small sharp transients with predominantly positive polarity at occipital electrodes (POSTS: Some examples are indicated by *#* marks) in stage I sleep. Also note a small sharp transient (V wave) with negative polarity at Cz electrode (V-wave transient indicated by asterisk marks). Both POSTS and V waves are less distinct in stage I as compared to those in stage II sleep (compare these with those of Fig. 7-42 same subject).

sleep toward the age of 5 years is replaced by POSTS after the age of 5 years. In some children, there may be large and predominantly negative slow wave transients (Fig. 7-38). POSTS are always bilaterally synchronous but could be asymmetric in amplitude between the O1 and O2 electrodes. If asymmetric, the amplitude on the right tends to be higher than on the left. The amplitude of POSTS is usually less than 50 µV but could reach 100 µV. When prominent, it resembles epileptiform activity, especially when followed by a prominent negative wave (Fig. 7-39A and B). The characteristic location and polarity should distinguish POSTS from epileptiform activity.

Vertex Sharp Wave Transients (V Waves)

V waves first appear in stage I sleep but usually have less amplitude and are less sharply contoured as compared to that seen in stage II. V waves generally consist of a diphasic wave with dominant surface negativity preceded by or followed by a small positive phase (Fig. 7-40A and B; see Figs. 7-37A and B, 7-38, and 7-45C). V wave is maximum at Cz and is symmetric and synchronous, though there may be some amplitude asymmetry on the two sides in a young child. V wave usually occurs singly in adults but may appear in a serial, repetitive fashion especially in a young child. In adults, the amplitude is usually 100 to 150 µV, and in children, it may reach 250 µV. A V wave is a primarily spontaneous phenomenon but can be induced by a light arousal stimulus. V waves can be recognized in infants at as early as 2 months of age. A consistently asymmetric amplitude of V waves greater than 50% raises the suspicion of an abnormality in the hemisphere of depression (see Fig. 15-43A and B).

In summary, low-voltage theta with POSTS, low-voltage V waves, and drifting horizontal eye movements with decreased muscle artifact denote stage I sleep.

STAGE II OR N2* SLEEP

As stage I sleep becomes stable, there will be a progressive increase of theta waves along with increased amplitude of V waves and POSTS, and eventually, sleep spindles appear in the frontal and central regions (Fig. 7-40A and B). V waves and POSTS become higher in amplitude and more distinct in stage II sleep than in stage I sleep. Theta activity becomes dominant, mixed with some small delta activity. The appearance of sleep spindles denotes the onset of stage II sleep. Widespread but frontal dominant K complexes also appear in stage II sleep, though K complex may be seen well before the appearance of sleep spindles (see Fig. 7-32B).

Sleep Spindles

Sleep spindles are rhythmic, 12 to 16 Hz, most commonly 14 Hz, fusiform waves appearing maximally at the frontocentral region (Fig. 7-40A and B; see also Fig. 7-45C). Frontal spindles may be slightly slower in frequency (10 to 12 Hz). The duration of sleep spindles is usually 1 to 2 seconds and the amplitude is usually less than 50 µV. Spindles are occasionally associated with V waves or K complexes (Fig. 7-41). The spindles are symmetric and synchronous in both children and adults, but commonly asynchronous before the age of 1 year (Fig. 7-42).[59] Asynchronous sleep spindles start to appear at the age of 6 to

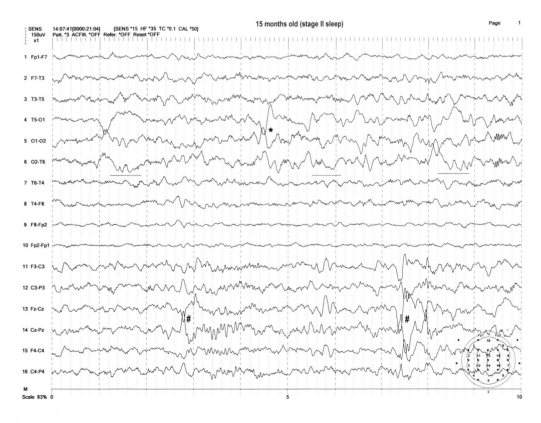

FIGURE 7-38 | Stage II sleep in a 15-month-old baby. Note prominent delta waves and sharp transients (marked by *) at occipital regions, characteristic of sleep in this age group. V waves are marked by #.

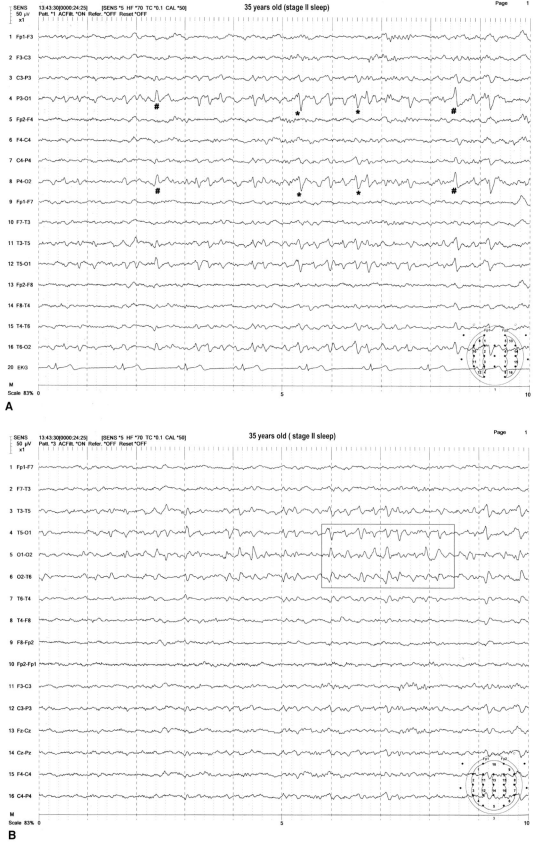

FIGURE 7-39 | Prominent POSTS of diphasic or triphasic configuration shown by the longitudinal **(A)** and circumferential **(B)** montages. Some POSTS are predominantly positive (# mark in **A**), while others have prominent negative component followed by small positive peak (* mark in **A**). Varieties of positive–negative phases of POST are also shown in **(B)** (*rectangular box*).

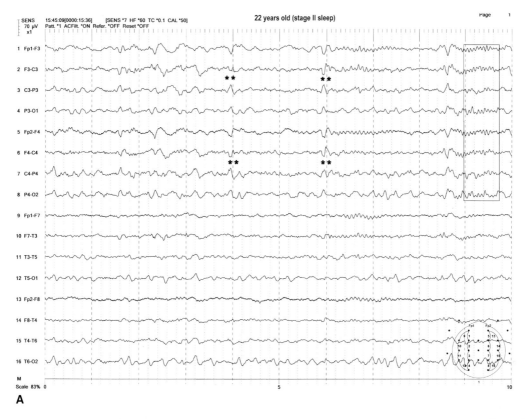

A

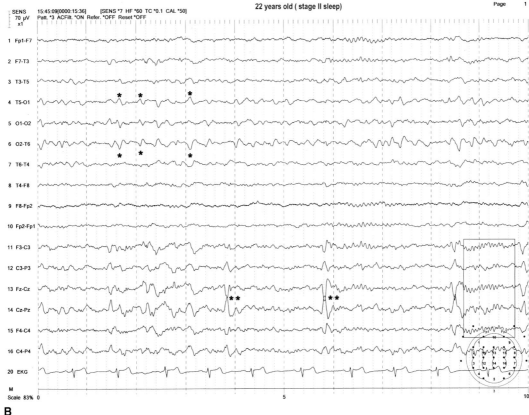

B

FIGURE 7-40 | Stage II sleep in a 22-year-old woman shown by the longitudinal **(A)** and circumferential **(B)** montages. Note the V-wave maximum at C3 and C4 in **(A)** and at vertex (Cz) electrode in **(B)**; examples are shown by *two asterisk marks*. POSTS are easier to identify in circumferential **(B)** than in longitudinal **(A)** derivation. Examples of POSTS are indicated by a *single asterisk mark* **(B)**. Examples of sleep spindles are shown by *rectangular box* **(A,B)**. (**A** and **B** are the same EEG samples.)

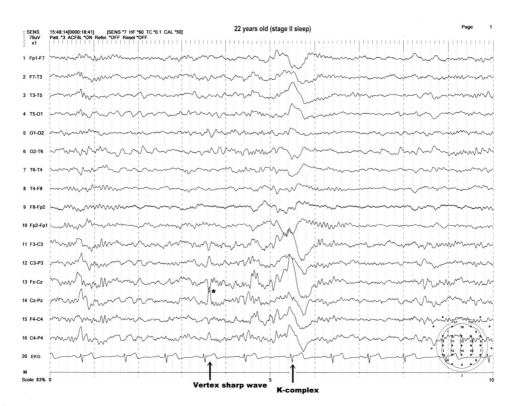

FIGURE 7-41 | K complex and V wave during stage II sleep in a 22-year-old man. Note the K complex consisting of large delta mixed with theta, spindles, and sharp waves with bifrontal dominance. Note the differences of wave form and distribution between K complex and V wave; K complex is complex waveform, whereas V wave is usually single sharp transient; K complex is maximum at frontal electrode, whereas V wave is maximum at vertex (Cz) region. Note phase reversal of V wave at Cz (indicated by *asterisk mark*) but not of K complex (this is the same subject with Fig. 7-36A and B).

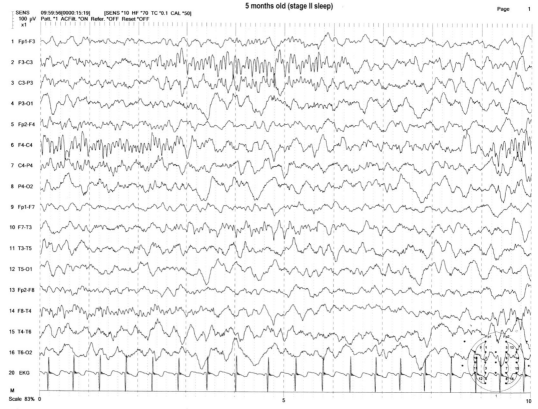

FIGURE 7-42 | Characteristic sleep spindles in babies less than 1 year of age shown by this 5-month-old baby. The spindles are asynchronous, appearing from left and right hemispheres independently. Also note characteristic waveform with mu-shaped configuration with pointed negativity.

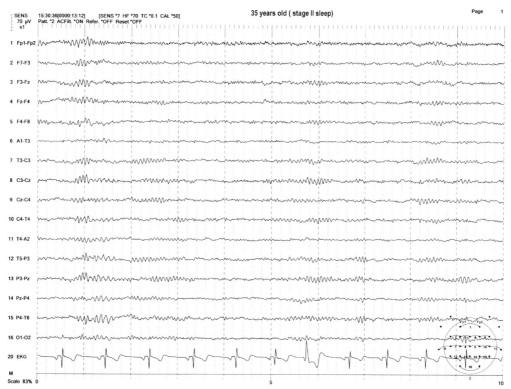

FIGURE 7-43 | Abundant sleep spindles induced by medication (Benzodiazepine) during stage 2 (N2) sleep. Note more or less continuous sleep spindles with scarcity of V waves.

8 weeks[59] and become progressively more synchronous toward 1 year of age. Asynchronous sleep spindles after the age of 2 years is considered to be abnormal. This may be seen in patients with agenesis of the corpus callosum, such as Aicardi's syndrome[60] (see Fig. 6-15) or hydrocephalus[61] (see Fig. 6-16). The spindles in infants and young children (<2 years old) have characteristic waveforms; they are sharply contoured with a surface-negative phase, resembling mu rhythm (Fig. 7-42).

Under sedative medications such as barbiturates or benzodiazepines, spindles become faster in frequency (18 to 22 Hz) and more abundant with lesser incidence of V waves (Fig. 7-43; see also Fig. 7-21B). In this condition, distinction between sleep spindles and beta activity may become difficult. Overdose of these medications is one condition, which results in diffuse, frontal dominant, and more or less continuous "spindling" called the "*spindle coma*" (see "Spindle Coma," Chapter 11; see also Figs. 8-4 and 11-16). The unilateral depression or slowing of sleep spindles is a reliable marker for focal pathology[62] (see Fig. 6-14B).

K Complex

K complex consists of a various mixture of delta–theta and sharp wave bursts often associated with sleep spindles (Fig. 7-44; see also Fig. 7-45C). K complexes start to appear in stage II (N2) sleep and continue in stage III/IV (N3) sleep. Although the term K complex has at times been interchangeably used with vertex sharp transients, a K complex is more frontally dominant than a vertex sharp transient, which is maximum at the Cz electrode.

K complexes also consist of variable and complex wave forms, but V waves are usually single monophasic or diphasic sharp transients. The waveform of K complexes varies within the same stage of sleep. K complexes occur spontaneously or could be induced by arousal stimuli such as a click sound or noise (Video 7-2). K complex is considered a part of an arousal response and is often followed by an arousal pattern with diffuse alpha or theta activity (Fig. 7-44; see also Fig. 7-32). The patient may show brief myoclonic jerking associated with K complex, which is referred to as hypnic jerks, sleep starts, or sleep twitches (Video 7-3).

STAGE III AND IV SLEEP (N3*)

As the sleep stage deepens, delta activity, usually less than 2 Hz, increases in amplitude as well as incidence. Stage III and IV sleep (N3), defined by the amount of delta activity, are often combined together and referred to as "*delta sleep*," or *slow wave sleep* (SWS) (see Fig. 7-45D and E). Unless the patient is sleep deprived or exceedingly somnolent, it is uncommon to record delta sleep in a routine EEG because the recording time for a routine EEG is usually not long enough (<30 minutes) to achieve delta sleep.

According to the standard for sleep staging defined by Rechtschaffen and Kales,[63] stages III and IV are based on the amount of delta activity larger than 75 µV, with greater than 25% and 50%, respectively, in one epoch (30 seconds) of polysomnography (PSG). K complexes and sleep spindles continue in stages III and IV. Sleep spindles become slightly slower in frequency (10 to 11 Hz) and more frontally dominant in stage III/IV sleep.

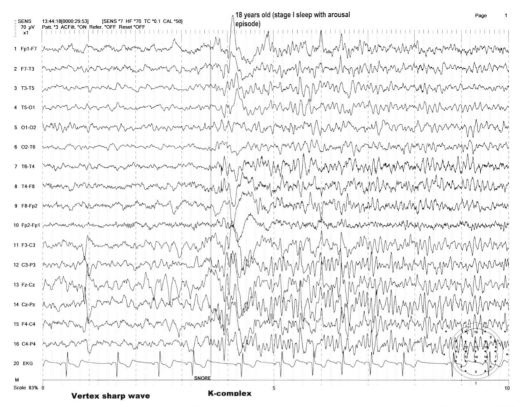

FIGURE 7-44 | K complex followed by arousal episode in 18-year-old man. Note K complex was induced by snoring, followed by diffuse bifrontal increased alpha activity with some mixture of theta–delta slow waves.

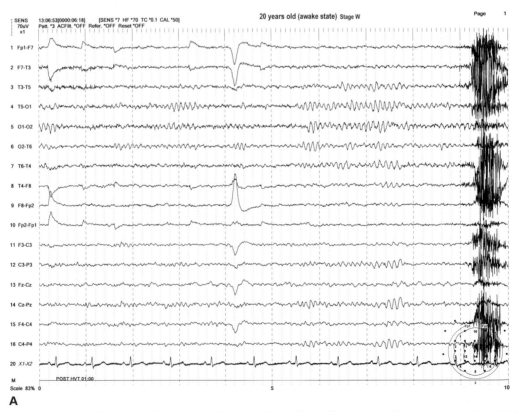

FIGURE 7-45 | Awake **(A)** and sleep stage changes in a 20-year-old man **(B to F)**. Note the V wave in stages I and II **(B,C)** and sleep spindles and K complex in stage II (N2*) **(C)**. Note the increase of delta in stage III (N3*) **(D)** and further increase in stage IV (N3*) **(E)**. REM sleep (R) **(F)** is characterized by low-voltage background activity consisting of mixture of alpha–theta rhythms and presence of rapid eye movements (shown by *rectangular box*). Note also "sawtooth" waves shown by *oval circle*.

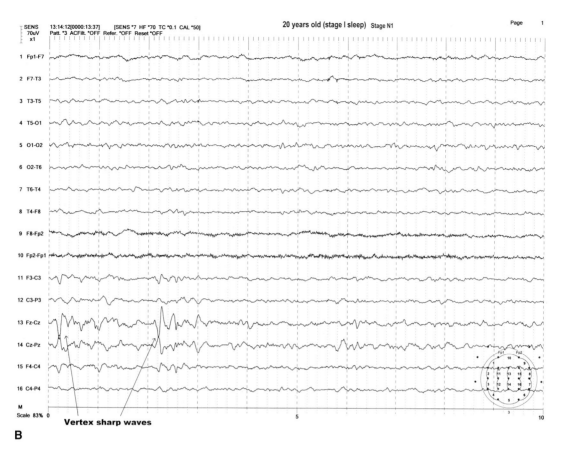

Vertex sharp waves

B

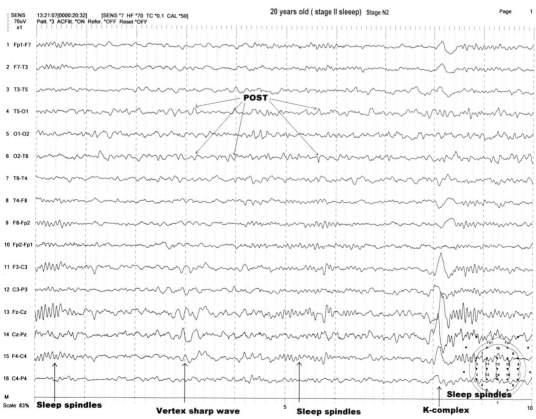

Sleep spindles   Vertex sharp wave   Sleep spindles   K-complex   Sleep spindles

C

FIGURE 7-45 | (*Continued*)

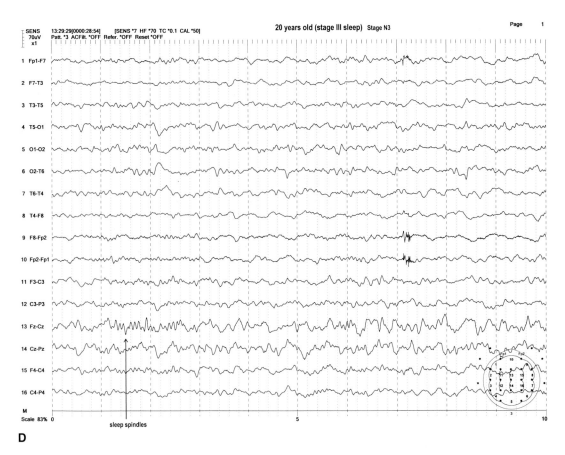

D

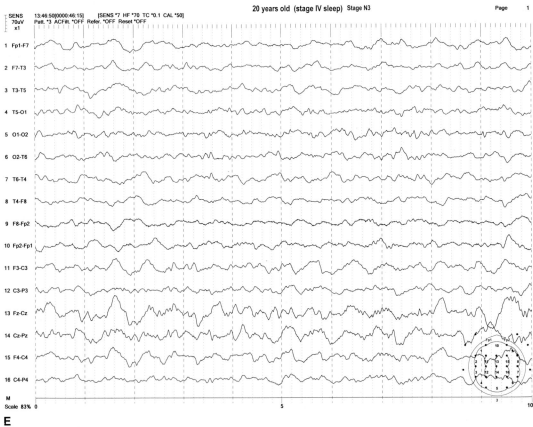

E

FIGURE 7-45 | (*Continued*)

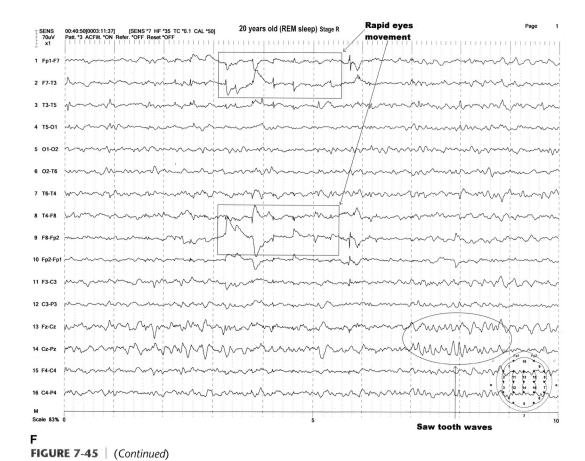

F

FIGURE 7-45 | (Continued)

REM SLEEP (R*SLEEP)

Aserinsky and Kleitman[64] first discovered an unusual sleep pattern, distinct from other sleep stages and often associated with dreaming. In a routine EEG recording, REM sleep is rarely observed because REM sleep usually appears approximately 90 minutes (80 to 110 minutes) after non-REM (stage I to IV) sleep. Early onset of REM sleep suggests narcolepsy, withdrawal from REM suppressant drugs or alcohol, sleep-deprived state, or disturbed sleep schedule. In an overnight recording, REM sleep episodes appear in approximately 60- to 90-minutes intervals with the longest REM episode being in the early morning.

The EEG pattern of REM sleep closely resembles stage I sleep or the transition from the awake state to stage I sleep. The EEG consists of relatively low-voltage theta and alpha activities (see Fig. 7-45F). No delta activity or sleep spindles are present, but serial V wave–like activity, called "*sawtooth waves*," is seen [this was named because of its appearance in slow sweep speed (30 mm/s)] on the polysomnographic recording. Concomitant with the EEG changes, muscle tone markedly decreases and prominent rapid eye movements (mostly horizontal) appear. Also, sporadic rapid muscle twitches increase. In PSG, EMG of the chin muscles and electrooculogram (EOG) with electrodes placed close to the

eyes are routinely monitored. Even without EMG or EOG monitoring, REM sleep can be easily recognized: low-voltage awake/drowsy-like (without slow waves or sleep spindles) EEG pattern, associated with rapid eye movements seen at F7 and F8 electrodes, absence of tonic muscle artifacts, and increased random muscle twitches indicate REM sleep. Other physiological features associated with REM sleep include irregular respiration, loss of temperature control, and penile erection.

Figure 7-45A–F shows progressive EEG change from awake to non-REM sleep and to REM sleep in one adult subject.

EEG Characteristics in Infancy and Childhood

Although the EEG patterns in infancy and childhood were described in previous sections, the overall characteristics are briefly summarized here. The interpretation of EEG in children and infants presents a number of special problems because of the wide range of normal variations and the factors of maturation. The EEG of a premature infant and neonate will be described in Chapter 16.

INFANCY

During the first few months of life, the basic waking background activity consists of a relatively low-amplitude delta and theta activity, with a frequency around 4 Hz (see Chapter 16);

---

*According to a new classification by American Academy of Sleep Medicine, stage 1 corresponds to N1 (non-REM sleep), stage 2 corresponds to N2, and combined stages 3 and 4 correspond to N3 and REM sleep or R sleep (Sleep 2009;32:139–149).

the amplitude progressively increases (up to 150 μV) toward 6 to 9 months of age. The theta components tend to be predominant in the central region. Continuous high-amplitude (>100 μV) delta activity in the awake state should be regarded as abnormal even in the neonate. By 6 months of age, rhythmic 4- to 5-Hz theta rhythm is established as the posterior rhythm. *Tracé alternant* (see Chapter 16, Fig. 16-3) in the slow-wave stage of sleep disappears by 1 month of age. REM sleep constitutes about 50% of sleep in neonates, and therefore, capturing REM sleep in a 1-hour routine EEG is not uncommon. Sleep spindles may appear at 2 to 3 months of age and should be seen by 6 months of age. The frequency of sleep spindles may be slightly slower than the 14 Hz typically seen in adults and occur asynchronously between the two hemispheres (Fig. 7-42). The waveform is more wicket-like or comb-like in appearance, resembling mu rhythm. V waves may be present by 2 to 3 months of age, and K complexes begin to occur at about 6 months of age.

CHILDHOOD EEG

Waking Pattern

There are progressive maturational changes from infancy to young adult age (see section of *Frequency of Alpha Rhythm* in this chapter). At about 1 and ½ years of age, the background activity starts to include a low-frequency alpha component mixed with a dominant theta rhythm (see Fig. 7-4). The mean frequency reaches 8 Hz at 3 to 4 years of age (see Fig. 7-5). With increasing age, the alpha rhythm becomes more persistent, but there is underlying delta activity with a superimposed alpha or theta rhythm or intermittent delta activity interrupting the alpha rhythm (*posterior slow waves of youth*) (see Figs. 7-5 to 7-7 and 7-25). The amplitude may reach 100 to 150 μV (measured at the occipital electrode with an ipsilateral ear reference). During the eyes-open state, the background activity is slower, consisting of an irregular delta–theta pattern (see Fig. 7-11). It is important to assess the background activity while the subject's eyes are closed, but during the fully awake state. If the subject is too young or mentally challenged and unable to follow the technologist's commands, eyes closed for 20 to 30 seconds must be recorded by the technologist holding the eyes closed. When the alpha rhythm reaches 10 Hz at about 15 years of age, underlying delta activity and posterior slow waves of youth diminish, and the amplitude becomes close to the adult range (40 to 60 μV) (see Figs. 7-7 and 7-8). In children and adolescents, frontocentral activity may be dominated by theta rhythm despite well-defined and dominant alpha rhythm posteriorly (see Fig. 7-23).

Sleep Pattern

Drowsiness (stage I sleep) is characterized by a strikingly rhythmic wave pattern; diffuse 5- to 6-Hz smoothly contoured theta bursts or frontal dominant 3- to 4-Hz delta–theta bursts (*hypnagogic hypersynchrony*) tend to be more common (see Figs. 7-34 and 7-35). These bursts are prominent until the age of 10 years and decrease thereafter. Similar bursts may be present when a child awakes from sleep before full alertness is regained (*hypnopompic hypersynchrony*) (see Fig. 7-36) and also during an arousal episode (see Fig. 7-33B). Sleep spindles

are typically asynchronous until 1 year of age (see Fig. 7-42). Asynchronous sleep spindles after 2 years of age, however, should be considered abnormal. Also, the waveform of sleep spindles is more mu shaped with a pointed negative wave. This waveform continues until age 2 to 3 years. There are no clear POSTS before the age of 5 years. Instead, large delta slow waves are dominant in the occipital region (see Fig. 7-38). In some children, bilaterally synchronous generalized and frontal dominant spike-wave bursts may be difficult to differentiate from physiological K complexes (see Fig 10-19A). In such cases, finding a clear and unequivocal spike discharge within the burst wave form is important to differentiate between spike-wave burst and K complex.

References

1. International Federation of Societies for Electroencephalography and Clinical Neurophysiology. A glossary of terms commonly used by clinical electroencephalographers. *Electroencephalogr Clin Neurophysiol* 1974;37:538–548.
2. Maulsby RL, Kellaway P, Graham M, et al. *The Normative Electroencephalographic Data Reference Library*. Final report, contract NAS 9–1200. Washington, DC: National Aeronautics and Space Administration, 1968.
3. Kellaway P, Noebels JL. *Problems and Concepts in Developmental Neurophysiology*. Baltimore, MD: The Johns Hopkins University Press, 1989.
4. Petersen I, Eeg-Oloffson O. The development of the electroencephalogram in normal children from the age of 1 through 15 years–nonparoxysmal activity. *Neuropadiatrie* 1971;2:247–304.
5. Eeg-Oloffson O. The development of the electroencephalogram in normal adolescence from the age of 16 through 21 years. *Neuropadiatrie* 1971;3:11–45.
6. Harvald B. EEG in old age. *Acta Psychiatr Scand* 1958;33:193–196.
7. Obrist WD. The electroencephalogram of normal aged adults. *Electroencephalogr Clin Neurophysiol* 1954;6:235–244.
8. Torres F, Faoro A, Loewenson R, et al. The electroencephalogram of elderly subjects revisited. *Electroencephalogr Clin Neurophysiol* 1983;56:391–398.
9. Arenas AM, Brenner RP, Reynolds CF III. Temporal slowing in the elderly revisited. *Am J EEG Technol* 1986;26:105–114.
10. Sulg IA, Cronqvist S, Schuller H, et al. The effect of intracardial pacemaker therapy on cerebral blood flow and electroencephalogram in patients with complete atrioventricular block. *Circulation* 1969;39:487–494.
11. Creutzfeldt OD, Arnold P-M, Becker D, et al. EEG change during spontaneous and controlled menstrual cycles and their correlation with psychological performance. *Electroencephalogr Clin Neurophysiol* 1976;40:113–131.
12. Chatrian GE. The low voltage EEG. In: Remond A, ed. *Handbook of Electroencephalography and Clinical Neurophysiology*. Vol. 6A. Amsterdam, The Netherlands: Elsevier, 1976:77–89.
13. Cobb WA. The normal adult EEG. In: Hill D, Parr G, eds. *Electroencephalography*. New York: Macmillan, 1963:232–249.
14. Leissner P, Lindholm L-E, Petersen I. Alpha amplitude dependence on skull thickness and measured by ultrasound technique. *Electroencephalogr Clin Neurophysiol* 1970;29:392–399.
15. Hoovey ZB, Heineman U, Creutzfeldt OD. Inter-hemispheric 'synchrony' of alpha wave. *Electroencephalogr Clin Neurophysiol* 1972;32:337–347.
16. Aird RB, Gastaut Y. Occipital and posterior electroencephalographic rhythms. *Electroencephalogr Clin Neurophysiol* 1959;11:637–656.
17. Picard P, Navarranne P, Laboureur P, et al. Confrontations des donnees de, l'elecroencephalogrmme et de l'examen psychologique chez 309 candidats pilotes a l'aeronautique. *Electroencephalogr Clin Neurophysiol Suppl* 1957;6:304–314.

18. Storm van Leewen W, Wieneke G, Spoelstra P, et al. Lack of bilateral coherence of mu rhythm. *Electroencephalogr Clin Neurophysiol* 1978;44:140–146.

19. Schoppenhorst M, Brauer F, Freund G, et al. The significance of coherence estimate in determining central alpha and mu activities. *Electroencephalogr Clin Neurophysiol* 1980;48:25–33.

20. Gastaut H, Terzian H, Gastaut Y. Etude d'une activite electroencephalographique meconnue: Le"rythme rolandique en arceau." *Marseille Med* 1952;89:296–310.

21. Jasper HH, Penfield W. Electrocorticogram in man: Effect of voluntary movement upon electrical activity of precentral gyrus. *Arch Psychiatry* 1949;183:163–174.

22. Chatrian GE, Petersen MC, Lazarte JA. The blocking of the rolandic wicket rhythm and some central changes related to movement. *Electroencephalogr Clin Neurophysiol* 1960;11:497–510.

23. Brechet R, Lecasble R. Reactivity of mu rhythm to flicker. *Electroencephalogr Clin Neurophysiol* 1965;18:721–722 (abst).

24. Klass D, Bickford RG. Observation on the rolandic anceau rhythm. *Electroencephalogr Clin Neurophysiol* 1957;9:570.

25. Yamada T, Kooi K. Level of consciousness and the mu rhythm. *Clin Electroencephalogr* 1975;6:80–88.

26. Kellaway P, Fox BJ. Electroencephalographic diagnosis of cerebral pathology in infants during sleep. I. Rationale, technique, and the characteristics of normal sleep in infants. *J Pediatr* 1952;41:262–287.

27. Cobb WA, Guiloff RJ, Cast J. Breach rhythm: The EEG related to skull defect. *Electroencephalogr Clin Neurophysiol* 1979;47:251–271.

28. Gibbs EL, Gibbs FA. Extreme spindles: Correlation of electroencephalographic sleep pattern in mental retardation. *Science* 1962;138:1106–1107.

29. Colgin LL, Denninger T, Fyhn M, et al. Frequency of gamma oscillations routes flow of information in the hippocampus. *Nature* 2009;462:353–357.

30. Berens P, Keliris GA, Ecker AS, et al. Feature selectivity of the gamma-band of the local field potential in primate primary visual cortex. *Front Neurosci* 2008;2:199–207.

31. Gold I. "Does 40-Hz oscillation play a role in visual consciousness?" *Conscious Cogn* 1999;2:186–195.

32. Bauer P, Paz R, Pare D. Gamma oscillation coordinate amygdalorhinal interactions during learning. *J Neurosci* 2007;29:9369–9379.

33. Gregoriou GG, Gotts SJ, Zhou H, Desimone R. "High frequency, long range coupling between prefrontal and visual cortex during attention." *Science* 2009;324:1207–1210.

34. Lutz A, Greischar LL, Rawlings NB, et al. Long-term meditators self-induced high-amplitudes gamma synchrony during mental practice. *Proc Natl Acad Sci U S A* 2004;101:16369–16373.

35. Williams S, Boksa P. Gamma oscillations and schizophrenia. *J Psychiatry Neurosci* 2010;35:75–77.

36. Cornelis JS, Anne Marie vCvW, Yolande A, et al. Generalized synchronization of MEG recordings in Alzheimer's disease: Evidence for involvement of the gamma band. *J Clin Neurophysiol* 2002;19:562–574.

37. Hughes JR. Gamma, fast, and ultrafast waves of the brain: Their relationship with epilepsy and behavior. *Epilepsy Behav* 2008;13(1):25–31.

38. Cohn R, Nardini JE. The correlation of bilateral occipital slow activity in human EEG with certain disorders of behavior. *Am J Psychiatry* 1958;115:44–54.

39. Faure J, Guerin A. Au subjet de l'electroencephalogramme des enfants caracteriels. *Rev Neurol (Paris)* 1958;99:209–219.

40. Garcia-Bardaracco J. EEG et psychisme: Les entretiens psychiatriques 1953. Paris: Collection. *Psyche Arche* 1953;140–165.

41. Lairy GC. EEG et neuropsychiatrie infantile. *Psychiatr Enfant* 1961;3:525–608.

42. Mundy-Castle AC. Theta and beta rhythm in electroencephalogram of normal adults. *Electroencephalogr Clin Neurophysiol* 1951;3:477–486.

43. Doose H, Gundel H. 4 to 7 cps rhythms in the childhood EEG. In: Anderson VE, Hauser WA, Penry JK, et al., eds. *Genetic Basis of the Epilepsies*. New York: Raven Press, 1982:83–93.

44. Gundel A, Baier W, Doose H, et al. Spectral analysis of EEG in the late course of primary generalized myoclonic—Astatic epilepsy. I. EEG and clinical data. *Neuropediatrics* 1980;12:62–74.

45. Ciganek L. Theta-discharges in the middle-line: EEG symptoms of temporal lobe epilepsy. *Electroencephalogr Clin Neurophysiol* 1961;13:669–673.

46. Westmoreland BF, Klass DW. Midline theta rhythm. *Arch Neurol* 1986;43:139–141.

47. Yamaguchi Y, Ishihara T, Mizuki Y. Frontal midline theta rhythm (Fm0). *Electroencephalogr Clin Neurophysiol* 1985;60:38.

48. Smith JR. The frequency growth of the human alpha rhythms during normal infancy and childhood. *J Psychol* 1941;11:177–198.

49. Jasper HH, Solomon P, Bradley C. Electroencephalographic analyses of behavior problem children. *Am J Psychiatry* 1938;95:641–658.

50. Lindsley DB, Cutts KK. Electroencephalogram of "constitutionally inferior" and behavioral problem children: Comparison with those of normal children and adults. *Arch Neurol Psychiatry* 1940;44:1199–1212.

51. Wiener JM, Delano JC, Klass DW. An EEG study of delinquent and nondelinquent adolescents. *Arch Gen Psychiatry* 1966;15:144–150.

52. Sutter C, Harrelson AB. Occipital slowing in the EEG of 5–15 year olds (teenage slow): A report on this finding in 237 child psychiatric patients. *Electroencephalalogr Clin Neurophysiol* 1966;20:624–625.

53. Cohn R, Nardini JE. The correlation of bilateral occipital slow activity in the human EEG with certain disorders of behavior. *Am J Psychiatry* 1958;115:44–54.

54. Hill D. Cerebral dysrhythmia: Its significance in aggressive behavior. *Proc R Soc Med* 1944;37:317–330.

55. Pavy R, Metcalfe J. The abnormal EEG in childhood communication and behavior abnormalities. *Electroencephalogr Clin Neurophysiol* 1965;19:414.

56. Gastaut Y. Un signe electroencephalographique peu connu: les pointes occipitales survenant pendant l'ouverture des yeux. *Rev Neruol (Paris)* 1951;84:640–643.

57. Roth M, Green J. The lambda waves as a normal physiological phenomenon in the human electroencephalogram. *Nature* 1953;172:864–866.

58. Barlow JS, Ciganek L. Lambda responses in relationship to visual evoked responses in man. *Electroencephalogr Clin Neurophysiol* 1969;26:183–192.

59. Kellaway P, Fox BJ. Electroencephalographic diagnosis of cerebral pathology in infants during sleep. I. Rationale, technique, and the characteristics of normal sleep in infants. *J Pediatr* 1952;41:262–287.

60. Fariello RC, Chun RWM, Doro JM, et al. EEG recognition of Aicardi's syndrome. *Arch Neurol* 1977;34:563–566.

61. Garvin JS, Gibbs EL. Electroencephalogram in hydrocephalus. *Clin Electroencephalogr* 1975;6:29–40.

62. Reeves AL, Klass DW. Frequency asymmetry of sleep spindles associated with focal pathology. *Electroencephalogr Clin Neurophysiol* 1998;106:84–86.

63. Rechtshaffen A, Kales A. *A Manual of Standardized Terminology, Techniques and Scoring System for Sleep Stages of Human Subjects*. Washington, DC: Government Printing Office, Public Health Service, 1968.

64. Aserinsky E, Kleitman N. Regularly occurring periods of eye mobility, and concomitant phenomena during sleep. *Science* 1953;118:273–274.

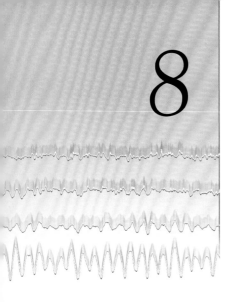

8

The Assessment of Abnormal EEG

THORU YAMADA and ELIZABETH MENG

General Assessment

Electroencephalograph (EEG) changes sensitively along with the state of consciousness in both physiological and pathological states. The alpha rhythm slows down in physiological sleep states and pathologically stuporous states. As the stage of sleep deepens or consciousness becomes more impaired, theta and then delta activities predominate. The EEG also changes dramatically with age, especially during infancy and early childhood, and there are many age-specific EEG patterns. There are also many inter- and intraindividual variables in both normal and abnormal states. Deciding whether the EEG is abnormal or normal depends on the qualitative and quantitative deviation from the normal state. The ordinary EEG interpretation by visual analysis, therefore, relies largely on the electroencephalographer's (EEGer) experience, knowledge, and subjective as well as objective judgment.

EEG interpretation is based on systematic visual inspection and multifactorial analyses of background activity and abnormal patterns by incidence, frequency, amplitude, morphology, topography, and reactivity and by their relationship to age and level of consciousness. Abnormalities may occur within the background activity alone, or with the appearance of abnormal patterns, or both. The abnormal EEG consists of slowing of the background (alpha) rhythm, the appearance of slow waves, paroxysmal activity, and/or varieties of specific patterns. These abnormalities may be (i) focal, (ii) bilaterally diffuse, or (iii) unilateral or lateralized. In a broad sense, slow background activity and slow waves imply cerebral dysfunction, whereas paroxysmal activity suggests an underlying seizure tendency. However, any EEG abnormality is rarely pathognomonic or specific for a certain diagnosis. Under certain clinical conditions, however, some EEG abnormalities help narrow the diagnostic possibilities.

Abnormal Background Activity

Background activity slower than 8 Hz during the fully awake state is abnormal in any age except for children less than 3 years old. When the alpha rhythm is replaced by slower rhythms, the background activity may be diffuse rather than the more typical occipital dominant pattern. Bilaterally diffuse or focally dominant slow background activity, even without another

abnormality, is a sensitive indicator of cortical dysfunction (see Fig. 6-10 and Fig. 11-1). In a focal cerebral lesion, however, the slower or depressed background activity is often associated with delta slow waves (Fig. 8-1; see also Fig. 6-11).

Amplitude asymmetry between homologous regions should be approached cautiously. This may be due to technical factors such as unequal interelectrode distance between the two homologous electrode pairs, especially, if this appears only in one bipolar montage but not in other montages (see Fig. 15-48A and B). An amplitude asymmetry noted on a bipolar recording must be confirmed by referential montage (see Fig. 15-47). Localized scalp edema, subgaleal collection of fluid, or a skull defect (i.e., craniotomy) can also cause amplitude asymmetry. This should be documented by the technologist.

Consistent amplitude asymmetry of the alpha rhythm greater than 50% may be clinically significant, especially when the amplitude is lower on the right side (since the alpha rhythm is generally of higher amplitude on the right in normal subjects). A *subdural hematoma* may have depressed background activity without accompanying other abnormalities (see Fig. 6-9). This is explained by the longer distance to the electrode from the cortex by the depressed cortex and increased impedance due to fluid collection. Amplitude accentuation ipsilateral to the lesion is rare, but this may occur with a *brain tumor* situated close to the cortex.[1] Focal accentuation of alpha and beta activities is a common finding in a patient with a *skull defect* (*Breach rhythm*) (see Fig. 7-20; see also Fig. 12-12).

The unilateral failure of alpha attenuation with eye opening is a rare finding and is termed *Bancaud's phenomenon*, which may be seen in a localized hemispheric lesion.[2] Although abnormal alpha rhythm without other abnormalities primarily represents cortical dysfunction, unilateral reduction of the alpha rhythm has been reported in patients with unilateral thalamic tumor[3] and subcortical cerebral infarct.[4]

Frequency asymmetry of background activity or alpha rhythm with or without amplitude depression is a more reliable finding than amplitude asymmetry alone, indicating focal pathology. Irrespective of amplitude difference, the side with slower frequencies is (more) abnormal (see Fig. 6-12).

Approximately 10% of normal subjects show a low-voltage (<20 **μ**V) background pattern that is difficult to measure.[5] There is some evidence that genetic factors play a role in determining the voltage pattern in a healthy person.[6] In some cases, it is difficult to differentiate if the low-voltage activity is abnormally

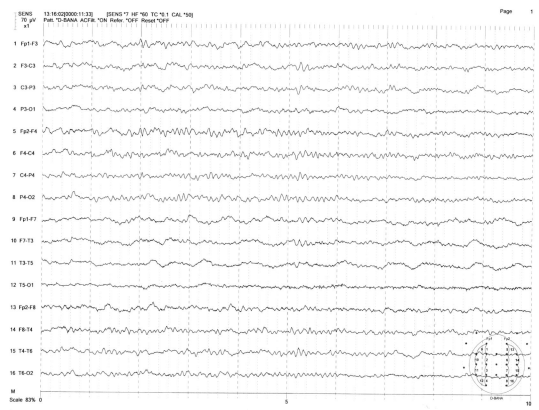

FIGURE 8-1 | A 69-year-old man with complaints of headache and dizziness after a fall hitting the head. MRI showed subdural hematoma on the left hemisphere and cerebral infarct on the left parietal region. EEG showed left polymorphic delta activity greater than right and depressed background activity on the left hemisphere.

suppressed or simply a normal variant. In some normal people, the background activity is low voltage initially but may show measurable alpha rhythm in the latter portion of the recording. The measurable alpha rhythm may also appear during hyperventilation. The normal low-voltage background pattern also tends to show well-defined and prominent photic driving responses with high-frequency photic stimulation. In some cases, it is not possible to determine the normality or abnormality unless a previous EEG is available for comparison. One clinical correlation of the low-voltage EEG pattern is *Huntington chorea* in which progressive voltage decline likely correlates with loss of cortical activity rather than indicating a desynchronized background that would be seen in normal people[7] (see Fig. 11-19).

Abnormal Beta Rhythm

A diffuse increase of beta activity is a common finding secondary to sedative, hypnotic, or anxiolytic *drug effect* (Fig. 8-2; see also Fig. 7-21A and B). The most common medications are benzodiazepines or barbiturates. The medication's effect is usually more prominent and distinct in sleep, characteristically showing abundant sleep spindles with a paucity of vertex sharp waves or K complexes (Fig. 8-3). The degree of beta accentuation varies considerably from one individual to another and is not dependent on the dose of medication; this alone should not be considered an abnormal finding. A prominent and diffuse beta activity in the form of sleep spindles can be seen in semicomatose or comatose patients after overdose or therapeutically induced by the hypnotic or anxiolytic

drugs (Fig. 8-4). This may be referred to as "*spindle coma*" (see "Spindle Coma," Chapter 11; see also Fig. 11-16).

An unusually prominent diffuse or localized beta activity may be seen in patients with grossly anomalous brain such as agyria (lissencephaly) or cortical dysplasia.[8] Unilateral or focal depression of beta activity is a reliable and sensitive indicator of focal cortical dysfunction (Fig. 8-5; see also Fig. 12-6).[9] This asymmetry may be accentuated when the patient is on a sedative or hypnotic drug, that is, the intact cortex can produce beta activity, while the impaired cortex cannot.

Beta and alpha activities can be focally enhanced in a patient who has a burr hole or skull defect, resulting in a "*breach rhythm*"[10] with a characteristic mu-shaped waveform (see Fig. 7-20; see also Fig. 12-12). This commonly occurs in central and midtemporal electrodes. The breach rhythm alone should not be regarded as abnormal because it is due to a physical effect, not cortical injury. In addition, EEG activity near the burr hole has a "sharper" or more "spiky" appearance than the activities from other areas. It is best to be conservative in determining these as spike discharges.

Focal or diffuse beta may signify the onset of an ictal event, which often shows progressive changes from low-voltage, faster- to slower-frequency waves with increasing amplitude as the seizure evolves (Fig. 8-6; see Fig. 10-7).

An unusual accentuation of fast activity in the form of sleep spindles is termed "*extreme spindle*." This is characterized by very frequent and high-amplitude (often >200 μV) sleep spindles, seen in children (<12 years old) with intellectual disability or cerebral palsy.[11] The spindle activity may be seen even in the awake state (Fig. 8-7).

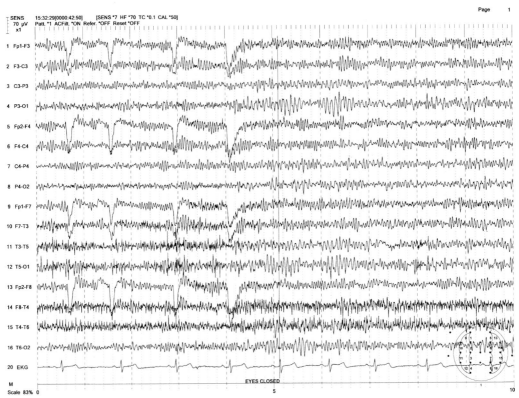

FIGURE 8-2 | Awake EEG in a 35-year-old woman taking benzodiazepine (diazepam) daily. Note prominent and diffuse beta activity.

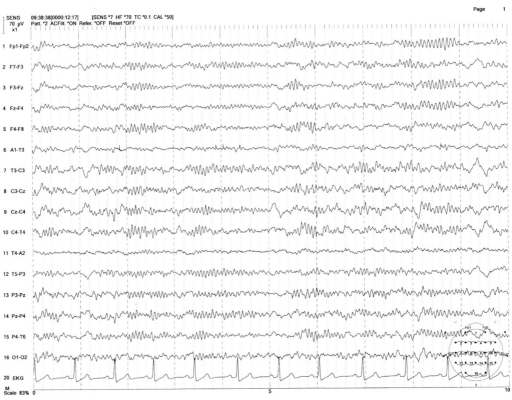

FIGURE 8-3 | Sleep EEG in a 40-year-old woman who takes benzodiazepine (clonazepam) daily. Note abundant 14-Hz sleep spindles occupying most of the 10-s EEG segment. Note also paucity of V sharp wave.

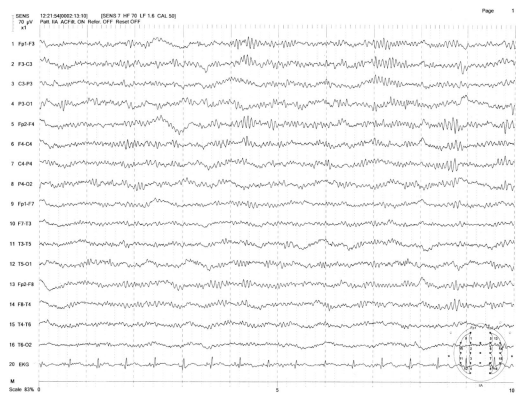

FIGURE 8-4 | An example of spindle coma recorded during therapeutic propofol infusion in a 20-year-old man. Note more or less continuous sleep spindles superimposed on delta slow waves.

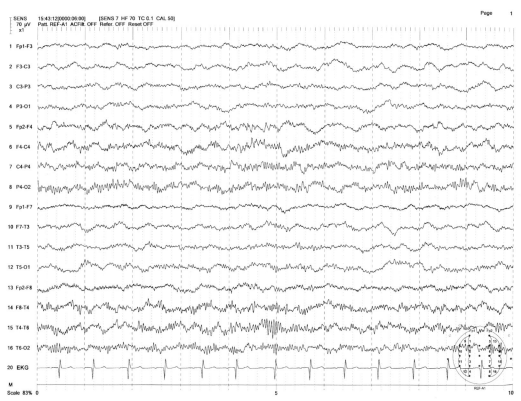

FIGURE 8-5 | EEG recorded during unresponsive state after a cluster of seizures in a 4-year-old patient with tuberous sclerosis. The patient received intravenous lorazepam just prior to EEG. Note bilaterally diffuse symmetrical delta but consistent depression of beta over the left hemisphere. MRI showed venous angiomatosis and atrophy of the left hemisphere.

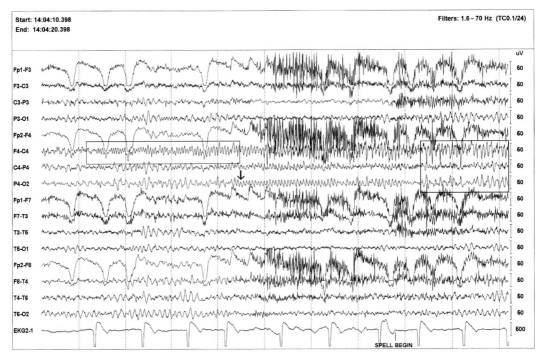

FIGURE 8-6 | The EEG of ictal onset in a 25-year-old male, with complaint of left face numbness spreading to left shoulder and arm. Note the onset of beta activity at the F4 to C4 derivation (shown by *left rectangular box*), which spreads to other electrodes (shown by *downward arrow*). As the ictal discharges evolve, beta activity changes to repetitive sharp discharges (shown by *right rectangular box*).

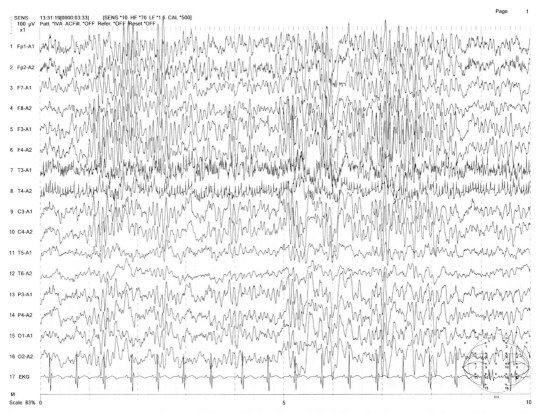

FIGURE 8-7 | Extreme sleep spindles in a 10-year-old boy with intellectual disability of unknown etiology. Note prominent and high-amplitude (>200 μV) sleep spindles.

Abnormal Gamma Rhythm

Activity with frequency faster than 30 Hz (gamma rhythm) is relatively rare in routine scalp EEG recordings but can be seen at the onset of seizure events (Fig. 8-8). Gamma rhythm recorded from intracranial subdural electrodes could demonstrate an accurate localization of seizure onset zone (Fig. 8-9).[12] Fast-frequency activity (close to gamma frequency) in association with rhythmic delta waves has been recognized as a unique diagnostic EEG pattern for patients with *anti-NMDA (N-methyl D-aspartate) receptor encephalitis* [13] (Fig. 8-10; see also Chapter 11 Fig. 11-21A and B).

Abnormal Slow Activity

There are two types of slow-wave activity. One is polymorphic delta or *arrhythmic delta activity* (ADA), which consists of an irregular wave form with a variable frequency and amplitude. The other is intermittently appearing rhythmic or monomorphic delta activity with a stereotyped waveform (*IRDA, intermittent rhythmic delta activity, or RDA*, rhythmic delta activity*). A single EEG may be characterized by either type or both. The ADA may have a focal, unilateral, or bilaterally diffuse appearance but is more commonly seen in focal brain dysfunction. The IRDA tends to be more bilaterally diffuse, representing diffuse cerebral dysfunction.

FOCAL ARRHYTHMIC DELTA ACTIVITY

Gray Walter was the first to describe focal ADA in patients with brain tumors.[14] Focal ADA is a reliable indicator of a focal supratentorial lesion or dysfunction mainly involving the white matter.[15] Focal theta slow waves have the same significance as ADA but imply a lesser degree of severity (i.e., the slower the frequency, the greater the dysfunction). It often accompanies other EEG abnormalities such as slowing of background activity or reduction of fast activity in the same region. Acute or severe cerebral dysfunction is characterized by slow and continuous delta with minimal or no accompanying background activity (Fig. 8-11A). With improved cerebral function, predominant delta activity changes (i) from continuous to intermittent, (ii) from slower- to faster-frequency delta with increase of theta activity (Fig. 8-11B), (iii) to an intermittent appearance or recovery of slow background activity (Fig. 8-11C), and, finally, (iv) to recovery of some alpha rhythm (Fig. 8-11D).

Focal ADA is generally better appreciated in the waking state than in sleep; in sleep, focal activity may become more bilateral or is obscured by the generalized increase in slow waves of sleep (see Fig. 6-13A compared with B; see also Fig. 12-14A compared with B). In the obtunded or semicomatose patient, it is important for the technologist to record at least a part of the EEG when the patient is at the highest level of consciousness; this may require stimulation in an attempt to arouse the patient.

Any focal structural lesion can produce focal ADA, but the field distribution of the focal abnormality could be much larger than the actual size of the lesion revealed by magnetic resonance imaging (MRI) or computerized tomography (CT) scan. Thus, the EEG is a useful measure to judge the extent of functional disturbance but not the actual size of the lesion. However, the EEG is relatively poor for accurate localization of the lesion (see Fig. 12-15). At best, EEG localization is

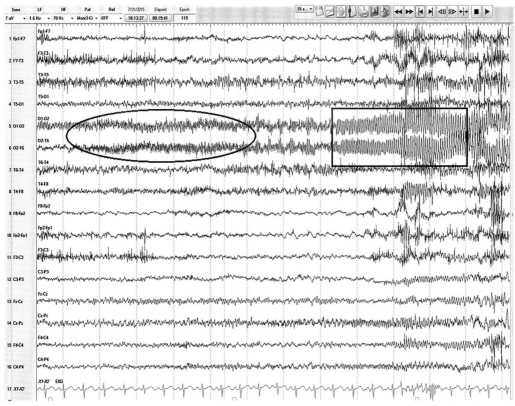

FIGURE 8-8 | Electrographic ictal event with the onset starting with gamma rhythm from O2 electrode (shown by *oval circle*), followed by beta rhythm (shown by *rectangular box*). This reliably indicates that the seizure arise from the cortex just underneath the O2 electrode.

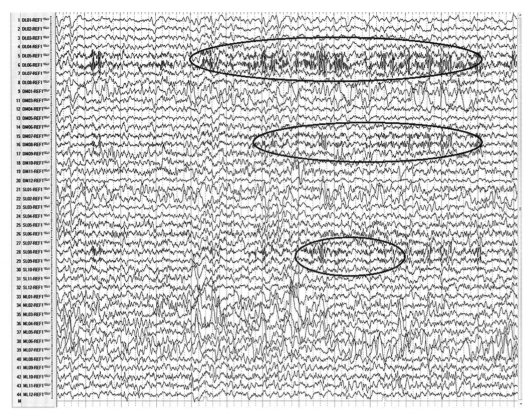

FIGURE 8-9 | Prominent gamma rhythm (shown by *oval circles*) recorded from multiple subdural cortical electrodes during presurgical evaluation for treatment of intractable epilepsy. This strongly suggests the seizure likely arises from these gamma zones.

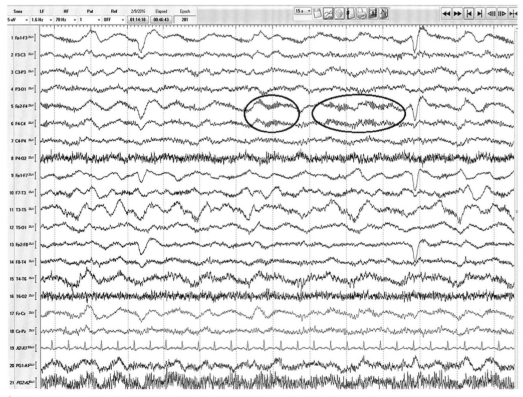

FIGURE 8-10 | The EEG in a patient with diagnosis of anti-NMDA encephalitis showing characteristic "*extreme delta brush*" consisting of semirhythmic delta associated with gamma rhythm (shown by *oval circle*).

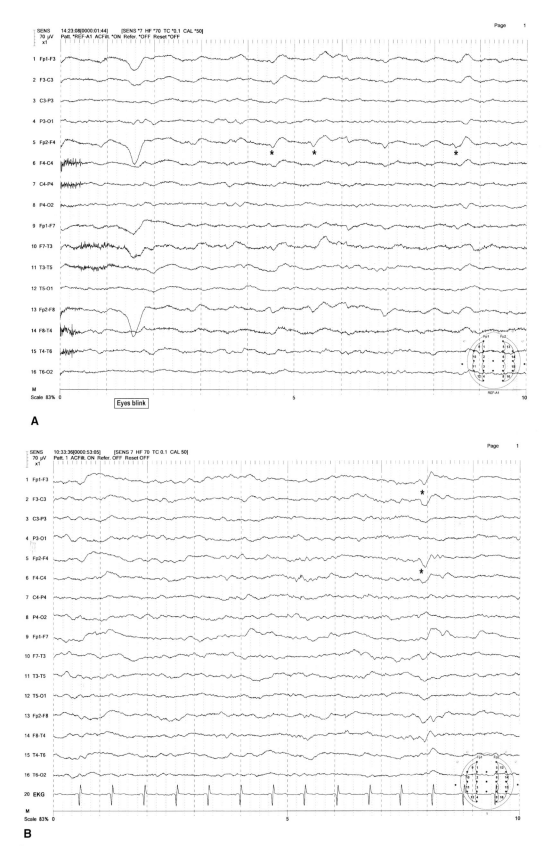

FIGURE 8-11 | Serial EEGs in a 43-year-old patient with acute encephalopathy secondary to drug (lithium) overdose. The first EEG **(A)**, recorded in semicomatose state, shows diffuse, relatively low-amplitude 1- to 1.5-Hz delta with minimal and very low-voltage theta background activity. Some low-voltage triphasic waves are also noted (shown by *asterisks*). The 2nd day EEG **(B)** shows slightly faster delta (2 to 3 Hz) and increased theta background activity (shown by *asterisks*). The 4th day EEG **(C)** shows greater amplitude of delta–theta slow waves, with intermittent triphasic sharp waves (shown by *asterisks*). The 7th day EEG **(D)** now shows background alpha rhythm, but there are still some delta waves remaining (shown by *underlines*).

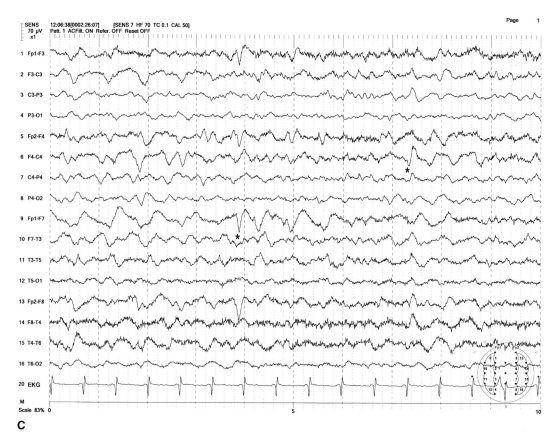

C

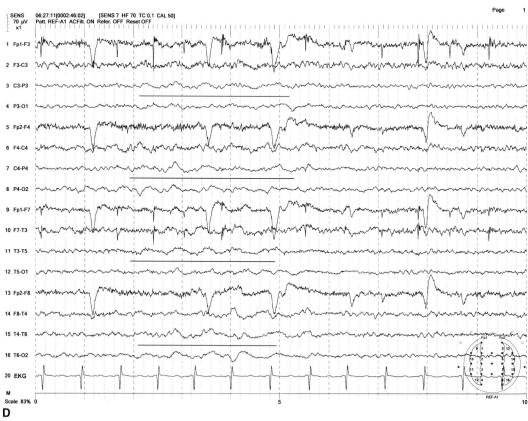

D

FIGURE 8-11 | *(Continued)*

limited to a left or right and posterior or anterior quadrant. For unknown reasons, changes in EEG activity are more sensitive in the temporal regions as compared to other regions. This, in turn, results in false-positive findings or false localizations to the temporal lobe. For example, a frontal or parietal lobe lesion may show maximum abnormality in the temporal electrodes.[16] On the other hand, false-negative findings are more common in parietal lobe or parasagittal lesions. If, however, the abnormalities are limited to the parietal region, this EEG localization is fairly accurate.

DIFFUSE ARRHYTHMIC DELTA ACTIVITY

Bilaterally diffuse ADA is a sign of diffuse disturbance of cerebral activity but is etiologically nonspecific. This may be seen in any diffuse cerebral dysfunction: toxic, metabolic, infectious, cerebral ischemia, or degenerative/demyelinating disorders. Diffuse white matter disease such as leukodystrophies can produce this pattern.[13] ADA may be associated with retained background activity (Fig. 8-12) or abnormally slow with absence of background activity (Fig. 8-13). The former implies primarily white matter disease, and the latter represents both cortical and white matter dysfunctions.

Diffuse ADA is addressed by amplitude, frequency, distribution, reactivity, and continuity and also by the presence or absence of abnormal background activity. Irrespective of amplitude, the slower the frequency, the worse the cerebral function. In cases of severe or acute cerebral dysfunction, there is paucity of background activity, and with improvement, there will be recovery of background activity superimposed upon or interspersed in between the delta activity. Continuous ADA without

a spontaneous or reactive change to stimulus is worse than ADA with a discontinuous or changing character. In a comatose patient having ADA with a mixture of theta waves, noxious stimulation may bring out higher-amplitude delta with reduction of theta activity (paradoxical arousal response) (see Fig. 6-19).

In comatose or stuporous patients, the EEG is a sensitive tool to determine the state of cerebral function, and serial EEGs are useful in evaluating the progress of the disease process or predicting the prognosis.

INTERMITTENT RHYTHMIC DELTA ACTIVITY

IRDA or RDA* consists of serial delta waves that appear intermittently with relatively consistent waveform and frequency.[17,18] IRDA is more commonly bilateral than focal or unilateral. If IRDA appears focally, one may consider it as possible epileptiform (ictal) activity. IRDA usually has frontal dominance [*FIRDA or frontally predominant GRDA* (*generalized rhythmic delta activity*)] (Fig. 8-14; see also Fig. 6-3) in adults but can be of *occipital dominance* (*OIRDA or occipitally predominant GRDA**), especially in children. OIRDA is common in children with absence seizures (Fig. 8-15; see video 10-6).[18,19] The difference in location from adults (FIRDA/frontally predominant GRDA*) to children (OIRDA/occipitally predominant GRDA*) is not related to the difference of pathology or lesion localization but simply appears to reflect an age-related variation.

FIRDA/frontally predominant GRDA* must be differentiated from the electrooculogram by vertical eye movement artifact or glossokinetic potential. In general, FIRDA/frontally predominant GRDA* can be distinguished from eye movement by its greater posterior spread as compared to the slow activity

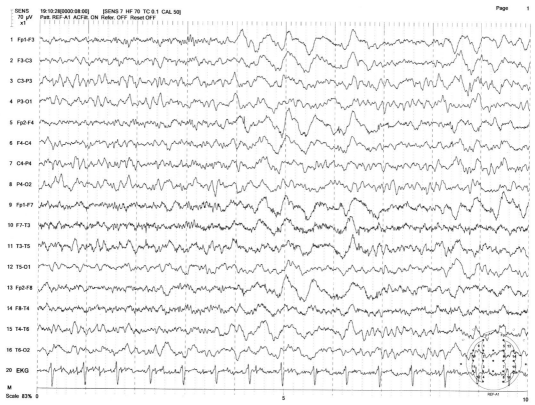

FIGURE 8-12 | Awake EEG in a 72-year-old woman with renal failure and dialysis. Note diffuse irregular delta activity but fairly well-presented background activity consisting of a mixture of alpha and theta rhythms.

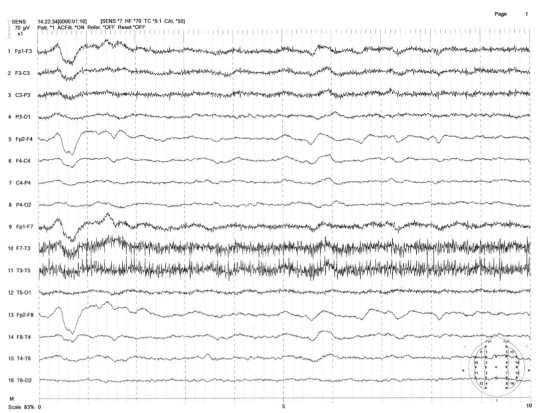

FIGURE 8-13 | EEG of a 57-year-old woman with acute encephalopathy of unknown etiology. The patient was obtunded at the time of EEG recording.

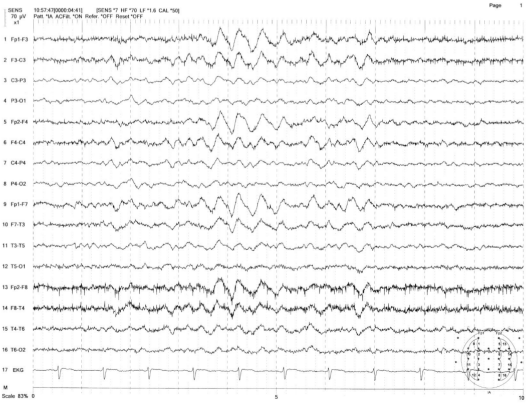

FIGURE 8-14 | An example of FIRDA in a 53-year-old man with moderate dementia with prominent impairment of language and visuospatial functions.

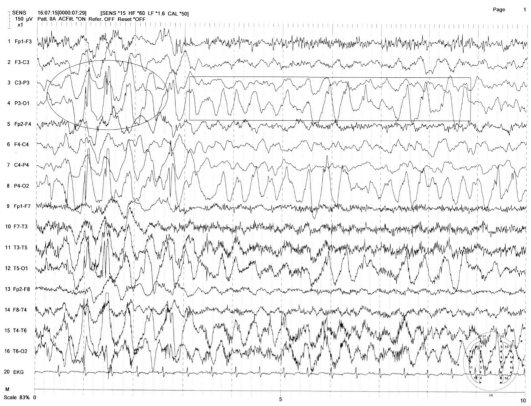

FIGURE 8-15 | An example of OIRDA in a 9-year-old boy with a history of absence seizures. Note occipital dominant 3-Hz spike–wave burst (shown by *oval circle*) mixed with 3-Hz OIRDA (shown by *rectangular box*).

produced by eye blinks (see Figs. 15-5 and 15-12A and B). In some cases, it is necessary to distinguish between the two by using additional electrodes placed on the infraorbital region; eye movement artifacts show an out-of-phase relationship between frontopolar (Fp1/Fp2) and infraorbital electrodes when referenced to ipsilateral ear electrode, whereas FIRDA activity is inphase. Both frontal delta and glossokinetic potentials are inphase, but frontal delta activity shows slightly higher amplitude at the frontopolar electrode than the infraorbital electrode, and the reverse is true for glossokinetic (Fig. 8-16A; see Chapter 15, "Eye Movement Artifacts" also Figs. 15-5, 15-11 to 15-13; and see also Video 15-3, 15-4). The lateral or horizontal eye movements also produce delta slow waves but can easily be differentiated from frontal delta or glossokinetic potential by opposite polarity between F7 and F8 electrodes for eye movement (see Fig. 7-29; see also Fig. 15-8). By placing eye monitor electrodes on each side of the outer cantus, one above and the other below a level horizontal line through the eye as shown in Figure 8-16B, all eye movements, either vertical or horizontal, show out-of-phase deflections between the two eye leads.

FIRDA is etiologically nonspecific and may be seen in any diffuse encephalopathy of various severities. If FIRDA is due to a hemispheric lesion, it more likely reflects a frontal lobe lesion.[20] In cases of mild encephalopathy, background activity is preserved, and in severe encephalopathy, background activity is suppressed. Earlier, FIRDA was thought to represent a "projecting rhythm" arising from increased intracranial pressure or deep midline or subcortical lesions.[21] This may be true in some cases, but FIRDA is more common in metabolic or other diffuse encephalopathies than in those with a focal deep seated lesion.

Because of the paroxysmal nature of this pattern, FIRDA may be difficult to differentiate from epileptiform activity in some cases, especially when associated with sharp or "spiky" components and appearing as a *triphasic wave*, which consists of initial sharply contoured negative–positive wave followed by negative slow (delta) waves. The triphasic pattern was first reported as a fairy specific pattern for the diagnosis of hepatic encephalopathy[22]; however, in reality, the pattern can be seen in many other metabolic/toxic encephalopathies or anoxic encephalopathy (see also Chapter 11, Triphasic waves). Triphasic patterns may vary from one case to another (Fig. 8-17A–C; see also Figs. 11-11 and 11-12). Some triphasic patterns may be difficult to differentiate from spike–wave discharges seen in epilepsy patients (Fig. 8-17D). The differentiation depends on the "spikiness" in the configuration of the initial negative potential (see Fig. 13-1B and C; see also Video 13-3A and B). Frontal dominant paroxysmal delta activity resembling FIRDA/frontal predominant GRDA* may be seen during the awake state in sleep-deprived individuals[22] or in normal elderly people.[23] Frontal dominant rhythmic delta activity is also seen during hyperventilation or during drowsiness in normal children.

IRDA in the temporal region, referred to as *TIRDA* (*temporal intermittent rhythmic delta activity or temporally predominant GRDA*), is often associated with temporal lobe epilepsy.[24]

Paroxysmal Activity

Paroxysmal activity is defined as discharges of abrupt onset and sudden termination that are clearly distinguishable from the ongoing background activity. These may appear in a single waveform (transient) arising either from a single focus or multiple independent foci (Fig. 8-18), serial arrhythmic (Fig. 8-19), or serial rhythmic waveform (burst)

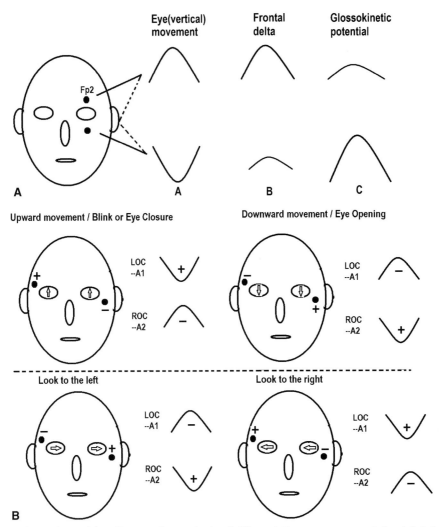

FIGURE 8-16 | **A:** Schematic model to illustrate the methods of differentiating eye movement, frontal delta (FIRDA), and glossokinetic potential. The two channel recordings in the top example from Fp1 or Fp2 and infraorbital electrodes, each referenced to the ipsilateral ear, show an "out-of-phase" relationship for vertical eye movement *(A)* but an "inphase" relationship for frontal delta *(B)*. Although tongue movement artifact (glossokinetic potential) also shows an "inphase" relationship, this shows greater amplitude of delta at infraorbital electrodes than at Fp1 or Fp2 electrode *(C)*. **B:** By placing the eye monitor electrodes at left and right outer cantus, one at above and the other below the eye level, as shown in the figure, all eye movements, either vertical or horizontal, shows "out of phase" relationship between the two electrodes.

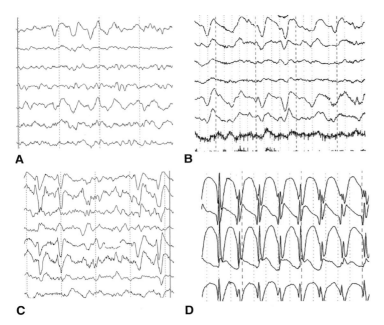

FIGURE 8-17 | Varieties of triphasic wave forms **(A–C)** from suggestive triphasic wave with minimal negative sharp discharge preceding delta wave **(A)** to distinct triphasic wave with prominent negative sharp followed by delta wave. **B:** Triphasic pattern with waveform in between **(A)** and **(C)**. **D:** Triphasic pattern but with typical spike–wave discharge. In some cases, distinction between triphasic sharp delta discharge and spike–wave discharge may not be clear.

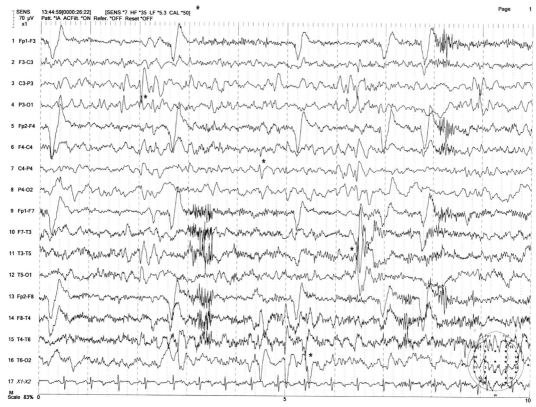

FIGURE 8-18 | Multifocal sharp and spike discharges in a 4-year-old boy with a history of partial complex seizure and generalized tonic–clonic convulsions. There are at least four spike foci appearing as single or repetitive transients from P3, C4, T3, and T6 electrodes (shown by *asterisk*) independently.

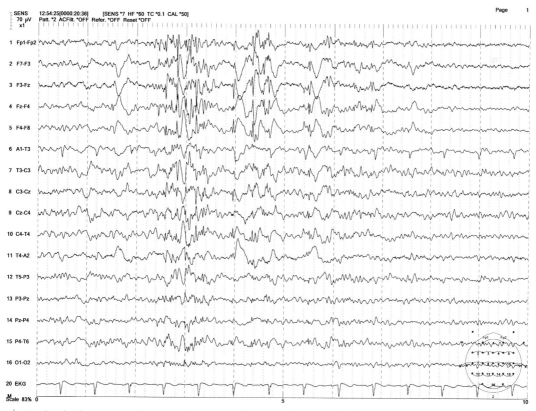

FIGURE 8-19 | Serial arrhythmic polyspike–wave bursts in a 25-year-old man with a history of myoclonic seizures.

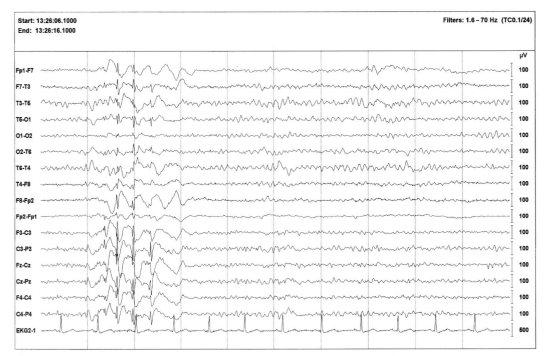

FIGURE 8-20 | Serial rhythmic 3-Hz spike–wave bursts in a 12-year-old girl with a history of absence seizures.

(Fig. 8-20). Paroxysmal activity generally implies potential seizure tendency and could be referred to as epileptiform activity. Some of the paroxysmal discharges are, however, physiological (e.g., vertex sharp waves and K complexes of sleep, delta bursts during hyperventilation, or drowsiness in children). Whether the pattern is normal or abnormal is dependent upon the spatial (frontal, temporal, occipital, etc.) and temporal (awake or sleep) relationship with given discharges (see "Temporal and Spatial Factor," Chapter 6; see also Fig. 6-7A and B, Fig. 6-8).

Paroxysmal activity consisting of spikes or spike–wave is more specific for a seizure diagnosis than that of sharp or other activities such as theta or delta waves. By definition, a spike is a transient with a pointed peak having a duration of 20 to 70 ms, and a sharp wave has a more blunted peak with duration of 70 to 200 ms (see Fig. 6-5A and B). In reality, distinction between the two is not always precise, and they have, therefore, been used interchangeably. Rather than duration of the discharge, waveform morphology, that is, the "sharpness" of the peak or slope (segmental velocity) by the EEGer's eyes, customarily defines the "spike" or "spike equivalent potential"(see Fig. 6-5C).[25] The morphology of a spike can be monophasic, diphasic, triphasic, or polyphasic (Fig. 8-21). A polyspike is defined as multiple spike complex. A spike followed by a wave is defined as a spike-and-wave complex.

The voltage topography of a spike on the scalp surface creates dipole fields. When the spike is generated at the crown of the cortex, it creates a radially (vertically) oriented dipole with maximum negativity just above the source with a positive field at a distant site, either deeper or in the opposite hemisphere (Fig. 8-22A). When the spike is generated

in the sulcus of the cortex, it yields tangentially (horizontally) oriented dipoles with fields of maximum negativity and positivity being displaced at either side of the source (Fig. 8-22B).

In epileptic conditions, cortical neurons change dramatically as the membrane potential changes from a resting state (at negative 70 to 80 mV) to sustained depolarization (positive 20 to 30 mV), thereby producing a group of action potentials. This is called *paroxysmal depolarization shift*

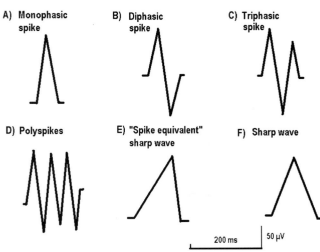

FIGURE 8-21 | Schematic models of morphology of various spikes and sharp discharges. Note the "spike equivalent potential" **(E)** having a steep declining phase (high segmental velocity).

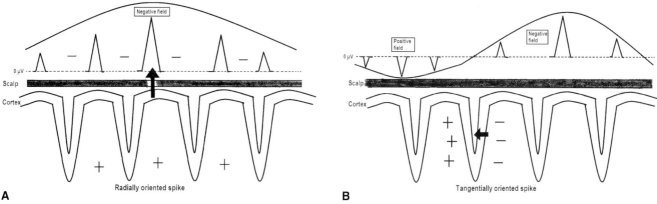

FIGURE 8-22 | Schematic models of spike orientation in relationship with the surface potential field. The radially oriented spike arising from the crown of cortex yields a maximum negative field just above the source of the spike and a positive field at a distance **(A)**. The tangentially oriented spike arising from the cortical sulcus creates surface-negative and surface-positive fields, posterior and anterior to the source, respectively, with maximum negativity and positivity being slightly displaced from the source. (The region closest to the source is actually "0" potential.) **(B)**.

(*PDS*).[26,27] This PDS originating from wide cortical regions is associated with spike discharges recorded from the scalp EEG (Fig. 8-23). In spike–wave complexes, a spike is the result of an *EPSP* (*excitatory postsynaptic potential*), whereas a wave is generated by an *IPSP* (*inhibitory postsynaptic potential*)[28] (see also Chapter 5: Cellular anatomy and physiology). Thus, the 3-Hz spike–wave bursts in absence seizures are viewed as alternating excitatory and inhibitory processes, whereas polyspike discharges represent sustained excitation. In tonic–clonic seizures, sustained muscle contraction during the tonic phase corresponds to polyspikes (i.e., sustained EPSP at the cellular level), and the clonic phase corresponds to spike-and-wave discharges (i.e., alternating EPSP and IPSP at the cellular level). The above are extremely simplified models; in reality, much more complex interactions, integration, and interfering actions occur among vast amount of excitatory and inhibitory neurons.

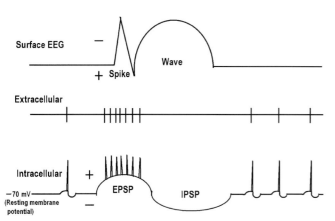

FIGURE 8-23 | Schematic relationship between intracellular and surface recording of spike discharges. The sustained depolarization of EPSP (paroxysmal depolarized shift) yields the group of action potentials, which correspond with surface "spike" discharges. This is followed by IPSP, corresponding with surface "wave." Isolated action potentials produce no change in cortical EEG.

References

1. Arfel G, Fischgold H. EEG-signs in tumours of brain. *Electroencephalogr Clin Neurophysiol Suppl* 1961;19:36–50.
2. Bancaud J, Hecaen H, Lairy GC. Modifications de la reactivite EEG, troubles de fonctions symboliques et troubles confusionnels dans les lesion hemispheriques localisees. *Electroencephalogr Clin Neurophysiol* 1955;7:179–192.
3. Jasper HH, Van Buren J. Interrelationship between cortex and subcortical structure: Clinical electroencephalographic studies. *Electroencephalogr Clin Neurophysiol* 1953;5:33–40.
4. Hammand EJ, Wilder BJ, Ballinger WE Jr. Electrophysiologic recording in a patient with a discrete unilateral thalamic infarction. *J Neurol Neurosurg Psychiatry* 1982;45:640–643.
5. Gibbs FA, Gibbs EL, Lennox WG. Electroencephalographic classification of epileptic patients and control subjects. *Arch Neurol Psychiatry* 1943;50:111–128.
6. Vogel F, Gotze W. Familienuntersurchungen zur genetik des normalen. Elektroenzephalogramms. *Dtsch A Nervenheilk* 1959;178:668–700.
7. Rosas HD, Koroshetz WS, Chen YI, et al. Evidence for more widespread cerebral pathology in early HD. *Neurology (Minneap)* 2003;60:1615–1620.
8. Dall Bernardina B, Perez-Jimenez A, Fontana E, et al. Electroencephalographic findings associated with cortical dysplasias. In: Guerrini R, Andermann F, Canapicchi R, et al., eds. *Dysplasias of Cerebral Cortex and Epilepsy*. Philadelphia, PA: Lippincott-Raven Publishers, 1996:235–245.
9. Gastaut H, Pinsard N, Raybaud C, et al. Lissencephaly (agyria-pachygyria): Clinical features and serial EEG studies. *Dev Med Child Neurol* 1987;29:167–180.
10. Cobb WA, Guiloff RJ, Cast J. Breach rhythm: The EEG related to skull defects. *Electroencephalogr Clin Neurophysiol* 1979;47:251–271.
11. Gibbs FA, Gibbs EL. *Atlas of Electroencephalography*. Vol. 3. Reading, MA: Addison-Wesley, 1964.
12. Worrell GA, Parish L, Cranstoun SD, et al. High-frequency oscillation and seizure generation in neocortical epilepsy. *Brain* 2004;149:1496–1506.
13. Schmitt SE, Pargeon K, Frechette ES, et al. Extreme delta brush: A unique EEG pattern in adults with anti-NMDA receptor encephalitis. *Neurology* 2012;79:1094–1100.
14. Walter WG. The localization of cerebral tumours by electroencephalography. *Lancet* 1936;2:305–308.
15. Gloor P, Kalabay O, Giard N. The electroencephalogram in diffuse encephalopathies: Electroencephalographic correlates of grey and white matter lesion. *Brain* 1968;91:779–802.

16. Joynt RJ, Cape CA, Knott JR. Significance of focal delta activity in adult electroencephalogram. *Arch Neurol (Chicago)* 1965;12:631–638.

17. Cobb WA. Rhythmic slow discharges in the electroencephalogram. *J Neurol Neurosurg Psychiatry* 1945;8:65–78.

18. Van der Drift JH, Magnus O. The value of the EEG in the differential diagnosis of cases with cerebral lesion. *Electroencephalogr Clin Neurophysiol Suppl* 1961;19:183–196.

19. Dalby MA. Epilepsy and 3 per second and wave rhythms: A clinical electroencephalographic and prognosis analysis of 346 patients. *Acta Neurol Scand Suppl* 1969;40:43.

20. Van der Drift JHA. *The Significance of Electroencephalography for the Diagnosis and Localization of Cerebral Tumours.* Leiden: H.E. Stenfert-Kroese, 1957.

21. Daly DD, Whelan JL, Bickford R, et al. The electroencephalogram in cases of tumor of the posterior fossa and third ventricle. *Electroencephalogr Clin Neurophysiol* 1953;5:203–216.

22. Rodin EA, Ludy ED, Gottlieb JS. The electroencephalogram during prolonged experimental sleep deprivation. *Electroencephalogr Clin Neurophysiol* 1962;14:544–551.

23. Torres F, Faoro A, Loeweson R, et al. The electroencephalography of elderly patients revisited. *Electroencephalogr Clin Neurophysiol* 1983;56:391–398.

24. Reiher J, Beaudry M, Leduc CP. Temporal intermittent rhythmic delta activity (TIRDA) and the diagnosis of complex partial epilepsy: Sensitivity, specificity and predictive value. *Can J Neurol Sci* 1989;16:398–401.

25. Kooi KA. Voltage-time characteristics of spike and other rapid electrographic transients: Semantic and morphological consideration. *Neurology (Minneap)* 1966;16:59–66.

26. Goldensohn ES, Purpura DP. Intracellular potentials of cortical neurons during focal epileptogenic discharges. *Science* 1963;193:840–842.

27. Matsumoto H, Marsan CA. Cortical cellular phenomena in experimental epilepsy: Ictal manifestation. *Exp Neurol* 1964;9:305–326.

28. Pollen DA. Intracellular studies of cortical neurons during thalamic induced wave and spike. *Electroencephalogr Clin Neurophysiol* 1964;17:398–406.

Activation Procedures

THORU YAMADA and ELIZABETH MENG

Activation procedures include various sensory and pharmacological stimulations to alter the physiological state. They are usually aimed at eliciting or enhancing abnormal activity, especially epileptiform activity. The most commonly used sensory stimulation is photic stimulation. Others include tactile or electrical stimuli for somatosensory stimulation and music or sounds for auditory stimulation. Pharmacological activation includes pentylenetetrazol to induce a seizure or benzodiazepine to attenuate one. The most routine activation procedures in any EEG laboratory are hyperventilation (HV), photic stimulation (PS), and sleep.

Hyperventilation

NORMAL HYPERVENTILATION RESPONSE

This procedure consists of deep and regular breathing at a rate of about 3 to 4 per 10 seconds for a period of 3 to 5 minutes. In young children, HV can be successfully performed by asking the child to blow on a pinwheel. A characteristic HV response consists of bilaterally diffuse and synchronous slow-wave bursts, initially with theta frequency and then progressing to delta frequency. This is called "HV buildup" (Figs. 9-1A and B and 9-2A and B). The amplitude may reach as high as 500 μV. Theta–delta buildup by HV is usually anterior dominant in adolescents or adults but may be posterior dominant in children. These occur in a serial semi-rhythmic fashion with fluctuating amplitude (Video 9-1). The effect is most prominent in children between the ages 8 and 12 years and progressively decreases toward adulthood (compare Figs. 9-1B and 9-2B); a clear HV response is seen in about 70% of children, but in adults, it may be less than 10%.[1] HV effects, however, vary considerably from one individual to another. Physiologically, HV reduces the carbon dioxide concentration (PCO_2), which causes vasoconstriction and reduction of cerebral blood flow. The reduction of PCO_2 (*hypocapnia*) is likely the major factor in producing HV buildup.[1] HV buildup is enhanced by a blood sugar level below 80 mg/100 mL.[2] Therefore, HV buildup may be more prominent when the patient is hungry or his/her last meal was some time ago. In subjects who show a low-voltage and poorly defined alpha rhythm, HV may bring out a better defined alpha rhythm.

Some delta bursts induced by HV may include "spiky" or spike-like discharges (small notched spikes preceding or mixed with theta–delta activity) especially in children. Unequivocal spikes or clear focal or lateralizing (focal) changes elicited by HV are considered to be abnormal. After cessation of HV, the patient may complain of numbness or tingling in the fingers and lips, transient blurring of vision, or ringing in the ears. Some may even show changes of consciousness or awareness. These symptoms are self-limiting and are not necessarily associated with EEG changes or related to the degree of buildup. Likewise, after cessation of HV, the slow waves disappear quickly and the EEG returns to the pre-HV state within 30 seconds. In some subjects, though, the effect may continue for a minute or longer. One should be cautious in interpreting a long-lasting post-HV effect, since some subjects may continue to hyperventilate even after being told to stop. The technologist should observe carefully to make sure that the patient did indeed stop HV. If the delta bursts appear longer than 1 minute in the post-HV period, they are not likely related to the HV effect. (An exception to this is seen in *moyamoya disease*.)[3,4]

ABNORMAL HYPERVENTILATION RESPONSE

HV is a well-known activation procedure for inducing absence seizures. HV activates more than 80% of untreated children with absence seizures.[5] It is important for the technologist to document clinical signs associated with an absence seizure. With a sudden onset of rhythmic (monomorphic) 3-Hz spike–wave bursts (Fig. 9-3; Video 9-2, also see Video 10-6), the patient usually stops HV and often stares into space, sometimes with eyelid or facial muscle twitches. If 3-Hz spike–wave bursts last longer than 5 seconds, the technologist is usually able to observe a clinical change by examining the patient's level of consciousness. An astute technologist will quickly ask the patient to remember words presented during the event and ask the patient after the event if he or she can recall the presented words. If the patient's communication or consciousness is impaired, the patient will not be able to recall the word spoken during the episode. A more accurate assessment may be made by testing reaction time; the patient is instructed to press a button (which makes a mark on the EEG recording) in response to an auditory signal given by the technologist during the event of 3-Hz spike–wave bursts. With cessation of the spike–wave

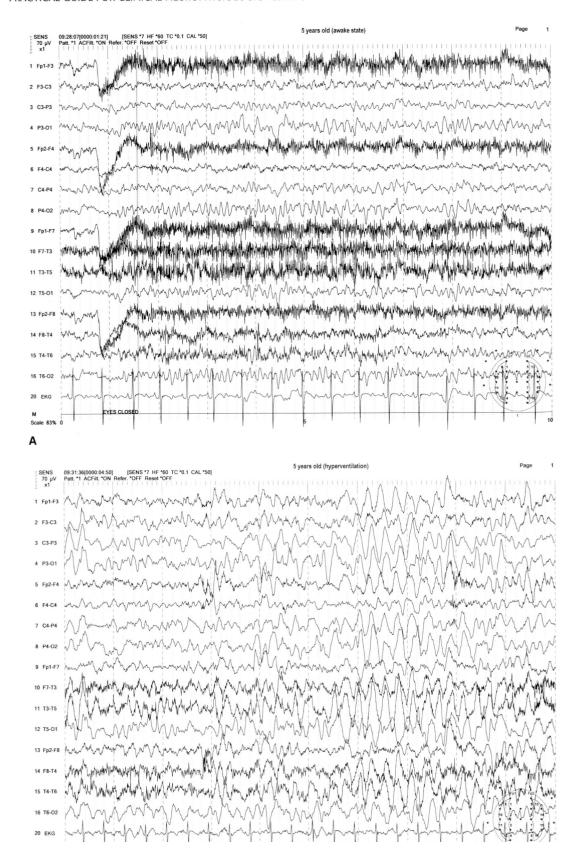

FIGURE 9-1 | Comparison of resting EEG in the awake state **(A)** and EEG during hyperventilation **(B)** in a 5-year-old boy. Note the increase of posterior delta waves (posterior slow waves of youth) and semirhythmic 3- to 4-Hz generalized delta–theta bursts during hyperventilation **(B)**.

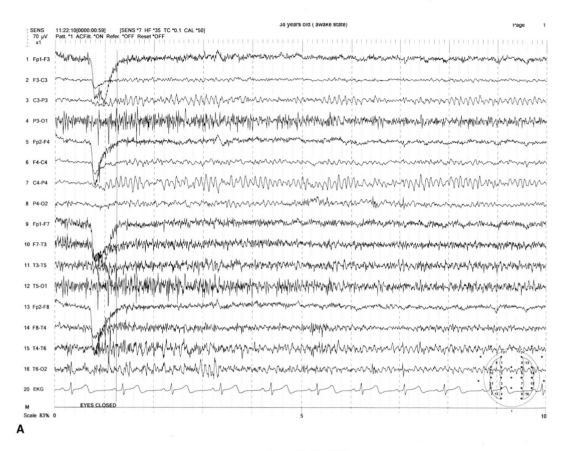

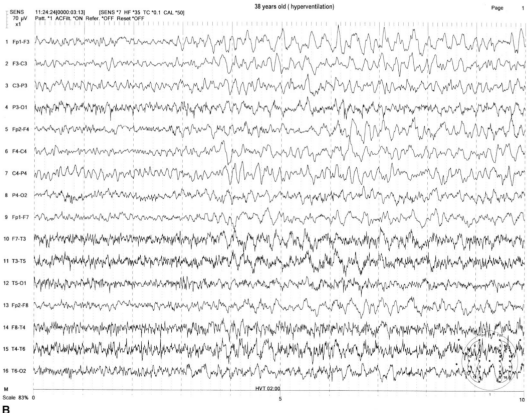

FIGURE 9-2 | Comparison of resting EEG in the awake state **(A)** and EEG during hyperventilation **(B)** in a 38-year-old man. Note the generalized bursts of 4- to 6-Hz theta waves. This is unusually prominent HV response in this age of patient. The frequency of bursts is faster than that seen in children (Fig. 9-1B).

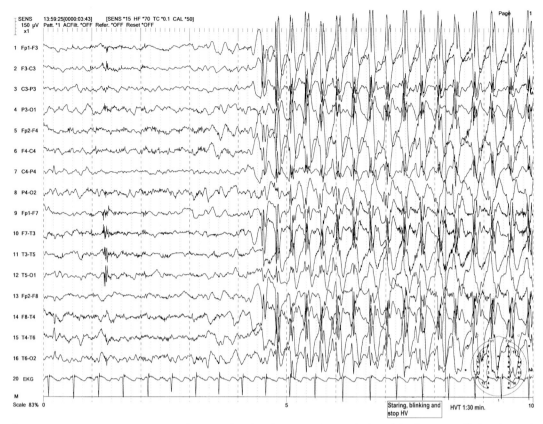

FIGURE 9-3 | Typical 3-Hz spike–wave bursts, characteristic for absence seizures, induced by hyperventilation in an 8-year-old girl. Apparently, a clinical seizure was associated with the event involving staring and blinking as noted by a technologist.

bursts, the patient usually resumes HV without being prompted by the technologist. There is no postictal confusion or impaired consciousness.

HV may also activate focal or other types of generalized seizures, or precipitate interictal epileptiform activity, though the incidence of such activation is far less (~5%) than that for absence seizures. Much more vigorous and prolonged HV is usually required to elicit partial seizures.[6]

HV may accentuate focal slowing, which is sometimes useful for verifying uncertain or subtle focal features observed in the resting EEG. One unique HV effect has been observed in *moyamoya disease* in which the delta bursts reappear 3 to 5 minutes after cessation of HV, called the "re-buildup" HV effect.[3,4]

CONTRAINDICATIONS OF HYPERVENTILATION

The American Clinical Neurophysiology Society (formerly American EEG Society)[7] recommended that HV should not be performed in certain clinical settings.

Included contraindications are acute stroke, recent intracranial hemorrhage, large-vessel stenosis, recent TIA, moyamoya disease, severe cardiopulmonary disorders, and sickle cell disease or trait. All these conditions are related to cerebrovascular problems.

Photic Stimulation

Photic stimulation is a routine activation procedure performed in most EEG laboratories. This is done primarily to elicit a

photoparoxysmal response for the diagnosis of photosensitive epilepsy. Photic stimulation provides other physiological responses but of less diagnostic value.

PROCEDURE

Photic stimulation commonly uses a stroboscope to deliver a repetitive, diffuse, flashing light of brief duration (10 to 30 ms). The repetitive rate is usually 1 to 30 Hz. The strobe light is placed directly in front of the patient's eyes at a distance of about 30 cm. The patient's eyes are usually closed during delivery of photic stimulation, but some laboratories prefer to have the eyes open at first and closed during the middle of photic stimulation (because this may enhance the incidence of the photoparoxysmal response).

The duration of each set of repetitive stimuli is usually 10 seconds, followed by 10 seconds of resting time before delivering the next set of stimuli. The stimulus rates vary according to laboratory protocols and technologist preference. It is typical to deliver a series of six to eight different frequencies. Some laboratories include crescendo type and decrescendo type of stimulus rates with a progressively increasing stimulus rate from 1 to 30 Hz and then a progressively decreasing stimulus rate from 30 to 1 Hz (see Fig. 7-26C).

PHOTIC DRIVING RESPONSE

The photic driving responses elicited by 5- to 30-Hz stimuli consist of occipital dominant rhythmic waves with a one-to-one frequency relationship with each flash (Fig. 9-4A).

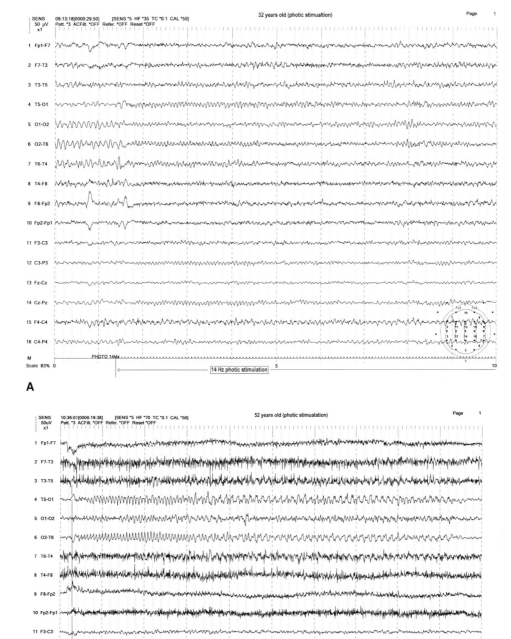

FIGURE 9-4 | Typical photic driving response with 14-Hz photic stimuli. Note the rhythmic activity with photic stimulation. The driving responses fade toward the end of the stimulation **(A)**. In some individuals, the frequency of the occipital response becomes half (sub-harmonic) of the frequency of photic stimuli **(B)**. In this individual, the driving response started with the same frequency as the stimulus frequency at first but became half the frequency in the middle of photic stimulation. Note the "on-response" by broad sharp transient occurring approximately 150 to 200 ms. after the onset of photic stimulation (indicated by *vertical line*).

Within one set of flashes, the driving response frequency may change from one-to-one to a harmonic or subharmonic pattern (Fig. 9-4B). The responses are usually most prominent at the flash frequency closest to the frequency of the individual's alpha rhythm. In a young child, the driving response may be elicited at theta frequency flashes. The amplitude of the photic driving response is generally higher in children and better visualized in adults with low-voltage background activity. The patients who have large lambda waves and/or POSTS tend to have large photic driving responses (see "Lambda Waves," Chapter 7; see also Fig. 7-26A–C). A photic driving response is absent in a blind person, but absence of a photic driving response per se is not an abnormal finding. It should be noted that the photic response with a slow frequency (<3 Hz) is not a driving response but rather an evoked potential elicited by each flash (Fig. 9-5). In some subjects, there are diffuse sharp discharges at the onset or offset of photic stimulation, called the on-response and off-response, respectively (see Fig. 9-4B).

PHOTOPAROXYSMAL RESPONSES

This was formerly referred to as the *"photoconvulsive response,"* but the use of this term is now discouraged. *Photoparoxysmal responses* (PPRs) typically consist of high-amplitude generalized irregular spike–wave or polyspike–wave bursts, with either bianterior or biposterior dominance (Figs. 9-6A and B and 9-7A and B; Videos 9-3; see also Video 10-7; Figs. 10-6B, 10-18B, and 10-21B). The most effective frequency is 15 to 20 Hz.[8] The incidence of PPR is highest between ages 6 and 15 and decreases with age.[9,10] PPRs correlate highly with a diagnosis of epilepsy; approximately 70% to 80% of patients with PPRs have epilepsy.[11,12] The seizure correlation is especially high in PPRs with spike–wave bursts that persist well beyond termination (>200 ms) of the flash stimulus (sustained PPR) (see Figs. 9-6A and 9-7B), as compared to the PPRs in which the spike–wave bursts cease at or before the termination of the flash stimulus[13] (self-limited PPR) (Fig. 9-6B). The frequency of PPRs is typically independent of the photic stimulus rates. Some of the atypical photic driving responses may consist of spike–wave-like discharges which are time locked and sustained in a one-to-one relationship with the stimulus rate. These should not be considered a PPR (Fig. 9-8).

The seizure type most often associated with PPR is *generalized tonic–clonic* (>80%). *Juvenile myoclonic epilepsy* (JME) has an incidence of PPR greater than 1/3.[14] Absence and *myoclonic seizures* represent less than 10% of all PPRs.[15] Partial seizures, especially temporal lobe seizures, associated with PPRs are extremely rare, if any, but may occur with occipital lobe seizures (see Fig. 10-6A and B).[16] If PPR is observed in a patient with complex partial seizure, this likely suggests that this patient has both types of seizures: primary generalized and complex seizures.

Some PPRs are more readily activated by a pattern such as dots or stripes. Overall, pattern stimulation is more effective for eliciting PPRs than a diffuse strobe light.[17] The color of photic stimulation also affects the degree of photosensitivity. A red color is more effective for eliciting PPRs than white flashes, and blue tinted sunglasses have been recommended for preventing

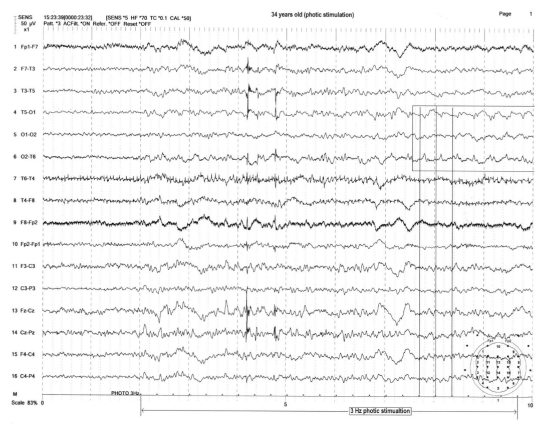

FIGURE 9-5 | Photic responses at slow-frequency rates. In some individuals, there may be a distinct response at slow-frequency (1- to 3-Hz) stimulation. Note the small sharp and wave complex in the occipital electrodes, time locked to, but slightly following, each flash. Examples are shown in the *rectangular box*. This is not a driving response but rather a photic-induced evoked potential.

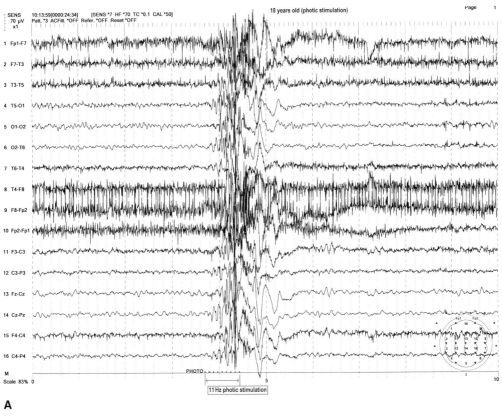

A

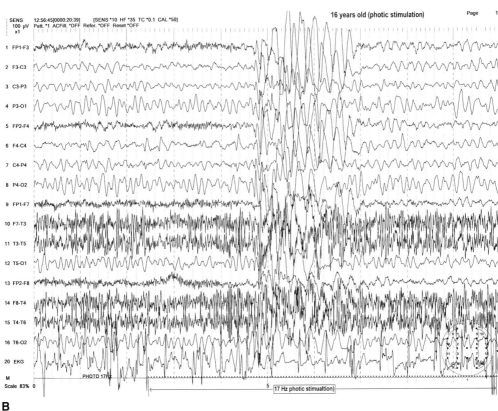

B

FIGURE 9-6 | Example of photoparoxysmal responses. In **(A)**, generalized irregular polyspike–wave bursts started immediately after the onset of 11-Hz photic stimulation. Spike–waves continued despite quick cessation of photic stimulation (unlimited photoparoxysmal response). In **(B)**, generalized irregular spike–wave bursts started in the middle of photic stimulation and ceased despite continuation of photic stimulation (self-limited photoparoxysmal response). A sustained photoparoxysmal response **(A)** is more epileptogenic and more likely associated with a history of seizure than the self-limited photoparoxysmal response **(B)**.

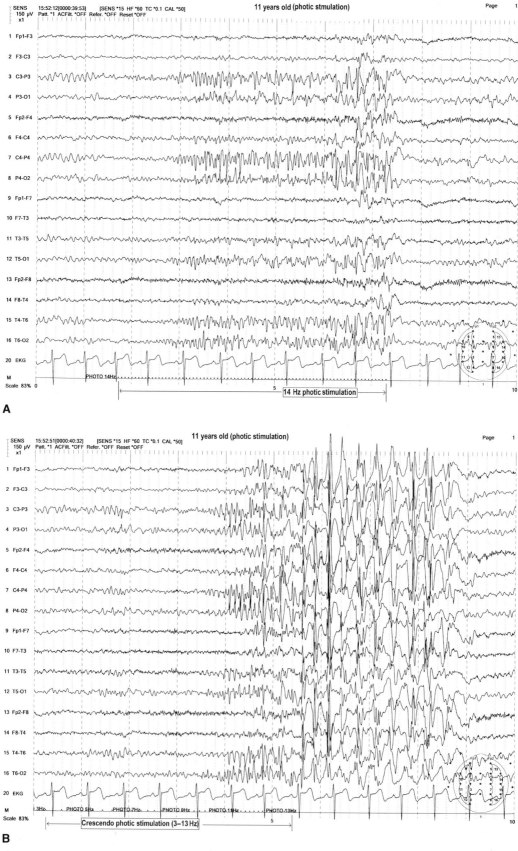

FIGURE 9-7 | Photoparoxysmal response with occipital onset in an 11-year-old girl. The photoparoxysmal response started in the occipital regions with frequency-dependent repetitive sharp discharges and became frequency-independent assuming spike–wave discharges toward the end of photic stimulation **(A)**. In crescendo photic stimulation, spike discharges started in the occipital electrodes at around 12-Hz photic stimuli and then evolved to generalized spike–wave bursts, which continued well after the cessation of photic stimulation **(B)**.

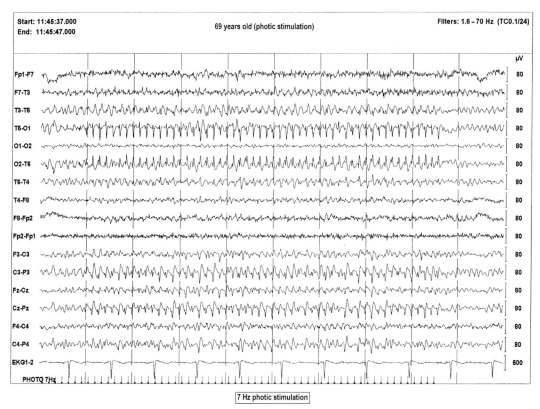

FIGURE 9-8 | Prominent photic responses in a 69-year-old woman. Note the repetitive spike–wave discharges consistently time locked with each flash. This is not a photoparoxysmal response.

seizure due to photosensitive epilepsy.[18] Technologists should be able to quickly identify the onset of a photoparoxysmal response (epileptiform activity) so that the stimulus may be stopped before provoking a clinical generalized tonic–clonic seizure. Once the technologist recognizes the PPRs, however, the same frequency of photic stimulation should be repeated to verify that the evoked epileptiform activity is indeed induced by photic stimulation and is not an incidental occurrence during photic stimulation. In this situation, the technologist must be extremely alert so as to stop photic stimulation immediately upon the onset of a photoparoxysmal response (see Fig. 9-6A). The technologist should also be able to differentiate a photoparoxysmal response from physiological variants of photic stimulation (see Fig. 9-8) or from a *photomyogenic response* (see "Photomyogenic Response"), which is not considered to be abnormal.

One remarkable incidence occurred in December 1997 in Japan; approximately 700 children throughout Japan had seizures almost simultaneously while watching a television cartoon program called pocket monster, or "Pokemon."[19] This was apparently caused by alternating red/blue frames flickering at 12 Hz on the TV screen. A photosensitive seizure may also be triggered by playing video games.[20]

The animal model of photosensitive epilepsy has been studied extensively in the photosensitive baboon, *Papio papio.*[21]

PHOTOMYOGENIC RESPONSE

The photomyogenic response (PMR) (formerly referred to as the "*photomyoclonic* response" [the term is now discouraged]) consists of EMG artifacts time locked with the flash frequency (Fig. 9-9A). These muscle potentials most often arise from frontal and orbicularis oculi muscles. Visible muscle twitches, time locked with the stimulus, may appear in the eyelids or face. In some occasions, muscle contractions progressively increase (Fig. 9-9B), involving larger muscle groups, spreading to the neck or upper body as the stimulus continues. This may appear clinically to be a generalized clonic seizure. In addition to the time-locked characteristics, stopping the stimulus will immediately stop the response in PMR. It is important for the technologist to note if there are any muscle twitches (often eyelid twitches) associated with the PMRs.

PMR may be enhanced with alcohol[22] or in a barbiturate withdrawal state.[23] However, PMR is essentially a nonspecific finding and should not be considered an abnormal response.

ATYPICAL PHOTIC RESPONSE

An asymmetric photic driving response (often right greater than left) is not an uncommon finding and should not be considered an abnormal response unless it is associated with another abnormality. If the photic driving response is asymmetric, POSTS and lambda waves are likely to show a similar asymmetry.

In patients who have slow background activity, a slow stimulus rate (1 to 3 Hz) may bring out delta activity, called "*delta driving*" (this is not an evoked potential),[24] enhancing the preexisting underlying slowing (Fig. 9-10). In some individuals, the photic stimulation elicits small spike–waves, which are time locked to the stimulus (see Fig. 9-8). This is an "exaggerated" evoked potential and should not be confused with a PPR. A relatively specific diagnostic pattern of photic stimulation is

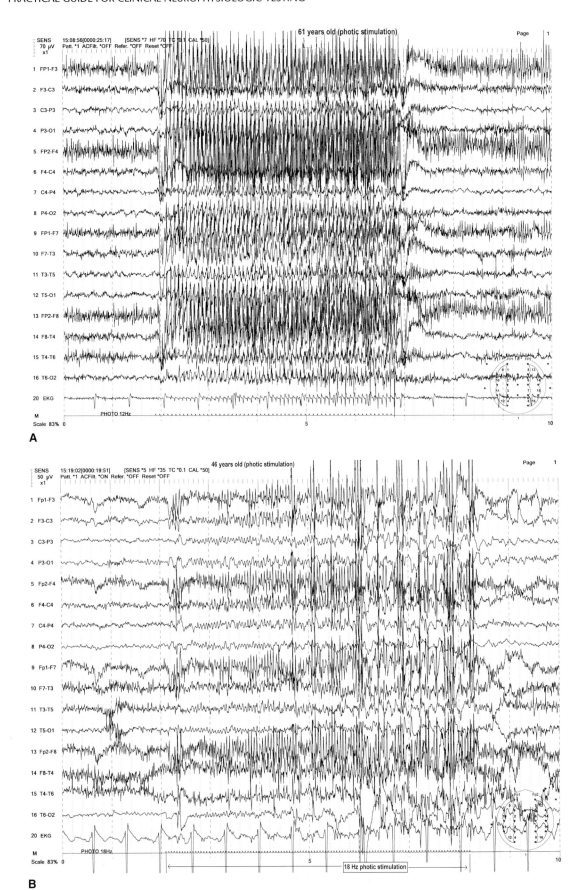

FIGURE 9-9 | Examples of the photomyogenic responses. Note EMG artifact time locked with the frequency of photic stimulation. In **(A)**, EMG artifacts started abruptly with the onset of photic stimulation and stopped abruptly with the cessation of photic stimulation, whereas in **(B)**, EMG gradually increased but abruptly stopped with the cessation of photic stimulation.

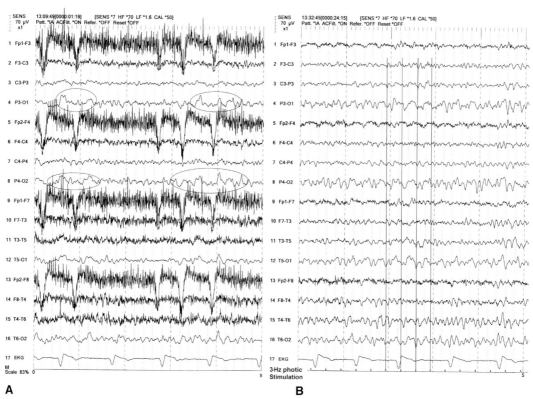

FIGURE 9-10 | "Delta driving" in a 65-year-old man. Waking background activity in this patient consisted of a mixture of theta and delta activities as shown by *oval circles* **(A)**. The 3-Hz photic stimulation introduced rhythmic 3-Hz delta activity in the occipital electrodes as indicated by *vertical lines* **(B)**.

high-amplitude spikes in the occipital region, time locked with a slow stimulus rate in a young child. This is a characteristic photic response for a patient with *ceroid lipofuscinosis* (*Batten's disease*) (Fig. 9-11).[25,26] In some individuals, a prominent *electroretinogram* (*ERG*), which ordinarily is recorded by a corneal electrode, may be seen at the Fp1 and Fp2 electrodes (see Fig. 15-14A and B). The ERG consists of two peaks, sharply contoured A and rounded B waves. These waves should also not be confused with spike–wave discharges.

Sleep Activation

Sleep is an essential tool for activating both generalized and focal *interictal epileptiform discharges* (*IEDs*). The technologist should always try to obtain a sleep record in patients with suspected seizures. If an awake-only EEG shows no IEDs or only questionable IEDs in suspected seizure patients, a repeat EEG with a sleep record should be justified. It is preferable to record an EEG after sleep deprivation so that a sleep record is achieved without sedation. If sedation is required, most EEG laboratories prefer chloral hydrate because the medication is relatively safe, does not increase beta activity, and does not attenuate IEDs. Benzodiazepines or barbiturates are not ideal for obtaining sleep recordings because they tend to produce excessive beta activity and may attenuate the IED.

In about one third of patients with partial complex seizures, no IEDs occur in the awake state and appear only in sleep.[27] Focal IEDs tend to be more generalized or may become multifocal in sleep. Since most sleep activation occurs in stage I or

II sleep, 20 to 30 minutes of stage I and II sleep recording will suffice to activate most IEDs.[28] In REM sleep, like during the awake EEG, IEDs are decreased or abolished.

Some epileptic syndromes have dramatically increased IEDs in sleep. Examples are *continuous spike–wave pattern during slow-wave sleep* (*CSWS*),[29] *Landau–Kleffner syndrome* (Fig. 9-12A and B),[30] and *benign epileptiform central midtemporal spikes* (*BECTS*)[31] (Fig. 9-13A and B) (see "Benign Epilepsy of Childhood with Central Midtemporal Spikes," Chapter 10, for further details).[31]

Sleep deprivation is an effective method for activating IEDs.[32] Sleep deprivation not only promotes sleep but also tends to enhance IEDs. In some patients, IEDs may appear in the awake state only after sleep deprivation.[33]

Pharmacological Activation

In order to evaluate a patient's seizures clinically as well as electrophysiologically, earlier studies used intravenous drugs to induce seizures. These include *pentylenetetrazole, methohexital, and bemegride* (*Megimide*). One problem associated with a drug-induced seizure is a false-positive seizure activation, or it may activate a seizure focus other than the focus related to the spontaneous seizures. Thus, IV drug activation is no longer routinely used.

Pharmacological activation, therefore, mainly focuses upon the withdrawal of antiepileptic drugs. Due to the risk of seizure recurrence, including status epilepticus, drug withdrawal has to be done in an inpatient setting and under close observation

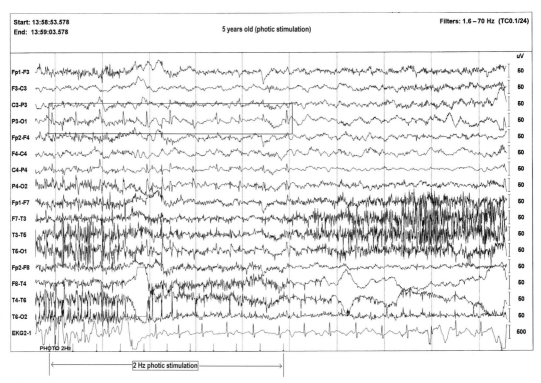

FIGURE 9-11 | Photic stimulation induced spikes in a 5-year-old boy with a diagnosis of Batten's disease. The time-locked spikes with slow photic stimulation are characteristic for this diagnosis as shown in *rectangular box*.

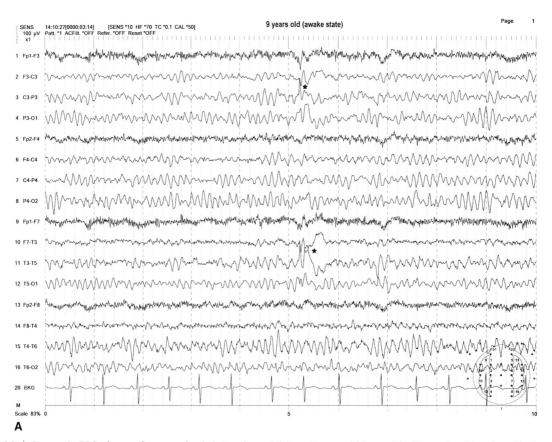

A

FIGURE 9-12 | Dramatic EEG change from awake **(A)** to asleep **(B)** in a 9-year-old boy with diagnosis of Landau–Kleffner syndrome. Note the sporadic sharp-wave discharges from the left hemisphere (indicated by *asterisk* in **A**) in the awake state and more or less continuous generalized spike–wave bursts becoming electrographic status epilepticus in sleep **(B)**.

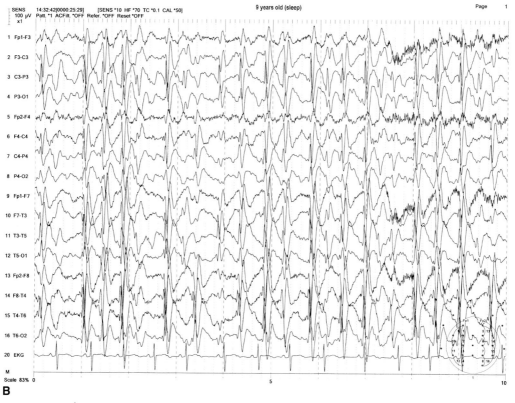

FIGURE 9-12 | (*Continued*)

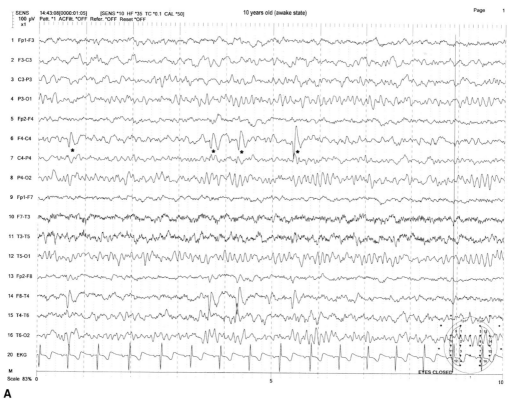

FIGURE 9-13 | Dramatic increase of spike discharges from awake (**A**) to asleep (**B**), characteristic for Rolandic spikes in a 10-year-old boy. In wakefulness, there were sporadic sharp–spike discharges from the right central and midtemporal regions (shown by *asterisk* in **A**). In sleep, there was a dramatic increase of sharp–spike discharges from the left and right central midtemporal regions independently.

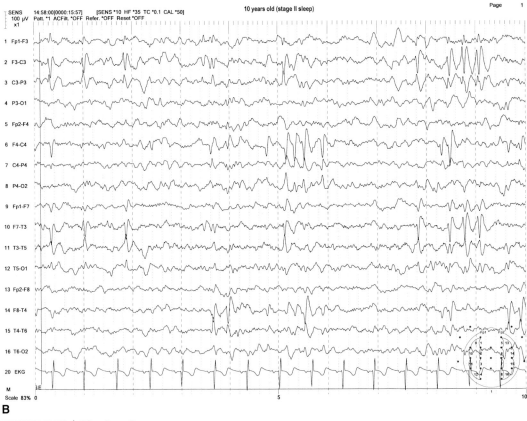

FIGURE 9-13 | (*Continued*)

in an epilepsy monitoring unit. Drug withdrawal may unmask (but not create) a seizure focus that was previously not evident or not in the same location of the habitual seizures.[34] Also, drug withdrawal may provoke generalized tonic–clonic convulsions in patients who previously did not have generalized seizures. Although it is unlikely that drug withdrawal may activate an entirely new focus, it is important to verify that the recorded seizures are clinically the same as the habitual seizures. This is especially important for localizing a seizure focus when planning epilepsy surgery.

Other Specific Activation Procedures

There are rare epileptic occurrences, which are triggered by specific stimulations, called "*reflex epilepsy*" and their stimulations include startle,[35,36] reading,[36,37] listening to music (musicogenic),[38] and tasks of decision-making.[36] Startle epilepsy can be triggered by a sudden, unexpected noise or touch. The EEG pattern may be vertex-dominant spikes or spike/waves. Reading epilepsy may be triggered by either silent reading or reading out loud. The EEG pattern is usually a generalized spike/wave or focal parietal spikes.

In musicogenic epilepsy, music of any type may be epileptogenic, but in some patients, only a specific tone or piece of music triggers a seizure. There may be additional emotional factors that potentiate seizures. The EEG may show anterior temporal spikes.

Decision-making–induced epilepsy may be triggered by, for example, chess playing, solving mathematical problems, or other forms of decision-making. The EEG pattern is usually generalized spike–wave bursts.

Other extremely rare activations include eating,[39] writing,[40] body or limb movement,[41] teeth brushing,[42] and tapping.[43] If the patient claims that a certain maneuver or stimulus tends to induce the "spell," it is important to try to reproduce the same maneuver or stimulus during EEG recording. One such example is vasovagal syncope (blackout spell), which is often triggered by standing up or coughing or a Valsalva maneuver. Although this is not a seizure, EEG usually shows dramatic diffuse delta slow waves associated with the spell (see Video 10-14). All these activating procedures should be performed with the attendance of a neurologist/electroencephalographer and with simultaneous video EEG recording.

References

1. Fisch BC, So EL. Activation methods. In: Ebersole JS, Pedley TA, eds. *Current Practice of Clinical Electroencephalography*. 3rd Ed. Philadelphia, PA: Lippincott Williams & Wilkins, 2003:246–270.
2. Davis H, Wallace WM. Factors affecting changes produced in electroencephalogram by standardized hyperventilation. *Arch Neurol Psychiatry* 1942;47:606–625.
3. Kodama N, Aoki Y, Hiraga H, et al. Electroencephalographic findings in children with moyamoya disease. *Arch Neurol* 1979;36:16–19.
4. Kameyama M, Shirane R, Tsurumi Y, et al. Evaluation of cerebral blood flow and metabolism in childhood moyamoya disease: An investigation into "re-build-up" on EEG by positron CT. *Child Nerv Syst* 1986;22:130–133.

5. Dalby MA. Epilepsy and 3 per second spike and wave rhythm: A clinical, electroencephalographic and prognostic analysis of 346 patients. *Acta Neurol Scand Suppl* 1969;40:1–80.

6. Schuler P, Claus D, Stegan H. Hyperventilation and transcranial magnetic stimulation: Two methods of activation of epileptiform EEG activity in comparison. *J Clin Neurophysiol* 1993;10:111–115.

7. ACNS Guidelines. Committee Guideline one: Minimal technical requirements for performing clinical electroencephalography. *J Clin Neurophysiol* 1994;112:4–5.

8. Panayiotopoulos CP. Effectiveness of photic stimulation on various eye—states in photosensitive epilepsy. *J Neurol Sci* 1974;23:165–173.

9. Jeavons PM, Harding GFA. *Photosensitive Epilepsy*. London: Heinemann, 1975.

10. Harding GF, Edson A, Jeavons PM. Persistence of photosensitivity. *Epilepsia* 1997;38:663–669.

11. Jayakar P, Chiappa KH. Clinical correlations of photoparoxysmal responses. *Electroencephalogr Clin Neurophysiol* 1990;75:251–254.

12. Watz S, Christen HJ, Doose H. The different patterns of photoparoxysmal response—a genetic study. *Electroencephalogr Clin Neurophysiol* 1992;83:138–145.

13. Reilly EW, Peters JF. Relationship of some varieties of electroencephalographic photosensitivity to clinical convulsive disorders. *Neurology* 1973;22:1040–1057.

14. Binnie CD. Simple reflex epilepsies. In: Engel J Jr, Pedley TA, eds. *Epilepsy: A Comprehensive Textbook*. Philadelphia, PA: Lippincott-Raven Publishers, 1997:2489–2505.

15. Janz D, Durner M. Juvenile myoclonic epilepsy. In: Engel J Jr, Pedley TA, eds. *Epilepsy: A Comprehensive Textbook*. Philadelphia, PA: Lippincott-Raven Publishers, 1997:2389–2400.

16. Ludwig BI, Marsan CA. Clinical ictal pattern in epileptic patients with occipital electroencephalographic foci. *Neurology* 1975;25:463–471.

17. Takakashi T, Tsukakara Y. Photoparoxysmal response elicited by flickering dot pattern stimulation and its optimal spatial frequency of provocation. *Electroencephalogr Clin Neurophysiol* 1998;106:40–43.

18. Takakashi T, Tsakakara Y. Usefulness of blue sun glasses in photosensitive epilepsy. *Epilepsia* 1992;33:517–521.

19. Takahashi T, Tsukahara Y. Pocket Monster incident and low luminance visual stimuli: Special reference to deep red flicker stimulation. *Acta Paediatr Jpn* 1998;40:631–637.

20. Harding GF, Fylan F. Two visual mechanisms of photosensitivity. *Epilepsia* 1999;40:1446–1451.

21. Killam KF, Killam EK, Naquet R. An animal model of light sensitive epilepsy. *Electroencephalogr Clin Neurophysiol* 1967;22:497–513.

22. Victor M, Brausch C. The role of abstinence in the genesis of alcoholic epilepsy. *Epilepsia* 1967;8:1–20.

23. Wikler A, Essig CF. Withdrawal seizure following chronic intoxication with barbiturates and other sedative drugs. In: Niedermeyer E, ed. *Modern Problems of Pharmacopsychiatry—Epilepsy*. Vol. 4. Basel, Switzerland: Karger, 1970:170–184.

24. Kooi, K. Electrographic signs of cerebral disorder. In: *Fundamentals of Electroencephalography*. New York: Harper & Row, 1971:114.

25. Pampiglione G, Harden A. Neurophysiological identification of a late infantile form of "neuronal lipidosis". *J Neurol Neurosurg Psychiatry* 1973;36:68–74.

26. Berkovic SF, So NK, Andermann F. Progressive myoclonus epilepsies: Clinical and neurophysiological diagnosis. *J Clin Neurophysiol* 1991;8:261–274.

27. Niedermeyer E, Rocca V. The diagnostic significance of sleep electroencephalogram in temporal lobe epilepsy. A comparison of scalp and depth tracing. *Eur Neurol* 1972;7:119–129.

28. Adachi N, Alarcon G, Binue C. Predictive value of interictal epileptiform discharges during non-REM sleep on scalp EEG recording for the lateralization of epileptogenesis. *Epilepsia* 1998;39:628–632.

29. Patry G, Lyagoubi S, Tassinari CA. Subclinical "electrical status epilepticus": Induced by sleep in children. A clinical and electroencephalographic study of six cases. *Arch Neurol* 1971;24:242–252.

30. Landau WM, Kleffner FR. Syndrome of acquired aphasia with convulsive disorder in children. *Neurology* 1957;7:523–530.

31. Blom S, Heijbel J. Benign epilepsy of children with centro-temporal EEG foci. Discharge rate during sleep. *Epilepsia* 1975;16:133–140.

32. Ellingson R, Wilken K, Bennet D. Efficacy of sleep deprivation as an activation procedure in epilepsy patients. *J Clin Neurophysiol* 1984;1:83–101.

33. Fountain N, Kim J, Lee S. Sleep deprivation activates epileptiform discharge independent of the activating effects of sleep. *J Clin Neurophysiol* 1998;15:69–75.

34. Marciani M, Gotman J. Effects of drug withdrawal on location of seizure onset. *Epilepsia* 1986;27:423–431.

35. Bejar M, Lai C-W, Zieglar DK. Sustained myoclonus in a woman with startle epilepsy. *Ann Neurol* 1985;18:101–103.

36. Forster FM. *Reflex Epilepsy, Behavioral Therapy and Conditional Reflexes*. Springfield, IL: Charles C. Thomas, 1977.

37. Bickford RG. Sensory precipitation of seizures. *J Mich Med Soc* 1954;53:1018–1021.

38. Joynt RJ, Green D, Green R. Musicogenic epilepsy. *JAMA* 1962;179:602–604.

39. Fiol ME, Mireles R, Leppik I, et al. Ictus emeticus: Clinical and electroencephalographic findings on surface and electrocorticography [abstract]. *Electroencephalogr Clin Neurophysiol* 1988;63:42p–43p.

40. Cirignotta E, Zucconi M, Mondisni S, et al. Writing epilepsy. *Clin Electroencephalogr* 1968;17:21–23.

41. Burger LJ, Lopez RI, Elliot FA. Tonic seizures induced by movement. *Neurology (Minneapolis)* 1972;22:656–659.

42. Holmes GL, Blair S, Eisenberg E, et al. Tooth-brushing induced epilepsy. *Epilepsia (New York)* 1982;23:657–661.

43. Negrin P, DeMarco P. Partial focal spike evoked by tactile somatotopic stimulation in sixty non-epileptic children: The nocturnal sleep and clinical and EEG evolution. *Electroencephalogr Clin Neurophysiol* 1977;43:312–316.

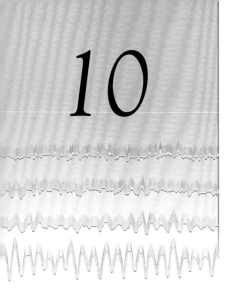

10

EEG and Epilepsy

THORU YAMADA and ELIZABETH MENG

Paroxysmal Discharges and Seizure Diagnosis

Since the introduction of CT (computerized axial tomography) in the early 1970s, neuroimaging diagnostic tests such as MRI (magnetic resonance image), fMRI (functional MRI), PET (position emission tomography), and SPECT (single photon emission computerized tomography) have made remarkable advancements in revealing the anatomical as well as functional disturbances of brain lesions. Despite these significant contributions to the diagnosis of various neurological disorders, EEG continues to play a pivotal role in the diagnosis and management of patients with epilepsy.

In evaluating the EEG of a patient with possible seizures, we may see *interictal epileptiform discharges* (IEDs) and/or nonspecific paroxysmal discharges, with or without focal or diffuse slowing. IEDs, represented by spike or spike-wave discharges, are the most sensitive and specific markers for the diagnosis of seizures. Other paroxysmal discharges represented sharp, alpha, theta or delta pattern is less specific for diagnosis of epilepsy. In a routine EEG (a recording of ~30 minutes), the chance of recording a clinical seizure (ictal) event is rather rare, unless the patient is having frequent seizures or is in status epilepticus. Thus, we often rely primarily on IEDs for the diagnosis of epilepsy.

The likelihood of detecting IEDs varies depending on seizure type, age, and seizure frequency. An EEG that includes sleep or that is recorded after sleep deprivation increases the yield of IEDs. Generally, greater seizure frequency is associated with a higher yield of IEDs.[1] IEDs are also recorded more often in children than in adults. Detection of IEDs differs depending on the origin of the epileptiform activity: if a relatively small area of the cortex is involved as the epileptogenic zone, IEDs may not be detected by scalp electrodes. Also, epileptiform activity arising from deep brain structures such as the medial temporal lobe, subfrontal lobe, or interhemispheric medial cortex may not be readily recorded using scalp electrodes.

The specificity of IEDs is determined by the incidence of IEDs in the normal populations (false positive) compared with that in patients with epilepsy. IEDs are found in 1.9% to 3.5% of healthy children[2,3] and 0.5% of healthy adults.[4] Specificity also varies depending on the type of IEDs: only about 40% of patients with benign Rolandic spikes of childhood or *BECTS* (*benign epilepsy of childhood with central midtemporal spikes*) and 50% of patients with *childhood epilepsy with occipital paroxysms* (*benign occipital spikes of childhood*) have a history of seizure.[5] Also, IEDs elicited by photic stimulation and generalized spike-wave discharges are less correlated with seizure history compared to focal spikes. Multifocal IEDs and focal IEDs, especially at the midline, frontal, and anterior temporal regions, are highly (75% to 95%) correlated with a history of seizures.[5,6] Overall, the incidence of detecting IEDs during the first EEG in adult epilepsy patients is about 30% to 50%.[7,8] In children less than 10 years old, the incidence is about 80%. Repeating the EEG once increases the yield by an additional 20% to 30%.[7,8]

A frequently asked question is whether anticonvulsant medication affects the incidence of IED detection. It is the general consensus that the use of oral *phenytoin (Dilantin)* or *carbamazepine (Tegretol)* does not decrease IEDs.[7] Thus, the patient does not need to discontinue anticonvulsants prior to having an EEG. However, valproate suppresses generalized spike-wave bursts and photoparoxysmal responses.[9] The intravenous administration of benzodiazepine such as *lorazepam (Ativan)*, *diazepam (Valium)*, or *clonazepam (Klonopin)* is a potent treatment regimen for status epilepticus abolishing generalized spike-wave discharges,[10] but oral administration of benzodiazepines has little effect on IED. The newer anticonvulsants such as *levetiracetam (Keppra)*,[11] *topiramate (Topamax)*,[12] and *lamotrigine (Lamictal)*[13] are reported to decrease IEDs, while *oxcarbazepine (Trileptal)*[14] and *vigabatrin (Sabril)*[15] may enhance generalized spike-wave discharges with an increase of generalized seizures in patients with focal seizure. The effects on IEDs by other anticonvulsants including *gabapentin (Neurontin)*, *pregabalin (Lyrica)*, *felbamate (Felbatol)*, and *zonisamide (Zonegran)* are still unclear. *Lacosamide (Vimpat)*, introduced recently for the treatment of pharmacoresistant epilepsy or status epilepticus, was reported to show no significant EEG changes in terms of power spectrum, mean frequency, and interictal abnormalities.

Although it is preferable to do the first EEG recording without anticonvulsants, these medications should not be discontinued for the purpose of an EEG study because abrupt discontinuation of the anticonvulsants may put the patient at increased risk of seizure, even worse, into status epilepticus. Therefore, withdrawing anticonvulsants for the purpose of capturing seizures, especially for poorly controlled seizure patients, must be done in an inpatient setting.

The Epilepsies

Certain forms of epileptic seizure disorders have special clinical and EEG characteristics irrespective of their etiologies. The International Classification of Epilepsies and Epileptic Syndromes was proposed by the Committee on Classification and Terminology of the International League Against Epilepsy.[16] This classification is based on two principles: distinguishing first between localized (focal) and generalized epilepsies and secondly between idiopathic and symptomatic etiologies. However, the classification, which includes detailed categories of the epileptic syndromes, has elicited some disagreement and controversy among epileptologists.

Normal or near-normal background activity is characteristic of *idiopathic epilepsy*, and slowing of background activity or multifocal epileptiform activity is suggestive of *symptomatic epilepsy*. Also, focal background abnormality and/or focal polymorphic delta activity is likely correlated with symptomatic epilepsy.

LOCALIZED (FOCAL) EPILEPSIES AND SYNDROMES

In the localized epilepsies and syndromes, examples of the idiopathic type include *benign childhood epilepsy* with *centrotemporal spikes* (*Rolandic spikes* or *BECTS*) and *childhood epilepsy with occipital paroxysms* (*benign childhood occipital lobe epilepsy*). Symptomatic localized epilepsies and syndromes include frontal or temporal lobe seizures that are secondary to focal pathology.

The localization of an epileptogenic focus often determines the character of the seizures. To some extent, it is possible to speculate on the clinical manifestation of seizures based on the localization and waveform of the epileptiform activity. Conversely, it may be possible to postulate the localization and waveforms of epileptiform activity based on clinical seizure types.

A focal spike or sharp wave commonly has surface-negative polarity associated with a distant field of positivity, thus forming a dipole field distribution. When spikes arise from the crown of a cortical gyrus, a radially oriented dipole is created with the negative field projecting to the cortical surface and positivity in the deeper areas of the brain (see Fig. 8-22A). When spikes arise from the sulcus of the cortical surface, a tangentially oriented dipole is created, with both positive and negative poles appearing on the cortical surface (see Fig. 8-22B). Discretely localized negative spikes likely arise from the cortical surface near the detecting electrodes, whereas widespread spikes may arise from the deeper structures. Unfortunately, predicting the source of spikes from scalp electrodes is limited because cortical spikes are much attenuated and the field distribution is distorted when detected at the scalp by intervening nonhomogeneous volume conductive media (scalp, skull, CSF, etc.) between the cortex and the scalp. In general, however, reasonable correlates exist between the partial seizure type and sites of interictal discharges.

Of the following sections in this category, the first and second sections are idiopathic and third through sixth are generally symptomatic.

Benign Epilepsy of Childhood with Central Midtemporal Spikes

Spikes maximally recorded from central or midtemporal electrodes have been described as BECTS or "benign Rolandic epilepsy." The term "benign" in this sense means a good prognosis for this seizure type. The waveform is more commonly "sharp" rather than a true spike, having a triphasic configuration with a prominent negative peak, preceded and followed by small positive peaks. The negative field centered at the central or midtemporal electrode is commonly associated with positive fields in the frontal region (Fig. 10-1A and B). These discharges are often unilateral, but one third of the patients have bilateral independent foci. Sleep (non-REM) greatly increases the spikes (see Fig. 9-13A and B) and about one third of the patients have spike discharges only in sleep.[17] Also, unilateral spikes in the awake state may progress to bilaterally independent spikes in sleep. Rolandic spikes tend to decrease progressively with age and eventually disappear by the midteen years.[18] The onset of seizures usually occurs between 4 years of age and adolescence. Consistent with the typical dramatic increase of spike discharges in sleep, about 80% of seizures occur exclusively in sleep.[17]

Clinically, seizures initially consist of unilateral paresthesias of tongue, lips, cheek, and gum and/or unilateral tonic–clonic activity of facial and pharyngeal/laryngeal muscles, contralateral to the side of the spike focus. The ictal discharges often start with an initial electrodecremental pattern (EEG flattening) followed by rhythmic spike bursts with subsequent spike-wave discharges. The seizure ends without postictal slowing unless the seizure evolves to a generalized tonic–clonic convulsion, which is not uncommon.

Not all spike discharges from central regions are benign. Some features help distinguish benign Rolandic epilepsy from symptomatic (non–benign) epilepsy. As shown in Figure 10-1A and B, benign Rolandic spikes are tangentially oriented (see Fig. 8-22B), with a negative field just behind the Rolandic fissure either at or close to the central or midtemporal electrode and a positive field over the frontal region. In symptomatic epilepsy, spikes often have a radially oriented distribution; thus, the negative field spreads diffusely over a wide scalp region (see Fig. 8-22A).[19] Focal slowing (corresponding to the side of spikes) is absent in benign Rolandic epilepsy but is often present in symptomatic epilepsy (Fig. 10-2). When a Rolandic spike is maximum at the midtemporal electrode, differentiation of temporal lobe epilepsy with spikes at the T3 or T4 electrode from benign Rolandic epilepsy can be more difficult. In this case, additional electrodes between C3 or C4 and T3 or T4 (C5 or C6 according to the expanded 10 to 20 system: see Fig. 2-4) help distinguish the two: Rolandic spikes are maximum at C5 or C6, whereas symptomatic temporal lobe seizures likely have a maximum at T3 or T4.[20]

Childhood Epilepsy with Occipital Paroxysms and Other Occipital Spikes

There are two types of seizures categorized in this entity: late onset, originally described by Gastaut[21] (Gastaut type), and early onset, more recently described by Panayiotopoulos,[22] and

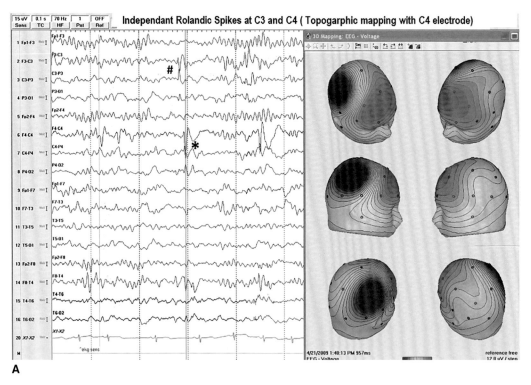

A

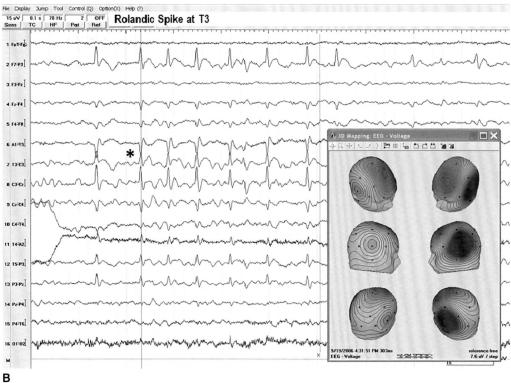

B

FIGURE 10-1 | A: BECTS in a 12-year-old girl with history of nocturnal generalized tonic–clonic convulsions with postictal aphasia and right arm weakness (Todd's paralysis). EEG showed spikes maximum at C3 (*marked by* #) and C4 (*marked by* *) independently. Topographic mappings are made at C4 spike peak. Note maximum negative (indicated by *blue*) field at C4 and positive (indicated by *red*) field at contralateral frontal regions shown by topographic mapping. This patient has an independent spike from C3 as well (*marked by* #). **B:** BECTS in a 10-year-old boy with history of nocturnal generalized tonic–clonic convulsions. EEG showed spikes maximum at T3 (*marked by* *). Note maximum negative field (*blue*) at T3 and positive field (*red*) at contralateral frontal region shown by 3D topographic mapping.

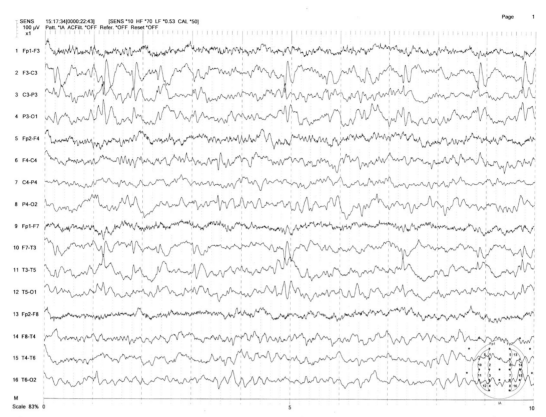

FIGURE 10-2 | Spike discharges at left central and midtemporal regions in a 6-year-old boy with history of focal seizure involving the right arm. Note the increased delta and decreased background activity over the left hemisphere. This is unlikely to be BECTS.

now referred to as *Panayiotopoulos syndrome.* Affected children are neurologically normal in both types. Family history of epilepsy is positive in more than one third of patients for the late-onset type but negative for the early-onset type. In the late-onset variant, age of seizure onset ranges from 15 months to 17 years with peak age of 7 to 9 years.[23] In the early-onset variant, onset is between 1 and 14 years with peak age of 3 to 6 years.[24]

In the late-onset type, seizures almost always begin with visual symptoms (blindness, scintillating scotoma, visual hallucinations, or illusions). The seizure is usually brief, lasting only a few to several seconds. Half of the patients complain of severe migraine-like headache associated with nausea and vomiting.[21] Thus, differentiation from migraine headache is sometimes difficult. The prognosis is good overall but less favorable than that of BECTS.

In the early-onset type, seizures lack characteristic visual symptoms but consist of a variety of autonomic symptoms including "feeling sick," paleness, nausea and vomiting, cyanosis, miosis or mydriasis, and cardiopulmonary irregularities. The seizure lasts much longer (5 to 10 minutes) than the late-onset type and often ends with a hemiconvulsion, Jacksonian march, or generalized motor activity. About one third of seizures occur in sleep. Nearly all patients become seizure free by age 12.[24]

EEG abnormalities are indistinguishable between these two types of seizures. Spikes consist of high-amplitude surface-negative spikes (200 to 300 μV), often followed by a

small positive and negative slow wave (Fig. 10-3). These occur singly or more commonly in serial, semirhythmic bursts with a unilateral or bilaterally independent appearance. Eye opening tends to abolish the spike wave, and eye closing may precipitate the burst. However, neither repetitive photic stimulation nor hyperventilation has an effect.[23] As with BECTS, sleep (NREM) increases the discharges, but less prominently.

About one fourth to one third of patients have other epileptogenic abnormalities including generalized spike wave or BECTS[23,25] (Fig. 10-4). The ictal EEG consists of rhythmic spike discharges starting from one occipital region, evolving into rhythmic theta–delta that spreads to the contralateral occipital region (Fig. 10-5).

Benign childhood occipital lobe epilepsy must be differentiated from other occipital spikes. Many patients with congenital or acquired amblyopia are found to have occipital spikes, but the morphology of the spike is much faster ("needle-like spike") than that of benign childhood occipital epilepsy.[26] Occipital spikes may also occur in idiopathic, generalized seizure patients with a photoparoxysmal response[27] (Fig. 10-6A and B). Irrespective of age, patients may have localization-related seizures with vivid visual hallucinations.[28] Although many "pure" partial/focal seizures fail to show ictal discharges, partial seizures of occipital origin tend to show well-localized ictal EEG activity, and the patient is often able to describe his or her visual hallucinatory event in detail (Fig. 10-7A–D; see Video 10-5A).

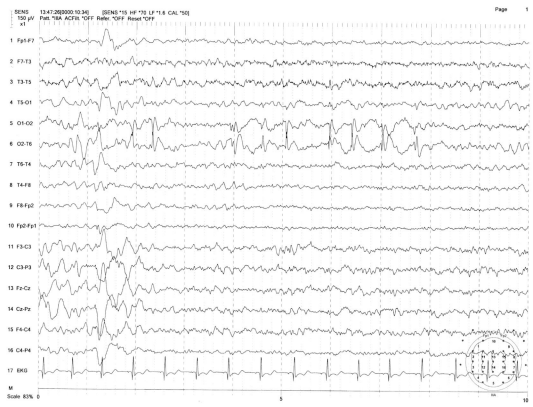

FIGURE 10-3 | Childhood epilepsy with occipital paroxysms (benign occipital lobe epilepsy) in a 4-year-old boy whose seizures manifest as seeing "flashing light." Note high-amplitude occipital spikes at O2 electrode.

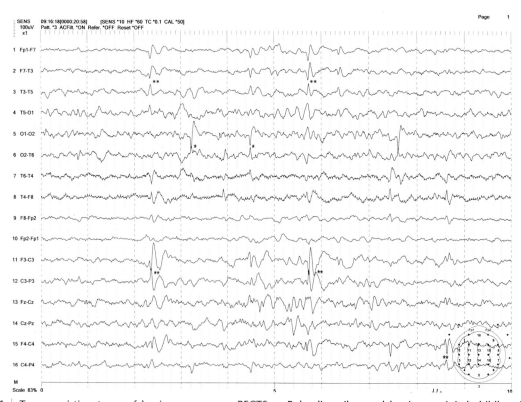

FIGURE 10-4 | Two coexisting types of benign paroxysm—BECTS or Rolandic spikes and benign occipital childhood epilepsy in a 10-year-old girl with history of generalized tonic–clonic seizures. Note two independent spikes left central/midtemporal (indicated by **) and occipital spikes (indicated by *) at O2 electrode.

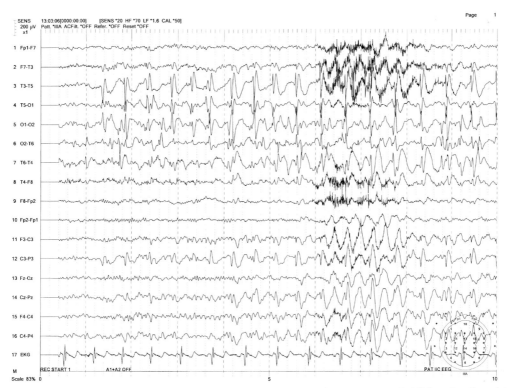

FIGURE 10-5 | Ictal discharges in childhood epilepsy with occipital paroxysm (benign occipital childhood epilepsy) in an 11-year-old girl with ictal manifestation of blindness, nausea, and migraine-like headache. Note rhythmic spike-wave discharges initially originating from O1 electrode with subsequent spread to other electrodes. Also, there were independent spikes at T6 electrode, which became synchronized with the occipital spikes as seizure progressed.

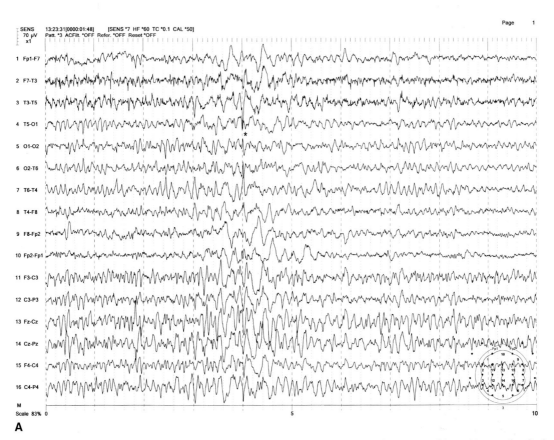

A

FIGURE 10-6 | Occipital spikes in a 34-year-old man with history of generalized tonic–clonic convulsions. Note spike discharges maximum at O1 electrode (indicated by*) **(A)**. This patient also had photoparoxysmal response at 17 Hz with the initial occipital polyspikes time-locked to the flashes, followed by generalized irregular spike-wave bursts **(B)**.

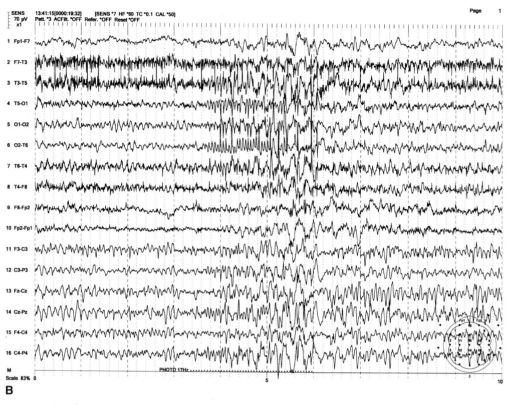

B

FIGURE 10-6 | (Continued)

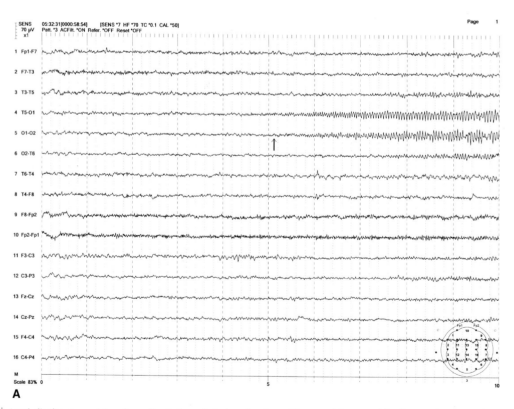

A

FIGURE 10-7 | Ictal discharges arising from the left occipital region in a 40-year-old man with diagnosis of anaplastic astrocytoma of the left parietal lobe, presenting with episodes of visual hallucination. Ictal discharges started with beta activity from the O1 electrode (*marked by arrow*) **(A)**. Beta activity progressively increased in amplitude as it spread to the other electrodes **(B)**. The ictal discharges then became progressively slower in frequency **(C)** and ended with semirhythmic sharp discharges and generalized theta–delta slowing in the occipital region **(D)**. The patient was conscious throughout the episode but became confused toward the end of the seizure. (**A** to **D** are consecutive recordings.)

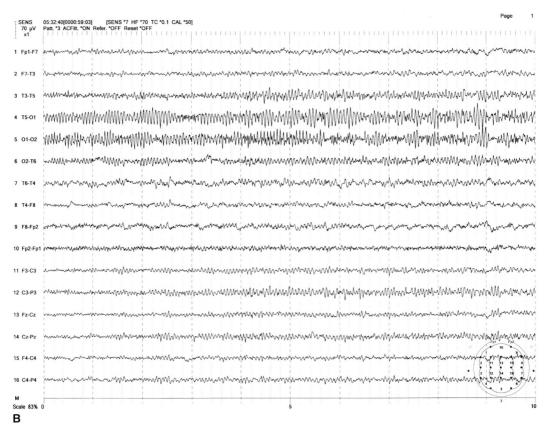

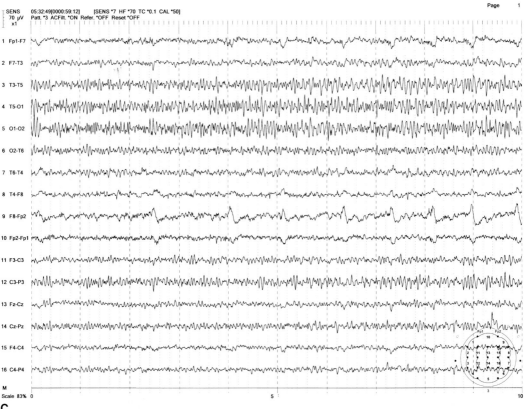

FIGURE 10-7 | (*Continued*)

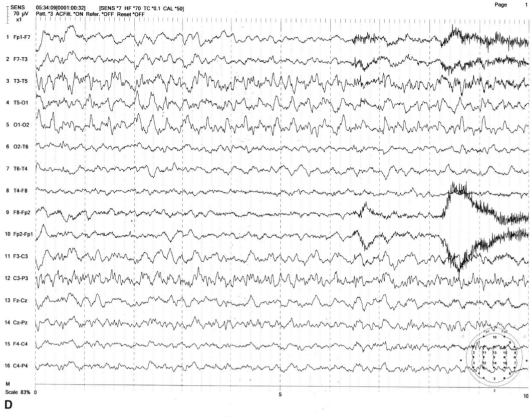

D

FIGURE 10-7 | *(Continued)*

Temporal Lobe Seizures

Temporal lobe seizures are far more common than any other seizure type. Clinical manifestation of temporal lobe seizures reflects the multitude of temporal lobe functions. In these seizures, the patient often maintains consciousness but has impaired awareness. A very common clinical finding is the presence of *automatisms*. Automatisms are stereotyped, repetitive movements such as picking at clothing, lip smacking, and chewing (Video 10-1 with Fig. 10-8). Because of characteristic psychic and motor symptoms, temporal lobe seizures were previously called "*psychomotor seizure*" but are now classified as "complex partial seizure" or "*focal seizure with impaired awareness.*[*]" Some patients may remain conscious and have

---

[*]Some of the EEG patterns are adopted from new ACNS Standardized Critical Care EEG Terminology (see Table in Chapter 13).

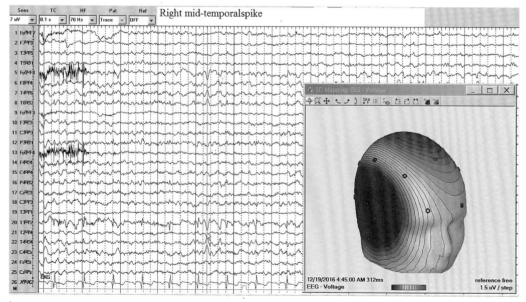

FIGURE 10-8 | Patient was a 30-year-old man with diagnosis of complex partial epilepsy (focal seizure with impaired awareness[†]) since age 14. MRI showed right hippocampal sclerosis. Interictal sharp discharges arose from the right temporal region. Topographic mapping showing maximum negativity (*blue*) was focused at T4 and positive field at the left parietal region. This patient's seizure is shown by Video 10-1.

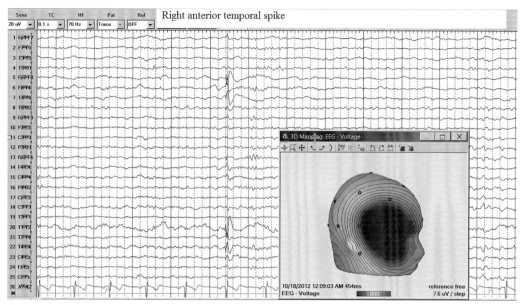

| Sens | TC | HF | Pat | Ref | Right anterior temporal spike |
| 20 uV | 0.1 s | 70 Hz | Trace | OFF | |

FIGURE 10-9 | Patient was a 62-year-old woman presenting with episodes of confusion, which started about 3 years ago. She was amnestic for these episodes. MRI was unremarkable. Interictal spikes arose from the right temporal region with maximum negativity at F8 (*blue*). EEG also showed polymorphic delta on the right temporal region. This patient's seizure is shown by Video 10-2.

seemingly normal behavior despite EEG showing widespread ictal discharges (Video 10-2 with Fig. 10-9).

Temporal lobe seizures can be divided into those originating in the mesial temporal lobe and those from the neocortex. Because many candidates for epilepsy surgery have temporal lobe seizures, it is important to differentiate these two foci before surgery. This may be difficult with scalp EEG alone, but there are some clinical and EEG features that help distinguish the two types.[29]

MESIAL TEMPORAL LOBE EPILEPSY. Details of the clinical manifestation of temporal lobe seizures are beyond the scope of this chapter. More than 80% of the patients with mesial temporal lobe epilepsy (MTLE) have a history of febrile seizures in early childhood. Seizures often begin with a variety of prodromal symptoms, that is, "aura," which most often consists of *gustatory* (e.g., a metallic taste) or *olfactory* (e.g., a smell of burning rubber) *hallucinations*. The patient may have a variety of illusional or hallucinatory experiences. An *illusion* is the distorted perception of an object, such as *microsopia* (e.g., an elephant looks as small as an ant), *macropsia* (e.g., a child looks as big as a giant), or another distortion of form. A *hallucination* is the perception of nonexisting objects. This may be visual, auditory, olfactory, or gustatory. Other relatively common symptoms are "*déjà vu*," in which unfamiliar objects or experiences seem familiar, and "*jamais vu*" in which familiar objects or experiences seem unfamiliar. Other relatively uncommon symptoms include "ideational symptomatology," which consists of sudden, forced thought processes, and "affective symptomology," which consists of states of extreme sadness or pleasure.

The interictal EEG of MTLE shows spike or sharp discharges of maximum negativity at the anterior temporal electrodes (F7/F8 or T1/T2). This relatively discrete negative field is accompanied by a more widespread positive field over the contralateral central–parietal region (Fig. 10-8). About one third of MTLE patients have bilateral IEDs that occur independently on the two sides.[30,31] MTLE is usually associated with mesial temporal sclerosis, which is often revealed by MRI.[32] Video 10-3 A&B show beta onset seizures arising from left or right temporal region independently secondary to mesial temporal sclerosis. The ictal EEG is often characterized by rhythmic theta or delta

discharges from anterior/midtemporal electrodes at the onset, with subsequent spread to other electrodes (see Videos 10-1 and 10-2). The onset of the ictal discharge usually starts within 30 seconds after the onset of clinical symptoms or signs.[33,34]

NEOCORTICAL TEMPORAL LOBE EPILEPSY. Clinical manifestations of neocortical temporal lobe epilepsy (NTLE) are less well characterized than those of MTLE. *Epigastric auras* are less common in NTLE, as are oroalimentary automatisms, visual and auditory hallucinations, head movement, and contralateral dystonic posturing.[35]

The interictal EEG features of NTLE are also less consistent and less specific than MTLE. Interictal spikes of NTLE tend to have a broader negative field and lack a positive field over the contralateral central–parietal regions.[36] An ictal onset with localized beta activity generally implies that seizure arises from the electrode nerby the beta onset zone. But this rule does not necessarily applies to NTLE as shown in Video 10-3 A&B. An example of NTLE secondary to a posterior temporal lesion is shown in Figure 10-10.

Distinction between MTLE and NTLE usually cannot be made with confidence based on scalp-recorded EEG alone because of the overlap in ictal or interictal EEG discharges between the two entities. Also, there are similarities in the seizure semiology. Some differences have been reported; history of febrile seizure and congenital malformation are more common in MTLE than NTLE.[37] Abdominal aura is more common in MTLE, while ictal dystonia is more common in NLTE. Maximum interictal spikes involving sphenoidal or F9 or F10 electrodes (modified 10 to 20 system nomenclature; see Fig. 2-4) occur more likely in MTLE. The maximum spike location in NTLE tends to be more posteriorly located, involving T7 or T8, TP7 or TP8, and P7 or P8 electrodes.[37] Despite some of these differences between MLTE and NLTE, the correct diagnosis must rely on the findings derived from EEG data recorded by subdural (cortical) and/or depth electrodes.

Frontal Lobe Seizures

The clinical symptoms of frontal lobe seizure are reflected by heterogenic functions of the frontal lobe and propagation of seizure

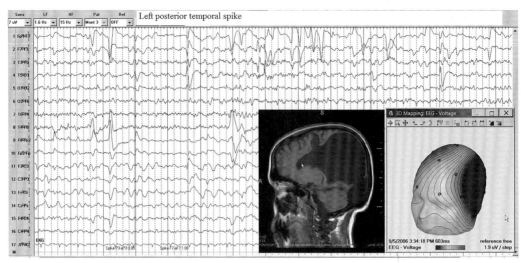

FIGURE 10-10 | Patient was a 35-year-old intellectually disabled woman with a long history of complex partial seizure and right static hemiparesis secondary to porencephalic cyst with enlarged posterior portion of the left lateral ventricle (shown by MRI). Interictal spikes arose from the left temporal region with maximum negativity (*blue*) at the posterior temporal to midtemporal electrode and positivity at the left parietal region.

activity from its origin to different areas of the frontal lobe. There are essentially four manifestations of frontal lobe seizures:

1. Simple partial seizures arising from the primary motor cortex manifesting as clonic twitching of contralateral muscles of the body, without loss of consciousness. According to the somatotopic arrangement of the precentral gyrus, the clonic movements are initially limited to the corresponding area of the body and then spread to other areas; for example, from finger to arm, to shoulder, and then to the face. This is known as a *Jacksonian march*.

2. Seizures arising from the supplementary motor cortex, consisting of deviation of head and eyes to one side (usually contralateral to the seizure focus), associated with tonic elevation of contralateral arm and downward extension of the ipsilateral arm. Thus, the patient appears to look at the raised arm. Depending on the extent of spread, the patient may or may not lose consciousness.

3. Immediate unconsciousness followed by a generalized tonic–clonic convulsion with minimal or no lateralizing signs. This may arise from the superior frontal region.

4. Complex motor manifestation characterized by vigorous body rocking, bicycling, dystonic posturing, repetitive movements, laughing, crying, etc. (Video 10-4). Because these movements or behaviors appear very bizarre and the EEG recording during seizures may not show any EEG change or ictal pattern, misdiagnosis as a nonepileptic spell or pseudoseizure is not uncommon. These seizures typically emanate from the medial frontal or orbital–frontal areas, but may arise anywhere within the frontal lobe.

As frontal lobe seizures often arise from the orbital–frontal cortex, interhemispheric convexity (medial frontal lobe), or cingulate cortex—all of which are relatively inaccessible to scalp EEG—it is not uncommon to miss interictal or even ictal discharges on scalp EEG. If IEDs are recorded, however, they may appear widespread and less localized because of the deep epileptogenic source. About two thirds of patients, especially those with medial frontal foci, show secondary bilaterally synchronous discharges.[38] Because spread from one hemisphere to the other is so rapid, it is not always possible to distinguish if the discharges are of frontal lobe origin or represent a primary generalized seizure. About half of the patients with frontal lobe epilepsy have IEDs in one frontal lobe only or with consistently unilateral dominance (Fig. 10-11A and B).[38,39]

The ictal EEG is nonlocalizing in more than half of the patients with frontal lobe epilepsy.[40] Even if there are ictal EEG changes associated with clinical seizures, they are often obscured by large muscle and movement artifacts that result from the seizure. This contrasts to temporal lobe epilepsy in which patients are typically quiet and motionless at the time of seizure onset; thus, artifacts are less problematic.

At the onset of a frontal lobe seizure, EEG often shows diffuse or bifrontal dominant voltage attenuation, which correlates with tonic posturing. This is followed by bilateral frontal or diffuse rhythmic theta–delta or spike-wave bursts correlating with clonic movements. In contrast, seizures of dorsolateral frontal origin are usually associated with focal or lateralizing rhythmic fast activity at seizure onset.[41]

Parietal Lobe Seizures

Parietal epilepsy is far less common than temporal or frontal lobe epilepsy. As with frontal lobe epilepsy, scalp EEG is often falsely negative, nonlocalizing, or falsely localizing.[42] Seizures of parietal origin have no typical clinical features. Seizures often present with visual disturbances such as scintillations or oscillopsia. If the seizure arises from the sensory cortex, symptoms may include a variety of sensations such as tingling, "pins and needles," numbness, pain, burning, or cold.[43] Strictly, sensory focal seizures are rather uncommon. Pain as an ictal sensation may be seen in temporal lobe seizures rather than in parietal lobe seizure.[44]

Occipital Lobe Seizures

Reflecting occipital lobe function, occipital lobe seizures may exhibit blindness or visual field loss or visual misconception such as macropsia, micropsia, misconception of spatial orientation, and hallucination such as seeing simple flashing light or color[45] or various more complex objects.[46] Interictal spikes

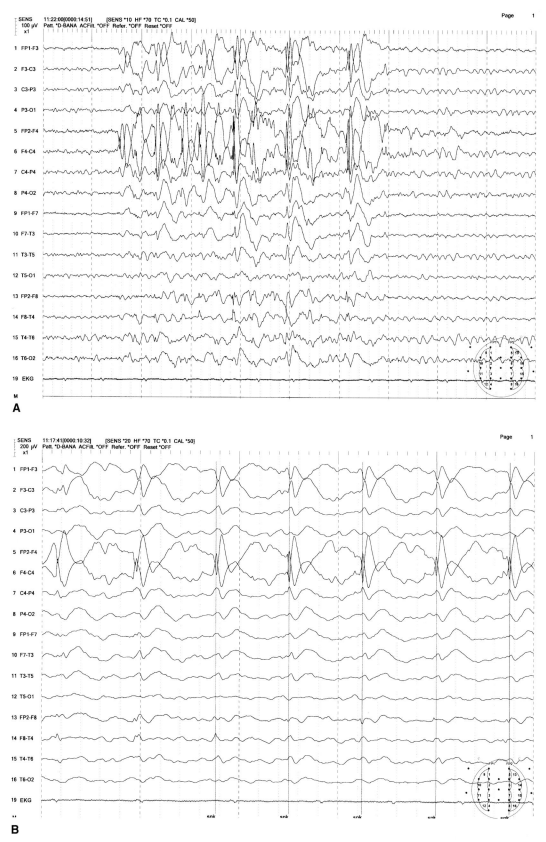

FIGURE 10-11 | Frontal lobe spikes in a 27-year-old woman with diagnosis of right frontal gliosis and intractable generalized tonic–clonic convulsions without aura. Note right-greater-than-left frontal dominant spike-wave discharges **(A)**. With routine sweep speed (10 s/page), spikes appear almost synchronous between left and right frontal regions, but with the faster sweep speed (5 s/page), right frontal spikes consistently preceded left frontal spikes **(B)**. (**A** and **B** are the same EEG samples.)

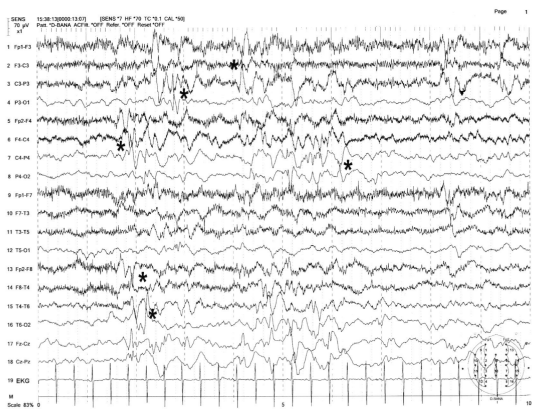

FIGURE 10-12 | Multifocal spikes in an 18-month-old baby boy with a history of generalized tonic–clonic convulsions with developmental delay. Note several epileptiform foci at F8, C3, C4, P3, P4, and T6 electrodes (*shown by * marks*).

are localized to the occipital electrodes, and ictal events often start with beta activity with progressive amplitude increase and slowing in frequency as ictal discharges spread to other region (see Figs. 8-8 and 10-7). Unlike other simple partial seizures, which often show no EEG change even when the patient is having a seizure, the simple partial occipital seizures often show electrographic ictal (seizure) patterns, and the patient is able to describe clearly what he or she is seeing (Video 10-5A and B).

Although most of photic induced spike-wave bursts (photoparoxysmal response) are associated with primary generalized seizures and not focal seizures, parieto-occipital spikes are exception (see Fig. 9-7). The seizure semiology is similar to other occipital seizures with a sequence of visual symptoms, but it is sometimes accompanied by headache and vomiting.[47] Therefore, this could be misdiagnosed as migraine headache with visual symptoms. Another type of occipital seizure is the benign nature of childhood epilepsy with occipital spikes (see Figs. 10-3 to 10-5; see also section of Occipital Epilepsy with Occipital Paroxysms and other occipital spikes in this chapter). The symptoms also include migraine-like headaches.[21–24] In some congenitally blind patients, occipital spikes with needle-like morphology can be observed, but these spikes are asymptomatic and usually disappear during childhood or adolescence.[26,48] Another rare condition showing interictal occipital spikes/polyspikes is *Dravet syndrome*, which presents with severe myoclonic seizures in infancy.[49,50] Occipital spikes eventually become generalized spike/polyspike. Some show photoparoxysmal response.

Other EEG Abnormalities Associated with Focal Epilepsy

MULTIFOCAL SPIKE DISCHARGES. Multifocal spikes, either within one hemisphere or from heterogeneous areas of each

hemisphere (Fig. 10-12; see also Fig. 8-18), generally correlate with multifocal or diffuse brain diseases such as the intellectually disabled or various neurological deficits. Slowing of the background rhythm as well as diffuse slow waves is common in these patients. The majority of patients have frequent seizures that are often intractable to treatment. Generally, increased spike frequency correlates with increased incidence of seizures and a greater degree of intellectual disability.[51] Multifocal spikes are also seen in patients with *West syndrome* (*infantile spasm with hypsarrhythmia*; see "Infantile Spasms, Salaam Spasms, West Syndrome" in this chapter; see Fig. 10-25A and B). In some cases, however, a strikingly abnormal EEG with multifocal spikes may be found in neurologically normal children with normal EEG background activity such as patients with BECTS and/or benign occipital epilepsy of childhood (see Fig. 10-4 and 10-5).[52]

Experimental animal studies clearly established that a seizure focus created by alumina cream or cobalt injection in the cortex results in the development of a secondary epileptogenic focus at the homotopic area of the contralateral hemisphere.[53] At first, spikes from the secondary focus (*mirror focus*) are dependent on the primary focus and disappear after the excision of the primary focus or after a corpus callosum resection. However, in time, spikes from the mirror focus become progressively more independent from the primary focus and can no longer be abolished with the resection of the primary focus. The existence of a mirror focus in human epilepsy has long been debated, but substantial evidence indicates that secondary epileptogenic foci exist in humans. For example, it is not uncommon to find bilateral independent interictal spike foci in both temporal lobes of patients who are evaluated for intractable seizure with

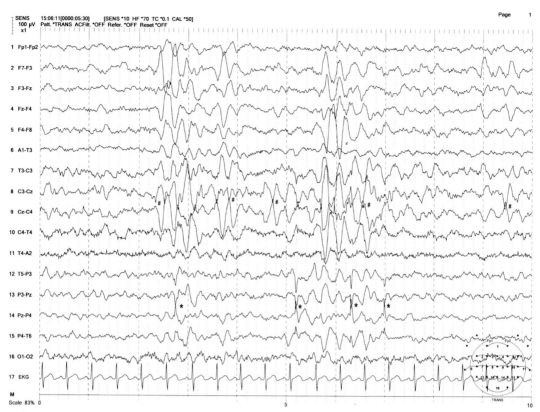

FIGURE 10-13 | Midline (Pz) spike in a 12-year-old girl with history of nocturnal generalized tonic–clonic seizures. Note spike discharges (indicated by * marks) at Pz, which can be easily differentiated from physiological vertex sharp waves of sleep (indicated by # marks).

implanted electrodes, even if ictal discharges arise only from one temporal lobe. Also, the patients with intractable epilepsy secondary to brain tumors occasionally showed additional independent spike foci in the hemisphere opposite the side of the lesion.[54]

MIDLINE SPIKES. Midline spikes appearing maximally at Fz, Cz, or Pz electrodes must be differentiated from physiologic K complexes or vertex sharp waves of sleep. A "spiky" waveform morphology or appearance during the awake state may assist in distinguishing between them. A Pz spike is relatively easy to differentiate from a vertex sharp wave (Fig. 10-13), but the differentiation is often difficult for Cz spikes (Fig. 10-14). These midline spikes are most likely a very localized expression of bilaterally symmetric, parasagittal dominant spikes or spike-wave discharges. Therefore, some patients have localized spikes at the midline as well as generalized and symmetric spikes or spike-wave discharges. Most of these patients, especially children, have generalized tonic–clonic seizures.[6] Midline spikes, especially in an adult, may correlate with structural lesions of the parasagittal regions or in the deeper mesial surface.[55]

GENERALIZED EPILEPSIES AND SYNDROMES

Idiopathic generalized epilepsies and syndromes include absence seizures (childhood and juvenile) and *juvenile myoclonic epilepsy (JME)*. *West syndrome* and *Lennox–Gastaut syndrome (LGS)* are examples of generalized epilepsy of a symptomatic type.

Generalized epileptiform discharges appear in both hemispheres simultaneously with similar configuration, symmetric amplitude, and synchronous timing between homologous electrodes. Timing between anterior and posterior discharges may differ slightly within the same hemisphere. When discharges have consistently higher amplitudes in one hemisphere or generalized discharges are consistently preceded by focal discharges, this may suggest a focal onset to a secondarily generalized seizure type, but clear-cut differentiation between a primary and secondary generalized seizure pattern is not always an easy task. Distinction between ictal and interictal patterns is also not as clear as that of a focal seizure. Often, the EEG associated with a clinical seizure may simply be a longer and more rhythmic repetition than interictal IEDs.

Absence Seizures

The discovery of 3-Hz spike-wave bursts associated with petit mal or absence seizures by Gibbs et al.[54] in 1935 was the first major epoch in the history of EEG and for the electrographic diagnosis of epilepsy. This is characterized by rhythmic cycles of spike and wave complexes at a frequency of about 3 Hz, usually lasting a few to several seconds. The spike-wave complexes are generally maximum in the frontal region and may start with 3 to 3.5 Hz and end with 2 to 3 Hz (Fig. 10-15; see also Figs. 6-6A and 9-3, Video 9-2). The initial complex may have a polyspike-wave pattern. Although the bursts seem to be synchronous between the two hemispheres, detailed analysis with a faster sweep recording shows that the spikes in one hemisphere may randomly precede those in the other hemisphere

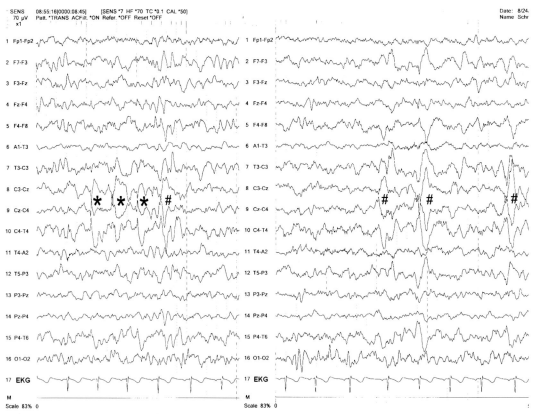

FIGURE 10-14 | Midline (Cz) spikes in a 6-year-old girl with spells of staring, rolling of head, and occasional incontinence. Sleep record showed localized spikes (indicated by * *marks*) at the Cz electrode, which had different waveform from physiological vertex sharp waves (indicated by # *marks*) of sleep, but some discharges were difficult to differentiate with certainty.

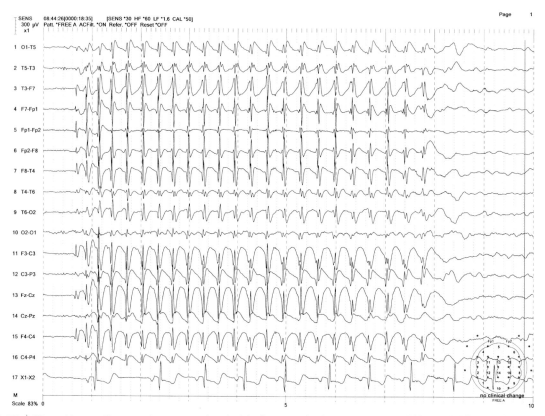

FIGURE 10-15 | Three-Hertz spike-wave bursts associated with absence of seizure in a 7-year-old boy (childhood absence). Note spike-wave bursts started with slightly faster than 3 Hz and ended with slightly slower than 3 Hz (see also Video 9-2).

by a few milliseconds.[55] The discharges tend to be inhibited by eye opening or increased vigilance. Hyperventilation can often precipitate the bursts associated with clinical absence seizures in 50% to 80% of patients[56–58] (see Video 9-2). Intermittent photic stimulation induces spike-wave bursts in about one fifth of the patients with absence epilepsy.[59] NREM sleep also increases the number of spike-wave complexes, which tend to become more irregular with polyspike-wave patterns.[60] REM sleep decreases the number of bursts to a frequency slightly less than the waking state.[60] Valproic acid and ethosuximide, commonly used medications for absence seizures, tend to decrease the number of spike-wave bursts[61] and also attenuate activation by photic stimulation.[62]

In patients with absence epilepsy, background activity is usually normal, but slowing can occur in a minority of patients. Generally, about 20% to 40% of patients with absence seizures show 3-Hz rhythmic delta bursts in the occipital regions (OIRDA, occipital intermittent rhythmic delta activity) (see Fig. 8-15; see also Video 10-6), and the incidence of OIRDA is much higher in children between 6 and 10 years old.[63] Visible clinical seizures can usually be observed when spike-wave bursts last more than 4 to 5 seconds. Symptoms are characterized by staring with impaired responsiveness and behavior arrest. Impaired responsiveness can occur with spike-wave bursts as short as 3 seconds. Responsiveness returns abruptly to normal at the end of the spike wave. Detailed psychophysiological testing of such patients found decreased reaction time even during a brief spike-wave burst without an associated overt clinical seizure.[64] Automatisms with lip smacking,

chewing, fumbling, or mild myoclonus (eyelid twitches) are common.[65] This may make it difficult to differentiate from temporal lobe seizures clinically. Some patients may have decreased postural tone. It is a technologist's role to examine the presence or absence of impaired responsiveness and to note the patient's behavior during spike-wave bursts. Absence seizures are classified into two types by age of onset.

CHILDHOOD ABSENCE EPILEPSY. Onset of seizures is from 3 to 12 years. EEG and clinical presentation can assist in predicting the prognosis. Patients with an EEG showing 3-Hz OIRDA have a smaller risk of developing tonic–clonic seizures in the future.[66] Absence seizures without myoclonus have a higher chance of remission than those with myoclonus.[58]

JUVENILE ABSENCE EPILEPSY (JAE). The onset of this type of epilepsy is around 9 to 13 years or even later. The spike-wave bursts tend to start with slightly faster frequency than 3 Hz and may have polyspike components (Fig. 10-16; Video 10-6). This group of patients is more likely to develop *JME* (see Fig. 10-21A and B).[59]

EYELID MYOCLONIA WITH ABSENCE (JEAVONS SYNDROME). Repetitive blinking is a common symptom during childhood absence seizures, but eyelid myoclonia typically occurs immediately after eye closure associated with brief generalized spike-wave bursts of 4 to 6 Hz. Photoparoxysmal discharges are common, inducing repetitive

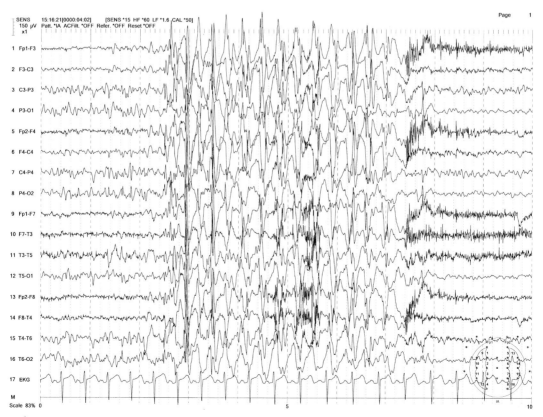

FIGURE 10-16 | Three-Hertz spike-wave burst with initial polyspike component in an 18-year-old girl (juvenile absence). The patient had absence seizures in the past and recently started having generalized tonic–clonic convulsions (see also Video 10-6).

eyes blinking (Video 10-7). The same patient may also have typical absence seizure with 3-Hz spike-wave bursts.[67]

Generalized Tonic–Clonic Seizures

Multiple spike-wave (polyspike-wave) bursts lasting less than one to several seconds are usually an interictal expression of a generalized seizure. The interictal EEG of idiopathic (primary) generalized tonic–clonic seizures consists of a variety of waveforms that are more irregular and of faster frequency than the 3-Hz rhythmic spike-wave discharges seen in absence seizures (Fig. 10-17A). In addition, spike-wave bursts often include multiple spikes (polyspikes) (Fig. 10-17B). Spike-wave bursts are usually, but not always, symmetric and synchronous. Asymmetric bursts do not necessarily exclude the possibility of primary generalized epilepsy. In fact, it is often difficult to differentiate primary from secondary generalized epilepsy, especially in the case of frontal lobe epilepsy. In some patients, focal spike discharges, such as "Rolandic spikes," may coexist with generalized spike-wave bursts. In such cases, it is not possible to determine if the patient has a seizure of focal onset with secondary generalization or has both partial and primary generalized epilepsies. There are two features that may help to point toward a diagnosis of primary generalized epilepsy. One is a photoparoxysmal response (Fig. 10-18A and B), and the other is generalized spike-wave bursts resembling K complexes (Fig. 10-19). Like K complexes, spike-wave bursts act as an arousal pattern and the patients may wake up or open their eyes coincident with the bursts. In some, generalized spike-wave bursts may be precipitated by arousal stimuli, similar to the K complex. In some patients, especially in children who tend to have "spiky" K complexes, it may be difficult to differentiate between the two. These features were studied in detail by Niedermeyer, who introduced the concept of "*dyshormia*," in which primary generalized spike-wave bursts and K complexes share the same generating mechanism, producing generalized burst activity.[68]

Onset of the ictal event in a generalized seizure consists of low-voltage rhythmic beta-range fast activity, with progressively increasing amplitude and decreasing frequency (Fig. 10-20A and B). This is followed by generalized spike-wave bursts, which become progressively slower in frequency and less rhythmic toward the end of the seizure. The EEG becomes suppressed during the immediate postictal period and is then followed by the appearance of postictal delta activity. Clinically, the initial fast activity corresponds to the tonic phase and the subsequent spike-wave bursts coincide with the clonic phase of the seizure. During the ictal events, both at onset and during the progress of the seizure, EEG activities are largely obscured by muscle and movement artifacts, making it difficult to recognize the EEG changes and to differentiate genuine seizure from pseudoseizure. The presence of postictal flattening or slowing provides evidence of genuine seizure (Video 10-8). Conversely, normal EEG immediately after the event favors pseudoseizure, especially if the patient remains unconscious or confused.

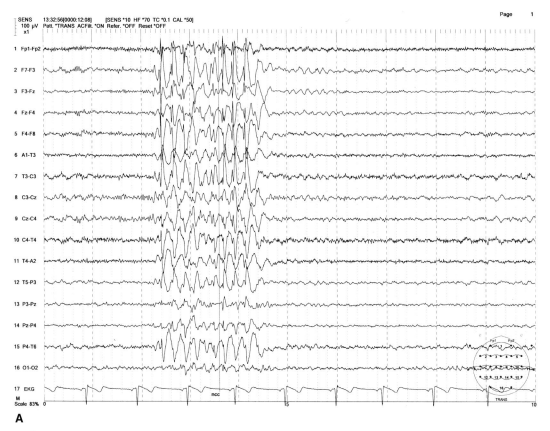

FIGURE 10-17 | Four- to six-Hertz, somewhat irregular, bilaterally synchronous generalized spike-wave bursts maximum at midline **(A)** in a 30-year-old woman with history of generalized tonic–clonic convulsion as well as myoclonic seizures. The patient also had more irregular polyspike-wave bursts during stage 2 sleep **(B)**.

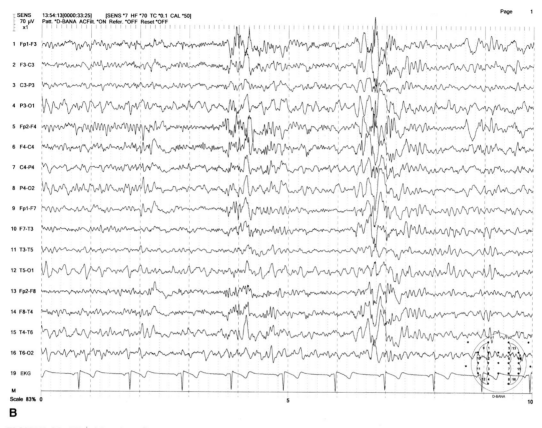

B

FIGURE 10-17 | (*Continued*)

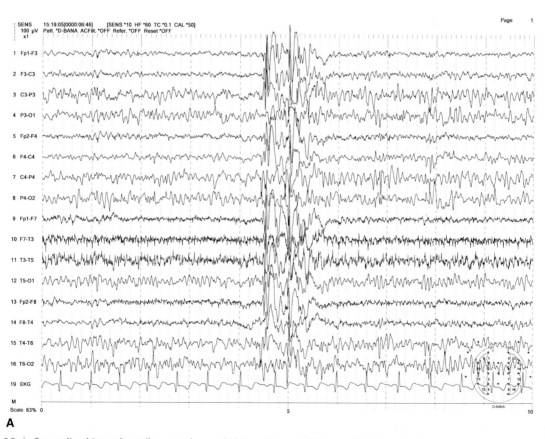

A

FIGURE 10-18 | Generalized irregular spike-wave bursts **(A)** in a 10-year-old boy with history of absence seizures and recent grand mal seizure. Photic stimulation produced photoparoxysmal response at 16-Hz frequency flashes with generalized irregular spike-wave bursts **(B)**.

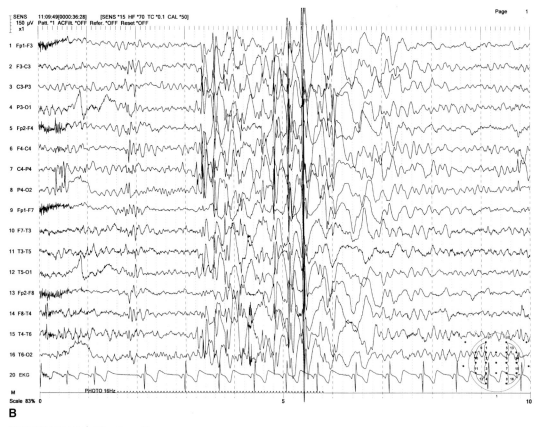

FIGURE 10-18 | (Continued)

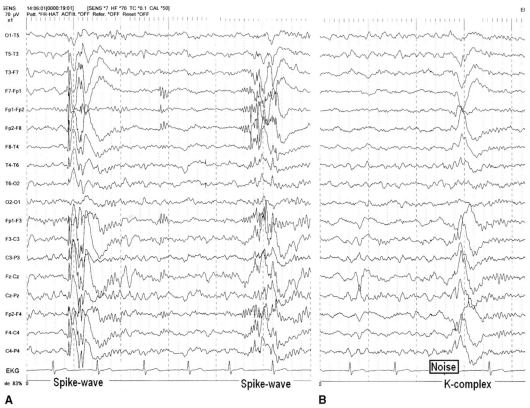

FIGURE 10-19 | This is an example of "dyshormia." Bilaterally diffuse synchronous and symmetric spike-wave bursts with bifrontal dominance in a 31-year-old man with history of grand mal seizures. Note that the spike and wave bursts were followed by spindles **(A)**. With exception of the spikes, the epileptiform bursts had similar wave form and distribution with K complex induced by noise **(B)**.

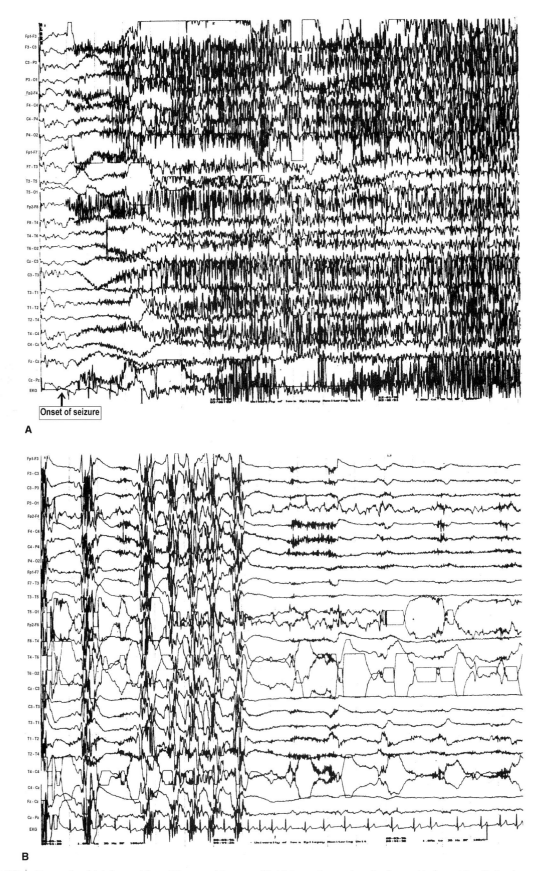

A

B

FIGURE 10-20 | Generalized ictal event in a 25-year-old man with history of grand mal seizure. Note sudden flattening of EEG activity at the onset, followed by beta activity peaking through the massive EMG (muscle) artifact during the tonic phase of seizure **(A)**. Toward the end of the seizure, ictal discharges changed to periodic spike-wave discharges, which were contaminated by muscle artifact (clonic phase). Afterward, there was postictal suppression of EEG activity **(B)** (see also Video 10-8).

Juvenile Myoclonic Epilepsy

This was originally described by Janz as "impulsive petit mal"[69] and may be referred to as "*juvenile myoclonic epilepsy of Janz.*" JME is the most common type of seizure among idiopathic generalized epilepsies. Close to half of the patients have a family history of epilepsy.[69] As the name implies, the seizures usually begin in adolescence. But many patients start with absence seizures at a younger age. The majority of patients (>90%) also have generalized tonic–clonic convulsions. Both myoclonic and generalized tonic–clonic convulsions tend to occur within 1 to 2 hours after awakening. A history of absence seizures coexists with or precedes myoclonic seizures in about one third of patients.[70]

Interictal EEG patterns consist of generalized polyspike and polyspike-wave discharges with frontocentral predominance (Fig. 10-21A). These patterns are not distinguishable from other idiopathic generalized epilepsies but may include more polyspike components. Like other idiopathic seizures, background activity is usually normal. Spike-wave or polyspike-wave bursts are usually faster than the typical 3-Hz spike waves seen in absence seizures, but in some patients, 2.5- to 3-Hz spike-wave bursts may occur that are indistinguishable from typical absence seizures (Fig. 10-21B).

Hyperventilation may activate epileptiform activity in JME but less often compared to absence seizures. About 30% to 40% of patients also have photoparoxysmal seizures (see Fig. 10-21B).[71] Photosensitive epilepsy is three to four times more common in girls than in boys.[71] In contrast to other types of epilepsy, epileptiform activity tends to decrease in sleep but markedly increase shortly after awakening.

The ictal pattern is indistinguishable from interictal epileptiform activity in most cases, but may have a greater number of polyspikes with higher amplitude and with a more rhythmic sequence.

Myoclonic Seizures

Myoclonus is characterized by sudden, brief involuntary muscle contractions, most predominantly in flexor muscles. These may be generalized or multifocal and synchronous or asynchronous. Myoclonus or myoclonic seizures are seen in a variety of clinical conditions including primary generalized epilepsy, focal epilepsy, infantile spasms with *hypsarrhythmia, LGS,* and various degenerative central nervous system (CNS) diseases such as *lipidosis, hereditary myoclonic epilepsy (Lafora–Unverricht–Lundborg), Creutzfeldt–Jakob disease (CJD), subacute sclerosing panencephalitis (SSPE), encephalitis, toxic/metabolic encephalopathy,* and *acute postanoxic cerebral insult.*

Three types of myoclonus have been proposed: (i) cortical reflex, (ii) reticular reflex, and (iii) primary generalized epileptic myoclonus.[72] In cortical reflex myoclonus,[73] the EEG usually fails to show cortical spikes associated with myoclonic jerks but computerized back-averaging ("jerk-locked" or "myoclonus-triggered" averaging; see Volume II, evoked potential section) could reveal time-locked spikes associated with myoclonus.[74] Reticular reflex myoclonus is due to hyperexcitability of the caudal brainstem reticular formation and, as such, does not

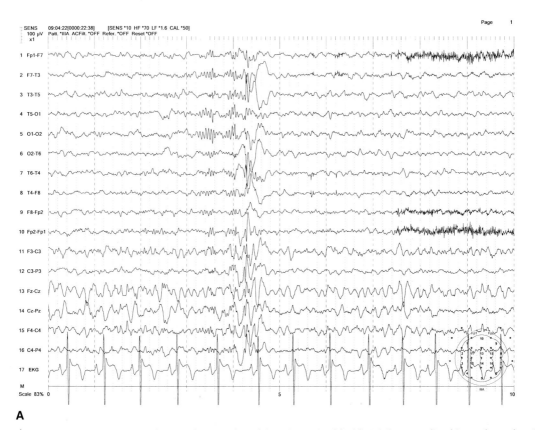

FIGURE 10-21 | An example of JME (juvenile myoclonic epilepsy) in a 14-year-old girl. Brief, generalized irregular polyspike-wave discharges were noted in sleep **(A)**. Photic stimulation induced 3-HZ rhythmic spike-wave bursts **(B)**.

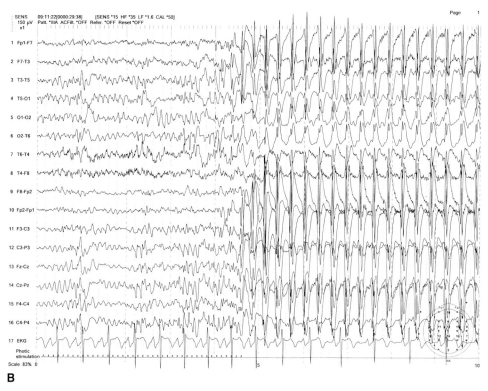

FIGURE 10-21 | (*Continued*)

show EEG changes.[75] Primary generalized epileptic myoclonus is associated with generalized spike and wave (usually irregular polyspike-wave burst) bursts, which may slightly precede the myoclonic jerk. This form of myoclonus can be seen in patients with primary generalized epilepsy, often associated with a photoparoxysmal response.

EEG correlates of myoclonus/myoclonic epilepsy vary between sudden flattening of EEG activity (desynchronized pattern) to irregular polyspike-wave bursts. The epileptiform discharges may be focal, associated with focal myoclonus (Fig. 10-22 and see also Video 13-8), or may be generalized, with irregular polyspike-wave bursts (which cannot be differentiated from the interictal discharges of generalized tonic–clonic epilepsy) (Fig. 10-23; see also Fig. 8-19). It should also be noted that myoclonus often occurs without detectable epileptiform activity.

Atonic Seizures

Atonic seizures are characterized by sudden loss of muscle tone, often associated with drop attacks, and lasting only a few seconds. Atonic seizures lasting a few minutes are referred to as "long form" and have been described as "inhibitory" seizures.[76] Epileptiform activity consists of brief, generalized, irregular polyspike-wave bursts, which are indistinguishable from interictal discharges seen in generalized tonic–clonic epilepsy or myoclonic seizures (Fig. 10-24). In the long form, discharges may be associated with slow (1.5- to 2-Hz) spike-wave activity.[76]

Infantile Spasms, Salaam Spasms, and West Syndrome

Gibbs and Gibbs[77] first termed "*hypsarrhythmia*" ("hyps" means mountainous) to characterize the EEG pattern of "very-high-voltage" (usually >500 µV), irregular, asynchronous delta slow waves associated with randomly occurring spikes from various locations (Fig. 10-25A). Spikes may be obscured by high-amplitude delta activity. The chaotic high-amplitude slow-wave activity may be intermittently replaced by a relatively low-amplitude pattern (partial flattening) lasting a few seconds. Because of exceedingly high-amplitude slow waves, waveforms are typically truncated in a recording using routine sensitivity. Also, spikes are often hidden among large slow waves, and multifocal spikes are better visualized by using a shorter time constant (higher low-frequency filter) (Fig. 10-25B). Typical hypsarrhythmia is common in younger infants, and over time, the degree of abnormality tends to lessen to produce more organized activity with greater synchrony and symmetry and lower amplitude.[78] The pattern may become modified, in which generalized sharp and slow-wave bursts become more synchronous within one hemisphere or between the two hemispheres.[79] In cases of large focal lesions such as cysts or porencephaly, the hypsarrhythmia pattern may be unilateral (asymmetric hypsarrhythmia) or associated with persistent focal spikes or sharp waves (Fig. 10-26). These variations may be classified as "*modified hypsarrhythmia.*" The hypsarrhythmic pattern is much more common in non-REM sleep than in the awake state or REM sleep.[80] In non-REM sleep, bursts may become associated with longer attenuation periods.

Hypsarrhythmia is commonly, but not always, associated with the clinical syndrome of "*infantile spasms.*"[81] Conversely, not all infantile spasms are associated with hypsarrhythmia. Infantile spasms are also seen in patients with *Aicardi's syndrome* with a distinct EEG pattern characterized by completely asynchronous burst suppression and multifocal spikes (see Fig. 6-15).[82] Seizures consist of brief flexion of the neck,

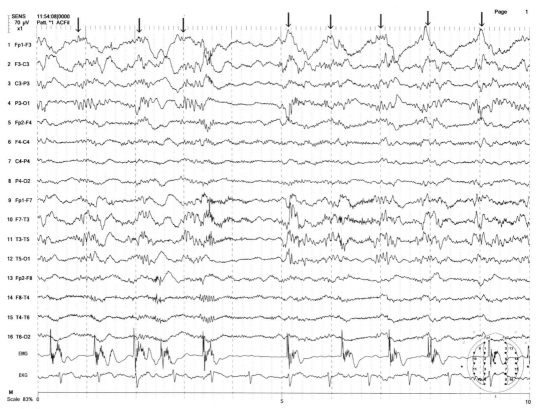

FIGURE 10-22 | Focal myoclonic seizure in a 42-year-old man presenting with recurrent jerking in the right leg. Periodic delta mixed with fast activities (PLEDs/LPD+F*) correlated consistently with EMG activity recorded from quadriceps muscles in EMG channel (indicated by *arrows*) (see also Video 13-7).

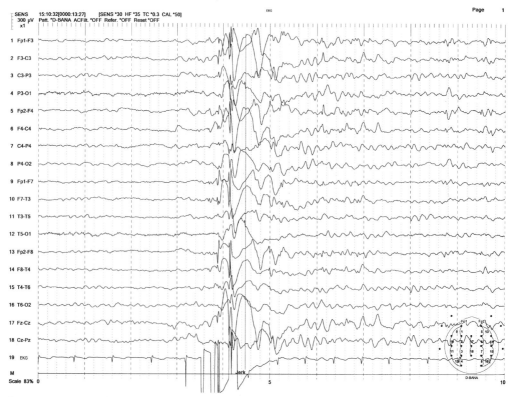

FIGURE 10-23 | Myoclonic seizure in a 10-year-old boy presenting with brief body jerking in sleep. EEG showed generalized irregular polyspike-wave bursts associated with movement artifacts recorded by the EKG channel.

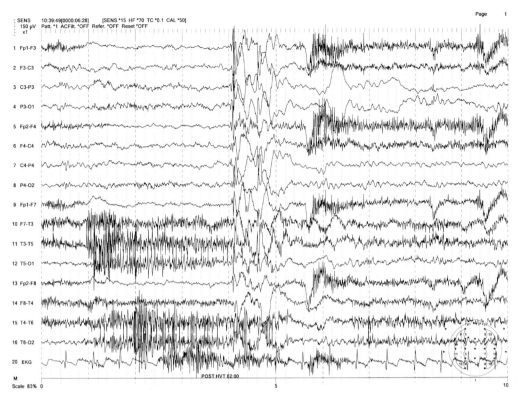

FIGURE 10-24 | Generalized irregular polyspike-wave bursts in 22-year-old woman with past history of absence seizures and recent "drop attacks," occasionally associated with loss of consciousness. Note the decrease of muscle artifacts during spike and wave bursts indicating the decrease of muscle tone.

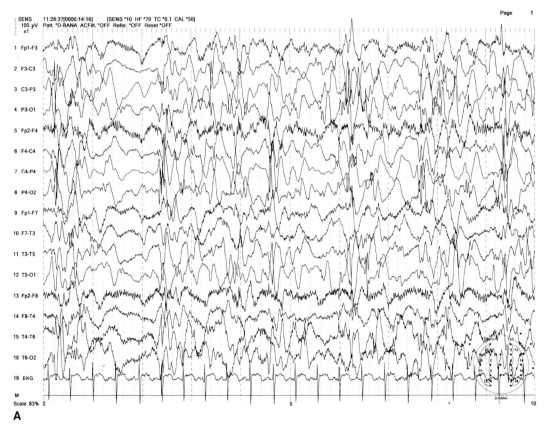

A

FIGURE 10-25 | Hypsarrhythmia in an 18-month-old microcephalic boy with infantile spasms. Note high-amplitude irregular delta activity mixed with multifocal spikes and characteristic brief episodes of quiescence between bursts **(A)**. The evidence of multifocal and scattered spikes are better visualized by eliminating slow waves using a shorter time constant (0.003 second) or lower filter setting of 5 Hz **(B)**. (**A** and **B** are the same EEG samples.)

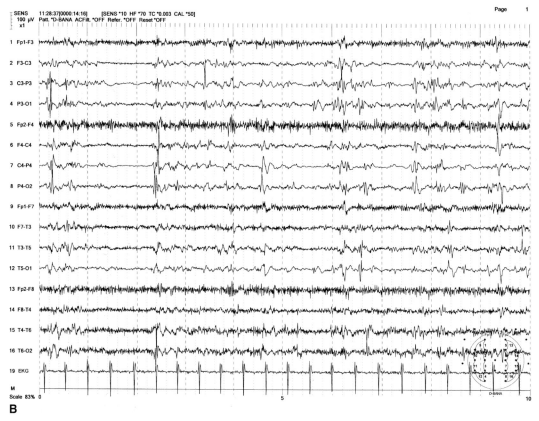

B

FIGURE 10-25 | (*Continued*)

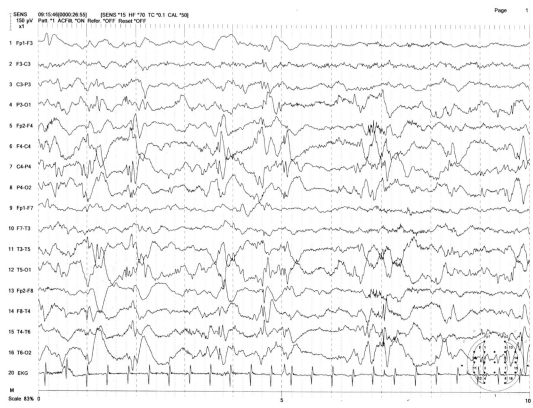

FIGURE 10-26 | Modified hypsarrhythmia in an 8-month-old girl with history of group B streptococcus meningitis at 2 weeks of age. The patient had frequent body jerks representing infantile spasms. Note the high-amplitude irregular spike-wave discharges from the right hemisphere, with brief quiescent periods between bursts (note sensitivity of 100 µV).

trunk, and extremities. This sudden flexed motion is called a *jackknife seizure or salaam attack*. Seizures tend to occur in clusters, shortly after awakening. The most common ictal EEG pattern associated with flexion spasms is sudden cessation of paroxysmal activity replaced by low-voltage fast activity or a flattening of EEG activity, termed an "*electrodecremental seizure*" (Fig. 10-27, Video 10-9). Other ictal patterns include frontal dominant, high-amplitude rhythmic delta bursts or, less commonly, generalized spike- or sharp-wave complexes.

The majority (>95%) of infantile spasms begin before the age of 1 year. Etiologies are diverse and include hereditary metabolic disorders, intrauterine infection, cerebral dysgenesis, tuberous sclerosis, hypoxic encephalopathy, etc. After adrenocorticotropic hormone (ACTH) or prednisone therapy, more than 60% of patients improved dramatically with normalization of the EEG.[83] Hypsarrhythmia disappears by 5 years; the EEG becomes normal in about half of the patients, while others continue to show various epileptiform discharges: either focal, multifocal, or evolve to generalized including a slow spike-wave pattern of Lenox–Gastaut syndrome (see next section). Normalization of the EEG does not necessarily indicate a normal neurologic state; nearly 90% of patients remain disabled by epilepsy and other neurological deficits including severe intellectual impairment.

Lennox–Gastaut Syndrome

Lennox[84] and later Gastaut[85] described the clinical and electroencephalographic features of this disorder. *LGS* represents a characteristic triad comprising (i) severe generalized seizures, (ii) intellectual disability, and (iii) an EEG showing slow spike and wave (SSW) complexes. The SSW complexes consist of biphasic or triphasic sharp or spike waves followed by high-voltage (generally 300 to 400 µV or greater) slow waves (Fig. 10-28). Frequency of SSW complexes is between 1.5 and 2.5 Hz and is slower and often more irregular than the 3-Hz spike-wave complexes associated with atypical absence epilepsy. The bursts are usually bilaterally synchronous but may show shifting or persistent asymmetries (Fig. 10-29A and B). Asymmetric bursts may be associated with a unilateral lesion.[86] In contrast to idiopathic absence epilepsy, which is usually associated with normal background activity, background activity in LGS is slow in more than 70% of the patients.[87] Unlike the 3-Hz spike-wave discharges of absence seizures, both hyperventilation and photic stimulation are less effective in eliciting spike-wave discharges.[88] In sleep, SSW complexes may become polyspike-wave discharges.[88] Also, paroxysmal fast activity is common during sleep.[89] In addition to the above characteristics of SSW complexes, focal or multifocal epileptiform discharges may be seen in some patients.[90]

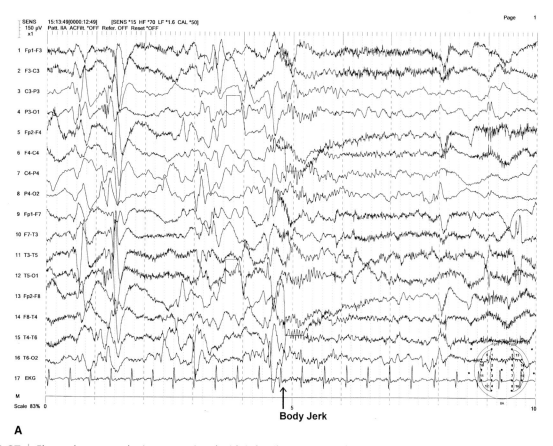

FIGURE 10-27 | Electrodecremental seizure associated with infantile spasms (ictal event) in a 2-year-old child. Five-year-old child with a history of hypoxic encephalopathy and severe developmental delay. Note sudden flattening of EEG activity accompanied by beta activity with concomitant increase of muscle tone artifact associated with body and arm jerks **(A)**. Interictal EEG consisted of extremely high-amplitude polymorphic delta (note sensitivity of 150) with scattered multifocal spikes and intermittent relative suppression periods, which are characteristic features of hypsarrhythmia **(B)** (see also Video 10-9).

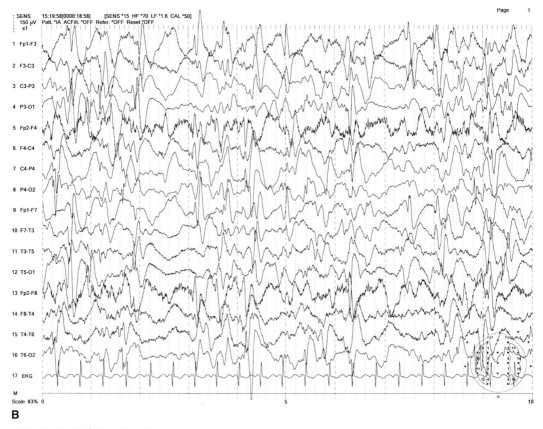

B

FIGURE 10-27 | (*Continued*)

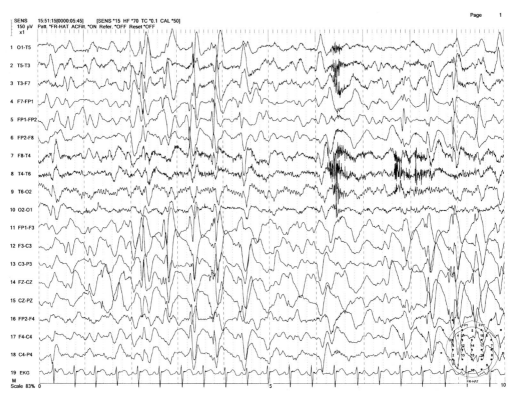

FIGURE 10-28 | Generalized 2-Hz spike-wave bursts in an 18-year-old intellectually disabled male patient with a history of intractable generalized tonic–clonic, tonic, and atypical absence seizures (Lennox–Gastaut syndrome). Note high-voltage slow (2-Hz) spike and wave complexes associated with abundant irregular delta–theta activity in this awake EEG.

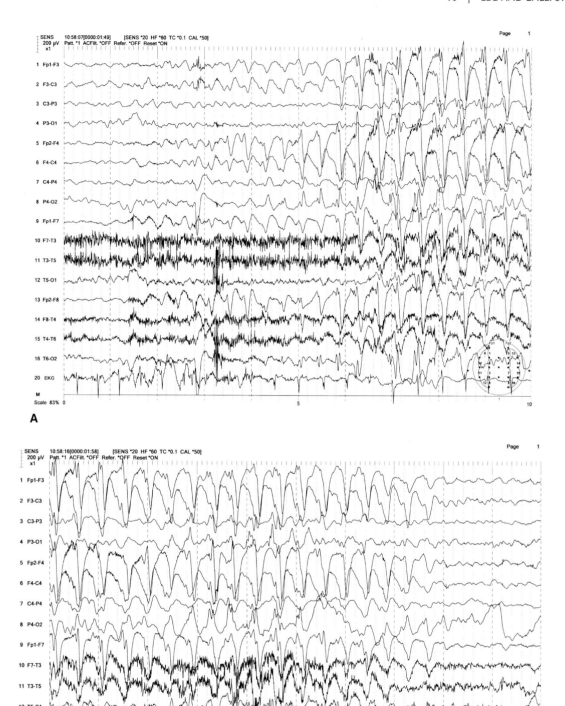

FIGURE 10-29 | **A and B:** Lennox–Gastaut syndrome associated with asymmetric slow (2-Hz) spike-wave bursts in a 7-year-old girl with diagnosis of *Angelman's syndrome.* The patient presented with a variety of intractable seizures including tonic, atypical absence, drop attack, and tonic–clonic types. Note the rhythmic, 2- to 2.5-Hz spike-wave discharges starting from the right hemisphere and then generalizing. This is likely an ictal (seizure) event. (**A** and **B** are consecutive recordings.)

Median age of seizure onset in LGS is about 1 year, and SSW complexes appear by 3 years. More than 75% of patients have more than one type of seizure. The most common seizures are tonic seizure and atypical absence. Tonic seizures tend to appear at an earlier age and consist of sudden flexion of the hips, upper trunk, and neck, as well as arm abduction, elevation, or semiflexion. Because the seizure resembles infantile spasms, it can be considered a mature form of infantile spasms.[91] Tonic seizures are associated with paroxysmal fast activity, often preceded by EEG flattening. The clinical distinction between typical and atypical absence seizures is not always clear, but some features distinguish them. With atypical absence, impairment of consciousness is incomplete, rendering the transitions between normal activity and seizure activity unclear. Other symptoms such as eyelid or mouth myoclonus, changes in muscle tone, excessive salivation, and automatisms are common with atypical absence.

Ictal EEG change with atypical absence may be difficult to distinguish from the interictal pattern because both are represented by slow spike-wave complexes. The ictal pattern, however, tends to be more rhythmic and more widely distributed and lasts longer than the interictal event.[88] Other seizure types in LGS include clonic or tonic–clonic, atonic, myoclonic, and infantile spasms. The least common seizure is partial complex seizure.

Progressive Myoclonic Epilepsy

There are several clinical entities that account for progressive myoclonic epilepsies. They are *myoclonic epilepsies with ragged red fibers (MERRF syndrome)*,[92] *Lafora disease*,[93] *Unverricht–Lundborg disease (Balic myoclonic epilepsy)*,[94] *neuronal ceroid lipofuscinosis (Batten's disease)*,[95] *sialidoses (cherry-red spot myoclonus syndrome)*,[96] and severe myoclonic epilepsy in infancy (Dravet syndrome).[49,50] These syndromes are characterized by myoclonic seizures, progressive ataxia, and dementia secondary to degenerative CNS disease with metabolic derangement. Other than myoclonic seizures, the patients may have generalized tonic–clonic seizures, atypical absence, and simple/complex partial seizures. In all forms of progressive myoclonic epilepsies, epileptiform activity consists of generalized spike wave, polyspike wave, and multifocal spikes. Background activity becomes progressively slower as the disease progresses. Photoparoxysmal responses are common in patients with Lafora disease, Unverricht–Lundborg disease, and Batten's disease. In Batten's disease, single or low-frequency intermittent photic stimulation characteristically produces prominent spike discharges at occipital electrodes with a one-to-one relationship with the light flash (see Fig. 9-11).

UNDETERMINED EPILEPSIES AND EPILEPTIC SYNDROMES

This category includes epileptic syndromes in which the focal or generalized nature of the seizure has not yet been determined. There are several diagnoses in neonate, infancy, and early childhood epilepsies that are categorized as epileptic syndromes. They are *benign neonatal seizure (BNS)*,[97,98] *early myoclonic encephalopathy (EME)*,[99] *early infantile epileptic encephalopathy (Ohtahara syndrome)*,[100] migrating partial seizures in infancy,[101] *benign myoclonic epilepsy in infancy*,[102] *benign infantile epilepsy*,[103] *severe myoclonic epilepsy in infants (Dravet syndrome)*,[49,50] and *myoclonic encephalopathy in nonprogressive disorders*.[104] Details of these disorders are beyond the scope of this chapter. All disorders with a "benign" character typically present normal interictal EEG. Some characteristic EEG features are generalized bursts of spike waves followed by suppression (bursts suppression pattern) seen in EME and Ohtahara syndrome. The photoparoxysmal responses are common in Dravet syndrome. In migrating partial seizure in infancy, EEG is characterized by nearly continuous electrographic seizures of multifocal origin. In many other syndromes, multifocal spikes and generalized spike-wave discharges are common epileptiform activity.

Landau–Kleffner Syndrome

Landau–Kleffner syndrome (LKS), first described by Landau and Kleffner,[105] is diagnosed based on characteristic clinical presentation and EEG abnormalities. LKS affects 3 to 9-year-old children who were previously in good health. The first clinical sign is dysphasia (speech difficulty), which progressively worsens. Speech becomes progressively less intelligible and is eventually limited to only a few words.[106] Hyperactivity and personality changes may appear as the aphasia worsens. About two thirds of patients have seizures of various types, including myoclonus, partial motor, akinetic/atonic, atypical absence, and generalized tonic–clonic convulsions.[107]

The EEG in LKS is characterized by abundant epileptiform activity that is extremely variable in both location and volume; because of the characteristic deterioration of speech function, one may assume that the dominant hemisphere (left) is primarily affected. In some cases, the epileptiform activity indeed affects preferentially the left temporal region. But surprisingly, the majority of cases show variable patterns ranging from unifocal, multifocal, and generalized spike wave. In the early stages of illness, epileptiform activity may appear only in sleep. As the disease progresses, EEG abnormalities change considerably in terms of location, abundance, and pattern. Eventually, spikes and spike-wave discharges become more or less continuous, resulting in an appearance of "*electrographic status epilepticus*" (see Fig. 9-12B). This EEG feature is similar to that seen in the *syndrome of continuous spike and wave during slow-wave sleep (CSWS)*.[108] In fact, LKS and CSWS overlap in both clinical and electrographic features.

Despite the severe degree of clinical and EEG abnormalities, many patients will recover with normal EEG and seizure remittance, but some degree of language dysfunction may persist.[107,109]

Continuous Spike and Wave during Slow-Wave Sleep

CSWS was first described by Patry.[109] The syndrome is characterized by continuous spike and wave activity during non-REM sleep[107,110] and is sometimes referred to as "*epilepsy with electrical status epilepticus during slow sleep*" (ESES) (Fig. 10-30A, compare with Fig. 10-30B).[110] The age of onset ranges from 1 to 12 years but is mostly around 8 years. Two thirds of patients are neurologically normal before onset. In time, most patients have

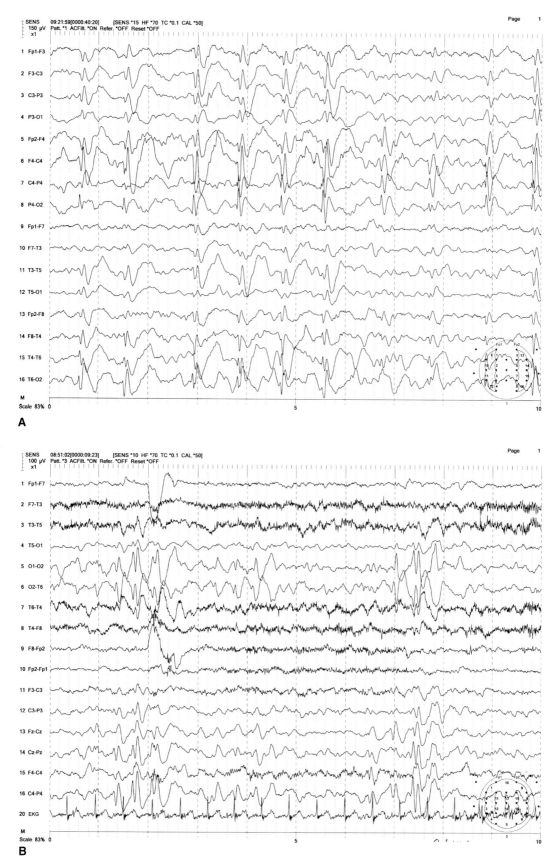

FIGURE 10-30 | Continuous spike and wave discharges during slow-wave sleep (CSWS) in a 7-year-old with history of generalized tonic–clonic seizures mostly during sleep and atypical absence associated with drop attacks. Note continuous right-greater-than-left parasagittal dominant spike-wave bursts in sleep **(A)**. These discharges are much less prominent in the awake state **(B)**.

frequent seizures (generalized tonic–clonic, atypical absence, and atonic) and have a significant decline in IQ with deterioration in language, impaired memory, reduced attention span, and behavioral changes with aggression or psychosis.[107,110]

Epileptiform activity consists of generalized slow (1.5 to 2.5 Hz) spike wave as well as focal or multifocal spikes, which are sporadic in the waking state. In sleep, spike-wave bursts become nearly continuous (CSWS pattern), occupying more than 85% of the total non-REM sleep time.[110] The CSWS pattern persists for one to several years. Similar to LKS, the EEG then tends to normalize and seizures remit spontaneously in most patients. However, recovery of neurological deficit and behavior is often incomplete and about half of the patients remain profoundly impaired.[107,110]

SPECIAL SYNDROMES

Febrile Seizures

This condition is categorized as a special syndrome by the International Classification. Febrile convulsions are the most common seizure disorder among infants and young children. Febrile seizures are classified into simple and complex types; the simple seizure consists of generalized convulsions and last less than 15 minutes. The complex type shows generally more focal features and last longer than 15 minutes or recur multiple times within 24 hours.[111] About 3% to 4% of all children have at least one febrile convulsion, usually between ages 6 months and 5 years. After the age of 5 years, a seizure occurring during fever is less likely to be an "uncomplicated" febrile seizure and more likely to be due to an underlying neurological problem.[112] In such cases, seizures associated with febrile illness must be differentiated from acute severe conditions such as encephalitis. Febrile seizure may be the presenting feature of Dravet syndrome or recently recognized clinical entity called febrile infection-related epilepsy syndrome (FIRES), which may later evolve into refractory status epilepticus.[111] With uncomplicated febrile seizures, the interictal EEG is normal and predicts favorable prognosis.[113] Conversely, an abnormal interictal EEG suggests an increased risk for a future epileptic disorder. Since Falconer's original description of high incidence of history of febrile convulsion in patients with mesial temporal lobe seizures,[114] the relationship between febrile seizure, especially complex febrile seizure, and later development of hippocampal sclerosis remains a topic of debate. The recent study has proposed temporal lobe epilepsy with history of febrile seizures as a distinctive subgroup among temporal lobe seizures.[115]

Other EEG Abnormalities Associated with Seizures

SECONDARILY GENERALIZED SPIKE AND WAVE DISCHARGES

In patients with tonic–clonic convulsions, predicting the seizure type (primary vs. secondary generalized) based on witness description is often inaccurate. Witness recall may be obscured by their surprise and fright. Additionally, they often do not see or notice the onset and may miss any focal manifestations. However, careful observation of seizure semiology such as the direction of head turning or arm/leg posturing may help to distinguish these two diagnoses (Video 10-10).

EEG helps distinguish primary from secondary generalized seizures in some cases but not always. Generally, bilaterally synchronous and symmetric spikes or spike-wave discharges represent a primary generalized seizure disorder. However, even in primary generalized epilepsy, spike waves may not be perfectly synchronous or symmetric. Conversely, epileptiform discharges arising from mesial or inferior aspects of the frontal lobe in one hemisphere may produce bifrontal dominant synchronous and symmetric discharges resembling generalized discharges.[116] It is, therefore, difficult to distinguish them even with the use of EEG. Some seizures spread relatively slowly from one hemisphere to the other and end in a generalized tonic–clonic convulsion (focal onset secondary generalized seizure) (Video 10-11).

The following features suggest secondary generalized seizures:

1. Spikes or spike-wave discharges in one hemisphere consistently preceding those in the other hemisphere. (This can be better visualized by increasing the sweep speed.) (See Fig. 10-31A and B; see also Fig. 10-11A and B.)
2. Amplitude of spikes or spike-wave discharges is consistently larger in one hemisphere.
3. In addition to bilaterally symmetric and synchronous discharges, focal spikes consistently appear in one location.
4. Morphology of focal interictal discharges is more variable in secondary than in primary generalized epilepsy.
5. Interictal discharges are multifocal.
6. Background activity is abnormal, either diffusely or focally.

PERIODIC DISCHARGES

There are several clinical conditions in which EEGs are characterized by periodically recurring paroxysmal discharges. Periodic discharges (PDs) usually reflect severe and acute or subacute CNS diseases. The discharges are comprised of a variety of waveforms including spikes, spike wave, sharp waves, and theta or delta slow waves or a mixture of these waves. Periodic discharges are usually of high amplitude, in the range of 100 to 300 μV, and may occur in a focal or lateralized [periodic lateralized epileptiform discharges (PLEDs/LPD)*] (see Figs. 10-37, 10-39, and 10-40) generalized periodic discharge (GPD*) (see Figs. 10-33D and 10-45A), bilaterally independent periodic discharge (BIPD*) (see Fig. 10-42) or multifocal periodic discharge (MfPD*) (see Fig. 10-41) pattern.

The following conditions are often associated with periodic discharge: subacute sclerosing panencephalitis, Creutzfeldt–Jakob disease, herpes simplex encephalitis, severe cerebral anoxia, and acute and severe cerebral infarct.

Diffuse Periodicity

SUBACUTE SCLEROSING PANENCEPHALITIS (SSPE). SSPE may be categorized in diffuse encephalopathy, but it is placed here because of the characteristic paroxysmal EEG pattern. SSPE is a sequel of the measles infection and has become extremely

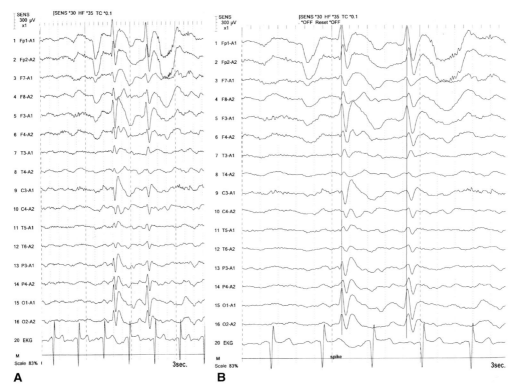

FIGURE 10-31 | Secondary generalized spike-wave discharges in an 8-year-old boy with diagnosis of fragile X syndrome and intellectual disability and with history of grand mal seizures **(A)**. Note left-sided frontal dominant spikes consistently precede right side spikes, which are better visualized by faster sweep speed **(B)**.

rare because of widely accepted immunization in the United States. The periodic burst activity in SSPE consists of high-amplitude slow waves mixed with sharp waves, occasionally including spike discharges, maximum in the frontocentral region (Fig. 10-32A and B). The bursts repeat at 4- to 15-second intervals[117] and tend to be more prominent during the awake state. Because of the relatively slow periodicity, a slower sweep speed (20 to 30 s/page) makes it easier to rate the repetition (Fig. 10-32B). Patients with SSPE often have myoclonus coinciding with the EEG bursts. Background activity becomes slow as the disease progresses. The origin of the periodic discharges has been debated as either thalamic[118] or cortical origin.[119]

CREUTZFELDT–JAKOB DISEASE. Creutzfeldt–Jakob disease can be also categorized in diffuse encephalopathy, but it is placed here because of its characteristic paroxysmal discharge pattern. The EEG plays an important role in the diagnosis of Creutzfeldt–Jakob disease (CJD). The clinical and neuropathological features of the disease were first described by Creutzfeldt[120] and Jakob.[121] The cardinal clinical signs are rapidly progressing dementia and myoclonus. Other symptoms include ataxia, visual signs and symptoms, extrapyramidal and/or pyramidal signs, and akinetic mutism. The disorder was initially thought to be due to a "slow virus infection" because the disease was transmitted from one chimpanzee to another by intracerebral inoculation.[122] The disease is now believed to be due to an abnormal isoform of the prion protein and is classified as a "*prion disease.*" This could be transmitted by tissue or medical instrument. It is therefore imperative to treat the electrodes according to infection control protocols.

Early EEG changes include reduction of normal background activity and an increase in slow waves. These slow waves are usually bilaterally diffuse but may start with a focal or lateralized prominence (Fig. 10-33A and B). As the disease progresses, diphasic or triphasic sharp and sharp wave discharges appear. Initially, the sharp discharges occur sporadically and may be focal or lateralized[123] (Fig. 10-33C). With further deterioration of the clinical picture, these paroxysmal discharges develop into a characteristic pattern with periodic and stereotyped sharp triphasic discharges of 100 to 600 ms duration in recurring intervals of 0.5 to 2 seconds[124,125] (Fig. 10-33D). The pattern is often indistinguishable from the EEG of nonconvulsive status epilepticus. Sometimes, periodic discharges appear in a lateralized fashion, assuming the form of PLEDs or LPD* before evolving to a bilateral generalized periodic pattern (GPD*). Evolution to the characteristic periodic pattern usually occurs within 12 weeks after the onset of disease. Therefore, serial EEGs are useful in confirming the diagnosis and monitoring the disease progression. Overall, EEG diagnosis has high sensitivity (~60%) and high positive predictive values (>90%).[126,127] Combining EEG and examination of the 14-3-3 protein in the cerebrospinal fluid increases the diagnostic probability of CJD.

Periodic discharges may be associated with clinical myoclonic jerks but, more often, they are not.[124] However, using innovative methods such as jerk-locked averaging techniques (evoked potential trigged by jerking and averaged by multiple jerking), Shibasaki et al.[128] found that the myoclonic jerks were associated with sharp discharges preceding the myoclonus by 50 to 85 ms recorded on the contralateral hemisphere. Toward the final stage of disease,

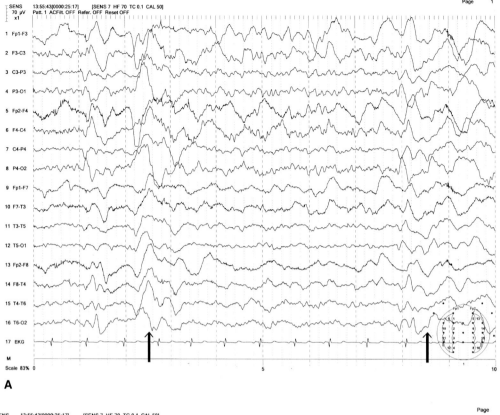

A

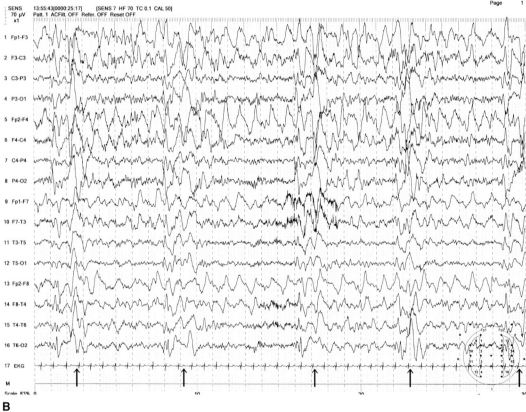

B

FIGURE 10-32 | Generalized periodic discharges in a 15-year-old boy with diagnosis of SSPE (subacute sclerosing panencephalitis). Note two bursts of irregular delta waves occurring in about 5-second intervals (indicated by *arrows*) **(A)**. Because of slow recurrence, the periodicity was not clear with routine sweep speed of 10 s/page, but this became more evident (indicated by *arrows*) with slower sweep speed of 30 s/page **(B)**. (First 10-second sample of **B** is the same sample with **A**.)

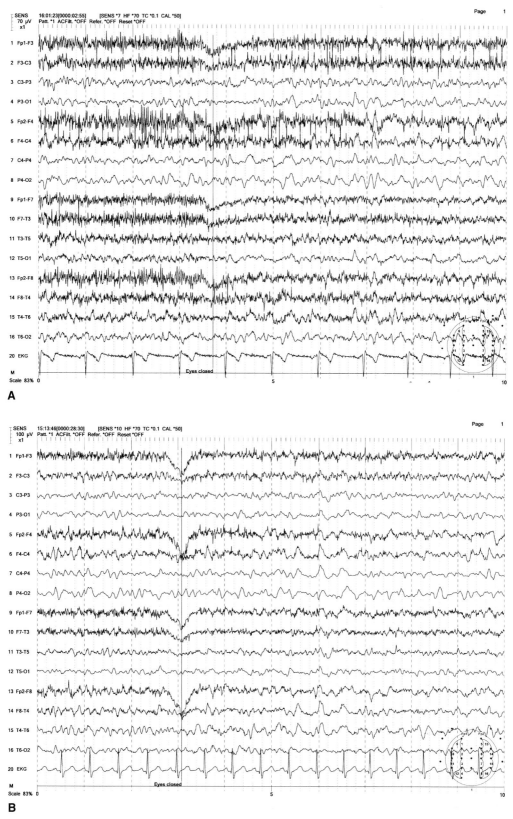

FIGURE 10-33 | Serial EEGs in a 60-year-old woman with a diagnosis of Creutzfeldt–Jakob disease, presenting with rapidly progressive dementia and myoclonus. The first EEG shows increased delta–theta slow waves, more prominent in the right posterior head region **(A)**. Two weeks later, delta slowing increases **(B)**. By the 4th week after the first EEG, the patient started to show myoclonic movements of her hands. At this time, the EEG shows intermittently periodic triphasic sharp discharges with right-greater-than-left posterior dominance (*shown by box in* **C**). At 3 months after the first EEG, periodically recurring diffuse triphasic sharp discharges at intervals of 1 to 1.5 seconds become evident **(D)**. The background activity initially consisted of a mixture of alpha and theta rhythms that progressively decreased.

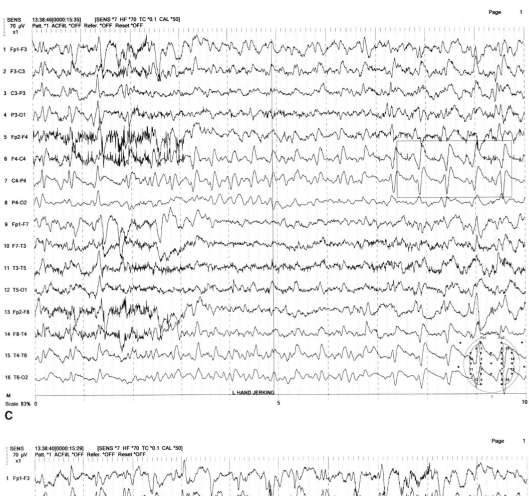

C

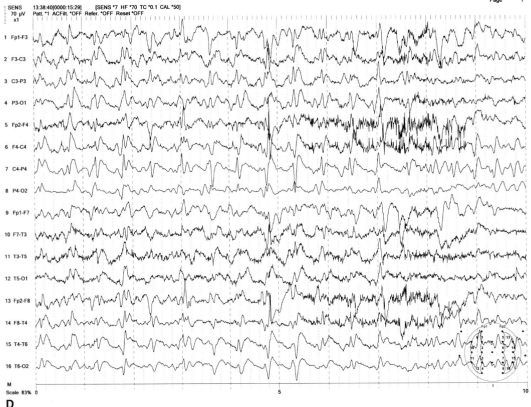

D

FIGURE 10-33 | (*Continued*)

the interval between sharp waves increases and their amplitude decreases. Eventually, the EEG becomes markedly suppressed.

Death usually occurs in a few to several months after the onset of periodic discharges. It should be noted that some patients with a confirmed diagnosis of CJD may not have a typical EEG picture, even with serial EEG recordings.

There is a variant of CJD, *Heidenhain's variant*, which predominantly affects the occipital lobes. The EEG often shows more focal slowing and periodic discharges over the posterior head regions.[129]

POSTANOXIC CEREBRAL INSULT. The EEG pattern after an anoxic event varies considerably, depending on the severity of the cerebral insult. The EEG may show diffuse slowing, frontal intermittent rhythmic delta activity (FIRDA, frontally predominant GRDA*), continuous spikes, periodic spikes, triphasic discharges, burst suppression pattern, alpha coma, severely depressed EEG activity, or electrocerebral silence. Periodic discharges may occur with lateralized (LPD*, bilaterally independent (BIPD*), or generalized (GPD*) form.

Periodic spikes or bursts are one of the patterns often encountered after severe postanoxic brain damage. The patient is invariably comatose. The periodic patterns vary from single spikes to more complex bursts consisting of various mixtures of theta–delta, sharps, and spikes. Between the periodic discharges, EEG activity is suppressed in various degrees from depressed activity to total flattening in between the bursts, forming a "*burst suppression pattern*" (Fig. 10-34A and B). Greater cerebral insults result in longer periods of suppression and lower amplitude of the bursts (compare Figs. 10-34A and 10-34B). Bursts or myoclonic jerks may be triggered by sensory stimuli.[130] The patient may exhibit a variety of myoclonic jerks which are often, but not always, time-locked to the bursts or spikes. If each movement is time-locked to the paroxysmal bursts, it is difficult or impossible to distinguish artifacts versus epileptiform activity. In this case, the patient should be paralyzed with muscle relaxant, assuming the patient is on artificial ventilation (Fig. 10-35A and B; see Video 13-7). In some patients, myoclonic twitches are totally independent from spikes or burst activities (Fig. 10-36, also compare with Fig. 10-22). Myoclonic jerks are often intractable to antiepileptic drugs. A decrease in bursts with longer

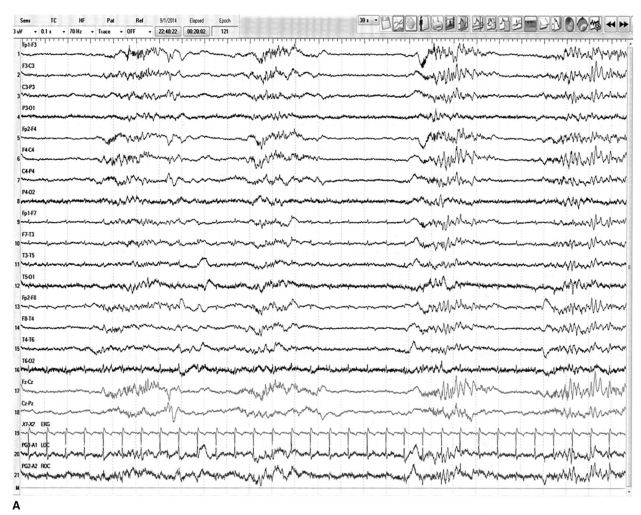

A

FIGURE 10-34 | Burst suppression pattern recorded 10 hours after an episode of cardiac arrest in a 68-year-old male. The burst consisted of mixture of diffuse beta/spindles/theta discharges of duration of 1 to 2 seconds, separated by 1- to 2-second suppression periods **(A)**. The following day, the burst became shorter with longer suppression periods **(B)**. This indicates either worsening cerebral function or increased sedation or deeper hypothermia if the patient is placed under hypothermia treatment.

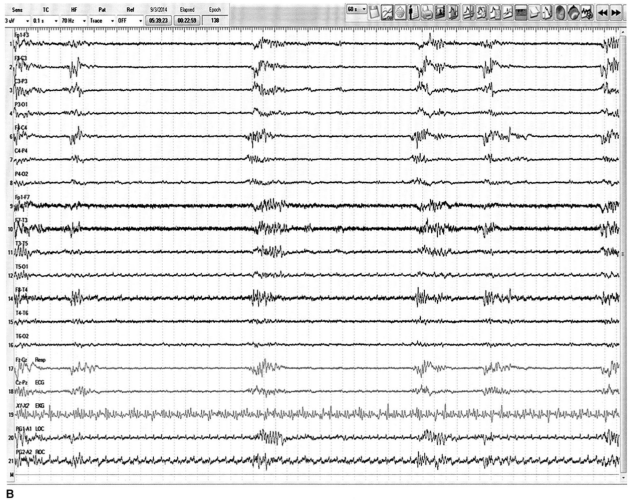

B

FIGURE 10-34 | *(Continued)*

suppression period indicates the deterioration of cerebral function or increased sedative drug effect (see Fig. 10-34A and B). Although most anoxic cerebral insult is bilaterally diffuse, some patients may show lateralized periodic lateralized discharges, PLEDs or LPD* (see next section, Fig. 10-37).

EEG can provide highly reliable prognostic value; the so-called malignant EEG patterns including low amplitude (<20 μV) or near electrocerebral silence, burst suppression pattern with or without generalized epileptiform activity, and electrographic status epilepticus were associated with poor outcomes (death) with false-positive predictive value of 3%.[131,132]

Another pattern, which also implies poor outcome, is alpha–theta coma pattern (see Alpha and Theta Coma Pattern in Chapter 11). Another commonly encountered EEG pattern in the postanoxic state is paroxysmal, periodic, or rhythmic ictal-like discharges named "*SIRPIDs*" (stimulus-induced rhythmic periodic or ictal discharges in comatose or semicomatose patients)[133] (Fig. 10-38A and B). This pattern is consistently induced by self-arousal or external stimuli by patient care activities (see SIRPID in this chapter; see also Video 13-3B). SIRPID likely has a better prognosis than the "malignant EEG patterns."[134] In any of the above EEG patterns after anoxic cerebral insult, the presence of reactive EEG changes

suggests a better prognosis than a nonreactive EEG (although it is extremely unlikely to see a reactive EEG in a very low voltage or in a burst suppression pattern).[135] It is, therefore, important for the technologist to stimulate the patient by calling his/her name or using nail bed pressure during an artifact-free recording period. Recently, therapeutic hypothermia has been introduced for the treatment of cerebral anoxic insult.[136] EEG monitoring was then recommended during the hypothermia (32°C to 34°C or 89.8°F to 93.2°F) because some patients show epileptiform discharges during the cooling phase or during the warming phase.[137] However, thus far, there has been no clear evidence that treating seizures improves the outcome.[137,138]

Periodic Lateralized Epileptiform Discharges (PLEDs)

PLEDs or LPD* (Lateralized Periodic Discharges) are periodically recurring paroxysmal discharges of sharp waves, spike waves, or complex discharges consisting of mixed theta–delta waves arising from one hemisphere or a relatively restricted area within one hemisphere (Fig. 10-39A and B; see Video 13-2A and B).

The discharges may repeat as fast as 3/s or as slow as 10/ min.[139] PLEDs or LPD* occur most often after acute, relatively large destructive cerebral lesions. The most common etiology

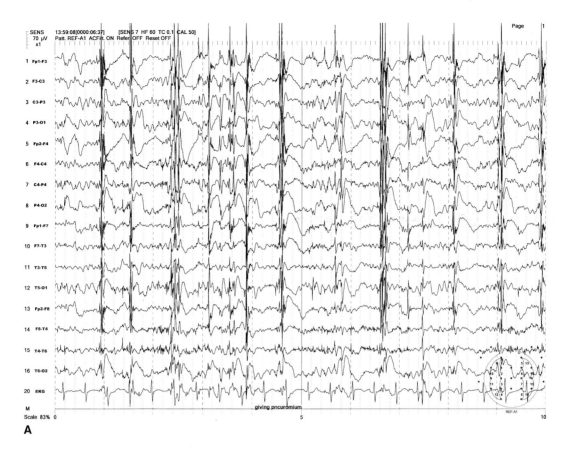

A

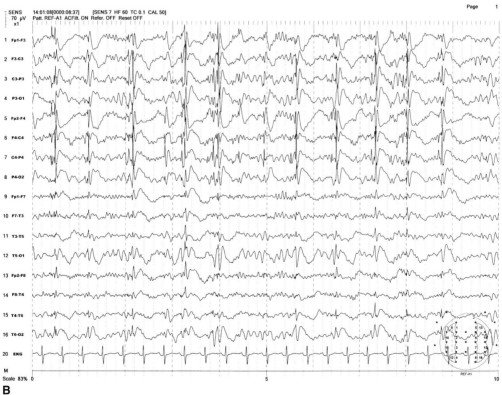

B

FIGURE 10-35 | EEG in a 65-year-old man in comatose state after postanoxic cerebral insult. The patient exhibited frequent facial muscle twitches, which contaminated the EEG **(A)**. Because it was not certain if the spike/polyspike discharge-associated twitches are of muscle or cerebral origin, the patient was paralyzed by pancuronium. Recurrent bursts of spike/polyspikes continued after the patient was pharmacologically paralyzed, verifying that the bursts were of cerebral origin, indicating that the patients was having myoclonic seizures **(B)** (see also Video 13-6).

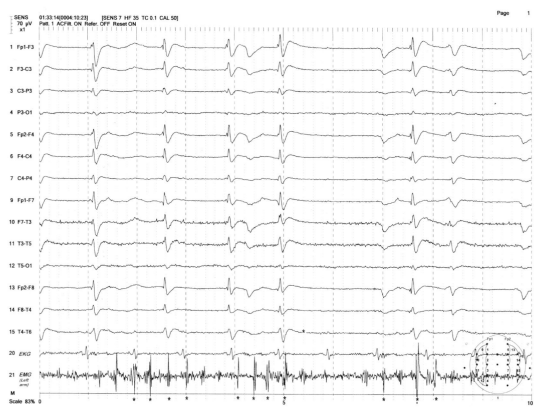

FIGURE 10-36 | Recurrent sharp discharges and suppression in a 72-year-old man in comatose state after postanoxic cerebral insult. The EEG showed recurrent, frontal dominant sharp discharges alternating with suppression periods. The patient showed repetitive left arm twitches, but they were not associated with EEG discharges. Note the dissociation of sharp discharges and EMG activity (*channel 21*) recorded from the left arm.

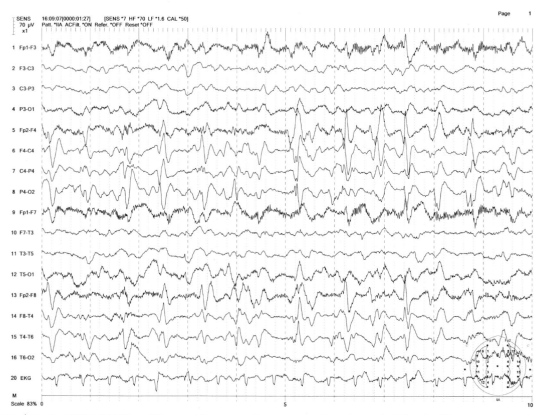

FIGURE 10-37 | Typical PLEDs/LPD* in a 77-year-old woman after severe postanoxic cerebral insult. CT scan was negative for cerebral infarct. Note periodically recurring sharp discharges at a rate close to one/s from right hemisphere.

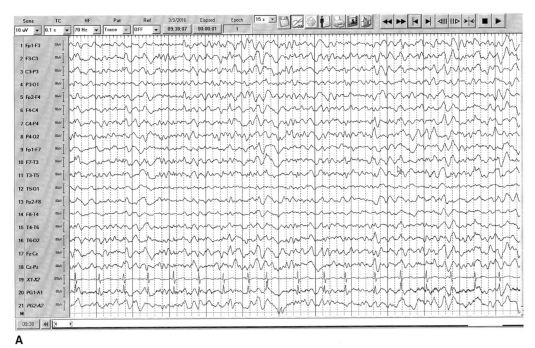

A

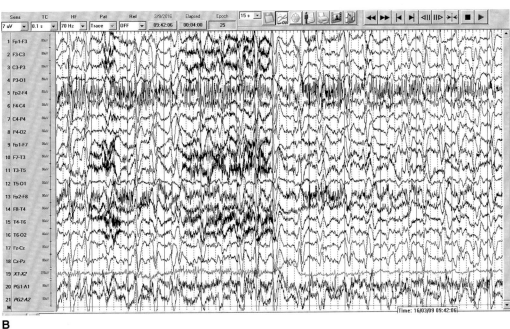

B

FIGURE 10-38 | Sixty-three-year-old female with diagnosis of lymphoma became confused 5 days after chemotherapy. EEG during quiet periods showed diffuse theta–delta slow waves **(A)**. Each time when the patient was aroused by ICU staff or self-aroused with increased muscle artifacts, EEG changed to periodically recurring triphasic sharp delta waves (SIRPID) **(B)**. Note the increased muscle artifacts indicating arousal episode in B (see also Video 13-3A and B).

is acute cerebral infarct (see Chapter 12, Cerebrovascular Accidents), especially of the watershed type. The second most common etiology is herpes simplex (HSV1) encephalitis.[140] HSV1 infection has a preference to involve the temporal lobe or frontotemporal region. Thus, PLEDs/LPD* are often focal to temporal electrodes. PLEDs are also reported in other types of encephalitis such as infectious mononucleosis[141] and Rasmussen encephalitis.[142]

PLEDs/LPD* may be associated with simultaneous contralateral focal motor seizures, called epilepsia partialis continua (focal motor status) (see Fig. 10-22; see also Video 13-8). In

this case, PLEDs (LPD*) are an expression of the focal ictal pattern, but most PLEDs are an interictal or postictal pattern. Once PLEDs (LPD*) are encountered, continuous EEG monitoring is highly recommended to find out if there is any episode or progressively changing pattern indicating ictal discharges (Fig. 10-39A and B; see Video 13-2A). The ictal pattern may be an electrographic expression only and may not be accompanied by clinical seizures. In some cases, PLEDs/LPD* may not readily be evident because the periodicity is exceedingly slow or the discharges consist mainly of slow waves (Fig. 10-40). Some PLEDs/LPD* may arise from two

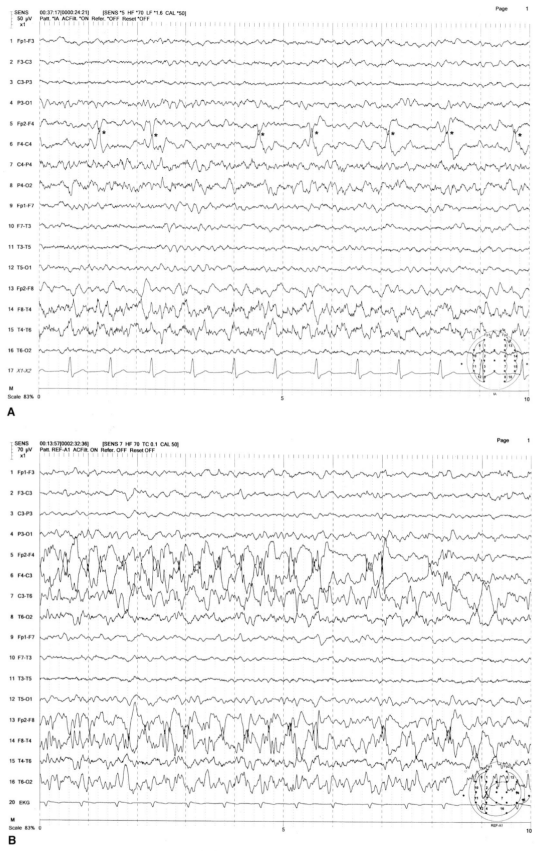

FIGURE 10-39 | Periodic lateralized epileptiform discharges (PLEDs/LPD*) in a 75-year-old woman with large, right intraparenchymal hemorrhage. The patient was comatose during EEG recording. Note periodic sharp discharges from the right hemisphere, most prominently at the right central region **(A)**. Long-term EEG monitoring revealed episodes of semirhythmic delta intermixed with fast activity involving the right hemisphere, representing an electrographic ictal (seizure) event without apparent clinical change **(B)** (see also Video 13-2A).

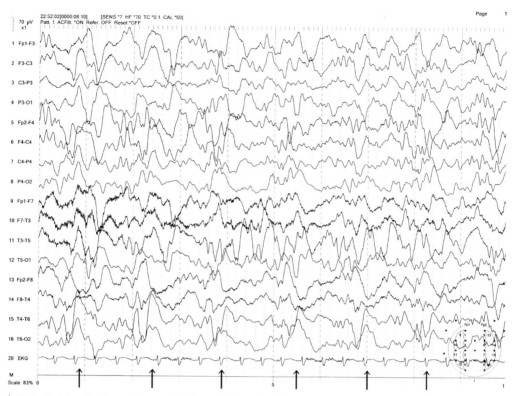

FIGURE 10-40 | Periodic lateralized epileptiform discharge (PLEDs/LPD*) in a 16-year-old boy with diagnosis of herpes simplex encephalitis. Unlike other PLEDs consisting mostly of sharp or spike epileptiform discharges, the periodic discharges in this case consist of delta mixed with sharp and theta discharges (indicated by *arrows*).

different locations within one hemisphere (Fig. 10-41A). In some PLEDs/LPD*, PLEDs from one region consistently lead PLEDs from another within one hemisphere (Fig. 10-41B; see also Video 13-2B).

PLEDs/LPD* may be a transient phenomenon and could change into other abnormalities. Some patients develop bilaterally independent periodic discharges, referred to as BiPLEDs (BIPD*) (Fig. 10-42A and B). These occur most often in herpes simplex encephalitis or severe anoxic encephalopathy.[143] BiPLEDs (BIPD*) are also present in children with acute CNS disease[144] including complex partial status epilepticus (CPSE).[145]

In the earlier stages of herpes simplex encephalitis, the EEG may show focal or unilateral polymorphic delta primarily in the temporal regions, but soon, periodically recurring sharp discharges of 100 to 500 μV amplitude occur with an interval of 2 to 4 seconds.

Ictal Discharges

ICTAL VERSUS INTERICTAL EPILEPTIFORM ACTIVITY

An important responsibility of the EEG technologist is recognizing an ictal event while recording an EEG. Once an ictal or suspected ictal event is recorded, a physician should be immediately notified before the recording is terminated.

In some cases, it is difficult to differentiate ictal discharges from interictal epileptiform activity based only on EEG findings. History and clinical observation may be correlated to determine if the recorded activity is an ictal (seizure) event. Four principles may help in characterizing an ictal pattern:

1. Sudden change of frequency. Onset of an ictal event is marked by a sudden change in frequency, often low-voltage fast (beta or gamma) activity, which is followed by progressively slower frequencies and higher-amplitude rhythmic activity (see Figs. 8-6, 8-8 and 10-7A–D, Video 10-12).
2. Sudden rhythmic activity. The sudden appearance of rhythmic activity of any frequency raises the possibility of an ictal event. The rhythmic activity may or may not show a progressive change in frequency or amplitude (see Videos 13-1 and 13-2). A seizure detection computer program measures the degree of rhythmicity as one of its criteria for an ictal event.
3. Sudden flattening of EEG activity. Some seizures, especially at the onset, show sudden flattening of EEG activity (desynchronization). This may be correlated with a tonic seizure, the tonic phase of a tonic–clonic seizure, or an electrodecremental seizure as seen in *West syndrome* (hypsarrhythmia) (see Fig. 10-27A; see Video 10-9).
4. Sudden appearance of rhythmic spike-wave discharges. A typical example of a sudden increase in amplitude is the 3-Hz spike-wave bursts associated with absence seizures (see Figs. 10-15, 10-16, 10-21B, and 10-29A and B; see also Videos 9-2 and 10-6). Generally, if the 3-Hz spike waves last longer than 4 to 5 seconds, the patient will likely show observable clinical changes, and then it is called ictal event. However, there is no clear definition or agreement how long the paroxysmal discharges should last to be called "ictal event." In fact, the EEG examples from Figures 10-11, 10-16, and 10-17A are difficult to decide if these represent an interictal or ictal pattern.

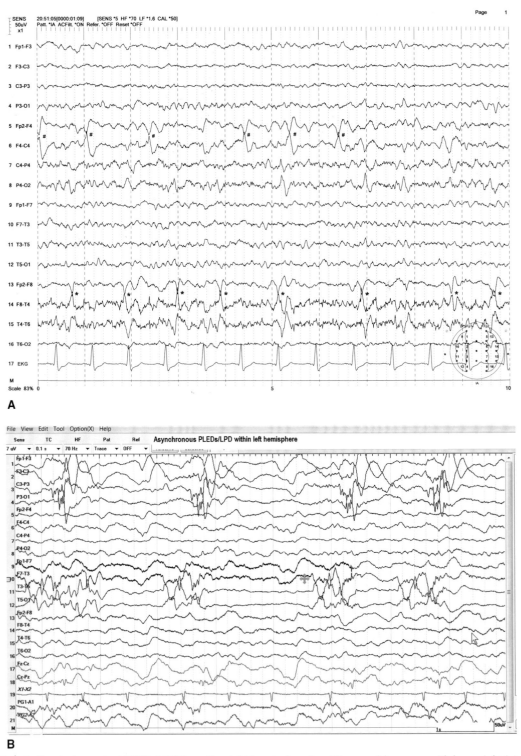

FIGURE 10-41 | **A:** Two independent PLEDs/LPD* from the right hemisphere in a 75-year-old woman with large right intraparenchymal hematoma. Note two independent PLEDs, one from F4 (indicated by #) and the other from F8 (indicated by *). **B:** Patient was a 57-year-old male with nontraumatic intracerebral hemorrhage. EEG was recorded a day after left hemicraniectomy for clot evacuation. There were asynchronous PLEDs within the left hemisphere, but PLEDs from the left temporal region consistently lead PLEDs from the left temporal region (see Video 13-2B ictal event for this patient).

Recently, the concept of *BIRD (brief ictal or interictal rhythmic discharges)*,[146] *BERD (brief electrographic rhythmic discharges)*,[147] or *BRD (brief rhythmic discharges* according to ACNS guideline) was initially described in critically ill neonates with seizures. Later, the same concept was applied to the adults and called *B(I)RD*, which stands for *brief potentially ictal rhythmic discharges*[148] (Fig. 10-43). The pattern is usually found in critically ill patients who undergo continuous bedside monitoring, mostly at an ICU setting (see Chapter 13). The discharges consist of brief (<10

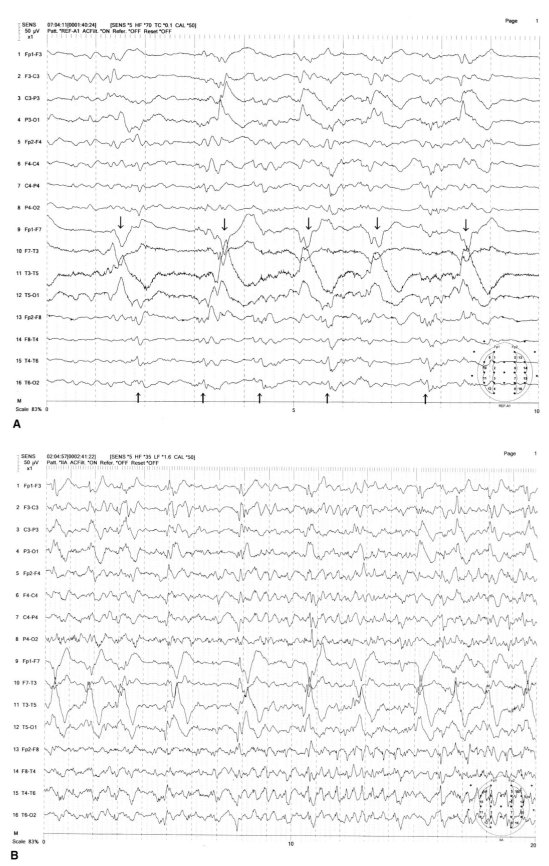

FIGURE 10-42 | Bilateral independent periodic lateralized epileptiform discharges (BiPLEDs, BIPD*) in a 62-year-old man with diagnosis of herpes simplex encephalitis. Two independent PLEDs from right and left temporal regions are evident; the left hemisphere shows periodic large delta activity (*downward arrows*), and the right hemisphere shows periodic sharp discharges (*upward arrows*) **(A)**. The periodicity was better visualized with slower sweep speed (20 s/page) **(B)**.

seconds) focal or generalized rhythmic or repetitive often sharply contoured activity of any frequency with our without progressive change, resembling ictal events and usually recur frequently during EEG monitoring (Fig. 10-43). This is usually seen in the EEG of diffuse slowing and/or definite electrographic ictal (seizure) events. As the above acronym with parenthesis implies, it is not certain if these brief events are ictal or interictal patterns. However, all agree that the presence of BIRD, B(I)RD, or BERD suggests a higher chance of the development of unequivocal clinical or subclinical seizure events and also a higher morbidity or mortality rate than the EEG without this pattern (see Video 13-5).

GENERALIZED SEIZURES

Absence Seizures or Generalized Absence†

There is essentially no difference between the ictal and interictal discharges in absence seizures except that generalized 3-Hz spike-wave bursts lasting longer than 3 to 4 seconds usually accompany a recognizable "absence" seizure clinically. The generalized spike-wave discharges begin abruptly with a frequency of 3.5 to 4 Hz at onset with gradual slowing to 2.5 to 3 Hz. The bursts terminate abruptly without postictal EEG change (see Fig. 10-15; see Video 9-2).

---

†Some of the nomenclature for seizure diagnoses are adopted from operational classification of seizure types by International League Against Epilepsy. www.uptodate.com/contents/ilae-classification-of-seizures-and-epilepsy

Juvenile Absence Seizures

This type of absence seizure generally affects older children (9 to 13 years old) more than childhood absence seizure. The ictal pattern is similar to that of childhood absence, although the bursts commonly include generalized polyspike components and consist of faster than 3 Hz spike waves (3.5 to 6 Hz) (see Fig. 10-16; see also Video 10-6).

Atypical Absence Seizures or Generalized Absence, Atypical†

Atypical absence seizures share the similar semiology with typical absence seizure such as blank stare or daydreaming, but the patients may be somewhat more responsive and show more pronounced motor symptoms such as stiffening, jerking, and/or automatism. Also, many patients have other types of seizure such as myoclonic and/or myoclonic astatic seizures (*Doose syndrome*). The ictal pattern is not typical 3-Hz spike-wave bursts but consists of rhythmic slow spike-wave activity (2 to 2.5 Hz) characterized by a more gradual beginning and ending than that of classical absence seizures (see Fig. 10-29A and B). Most patients are intellectually disabled and could be associated with LGS.

Myoclonic and Atonic Seizures or Generalized Myoclonic† and Generalized Atonic†

The EEG patterns of atonic and myoclonic seizures may be indistinguishable (see and compare Figs. 10-23 and 10-24). The ictal pattern consists of high-amplitude, rapid (10 to 15 Hz) polyspikes with or without accompanying slow waves. This may be followed by a brief electrodecremental period.

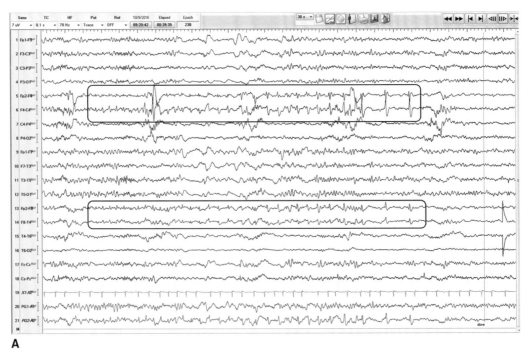

A

FIGURE 10-43 | Example of B(I)RD **(A)** and nonconvulsive focal seizure **(B and C)** in 73-year-old female with right frontal craniotomy for intracerebral hemorrhage. The patient showed recurrent episodes of brief (~25 seconds in full scale of 30 seconds page) with repetitive small spikes involving Fp2, F4, and F8 electrodes (shown by *rectangular box*) with some progression, consistent with B(I)RD. This patient also showed occasional episodes of clear electrographic ictal pattern (nonconvulsive) with repetitive spikes involving the same electrodes as those of B(I)RD. The ictal event consisted of much faster frequency and progressively larger spikes with slower frequency (Fig. 10-43B–E). The ictal event lasted about 5 minutes (see also Video 13-5).

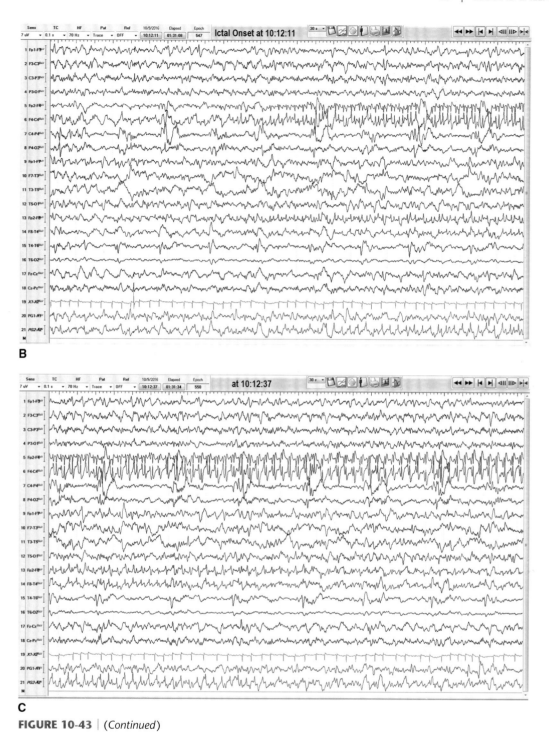

B

C

FIGURE 10-43 | (Continued)

Generalized Tonic–Clonic Seizures

The seizure often commences with a brief period of extreme "flattening" of EEG activity with or without superimposed low-voltage beta activity. But this portion of EEG recording is usually obscured by muscle artifacts (see Fig. 10-20A and B; see also Video 10-8). This evolves to progressively higher amplitude and slower frequency at about 10 Hz. The fast activity is associated with the tonic phase of the seizure. It is followed by rhythmic slow activity blending with polyspike or spike-wave discharges, which progressively become slower in frequency toward the end of the seizure (see Fig. 10-20B; see also Video 10-8). The rhythmic slow-wave and polyspike and wave discharges are associated with the clonic phase of the seizure. When the seizure is finished, the patient is usually unresponsive and limp. The postictal phase consists of profound voltage suppression, which is gradually replaced by low-voltage delta that increases in amplitude and frequency until full recovery of the background activity. If the seizure is less severe, the postictal pattern consists of diffuse delta slow waves, which gradually recover to the preseizure state. Noticing postictal EEG change is important to confirm the seizure and to differentiate from non-epileptic seizure because the EEG could be totally obscured by muscle and movement artifacts throughout

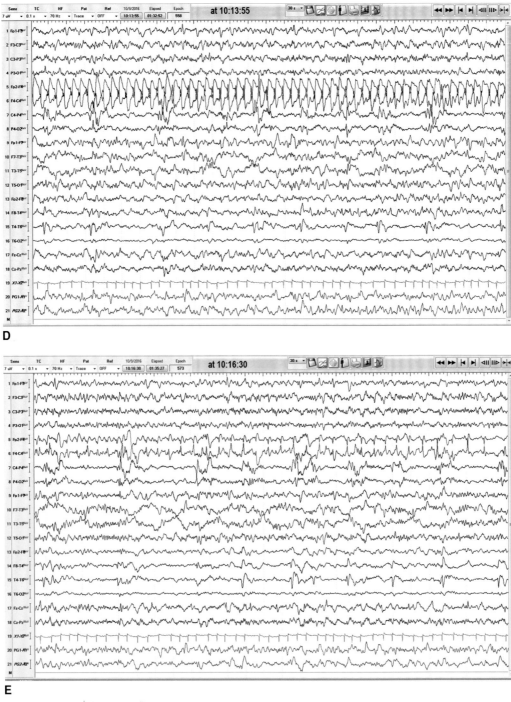

FIGURE 10-43 | (Continued)

the entire event. Duration of the postictal phase is usually brief (less than a few minutes) but varies considerably depending on the duration, severity, recurrence, and type of seizures.

FOCAL SEIZURES

In contrast to some generalized seizures (absence) in which the ictal pattern shows little change throughout the seizure (isomorphic seizure pattern) and is similar to the interictal epileptiform pattern, a focal ictal pattern changes progressively during the seizure and is dissimilar from the interictal epileptiform activity. The ictal pattern is characterized by sustained rhythmic activity with frequency between 3 and 20 Hz and starts focally or unilaterally with progressive change in amplitude, frequency, and spatial distribution.

Simple Partial Seizures or Focal Aware (Seizures)[†]

It is not uncommon for simple partial seizures to occur without any detectable scalp EEG change. This is because the area involved in the epileptic discharge is too small or distant to be detected by scalp electrodes. EEG expression of an ictal event may only be local attenuation of background or interictal epileptiform activity. One should be aware that a negative EEG recorded while the patient is having a simple partial seizure does not rule out a seizure diagnosis. In general, it is our experience that partial seizures arising from the occipital lobe frequently show a progressive ictal pattern (see Fig. 10-7A–D). EEG will likely show a change when a simple partial seizure evolves to a complex partial or secondary generalized seizure (see Videos 10-5a and 10-5B).

Complex Partial Seizures/Focal with Impaired Awareness† (Seizures)

As surgical treatment for medically intractable epilepsy has become increasingly popular in recent years, the knowledge gained from implanted electrodes has brought better understanding of scalp-recorded ictal patterns.

The ictal pattern in partial complex seizures starts with rhythmic waves of any frequency. In general, fast frequency activity at the onset suggests that the seizure origin is close to the detecting electrode (see Figs. 8-6, and 10-7A–D see also Video 10-12). Slow-frequency activity (theta or delta) usually implies a more distant seizure focus that has already spread to a wider area (see Videos 10-1 and 10-2). In some cases, there is attenuation of ongoing EEG activity, including interictal spikes prior to the onset of rhythmic discharges. If the attenuation is limited to a focal region, this could be a reliable sign in localizing the seizure onset.

Rhythmic discharges at onset become progressively larger in amplitude and slower in frequency, spreading to other areas, and may or may not include sharp or spike discharges. The postictal phase consists of diffuse or lateralized delta activity which progressively diminishes until the return to a baseline background activity. The clinical seizure usually starts well before the onset of EEG changes. Because the onset of ictal discharge is discretely localized to a small region or deep source, scalp-recorded EEG begins to show the ictal discharges only when the ictal activity involves sufficiently large areas. Implanted electrodes placed close to the region of origin often show discretely localized low-voltage fast activity which often coincides with the onset of the aura or clinical seizure. EEG may show no clear EEG changes in about 5% during a complex partial seizure,[149] especially a seizure originating from mesial frontal lobe.[150]

Status Epilepticus

Status epilepticus is a condition in which prolonged or recurrent seizures accompany persistent alteration of the neurological state. The International League Against Epilepsy (ILAE) traditionally defines epileptic status as "a single epileptic seizure lasting more than 30 minutes or a series of epileptic seizures during which function is not regained between ictal events in a 30 minute period."[151] However, the recent report from ILAE has defined a seizure lasting longer than 5 minutes as "status epilepticus,"[152] primarily because the initiation of treatment should not wait for ½ hour when a continual seizure is encountered, especially for a generalized tonic-clonic seizure. Prompt EEG recording and examination is essential for appropriate determination and management of the condition. The clinical expression of status epilepticus, especially nonconvulsive status, may be subtle or unrecognizable in some patients. EEG may be the first diagnostic tool that leads to the correct diagnosis. If the technologist suspects status epilepticus from the clinical as well as EEG findings, he or she should initiate prompt communication with the electroencephalographer/neurophysiologist and/or referring physician because status epilepticus is a medical emergency.

GENERALIZED CONVULSIVE STATUS EPILEPTICUS

Generalized tonic-clonic status epilepticus is a serious condition having a fairly high mortality rate if not treated promptly. Most (95%) of these cases are due to focal epilepsy with secondary generalization.[153] In more than 50% of patients, status epilepticus may be the first epileptic manifestation.[153] The most frequent etiologies of focal onset generalized status are brain tumor,[153,154] cerebrovascular disease,[155] and head trauma.[154] A frontal focus is particularly prone to induce convulsive status.[155] Most patients are in a coma or a stuporous state, both during and between seizures.

The EEG shows focal or diffuse flattening followed by low-voltage fast activity, which is associated with the tonic phase. This progresses to rhythmic spike-wave or delta activity, corresponding to the clonic phase. In most cases, however, the EEG is obscured by intense muscle artifact from the start of the seizure (unless the patient is pharmacologically paralyzed). The only reliable EEG findings may be in the postictal state, when the EEG shows initial flattening and subsequent delta activity, which progressively evolves to faster frequency and greater amplitude activity coupled with recovery from the postictal state. The next seizure starts before the EEG recovers to the preseizure state. As generalized convulsive status progresses, clinical manifestation becomes less dramatic and spike-wave bursts become less continuous.

Other types of generalized convulsive status include myoclonic, tonic, and clonic seizures. The mortality of all types of status epilepticus, though most are generalized convulsive status, is about 20% to 25%.[156] However, most of the mortality derives from the underlying illness causing status rather than status itself.[157]

ABSENCE STATUS EPILEPTICUS (PETIT MAL STATUS)/NONCONVULSIVE STATUS EPILEPTICUS

This is often categorized as "nonconvulsive status epilepticus." The first description of this condition was reported by Lennox.[158] Although the term "absence status" appears to imply prolonged or recurrent absence seizures, clinical presentations are quite different from the typical absence seizure. Unlike absence seizures which mostly affect children and adolescents, absence status is more often seen in adults between 20 and 70 years old and might even be a first seizure in old age.[159] The patient usually presents in an obtunded state. Impairment of consciousness varies from slow mental function and confusion to mutism.[160] The patient may show subtle myoclonic twitches

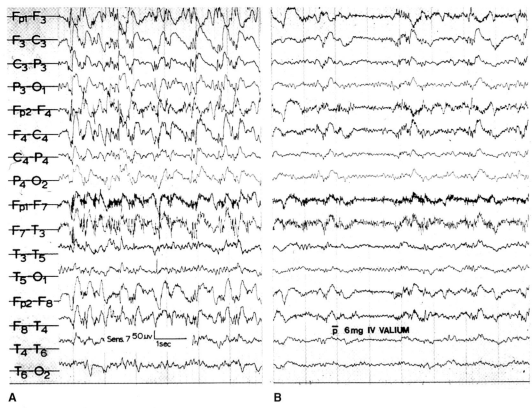

FIGURE 10-44 | Nonconvulsive status epilepticus in a 47-year-old woman who has history of grand mal seizures in her youth. The patient was awake but confused with minimal verbal communication and echolalia (the patient repeated the same sentence as the examiner's questions). The EEG showed continuous, semirhythmic 1.5- to 2-Hz spike-wave and polyspike-wave bursts with bifrontal dominance **(A)**. Diazepam administration promptly attenuated the epileptiform bursts and the patient recovered to her normal state within 5 minutes **(B)**.

in the eyelids, face, mouth, or fingers. The seizure may last from as short as 10 to 15 minutes to as long as days or weeks. Some patients may develop generalized tonic-clonic seizures during the height of status.

The EEG during ictal episodes varies from classical 3-Hz spike wave to more irregular but repetitive spike wave, polyspike wave, and sharp triphasic waves (Fig. 10-44A and B). Because the discharges are not always spikes or spikes and waves, but often repetitive sharp triphasic waves, it is difficult to differentiate status epilepticus from toxic/metabolic encephalopathy (Fig. 10-44A and B, compare with Fig. 11-11, also compare Fig. 13-1B and C; see also Fig. 8-17). Prompt resolution of the discharges by a small dose of intravenous benzodiazepine favors the seizure rather than metabolic encephalopathy (Fig. 10-45A and B).

The termination of the seizure is usually sudden and abrupt, and the patient then quickly returns to his or her baseline normal state without postictal confusion or sleepiness. Intravenous administration of benzodiazepines is often effective in dramatically attenuating epileptiform activity and normalizing both the EEG and neurologic state, although this rule may not always be true; nonconvulsive status epilepticus in patients with coma or stupor secondary to various encephalopathies will not awaken the patients immediately after IV administration of benzodiazepine even if epileptiform activity disappear (Fig. 10-45A and B).

COMPLEX PARTIAL STATUS EPILEPTICUS

Absence status is relatively rare but CPSE is even more so. CPSE is also categorized as nonconvulsive status epilepticus. Clinically, there are two types of CPSE: one is recurrent, discrete, complex partial seizures with partial recovery of consciousness between seizures, and the other is continuous, long-lasting confusion or psychiatric or psychotic behavior with or without automatisms.[161] Absence status and CPSE share a similar clinical picture in some cases, and the distinction between the two may be difficult. The EEG is useful in differentiating the two because CPSE shows a more focal pattern.[162] CPSE of frontal lobe origin, however, tends to show bilateral epileptiform discharges with generalized spike-wave or polyspike-wave discharges during the ictus.[163,164] The presence of focal interictal discharges aids in differentiating CPSE from generalized status epilepticus.

FOCAL STATUS EPILEPTICUS

Focal status epilepticus consists of varieties of clinical symptoms like focal motor, focal sensory, autonomic, psychic, speech, or other cognitive dysfunctions. The most common etiologies of focal status are vascular and infectious causes, but it could be seen in other focal disturbances such as brain tumor, head trauma, multiple sclerosis, degenerative disorder, etc.[165]

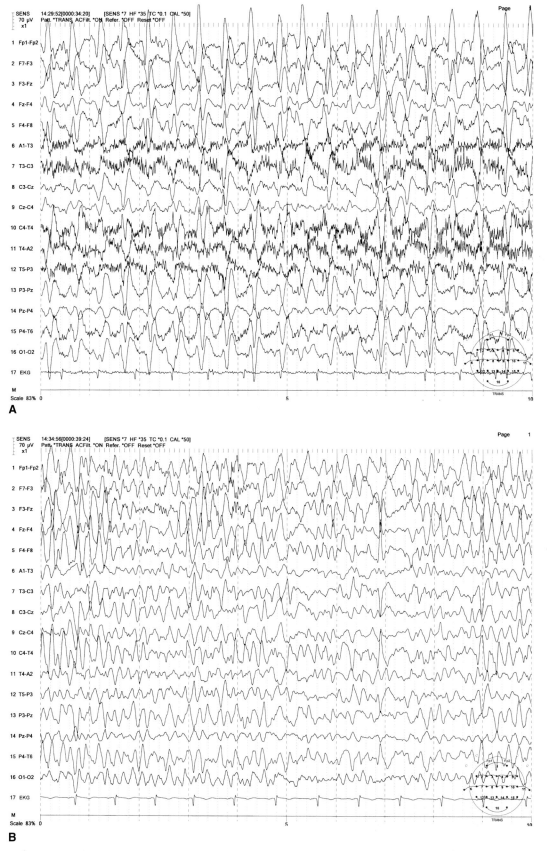

FIGURE 10-45 | Nonconvulsive status epilepticus in a 73-year-old woman with diagnosis of bilateral subarachnoid and intraventricular hemorrhage. The EEG was recorded 2 days after endovascular embolization. The patient was confused and showed continuous diffuse sharp triphasic waves **(A)**. Ativan attenuated these discharges but no change in mental status was noted **(B)**.

Because seizure discharges involve limited volume of brain tissue, only 20% to 30% of ictal events are detected by scalp electrodes.[166] A special form of focal status seizure is *epilepsia partialis continua,* which is defined as more or less continuously repeating muscle twitching in a part of the body (see Video 13-8). Vascular etiology (hemorrhagic, ischemic) is common in adults. Other causes include various infections, congenial cortical anomalies, or head trauma.[167] Many seizures are associated with PLEDs/LPD.[*,168] In this case, PLEDs/LPD* are an ictal pattern instead of interictal pattern.

OTHER NONCONVULSIVE STATUS EPILEPTICUS

Electroencephalographically, there are three forms of nonconvulsive status epilepticus. The first two are absence status and complex partial status (CPSE) as described above. The third form shows repetitive, at times periodic, spikes, polyspikes, or spike-wave discharges, which often occur after severe anoxic or other significant acute cerebral insults. These EEG patterns are similar to other types of status epilepticus, but it is debatable if this third form of status should be categorized as nonconvulsive status epilepticus. Unlike those patients with absence status or CPSE, who are usually awake or at least readily arousable, the patient with the third form is invariably comatose or, at best, stuporous (see Chapter 13; Bedside EEG monitoring). The IV anticonvulsant drugs are often effective to normalize the EEG and clinical state promptly in the first and second forms, but the third form of status is usually intractable to multiple medications. Even if epileptiform activity is abolished by the medication, the patient's level of consciousness remains unimproved. The prognosis of this condition is usually grave.

EEG Patterns Resembling Ictal Discharges

Any sudden alteration of the EEG pattern, especially with rhythmicity, should raise the suspicion of ictal discharge. However, some normal patterns or nonspecific patterns resemble electrographic ictal events. These include prolonged episodes of rhythmic midtemporal theta of drowsiness (RMTD) (see Figs. 14-12 and 14-13), hypnogogic or hypnopompic theta–delta bursts (see Figs. 7-34 to 7-36), arousal bursts (see Fig. 7-33A and B) in children, recurrent POSTs (Fig. 7-39A and B; see also Video 7-1B), rhythmic alpha variant (especially if unilateral) (see Fig. 7-16B), and SREDA (subclinical rhythmic EEG discharge of adults) (see Fig. 14-15A-D). Also, there are artifacts that resemble ictal events, such as those induced by rhythmic body or head movement or tremor. Electrode "pop" may also resemble an ictal pattern (see Fig. 15-26B). Several nonepileptic patterns may resemble IEDs. These include SSSs (small sharp spikes) or BETS (benign epileptiform transients of sleep) (see, Figs. 14-6 and 14-7), wicket spikes (see Figs. 14-10 and 14-11), 14- and 6-Hz positive spikes (see Fig. 14-1 through 14-5),

and phantom spike wave (see Figs. 14-8 and 14-9). These are discussed in Chapters 13 and 14.

Miscellaneous diagnoses

Of the miscellaneous diagnoses are the reflex epilepsies which are discussed in Chapter 9, Section "Other specific activation procedures." Here, we present a few unusual spells.

GELASTIC SEIZURE

Gelastic seizure is a rare but well-recognized syndrome affecting mainly children. As the term "gelastic" in Greek word means "laughter," the patient exhibits a sudden uncontrollable smiling, giggling, or laughing without apparent reason. Other associated clinical signs include automatism such as lip smacking, mumbling, or fidgeting of the hands (Video 10-12). The seizure usually lasts less than 1 minute. Varieties of etiologies have been reported, but the most common cause is hamartoma or astrocytoma in the hypothalamus, especially in patients who show precocious puberty. Many patients have other types of seizures including tonic–clonic convulsions and/or atonic seizures.[169,170]

SUDDEN UNEXPECTED DEATH IN EPILEPSY

Sudden unexpected death in epilepsy (SUDEP) is a fatal complication of epilepsy without identifiable cause such as trauma, toxic, metabolic, or vascular origin. Other than epilepsy, the patients are usually healthy, but SUDEP tends to occur in poorly controlled epilepsy patients. Each year, 1 out of 1,000 epilepsy patients die with SUDEP. The causes of SUDEP are likely multifactorial; cardiac arrhythmias (Video 10-13) or respiratory suppression or autonomic dysregulation has been proposed.[171,172]

VASOVAGAL SYNCOPAL ATTACKS

Although the vasovagal syncope is not seizure or epilepsy, this must be differentiated from seizure. EEG with simultaneous EKG recording is useful for differentiation. This is also called a *neurocardiogenic syncope.* The patient complains of blackout spell often upon standing, breath-holding, micturition, seeing blood, or extreme emotion. The spell is associated either with bradycardia or asystole (cardioinhibitory) or drop in blood pressure (vasodepressor) or both, secondary to enhancement of parasympathetic (vagus nerve) tone.[173] The patient may have myoclonic jerks, resembling seizure. EEG shows diffuse theta followed by prominent delta with bifrontal dominance. The EEG changes are preceded by or followed by bradycardia or even asystole in severe case (Fig. 10-46A–D). The patient can be examined by creating conditions that can trigger the spell, such as standing up from supine position (Video 10-14) or breath-holding with Valsalva maneuver.

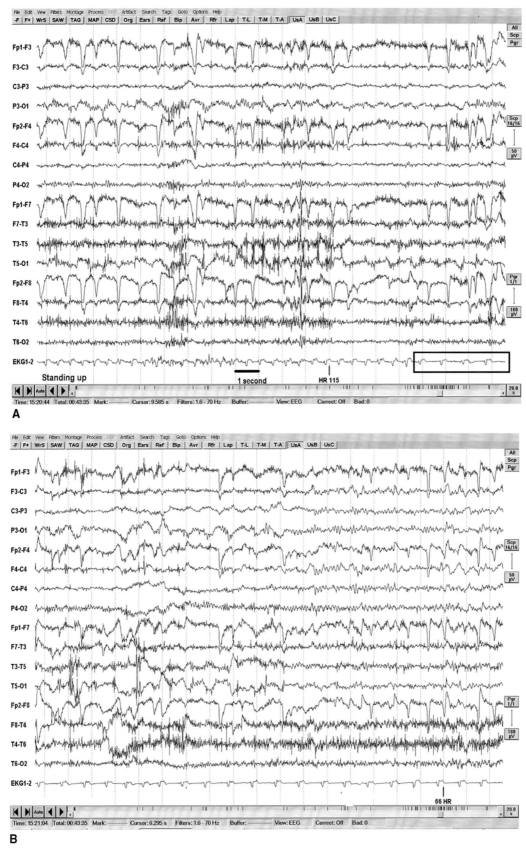

FIGURE 10-46 | Forty-four-year-old female with complaint of syncopal attack, especially when standing up. EEG was normal before the spell. Sixteen seconds after standing up, EKG rate started to slow down (shown by *rectangular box*) **(A)**. EKG rate dropped to 66 from 115/min with appearance of small delta toward the end of this page **(B)**. Subsequent EEG showed progressive increase of diffuse delta with bifrontal prominence associated with bradycardia with rate down to 56/min. The patient became unresponsive toward the end of this page **(C)**. After sitting down, EEG promptly recovered but bradycardia recovered slowly **(D)** (**A** to **D** were consecutive tracings) (see also Videos 10-15 and 10-16).

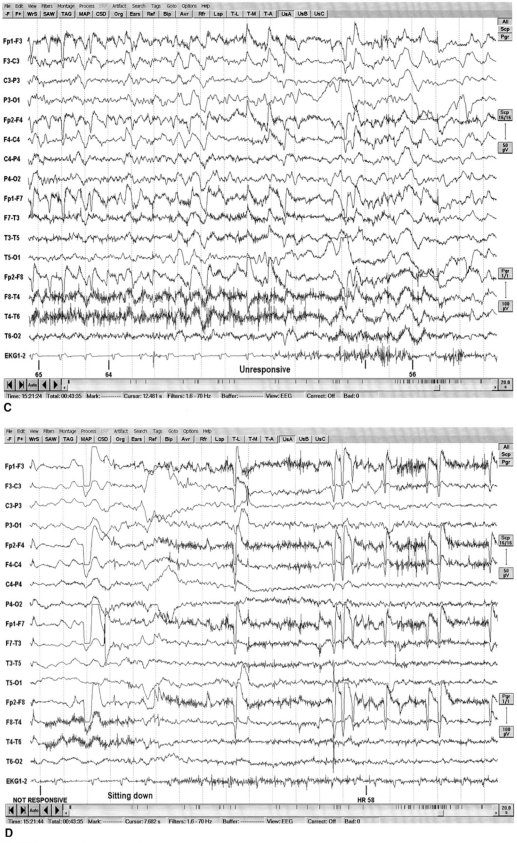

FIGURE 10-46 | (Continued)

References

1. Gotman J, Marciani MG. Electroencephalographic spiking activity, drug levels, and seizure occurrence in epileptic patients. *Ann Neurol* 1985;17:597–603.
2. Eeg-Olofsson O, Petersen I, Sellden U. The development of the electroencephalogram in normal children from the age of 1 though 15 years. Paroxysmal activity. *Neuropediatrics* 1971;2:375–404.
3. Cavazzuti GB, Cappella L, Nalin A. Longitudinal study of epileptiform EEG patterns in normal children. *Epilepsia* 1980;21:43–55.
4. Bennet DR. Spike wave complexes in normal flying personnel. *Aerosp Med* 1967;38:1276–1282.
5. Kellaway P. The incidence, significance, and natural history of spike foci in children. In: Henry CE, ed. *Current Clinical Neurophysiology: Update on EEG and Evoked Potentials.* Amsterdam, The Netherlands: Elsevier, 1981:151–175.
6. Ehle A, Co S, Jones MG. Clinical correlates of midline spike. An analysis of 21 patients. *Arch Neurol* 1981;38:355–357.
7. Ajimone-Marsan C, Zivin LS. Factors related to the occurrence of typical paroxysmal abnormalities in the EEG records of epileptic patients. *Epilepsia* 1970;11:361–381.
8. Salinsky M, Kanter R, Dasheiff RM. Effectiveness of multiple EEGs in supporting the diagnosis of epilepsy: An operation curve. *Epilepsia* 1987;28:331–334.
9. Bruni J, Wilder BJ, Bauman AW, et al. Clinical efficacy and long-term effects of valproic acid therapy on spike-and-wave discharges. *Neurology* 1980;30:42–46.
10. Riss J, Cloyd J, Gates J, et al. Benzodiazepines in epilepsy: Pharmacology and pharmacokinetics. *Acta Neurol Scand* 2008;118:69–86
11. Stodieck S, Steinhoff BJ, Kolmsee S, et al. Effect of Levetiracetam in patients with epilepsy and interictal epileptiform discharges. *Seizure* 2001;10:583–587.
12. Placidi F, Tombini M, Romigi A. Topiramate: Effect on EEG interictal abnormalities and background activity in patients affected by focal epilepsy. *Epilepsy Res* 2004;58(1):43–52.
13. Marciani MG, Spanedda F, Bassetti MA, et al. Effect of lamotrigine on EEG paroxysmal abnormalities and background activity: a computerized analysis. *Br J Clin Pharmacol* 1996;42(5):621–627.
14. Vendrame M, Khurana DS, Cruz M, et al. Aggravation of seizures and or/EEG features in children treated with oxcarbazepine monotherapy. *Epilepsia* 2007;48(11):1528–1167.
15. Marciani MG, Stanzione P, Maschio M, et al. EEG changes induced by vigabatrin monotherapy in focal epilepsy. *Arch Neurol Scand* 1997;95(2):115–120.
16. Fisher RS, Cross JH, French JA, et al. *Operational classification of seizure types by the International League Against Epilepsy.* 2016. Available at: http://www.ilae.org/Visitors/Centre/documents/Classifi
17. Blom S, Heijbel J. Benign epilepsy of children with centro-temporal EEG foci: Discharge rate during sleep. *Epilepsia* 1975;16:133–140.
18. Loiseau P, Duche B, Cordova S, et al. Prognosis of benign childhood epilepsy with centrotemporal spikes: A follow-up study of 168 patients. *Epilepsia* 1988;29:229–235.
19. Gregory DL, Wong PK. Topographic analysis of the centrotemporal discharges in benign rolandic epilepsy of childhood. *Epilepsia* 1984;25:705–711.
20. Legarda S, Jayakar P, Duchowny M, et al. Benign rolandic epilepsy: High central and low central subgroups. *Epilepsia* 1994;35:1125–1129.
21. Gastaut H. A new type of epilepsy: Benign partial epilepsy of childhood with occipital spike-waves. *Clin Electroencephalogr* 1982;13:13–22.
22. Panayiotopoulos CP. Benign childhood epileptic syndromes with occipital spikes: New classification proposed by the International League Against Epilepsy. *J Child Neurol* 2000;15:548–552.
23. Gastaut H, Zifken BG. Benign epilepsy of childhood with occipital spike and wave complexes. In: Andermann F, Lugaresi E, eds. *Migraine and Epilepsy.* Boston, MA: Butterworth, 1987:47–81.
24. Panayiotopoulos CP. Early-onset benign childhood occipital seizure susceptibility syndrome: Syndrome to recognize. *Epilepsia* 1999;40:621–630.
25. Ferrie CD, Beaumanoir A, Guerrini R, et al. Early-onset benign occipital seizure susceptibility syndrome. *Epilepsia* 1997;38:285–293.
26. Kellaway P. The incidence, significance and natural history of spike foci in children. In: Henry CE, ed. *Current Clinical Neurophysiology: Update on EEG and Evoked Potentials.* Amsterdam, The Netherlands: Elsevier, 1981:151–175.
27. Guerrini R, Dravet C, Genton P, et al. Idiopathic photosensitive occipital lobe epilepsy. *Epilepsia* 1995;36:883–891.
28. Cooper GW, Lee SI. Reactive occipital epileptiform activity: Is it benign? *Epilepsia* 1991;32:63–68.
29. Ebersole JS, Wade PB. Spike voltage topography identifies two types of frontotemporal epileptic foci. *Neurology* 1991;41:1425–1433.
30. Chung MY, Walczak TS, Lewis DV, et al. Temporal lobectomy and independent bitemporal interictal activity: What degree of lateralization is sufficient? *Epilepsia* 1991;32:195–201.
31. Engel J Jr, Williamson PD, Wieser HG. Mesial temporal lobe epilepsy. In: Engel J Jr, Pedley TA, eds. *Epilepsy: A Comprehensive Textbook.* Philadelphia, PA: Lippincott-Raven Publishers, 1997:2417–2426.
32. Jackson GD, Berkovic SF, Tress BM, et al. Hippocampal sclerosis can be reliably detected by magnetic resonance imaging. *Neurology* 1990;40:1869–1875.
33. Risinger MW, Engel J Jr, Van Ness PC, et al. Ictal localization of temporal lobe seizures with scalp/sphenoidal recordings. *Neurology,* 1989;39:1288–1293.
34. Walczak TS, Radke RA, Lewis DV. Accuracy and interobserver reliability of scalp ictal EEG. *Neurology* 1992;42:2279–2285.
35. Saygi S, Spencer SS, Scheyer R, et al. Differentiation of temporal lobe ictal behavior associated with hippocampal sclerosis and tumors of temporal lobe. *Epilepsia* 1994;35:737–742.
36. Ebersole JS, Pacia SV. Localization of temporal lobe foci by ictal EEG pattern. *Epilepsia* 1996;37:386–399.
37. Pfander M, Arnold S, Henkel A, et al. Clinical feature and EEG findings from neocortical temporal lobe epilepsy. *Epilepsia* 2002;4:189–195.
38. Rasmussen T. Characteristics of a pure culture of frontal lobe epilepsy. *Epilepsia* 1983;24:482–493.
39. Salanova V, Morris HH III, VanNess PC, et al. Comparison of scalp electroencephalogram with subdural electrocorticogram recordings and functional mapping in frontal lobe epilepsy. *Arch Neurol* 1993;50:294–299.
40. Lee SK, Kim JY, Hong KS, et al. The clinical usefulness of ictal surface EEG in neocortical epilepsy. *Epilepsia* 2000;41:1450–1455.
41. Bautista RE, Spencer DD, Spencer SS. EEG findings in frontal lobe epilepsies. *Neurology* 1998;50:1765–1771.
42. Williamson PD, Boon PA, Thadani VM, et al. Parietal lobe epilepsy: Diagnostic consideration and results of surgery. *Ann Neurol* 1992;31:193–201.
43. Russell WR, Whitty CWM. Studies in traumatic epilepsy, part II. Focal motor and somatic sensory fits: A study of 85 cases. *J Neurol Neurosurg Psychiatry* 1953;16:73.
44. Sahota PK, Stacy MA. Pain as a manifestation of seizure disorder. *Clin Electroencephalogr* 1993;24:63–65.
45. Salanova V, Andermann F, Oliver A, et al. Occipital lobe epilepsy: electroclinical manifestation, electrocorticography, cortical stimulation and outcome in 42 patients treated between 1930 to 1991. *Brain* 1992;115:1655–1680.
46. Sowa MV, Pituck S. Prolonged spontaneous complex visual hallucination and illusion as ictal phenomena. *Epilepsia* 1989;30:524–526.
47. Yalcin AD, Kaymaz A, Forta H. Reflex occipital lobe epilepsy. *Seizure* 2000;9:436–441.
48. Lairy GC, Harrison A, Leger EM. Foyers EEG bi occipitaux asynchrones de pointes chez l'enfant mal voyant et aveugle d'age scolaire. *Rev Neurol (Paris)* 1964;111:351–389.
49. Dravet C. Les Epilepsies graves de l'efant. *Vie Med* 1978;8:543–548.
50. Dalla Bernardina B, Dulac O, Bureau M, et al. Encephalopathie myoclonique precoce avec epilepsie. *Rev EEG Neurophysiol* 1982;12:8–14.

51. Blume WT. Clinical and electrographic correlates of the multiple independent spike foci pattern in children. *Ann Neurol* 1978;4:541–547.

52. Hauser WA, Rich S, Anderson VE. The multifocal spike pattern and sibling risk for epilepsy. *Electroencephalogr Clin Neurophysiol* 1984;57:44–45 (abst.).

53. Morrell F. Physiology and histochemistry of the minor focus. In Jasper HH, Ward AA Jr, Pope A, eds. *Basic Mechanism of the Epilepsies*. Boston, MA: Little Brown, 1969:370.

54. Morrell F. Secondary epileptogenics in man. *Arch Neurol* 1985;42:318–335.

55. Kennedy WA. Clinical and electroencephalographic aspects of epileptogenic lesions of the medial surface and superior border of the cerebral hemisphere. *Brain* 1959;82:147–161.

56. Gibbs FA, Davis H, Lennox WG. The electroencephalogram in epilepsy and in conditions of impaired consciousness. *Arch Neurol Psychiat* 1935;34:1133–1148.

57. Rodin E, Ancheta O. Cerebral electrical fields during petit mal absences. *Electroencephalogr Clin Neurophysiol* 1987;66:457–466.

58. Sato S, Dreifuss FE, Perry JK, et al. Long-term follow-up of absence seizures. *Neurology* 1983;33:1590–1595.

59. Wolf P. Juvenile absence epilepsy. In: Roger J, Bureau M, Dravet C, et al., eds. *Epileptic Syndrome in Infancy, Childhood and Adolescence*. London: John Libbey, 1992:307–312.

60. Sato S, Dreifuss FE, Penry JK. The effect of sleep on spike-wave discharge in absence seizures. *Neurology* 1973;23:1335–1345.

61. Sato, White BG, Penry JK, et al. Valproic acid versus ethosuximide in the treatment of absence seizures. Neurology 1982;32:157–163.

62. Harding GF, Herrick CE, Jeavons PM. A controlled study of the effect of sodium valproate on photosensitive epilepsy and its prognosis. *Epilepsia* 1978;19:555–565.

63. Holmes GL, McKeever M, Adamson M. Absence seizures in children: Clinical and electroencephalographic features. *Ann Neurol* 1987;21:268–273.

64. Browne TR, Penry JK, Proter RJ, et al. Responsiveness before, during and after spike-wave paroxysms. *Neurology* 1974;24:659–665.

65. Penry JK, Dreifuss FE. A study of automatisms associated with the absence of petit mal. *Epilepsia (Amsterdam)* 1969;10:417–418 (abst.).

66. Loiseau P. Childhood absence epilepsies. In: Roger J, Dravet C, Bureau M, et al., eds. *Epileptic Syndrome in Infancy, Childhood and Adolescence*. London: John Libbey, 1985:106–120.

67. Camfield CS, Camfield PR, Sadler M, et al. Paroxysmal eyelid movements: Paroxysmal eyelid movement: confusing feature of generalized photosensitive epilepsy. *Neurology* 2004;63:40–42.

68. Niedermeyer E. Generalized seizure discharges and possible precipitating mechanisms. *Epilepsia (Amsterdam)* 1966;7:23–29.

69. Janz D, Christian W. Impulsive–petit mal. *Dtsch Z Nervenheilk* 1957;176:346–386.

70. Delgado-Escueta AV, Enrile-Bascal F. Juvenile myoclonic epilepsy of Janz. *Neurology (Chicago)* 1984;34:285–294.

71. Wolf P, Groosses R. Relation of photosensitivity to epileptic syndrome. *J Neurol Neurosurg Psychiatry* 1986;49:1386–1391.

72. Hallett M. Myoclonus: Relation to epilepsy. *Epilepsia* 1985;26:S67–S77.

73. Shibasaki H, Yamashita Y, Kuroiwa Y. Electroencephalographic studies of myoclonus. Myoclonus-related cortical spikes and high amplitude somatosensory evoked potentials. *Brain* 1978;101:447–460.

74. Shibasaki H, Kuroiwa Y. Electroencephalographic correlates of myoclonus. *Electroencephalogr Clin Neurophysiol* 1975;39:455–463.

75. Halliday AM. The neurophysiology of myoclonus—a reappraisal. In: Charlton MH, ed. *Myoclonic Seizures*. Amesterdam, The Netherlands: Excerpta Medica, 1975:1–29.

76. Gastaut H, Broughton R. *Epileptic Seizures*. Springfield, IL: Charles C Thomas, 1957

77. Gibbs FA, Gibbs EL. *Atlas of Encephalography*. Cambridge, MA: Addison–Wesley, 1952.

78. Kellaway P, Frost JD Jr, Hrachovy RA. Infantile spasms. In: Morselli PD, Pippinger KF, Penry JK, eds. *Antiepileptic Drug Therapy in Pediatrics*. New York: Raven Press, 1983:115–136.

79. Hrachovy RA, Frost JD Jr, Kellaway P. Hypsarrhythmia: Variations on them. *Epilepsia* 1984;25:317–325.

80. Watanabe K, Negoro T, Aso K, et al. Reappraisal of interictal electroencephalogram in infantile spasms. *Epilepsia* 1993;34:679–685.

81. West WJ. On a particular form of infantile convulsions. *Lancet* 1841;1:724–725.

82. Fariello RG, Chen RW, Doro JM, et al. EEG recognition of Aicardi's syndrome. *Arch Neurol* 1977;34:563–566.

83. Hrachovy RA, Frost JD Jr, Kellaway P, et al. Double-blind study of ACTH vs prednisone therapy in infantile spasms. *J Pediatr* 1983;103:641–645.

84. Lennox WG. *Epilepsy and Related Disorders*. Boston, MA: Little Brown, 1960.

85. Gastaut H, Broughton R. *Epileptic Seizures*. Springfield, IL: Charles C Thomas, 1972.

86. Gastaut H, Roger J, Soulayrol R, et al. Epileptic encephalopathy of children with diffuse slow spikes and waves (alias "petit mal variant") or Lennox syndrome. *Ann Pediatr (Paris)* 1966;13:489–499.

87. Blume WT. Lennox-Gastaut syndrome. In: Luders H, Lesser RP, eds. *Epilepsy: Electroclinical Syndromes*. London: Springer-Verlag New York, 1987:73–92.

88. Markand ON. Slow spike-wave activity in EEG and associated clinical feature: Often called "Lennox" or "Lennox-Gastaut" syndrome. *Neurology (Chicago)* 1977;27:746–757.

89. Beaumanoir A. The Lennox-Gastaut syndrome: A personal study. *Electroencephalogr Clin Neurophysiol Suppl* 1982;35:85–99.

90. Blume WT, David RB, Gomez MR. Generalized sharp and slow wave complexes. Associated clinical features and long-term follow up. *Brain* 1973;96:289–306.

91. Egli M, Mothersill I, O'Kane N, et al. The axial spasm—the predominant type of drop seizure in patients with secondary generalized epilepsy. *Epilepsia* 1985;26:401–415.

92. Ohtsuka Y, Amano R, Oka E, et al. Myoclonus epilepsy with ragged-red fibers: A clinical and electrophysiological study on two siblings cases. *J Child Neurol* 1993;8:366–372.

93. Reese K, Toro C, Malow B, et al. Progression of the EEG in Lafora-body disease. *Am J EEG Technol* 1993;33:229–235.

94. Roger J, Genton P, Bureau M, et al. Progressive myoclonus epilepsies in childhood and adolescence. In: Roger J, Bureau M, Dreifus FF, et al., eds. *Epileptic Syndromes in Infancy, Childhood and Adolescence*. 2nd ed. London: Libbey, 1992:381–400.

95. Pampiglione G, Harden A. So-called neuronal ceroid lipofuscinosis. Neurophysiological studies in 60 children. *J Neurol Neurosurg Psychiatry* 1977;40:323–330.

96. Engel J Jr, Rapin I, Giblin DR. Electroencephalographical studies in two patients with cherry red spot-myoclonus syndrome. *Epilepsia* 1977;18:73–87.

97. Aso K, Watanabe K. Benign familial neonatal convulsions: generalized epilepsy? *Pediatr Neurol* 1992;8:226–228.

98. Bye AM. Neonate with benign familial neonatal convulsion recorded generalized and focal seizures. *Pediatr Neurol* 1994;10:164–165

99. Aicrdi J, Goutieres F. Encephalopathie myoclonique neonatale. *Rev EEG Neurophysiol* 1978;8:99–101.

100. Ohtahara S, Ishida T, Eiji OKA, et al. On the specific age-dependent epileptic syndrome. The early infantile epileptic encephalopathy with suppression-burst. *No-to-Hattatsu (Tokyo)* 1976;8:270–280.

101. March E, Melamed SE, Barron T, et al. Migrating partial seizures in infancy; expanding the phenotype of a rare seizure syndrome. *Epilepsia* 2005;46:569–572.

102. Darra F, Fiorini E, Zoccante L et al. Benign myoclonic epilepsy of infancy (BMEI): a longitudinal electroclinical study of 22 cases. *Epilepsia* 2006;47(Suppl 5):31–35.

103. Specchio N, Vigevano F. The spectrum of benign infantile seizures. *Epilepsy Res* 2006;70(Suppl 1):156–167.

104. Caraballo RH, Cersosimo RO, Espeche A, et al. Myoclonic STATus in nonprogressive encephalopathies : study of 29 cases. *Epilepsia* 2007;48:107–113.

105. Landau WM, Kleffner FR. Syndrome of acquired aphasia with convulsive disorder in children. *Neurology (Chicago)* 1957;7:523–530.

106. Beaumanoir A. EEG data. In: Beaumanoir A, Bureau M, Deonnat T, et al., eds. *Continuous Spike and Waves During Slow Sleep Electrical Status Epileptics During Slow Sleep.* London: John Libbey, 1995:217–223.

107. Hirsch E, Marescaux C, Maquet P, et al. Landau–Kleffner syndrome: A clinical and EEG study of five cases. *Epilepsia* 1990;31:756–767.

108. Deonna T, Peter C, Ziegler AL. Adult follow-up of the acquired aphasia—epilepsy syndrome in childhood. Report of 7 cases. *Neuropediatrics* 1989;20:132–138.

109. Patry G, Lyagoubi S, Tassinari CA. Subclinical "electrical status epilepticus" induced by sleep in children. A clinical and electroencephalographic study of six cases. *Arch Neurol* 1971;24:242–252.

110. Tassinari CA, Bureau M, Dravet C, et al. Epilepsy with continuous spikes and waves during slow wave sleep—otherwise described as ESES (epilepsy with electrical status epilepticus during slow sleep). In: Roger J, Bureau M, Dravet C, et al., eds. *Epileptic Syndrome in Infancy, Childhood and Adolescence.* London: John Libbey, 1992:245–256.

111. Joshi CN, Yamada T. Pediatric Febrile Seizures. In Galloway GM, ed. *Clinical Neurophysiology in Pediatrics.* New York: Demo Meical Pub, 2016:21–28.

112. Beaumanoir A. Les epilepsies infantiles. *Problemes de Diagnostic et de Traitement.* Basel, Switzerland: Editiones Roche, 1976.

113. Yamatogi Y, Ohtahara S. EEG in febrile convulsion. *Am J EEG Technol* 1990;30:267–280.

114. Falconer MA, Serafetinides EA, Corsellis JA. Etiology and pathogenesis of temporal lobe epilepsy. *Arch Neurol* 1964;10:233–248.

115. Heuser K, Cvancarova M, Gjestad L, et al. Is temporal lobe epilepsy with childhood febrile seizures a distinctive entity? A comparative study. *Seizure* 2011;20(2):163–166.

116. Penfield W, Jasper HH. *Epilepsy and the Functional Anatomy of the Human Brain.* Boston, MA: Little Brown, 1954.

117. Rabending G, Radermecker FJ. Subacute sclerosing panencephalitis (SSPE). In: Remmon A, ed. *Handbook of Electroencephalopathy and Clinical Neurophysiology.* Vol. 15A. Amsterdam, The Netherlands: Elsevier, 1977:28–35.

118. Radermecker J, Poser CM. The significance of repetitive paroxysmal electroencephalographic pattern. Their specificity in subacute sclerosing leukoencephalitis. *World Neurol* 1960;1:422–433.

119. Storm van Leeuwen W. Electroencephalographical and neurophysiological aspects of subacute sclerosing leuco-encephalitis. *Psychiatr Neurol Neurochir (Amsterdam)* 1964;67:312–322.

120. Creutzfeldt HG. Uber eine eigenartige herdformige Erkrankung des Zentralnervensystems. *Z Ges Neruol Psychiat* 1920;57:1.

121. Jakob A. Uben eigenartige Erkrankungen des Zentralnervensystems mit bemerkenwerten anatomischen Befunden (spastische Pseudosklerose, Encephalomyelopathie mit disseminierten Degenerations beschwerden). *Deutsch Z Nervenheilk* 1921;70:132.

122. Gibbs CJ Jr, Gajdusek DC. Infection as the etiology of spongiform encephalopathy (Creutzfeldt–Jacob disease). *Science* 1969;165:1023–1025.

123. Burger LJ, Rowan AJ, Goldensohn E. Creutzfeldt-Jakob disease. An electroencephalographic study. *Arch Neural* 1972;26:428–433.

124. Radermecker FJ. Infection and inflammatory reaction, allergy and allergic reaction. In: Remond A, ed. *Degenerative Disease/Handbook of Electroencephalography and Clinical Neurophysiology.* Vol. 15, part A. Amsterdam, The Netherlands: Elsevier, 1977.

125. Jones DP, Nevins S. Rapidly progressive cerebral degeneration (subacute vascular encephalopathy) with mental disorder, focal disturbances, and myoclonic epilepsy. *J Neurol Neurosurg Psychiatry* 1954;17:148–159.

126. Steinhoff BJ, Zerr I, Glatting M, et al. Diagnostic value of periodic complexes in Creutzfeldt-Jakob disease. *Ann Neurol* 2003;56:702–708.

127. Zerr I, Pocchiari M, Collins S, et al. Analysis of EEG and CSF 14-3-3 proteins as aids to the diagnosis of Creutzfeldt–Jacob disease. *Neurology* 2000;55(6):811–815.

128. Shibasaki H, Yamashita Y, Neshige R. Electroencephalographic correlates of myoclonus. *Adv Neurol* 1986;43:367–372.

129. Furlan AJ, Henry CE, Sweeney PJ, et al. Focal EEG abnormalities in Heidenhain's variant of Creutzfeldt-Jakob disease. *Arch Neurol* 1981;38:312–314.

130. Niedermeyer E, Bauer G, Burnite R, et al. Selective stimulus—sensitive myoclonus in acute cerebral anoxia—a case report. *Arch Neurol* 1977;34:365–368.

131. Wijdicks EFM, Hijdra A, Young B, et al. Practice parameter: prediction of outcome in comatose survivors after cardiopulmonary resuscitation (an evidence-based review): report of the Quality Standards Subcommittee of American Academy of Neurology. *Neurology* 2006;67:203–210.

132. Alvarez V, Rossetti AO. Prognosis after cerebral anoxia in Adults: What's the Role of EEG Specialist. *Epileptologie* 2012;29:218–224.

133. Hirsch LJ, Classen J, Mayer SA, et al. Stimulus-induced rhythmic, periodic or ictal discharges (SIRPIDs): a common EEG phenomenon in the critically ill. *Epilepsia* 2004;45:109–123.

134. Alvarez V, Oddo M, Rossetti AO. Stimulus-induced rhythmic, periodic or ictal discharges (SIRPIDs) in comatose survivors of cardiac arrest: Characteristics and prognostic value. *Clin Neurophysiol* 2013;124:204–208.

135. Wijdicks EFM, Hijdra A, Young B, et al, Practice parameter: prediction of outcome in comatose survivors after cardiopulmonary resuscitation (an evidence-based review): report of the Quality Standards Subcommittee of American Academy of Neurology. *Neurology* 2006;67:203–210.

136. ECC Committee, Subcommittees and Task Forces of the American Heart Association. American Heart Association Guidelines for Cardiopulmonary Resuscitation and Emergency Cardiovascular Care. *Circulation* 2005;112:IV1–IV203.

137. Rossetti AO, Urbano LA, Delodder F, et al. Prognostic value of continuous EEG monitoring during therapeutic hypothermia after cardiac arrest. *Crit Care* 2010;14(5):R173.

138. Jehi LE. The role of EEG after cardiac arrest and hypothermia. *Epilepsy Curr* 2013;13(4):160–161.

139. Chatrian GE, Shaw C-M, Leffman H. The significance of periodic lateralization epileptiform discharges in EEG: An electrographic, clinical and pathological study. *Electroencephalogr Clin Neurophysiol* 1964;17:177–193.

140. Illis LS, Taylor FM. The electroencephalogram in herpes simplex encephalitis. *Lancet* 1972;299:718–721.

141. Aminoff MJ, Greenberg DA, Wiekle DJ. Periodic EEG complexes in infectious mononucleosis encephalitis. *Electroencephalogr Clin Neurophysiol* 1982;53:28 (abst.).

142. Beach RL, Barkan H, Deperalta E. The EEG in Inflammatory CNS Conditions. In: Shomer D, Lopes de Silva FH, eds. *Niedermeyer's Electroencephalography. Basic Principle, Clinical Applications, and related Fields.* 6th Ed. Philadelphia, PA: Lippincott Williams and Wilkins, 2011:331–393.

143. De la Paz D, Brenner RP. Bilateral independent periodic lateralized epileptiform discharges—Clinical significance. *Electroencephalogr Clin Neurophysiol* 1982;53:27 (abst.).

144. Andriola M. PLEDs and bi-PLEDs in children. *Electroencephalogr Clin Neurophysiol* 1982;53:88 (abst.).

145. Ritaccio AL, March G. The significance of BIPLEDs in complex partial status epilepticus. *Am J EEG Technol* 1993;33:27–34.

146. Shewmon DA. What is neonatal seizure? Problems in definition and quantification for investigative and clinical purposes. *J Clin Neurophysiol* 1990;7:315–368.

147. Nagarajan L, Palumbo L, Ghosh S. Brief Electroencephalographic Rhythmic Discharges (BERDs) in the neonate with seizures: Their significance and prognostic implications. *J Child Neurol* 2011;26(2):1529–1533.

148. Yoo JY, Rampal N, Petroff OA, et al. Brief potentially ictal rhythmic discharges in critically adults. *JAMA Neurol* 2014;71(4):454–462.

149. Gastaut H, Broughton R. *Epileptic Seizures.* Springfield, IL: Chales Thomas, 1957.

150. Salanova V, Morris HH, Van Ness P, et al. Frontal lobe seizures: Electroclinical syndromes. *Epilepsia* 1995;36:16–24.

151. Commission on Epidemiology and Prognosis. International League Against Epilepsy. Guideline for Epidemiologic Studies on Epilepsy. *Epilepsia* 1993;34:592–596.

152. Trinka E, Cook H, Hesdorffer D, et al. A definition and classification of status epileptics-Report of ILAE Task Force of Status Epileptics. *Epilepsia* 2015;56(10):15–23.

153. Gastaut H, Poire R, Roger J, et al. Les etats de mal generalises tonico-cloniques. In: Gastaut H, Roger J, Lob H, eds. Les Etas de Mal Epile*ptiques*. Paris: Masson, 1967:11–43.

154. Heintel H. *Der Status Epilepticus*. Stuttgart, Germany: Fisher, 1972.

155. Celesia CG. Modern concepts of status epilepticus. *JAMA* 1976;235:1571–1574.

156. DeLorenzzo RJ, Hauser WA, Tomne AR, et al. A prospective, population-based epidemiologic study of status epilepticus in Richmond, Virginia. *Neurology* 1996;46:1029–1035.

157. Hauser WA. Status epileptics: epidemiologic considerations. *Neurology* 1990;40 (Suppl 2):9–13.

158. Lennox WG. The petit mal epilepsies: Their treatment with tridione. *JAMA* 1945;129:1069–1074.

159. Lob H, Roger J, Soulayrol R, et al. Les etats de mal generalises a expression confusionnelle. In: Gastaut H, Roger J, Lob H, eds. *Les Etas de Mal Epileptiques*. Paris: Masson, 1967:91–109.

160. Dongier S. A propos des etats de mal generalises a expression confusionelle Etude psychologique de la conscience au cours de l'etat de petit mal. In: Gastaut H, Roger J, Lob H, eds. *Les Etas de Mal Epileptiques*. Paris: Masson, 1967:110–118.

161. Wieser HG. Temporal lobe or psychomotor status epilepticus. A care report. *Electroencephalogr Clin Neurophysiol* 1980;48:558–572.

162. Grand'Maison F, Reiher J, Leduc CP. Retrospective inventory of EEG abnormalities in partial status epilepticus. *Electroencephalogr Clin Neurophysiol* 1991;79:264–270.

163. Williamson PD, Spencer DD, Spencer SS, et al. Complex partial status epilepticus: A depth electrode study. *Ann Neurol* 1985;18:647–654.

164. Lee SI. Non-convulsive status epilepticus. Ictal confusion in later life. *Arch Neurol* 1985;42:778–781.

165. Shormer DL. Focal status epilepticus and epilepsia partialis continua in adult and children. *Epilepsia* 1993;34(Suppl 1):529–536.

166. Devinsky O, Kelley K, Porter RJ, et al. Clinical and electroencephalographic features simple partial seizures. *Neurology* 1988;38:1347–1352.

167. Cockerell OC, Rothwell J, Thompson PD, et al. Clinical and physiologic features of epilepsia partialis continua. Cases ascertained in the UK. *Brain* 1996;119(Pt 2):393–407.

168. Thomas JE, Reagan TJ, Klass DW. Epilepsia partialis continua. A review of 32 cases. *Arch Neurol* 1966;34:266–275.

169. Tellez-Zenteno J, Serrano-Almeida C, Moien-Afshari F. Gelstic seizures associated with hypothalamic hamartomas. An update in the clinical presentation, diagnosis and treatment. *Neuropsychiatr Dis Treat* 2008;4(6):1021–1031.

170. Utribe-San-Martin R, Ciampi E, Lawson-Peralta B. Gelastic epilepsy: Beyond hypothalamic hamartomas. *Epilepsy Behav Case Rep* 2015;4:70–73.

171. Ryvlin P, Nashef L, Tomson T. "Prevention of sudden unexpected death in epilepsy: a realistic goal?" *Epilepsia* 2013;54(Suppl 2):23–28.

172. Devinsky O. Sudden unexpected death in epilepsy. *N Engl J Med* 2011;365:1801–1811.

173. Aydin MA, Salukhe TV, Wilke I, et al. Management and therapy of vasovagal syncope. *World J Cardiol* 2010;2:308–315.

11

Diffuse EEG Abnormalities

THORU YAMADA and ELIZABETH MENG

General Features of Diffuse EEG Abnormalities

Any clinical condition that causes clouding of consciousness is usually accompanied by diffuse EEG abnormalities. The degree of impaired consciousness is categorized as follows:

1. *Delirium* is characterized by a severe degree of confusion with disorientation to time, place, and/or person. The patient may be restless and hyperkinetic with psychic symptoms including incoherence, hallucinations, and delusion.
2. *Confusion* is a state in which there is a mild reduction in the level of consciousness. The patient with a defect in attention span reacts normally to ordinary stimulation but is disoriented to time, place, and/or person.
3. *Lethargy* or *hypersomnia* is a severe degree of drowsiness in which the patient can be awakened with ordinary stimulation but may fall back to sleep as soon as the stimulus is removed.
4. *Stupor* or *semicoma* is a state of partial loss of response in which the patient can be temporarily aroused with vigorous stimulation but lapses into an unresponsive state when not stimulated.
5. *Coma* is defined as a state of complete or almost complete loss of consciousness from which the patient cannot be aroused, even by powerful stimuli.

More detail in degree of consciousness can be measured by a Glasgow Coma Scale.[1] It is based on three measures: (1) eye opening (E), (2) verbal response (V), and (3) motor response (M). The scales are 1 to 4 for E where 4 is spontaneous and 1 is none, 1 to 5 for V where 5 is normal conversation and 1 is none, and 1 to 6 for M where 6 is normal and 1 is none. Using the Glasgow Coma Scale, the overall degree of impaired consciousness can be categorized as severe for GSC 3 to 8, moderate for GCS 9 to 12, and mild for GCS 13 to 15. (For children who are too young to have reliable language skills, modified scales can be used for verbal response.)

Diffuse cerebral dysfunction could be secondary to metabolic, toxic, or inflammatory illnesses, and demyelinating or degenerative diseases. EEG can provide an objective measure of severity of these pathological processes. It can also aid in prognostication. EEG changes are, however, rarely specific for the diagnosis. Nevertheless, the EEG assists to narrow down the diagnostic possibilities when combined with appropriate clinical information.

Diffuse EEG "slowing" can be categorized into three basic patterns:

1. Background slowing without accompanying theta or delta slow waves (Fig. 11-1)
2. Diffuse theta and delta activity associated with normal background activity (Fig. 11-2)
3. Slow background activity along with diffuse theta and delta activity (Fig. 11-3)

In general, slowing of background activity implies cortical dysfunction. Delta–theta slow waves signify white matter disease. Delta–theta slow waves, along with slow background activity, represent dysfunction of both the cortex and the white matter.

The degree of diffuse EEG abnormalities correlates fairly well with the level of consciousness. EEG grades can be classified as follows:

Grade IA: Mild slowing of background activity (7 to 8 Hz) without significant increase of theta–delta slow waves (Fig. 11-4A)

Grade IB: Moderate slowing of background activity (4 to 6 Hz) without significant increase of theta–delta slow waves (Fig. 11-4B)

Grade IIA: Dominant theta activity with some delta slow waves associated with normal or near-normal background activity (Fig. 11-5A)

Grade IIB: Dominant theta activity with some delta slow waves associated with slow background activity (Fig. 11-5B)

Grade IIIA: Dominant delta activity associated with normal or near-normal background activity (Fig. 11-6A)

Grade IIIB: Dominant delta activity associated with slow background activity (Fig. 11-6B)

Grade IVA: Moderate to high-amplitude (>50 μV) delta activity with minimal or no background activity (Fig. 11-7A)

Grade IVB: Low-amplitude (<50 μV) delta activity with minimal or no background activity (Fig. 11-7B)

Grade VA: Burst suppression pattern with suppression period of less than 5 seconds (Fig. 11-8A)

Grade VB: Burst suppression pattern with suppression period of greater than 5 seconds (Fig. 11-8B)

Grade VIA: Near electrocerebral inactivity (Electro-Cerebral Inactivity or ECI) (Fig. 11-9A and B)

Grade VIB: ECI (Fig. 11-9C and D)

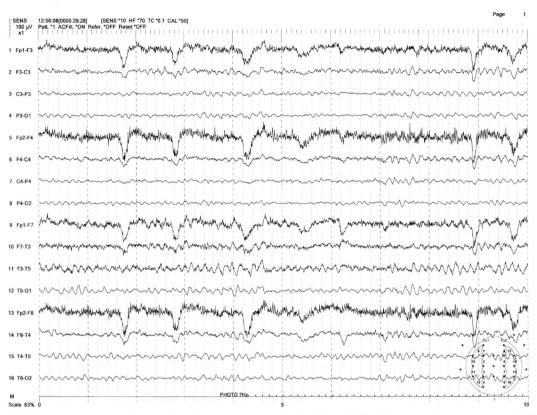

FIGURE 11-1 | An example of slight slowing of waking background activity (7 to 8 Hz) without significant increase of delta–theta slow waves. This is grade IA abnormality.

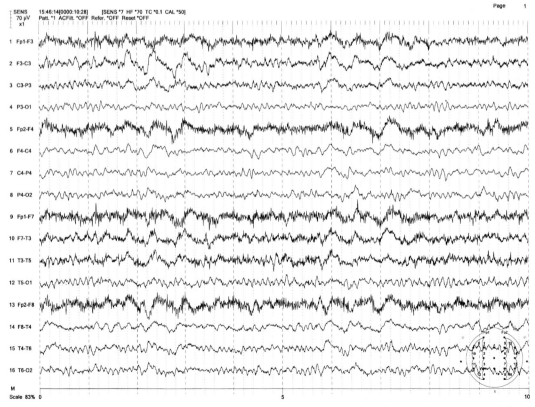

FIGURE 11-2 | An example of excessive irregular diffuse delta slow waves associated with normal 9- to 10-Hz alpha rhythm. This is grade IIA abnormality.

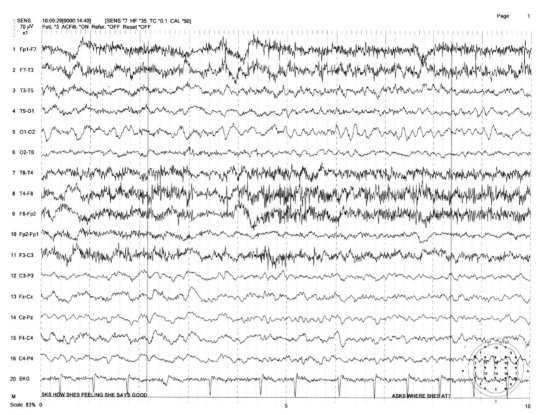

FIGURE 11-3 | An example of slow background activity (5 to 7 Hz) associated with diffuse delta–theta slow waves. This is grade IIB abnormality.

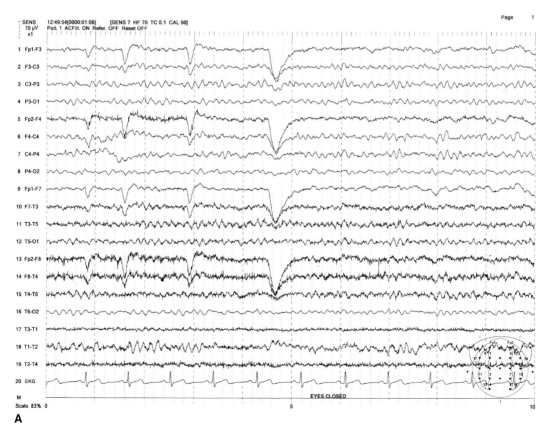

A

FIGURE 11-4 | **A:** Grade IA with slight slowing of background activity (7 to 8 Hz) without significant delta–theta slow waves. **B:** Grade IB with moderate slowing of background activity (6 to 7 Hz) without significant delta–theta slow waves.

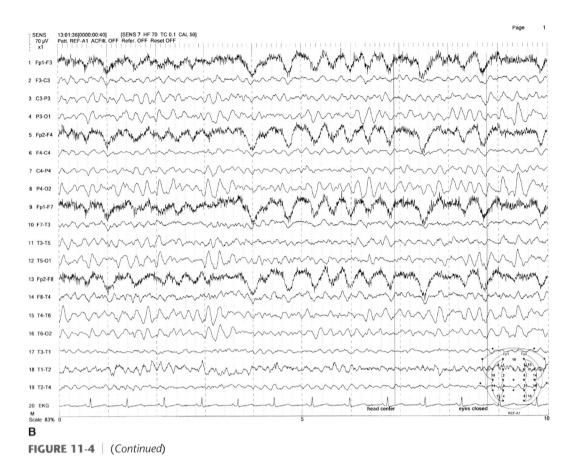

B

FIGURE 11-4 │ (*Continued*)

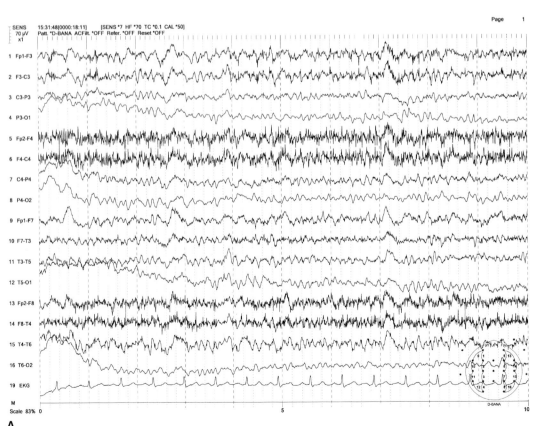

A

FIGURE 11-5 │ **A:** Grade IIA with background activity of mostly alpha rhythm associated with interspersed theta–delta slow waves. **B:** Grade IIB with background activity of 5 to 6 Hz associated with mixture of theta–delta slow waves.

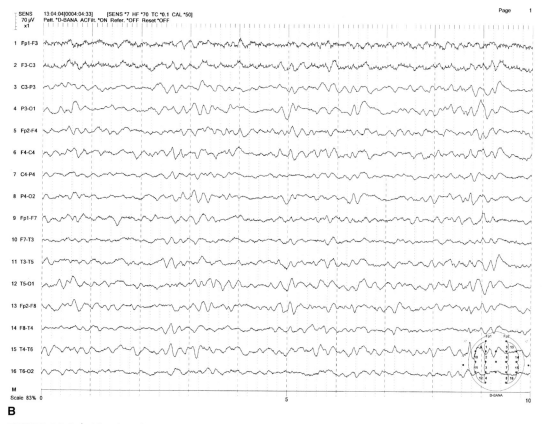

B

FIGURE 11-5 | (*Continued*)

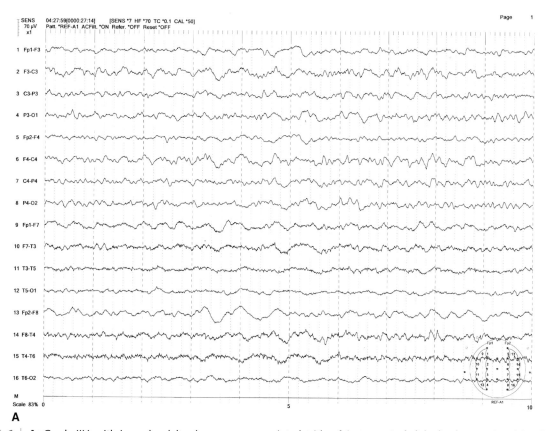

A

FIGURE 11-6 | **A:** Grade IIIA with irregular delta slow waves, associated with a fair amount of alpha background activity. **B:** Grade IIIB with irregular delta slow waves, associated with slow background activity consisting of 5- to 7-Hz theta activity.

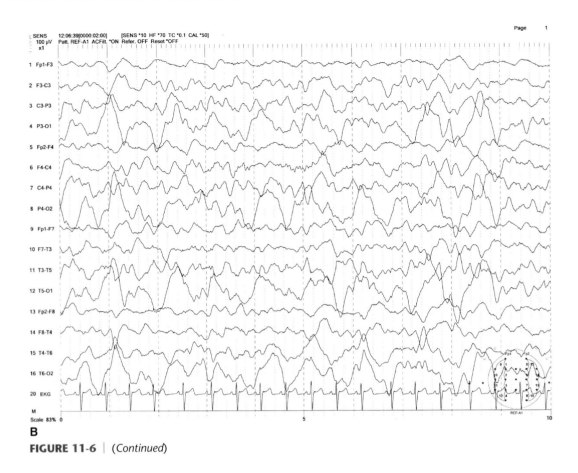

B

FIGURE 11-6 | (*Continued*)

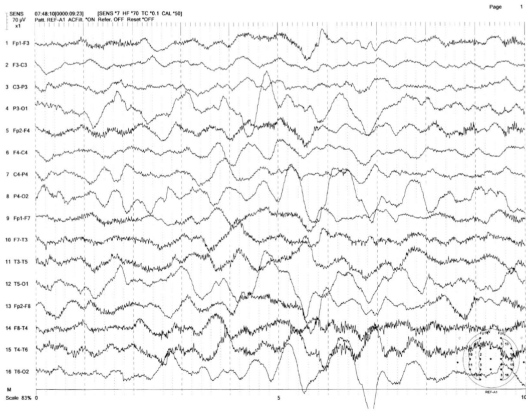

A

FIGURE 11-7 | **A:** Grade IVA with high-amplitude prominent, irregular delta slow waves with minimal alpha or theta background activity. **B:** Grade IVB low-amplitude irregular delta slow waves with minimal or no alpha or theta background activity.

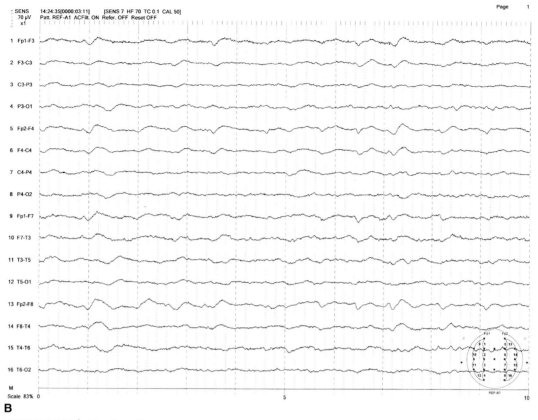

B

FIGURE 11-7 | (Continued)

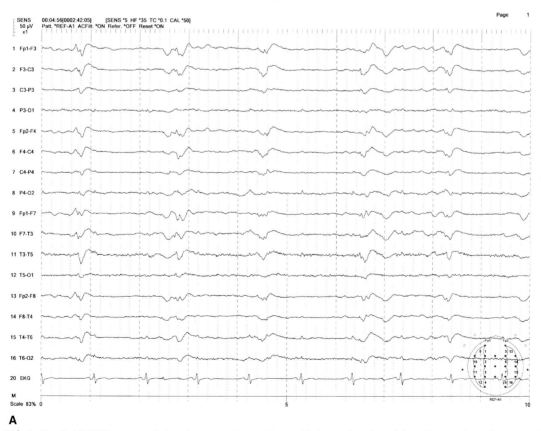

A

FIGURE 11-8 | **A:** Grade VA EEG represents burst suppression pattern with burst duration of 1 to 2 seconds and suppression period of 0.5 to 1 seconds. **B:** Grade VB EEG with prolonged suppression period of more than 5 seconds and short burst duration.

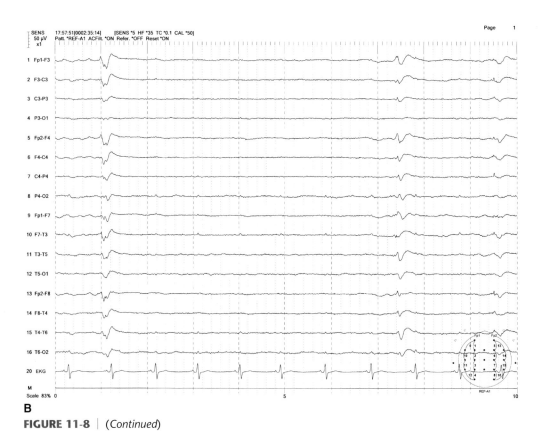

B

FIGURE 11-8 | (Continued)

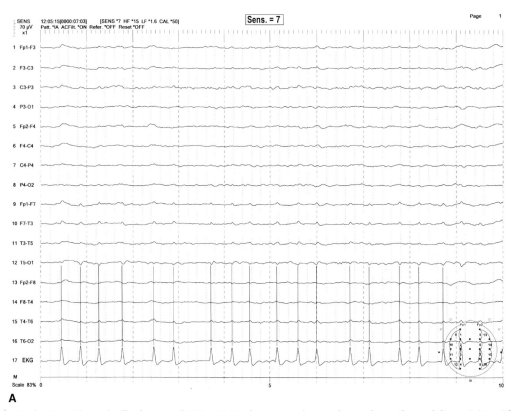

A

FIGURE 11-9 | Grade VIA with markedly depressed EEG activity showing only very-low-voltage theta–delta activity with a sensitivity of 7. Note EKG contamination on the EEG tracings (shown by *vertical lines*) **(A)**. With increased sensitivity (*S* = 2), however, the presence of EEG activity in between EKG artifacts becomes clear **(B)**. **C, D:** Grade VIB with ECS recorded with ECS montage including long inter-electrode distance at channels 1 and 2 (Fp1–O2 and Fp2–O1). With regular sensitivity (*S* = 7), tracings are "flat," only showing small EKG artifacts **(A)**. Cerebral inactivity (ECS or ECI) is verified with increased sensitivity (*S* = 2), only showing EKG artifacts (QRS and T waves) and intrinsic "noise" (low-voltage fast activity) **(B)**.

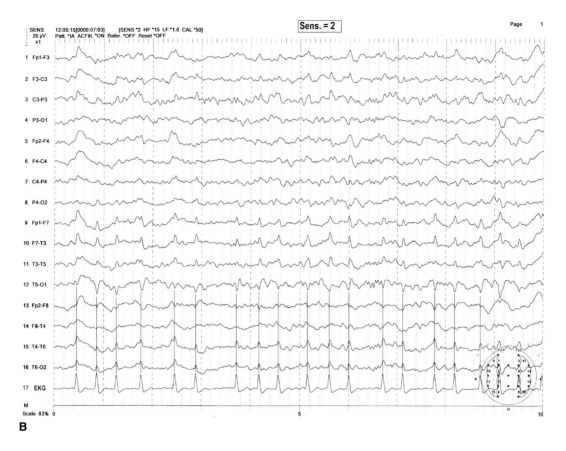

B

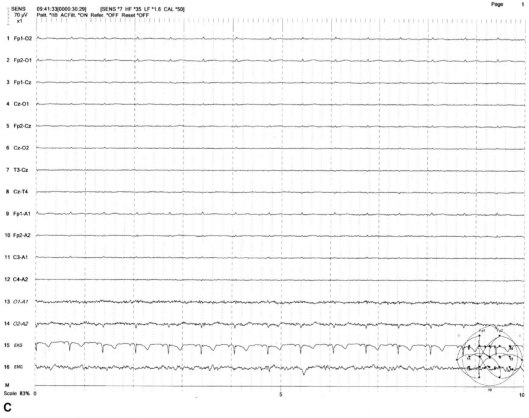

C

FIGURE 11-9 | (Continued)

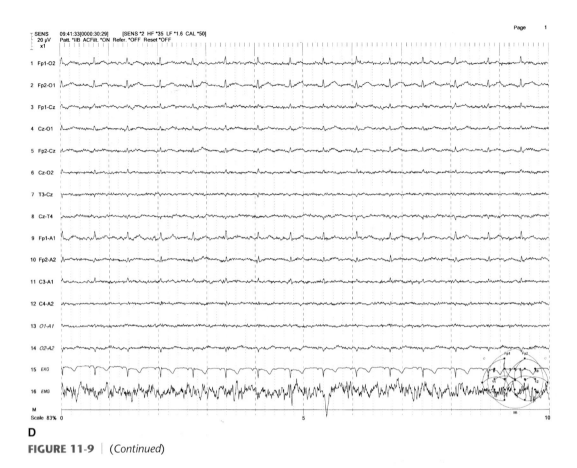

FIGURE 11-9 | (Continued)

In general, the degree of diffuse cerebral dysfunction correlates with the above grades, progressively worse from grade I to VI, and B is worse than A within the same grade.

In grade I, the EEG shows only slight slowing of alpha rhythm, and consciousness may not be altered. As the degree progresses to II, the patient may be awake but may be slow in responding or somewhat lethargic. At grade III, the patient is likely to be stuporous, but external stimuli shows reactive EEG changes with increased faster-frequency activity. In some cases, stimulus brings out slower activity with generalized high-voltage delta bursts, which is termed *paradoxical arousal response* (see Fig. 6-19). As delta activity becomes more dominant, correlating clinically with a semicoma or coma state, there will be less reactive EEG changes when stimulated. In addition to slowing of the background activity and increased theta–delta slow wave activity, some diffuse EEG abnormalities may also include paroxysmal activity like sharp waves, theta, delta bursts, or spike discharges. Grade IV or V is usually associated with a comatose state. The patient may show a reactive EEG change to external stimulus in grade IV but usually not in grades V or VI. In evaluating the course of the disease process, serial EEGs are useful. An example of this progressive EEG improvement is shown in Figure 11-10A–D. The frequency change is more reliable than the amplitude change; slower-frequency and lower-amplitude delta waves are worse than faster-frequency and higher-amplitude delta activity. Spontaneously fluctuating EEG patterns (e.g., alternating theta–delta dominant pattern and alpha–theta dominant pattern) or the presence of reactive EEG to external stimuli suggests a better prognosis than those of nonreactive, relentless EEG. Despite close correlation between the degree of EEG abnormality and the level of consciousness, EEG change may precede clinical deterioration of mental status. Conversely, EEG improvement may lag during the process of clinical recovery.

EEG Patterns that Reflect Diffuse Cerebral Dysfunction

Other than diffuse slowing, there are some EEG patterns that characterize the EEG abnormalities in relation to diffuse encephalopathy. They are triphasic waves, frontal intermittent rhythmic delta activity (FIRDA) (frontally predominant GRDA*) or occipital intermittent rhythmic delta activity (OIRDA) (occipitally predominant GRDA*), periodic patterns, burst suppression pattern, alpha–theta coma, spindle coma, and ECI.

TRIPHASIC WAVES

Triphasic waves consist of an initial small negative sharp discharges followed by large positive sharp discharges with subsequent negative wave. The typical triphasic pattern of more or less continuous, stereotyped waveforms was classically described in patients with hepatic coma[2] (Fig. 11-11; see also "Hepatic Encephalopathy" in this chapter). Atypical triphasic patterns consisting of less continuous and less stereotyped waveforms may be seen in other toxic–metabolic encephalopathies (i.e., uremic encephalopathy, anoxic encephalopathy, lithium toxicity, and other metabolic derangements) (Fig. 11-12).[3–7] Triphasic waves usually occur in patients with

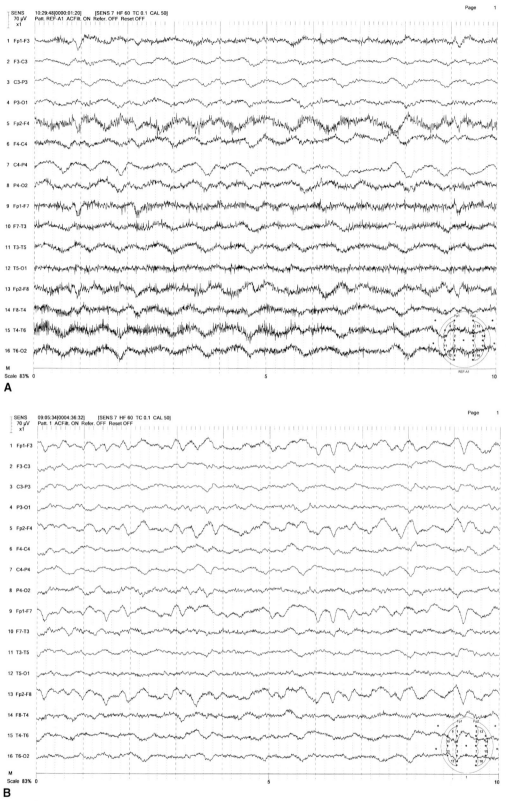

FIGURE 11-10 | A 38-year-old patient with diagnosis of viral encephalitis. On admission, the patient was stuporous with EEG showing diffuse semirhythmic 1.5- to 2-Hz delta activity with no appreciable background activity **(A)**. Within 2 days, EEG started to show improvement with faster-frequency delta activity **(B)**. On the 5th day, EEG further improved consisting of a mixture of delta and theta activities and the patient became arousable **(C)**. On the 7th day, patient was awake and EEG showed 7- to 8-Hz background activity mixed with some delta–theta slow waves **(D)**.

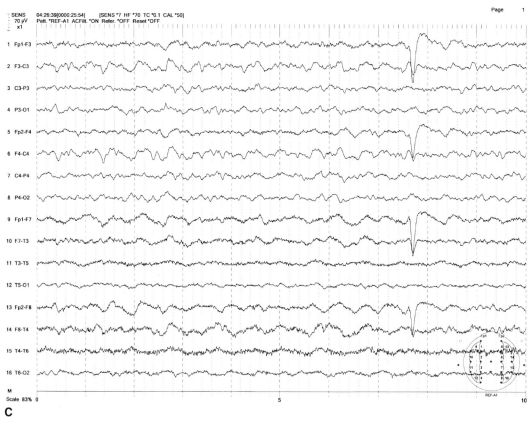

C

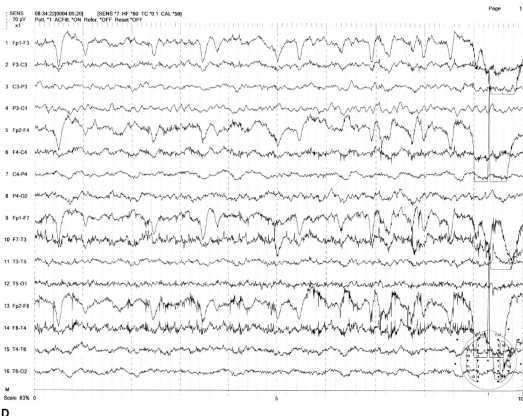

D

FIGURE 11-10 | *(Continued)*

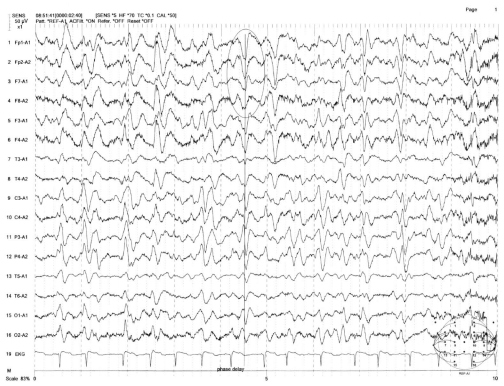

FIGURE 11-11 | A 54-year-old patient with diagnosis of hepatic encephalopathy secondary to cirrhosis of liver with EEG showing fairly rhythmic triphasic waves (*examples are circled*). Note a phase lag of the triphasic waves from the front to the back of the head.

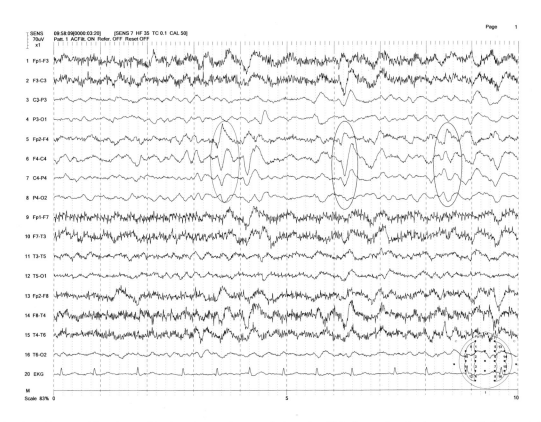

FIGURE 11-12 | A 49-year-old patient with chronic uremic encephalopathy. EEG shows slow background activity consisting of 4- to 6-Hz theta background activity and irregular delta slow waves. Note intermittent triphasic waves (shown by *circles*) that were less stereotypical and less rhythmic as compared to those seen in hepatic encephalopathy (see Fig. 11-11).

a mild to moderate impairment of consciousness but may also be seen in fully awake patients. Some triphasic discharges secondary to encephalopathy are difficult to differentiate from nonconvulsive status epilepticus (see Figs. 8-17 and 10-33B; see also Fig. 13-1B and C).

FIRDA (FRONTALLY PREDOMINANT GRDA*)/ OIRDA (OCCIPITALLY PREDOMINANT GRDA*)

FIRDA/frontally predominant GRDA or OIRDA/occipitally predominant GRDA can also be seen in patients with encephalopathy or seizures. This was described in detail in "Intermittent Rhythmic Delta Activity," Chapter 8.

PERIODIC PATTERNS

Periodic patterns consist of repetitive and fairly stereotyped waveforms appearing in regular (or nearly regular) intervals. Examples are seen in Creutzfeldt–Jakob disease (CJD) (see Fig. 10-33A–D), subacute sclerosing panencephalitis (SSPE) (see Fig. 10-32A and B), and also in postanoxic cerebral insult (see Figs. 10-34B and 10-35B; see also Video 13-1). If periodic discharges occur in a focal or lateralized prominence, they are referred to as *periodic lateralized epileptiform discharges* (*PLEDs*) or (*LPD* = lateralized periodic discharges) (see Figs. 10-39 to 10-41). If they occur in a bilaterally independent fashion, they are called *bilateral independent periodic lateralized epileptiform discharges* (*BiPLEDs*) (*BIPD* = bilateral independent periodic discharges) (see Fig. 10-42A and B). PLEDs are commonly seen in patients with acute or subacute, severe and focal destructive lesions such as massive cerebral infarction, acute exacerbation of a brain tumor, or herpes simplex encephalopathy. PLEDs may also be seen in patients with *epilepsia partialis continua* (see Video 13-8). These are described in more detail in "Periodic Lateralized Epileptiform Discharges," Chapter 10.

BURST SUPPRESSION PATTERN

Burst suppression pattern consists of recurrent, at times periodic or pseudoperiodic, bursts associated with an EEG suppression period of variable duration. The suppression period is of either no or very-low-amplitude (<10 µV) cerebral activity (Fig. 11-8A and B; see also Fig. 10-34A and B). Burst suppression pattern may be categorized as a subset of periodic or pseudoperiodic pattern. The bursts can be a mixture of a variety of all types of waveforms including sharp, spike, alpha, beta, theta, and delta activities. The suppression period commonly lasts from 2 to 10 seconds but could be longer than 10 to 20 minutes. This is one of the reasons why an EEG recording requires a minimum of 30 minutes to determine brain death. The burst suppression pattern induced by anesthetic drugs may last as long as several hours, which can still be recovered after cessation of drugs. Burst suppression implies the deepest level of a coma state before brain death. It is commonly seen in patients with an acute and severe degree of cerebral insult, most commonly in severe anoxic encephalopathy,[8,9] acute intoxication of CNS-suppressant drugs,[10,11] and severe hypothermia.[12] Some patients may have myoclonic twitches associated with the bursts (see Fig. 10-35A and B; also see Video 13-7).

Longer suppression periods, along with shorter duration and smaller amplitude bursts, are associated with a worse degree of cerebral insult (see Fig. 11-8A and B). Most conditions with burst suppression pattern, especially in a postanoxic cerebral insult, indicate a grave prognosis. However, recoverable burst suppression pattern can be induced therapeutically by various anesthetic agents including barbiturates,[13,14] propofol,[15] (see Video 11-2), etomidate,[14] and isoflurane.[16] A suppression period of several hours induced by deep anesthesia can be recovered.

ALPHA-COMA AND THETA-COMA PATTERN

In a coma state, EEG is expected to show diffuse, generally low-voltage slowing or burst suppression pattern. In contrast to this expectation, there is a pattern that is paradoxically represented by abundant alpha activity with little or no slow waves in comatose patients (Fig. 11-13). This pattern is termed *alpha coma*. The alpha activity is often diffuse or more anteriorly dominant than that seen in a normal condition. It is also nonreactive to external stimuli. This pattern is most frequently seen in severe anoxic encephalopathy and generally suggests an extremely poor prognosis.[17,18] However, some studies have reported cases of recovery from alpha coma.[19] Alpha coma may be a transient phenomenon in a postanoxic state.[18] We have experienced a case of postanoxic encephalopathy where continuous EEG monitoring started with burst superstition pattern changing progressively to faster background activity through theta then to alpha and eventually became low-voltage pattern before death (Fig. 11-14A–D). Alpha coma has been reported in other conditions including patients with brainstem lesions limited to the pontomesencephalic level,[18,20] high-voltage electrical injury,[21] and Reye's syndrome.[22] Alpha coma in these conditions has a better prognosis than that of postanoxic cerebral insult.

Theta coma is analogous to alpha coma but has a slightly slower frequency than alpha coma (Fig. 11-15).[23]

SPINDLE COMA

Some comatose patients display a sleep pattern including spindles, vertex sharp waves, and/or K complexes mixed with theta–delta slow waves, but the patient is not arousable (Fig. 11-16; see also Fig. 8-4). This is referred to as *spindle coma*. This pattern has most often been described in patients with head injury[24–27] and has been reported in other conditions including acute cerebral anoxia,[28,29] viral encephalitis,[30] thalamic or brainstem lesion,[28,29] subarachnoid hemorrhage,[28] and drug intoxication.[28]

A functional disturbance of anatomical lesions involving the midbrain, hypothalamus, or pons has been postulated for generation of spindle coma but pathological confirmation has not been made. Some coma or vegetative state patients may show diurnal EEG changes with alternating awake and sleep patterns.[24]

Spindle coma, especially secondary to posttraumatic coma, carries a relatively benign outcome.[24,26] Reactive EEG changes including K complexes by external stimuli also suggest favorable outcomes.[27–31] Recent review of studies has shown overall mortality of 23% in spindle coma patients compared to mortality exceeding 65% in comas associated with other EEG patterns including burst suppression, periodic pattern, and alpha-coma pattern.[32] The appearance of sleep spindles following diffuse slowing during a coma or a semicoma state during long-term recording suggests improvement of cerebral function.

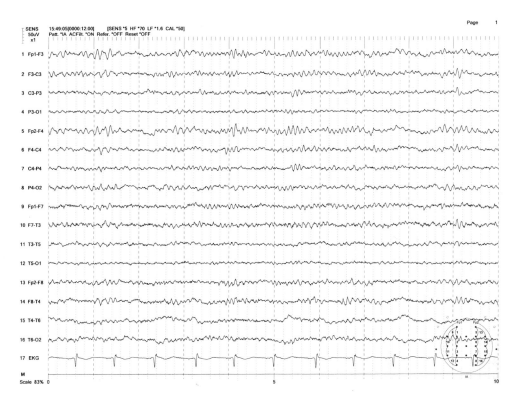

FIGURE 11-13 | A 52-year-old comatose patient after anoxic cerebral injury. EEG showed diffuse and bianterior dominant 10- to 11-Hz alpha activity, representing alpha-coma pattern. Some underlying delta slow waves are also seen.

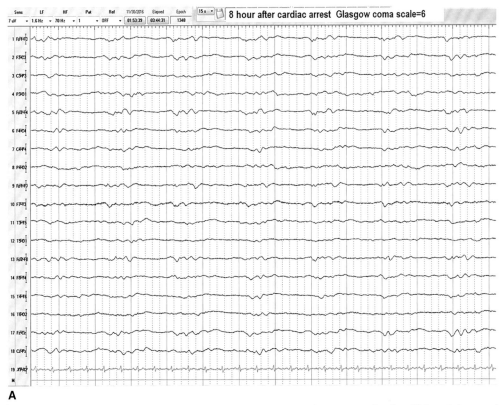

FIGURE 11-14 | A 65-year-old male with postanoxic cerebral insult after cardiac arrest. The first EEG at 8 hours after cardiac arrest showed intermittent diffuse low-voltage theta interrupted by some brief suppression periods **(A)**. EEG then showed progressively faster frequency **(B)** and background activity reaching alpha frequency, that is, alpha-coma state **(C and D)**, which seemingly was improving from the earlier EEG despite Glasgow Coma state remained the same.[6] EEG then changed to the low-voltage pattern when Glasgow Come Scale changed from 6 to 3 **(D)**. The patient expired several hours after this EEG.

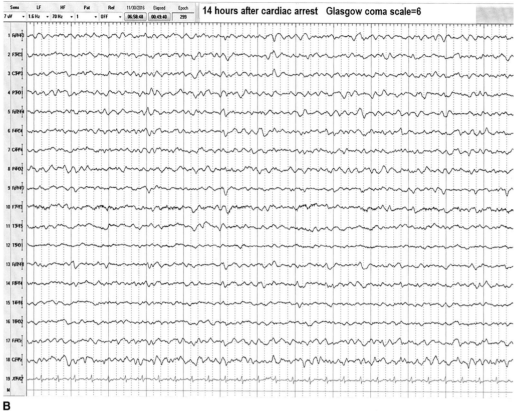

B

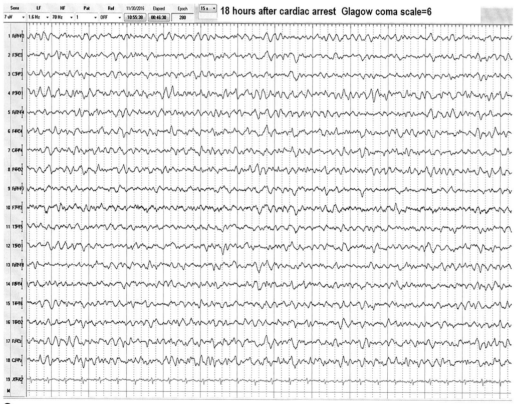

C

FIGURE 11-14 | (Continued)

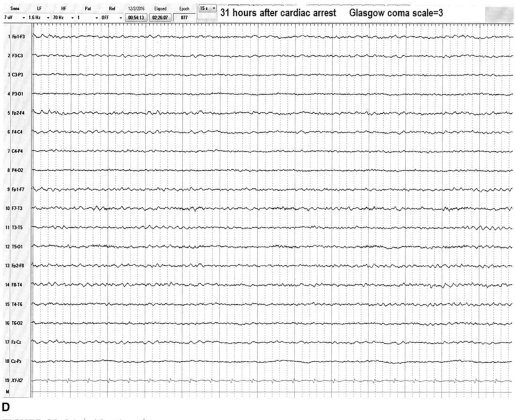

D

FIGURE 11-14 | (Continued)

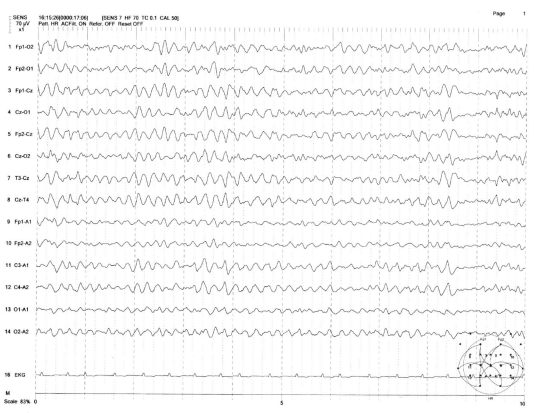

FIGURE 11-15 | A 45-year-old comatose patient following a cardiac arrest. Diffuse theta activity, representing theta-coma pattern.

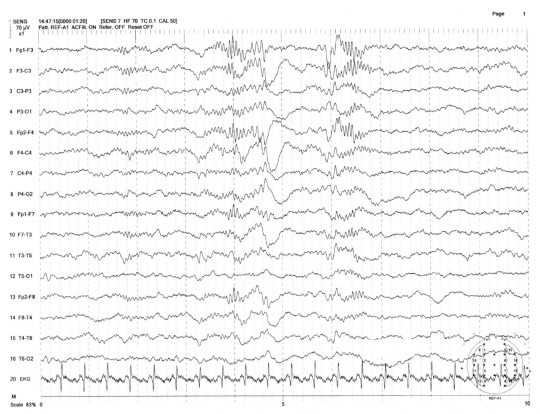

FIGURE 11-16 | A 15-year-old patient after nonpenetrating head injury. EEG showed sleep spindles and K complex resembling normal sleep pattern, but the patient was not arousable. This represents spindle coma.

ELECTROCEREBRAL SILENCE (ECS) OR ELECTROCEREBRAL INACTIVITY (ECI)

The definition of brain death may differ depending on social, religious and ethical backgrounds, and traditional custom and philosophical concept. In the United States, brain death is defined as "irreversible loss of function of the brain including brainstem."[33] This can be diagnosed by clinical evaluation, which demonstrates signs of unresponsiveness, total absence of brainstem reflexes, and apnea. Before determining the brain death, reversible medical conditions that may mimic brain death must be excluded. These include hypothermia with a core temperature below 32°C (although to make an EEG "flat" in normal conditions requires 20°C or less), drug intoxication especially by barbiturate or other sedative drugs, and severe metabolic and endocrine derangements. EEG and neuroradiologic examinations are used as ancillary tests. In the United States, the ancillary tests are no longer mandatory if a clinical examination and history are solid and meet the clinical criteria of brain death. Guidelines of American Clinical Neurophysiology Society (ACNS) define ECS or ECI as "no EEG activity over 2 µV when recorded from scalp electrode pairs 10 or more centimeters apart with interelectrode impedances under 10,000 Ohm" (see Fig. 11-9C and D). The following are recommended for EEG recording for determination of ECII[34]:

1. A full set of scalp electrodes should be utilized: the electrodes should include Fz, Cz, and Pz. Additionally, a ground electrode is required, though double grounding should be avoided.
2. Interelectrode impedance should be under 10,000 Ω but over 100 Ω: extremely high- and extremely low-electrode impedance attenuates the potential. Extreme low impedance (<100 Ω) suggests shorting (electrodes "salt bridge") of two electrodes.
3. The integrity of the entire recording system should be tested: this can be accomplished by observing artifacts introduced by touching each electrode.
4. Interelectrode distance should be at least 10 cm: this is to avoid a cancellation effect of short interelectrode distance, especially when dealing with extremely low-amplitude activity. Double interelectrode distances compared to routine electrode placement, for example, Fp1 to C3 (instead of Fp1–F3) are commonly used. The longest interelectrodes (Fp1–O2 or Fp2–O1) may also be included.
5. Sensitivity must be increased from 7 µV/mm to at least 2 µV/mm for at least 30 minutes of the recording, with inclusion of appropriate calibration. This is necessary to delineate low-voltage activity (Fig. 11-9C and D). A calibration signal of 10 to 20 µV is appropriate for a sensitivity of 2 µV/mm.
6. Filter setting should be appropriate for assessment of ECS: the high filter (low-pass filter) should not be below 30 Hz and the low filter (high-pass filter) should not be higher than 1 Hz. The use of the 60-Hz notch filter is allowed if necessary. One may include a low filter (high-pass filter) setting of 0.3 Hz for part of the recording to enhance slow waves, but that filter is not required.
7. Additional monitoring techniques should be employed when necessary to clarify the record: this include EKG and respiration monitoring. Additional electrodes placed over the dorsum of the hand may help to monitor

environmental electrical artifacts. If excessive EMG (muscle tone) artifacts interfere with a reliable interpretation of the EEG, the use of a short-acting muscle relaxant is allowed.

8. There should be no EEG reactivity to intense somatosensory, auditory, or visual stimuli: this can be accomplished by calling the patient's name, pinching the nail bed, and/or delivering photic stimulation. Photic stimulation may elicit *ERG* (*electroretinogram*) at Fp1 or Fp2 but should not yield photic evoked response or driving response at occipital electrodes.

9. Recording should be made only by a qualified technologist: because ECI is recorded in an "electrically hostile" ICU setting where many electrical and mechanical pieces of equipment are attached to the patient, the EEG is often contaminated by a variety of artifacts. This is further aggravated by the increased sensitivity (gain) required for ECS determination. Identifying and eliminating artifacts that interfere with the accurate interpretation depends on the skill, knowledge, and experience of the technologist (R. EEG T.) and also of the interpreting EEGer (Electroencephalographer or clinical neurophysiologist).

10. A repeat EEG should be performed when ECI is in doubt. Before 1980, repeating the EEG 24 h after the first ECS recording was mandatory in order to determine brain death. However, accumulated evidence indicates that no patients survived for more than a short period after one EEG showed ECI.[35] Therefore, a repeat EEG is no longer required for adult patients. Although this can apply to term neonates and children, an EEG cannot substitute for a neurological examination in brain death evaluation. If there is any doubt, question, or uncertainty from either a technical or clinical perspective, the EEG should be repeated after an interval, for example, of 6 hours.

11. Physiological variables and medication should be documented. This is because severe hypothermia, low blood pressure, or low oxygen saturation can cause cerebral inactivity or severe suppression EEG activity, which may be reversible by correcting these variables. Also, it is important to record all medications, especially sedative or anesthetic drugs such as barbiturates, benzodiazepine, propofol, or narcotics.

EEG or another ancillary test is also required for pediatric patients greater than 37 weeks gestational age to 18 years only when other clinical tests for determinations of brain death are not definitive or in doubt. The Task Force for Determination of Brain Death in Children[36] recommends a repeat EEG 24 hours after the first ECI for newborns of 37 weeks gestation to 30 days. For age of 30 days to 18 years, 2 EEG examinations 12 hours apart are recommended.

Because of the electrically "noisy" environment in the ICU and the high sensitivity used in the recording, artifact contamination in EEG is inevitable. The most common artifact is EKG. In fact, if EKG artifact is not present in an ECI recording, the technologist should check the integrity and parameters of the recording system. At times, an exceedingly high-amplitude EKG prevents appropriate EEG interpretation. In this case, selecting or creating a different montage may reduce the artifact. Repositioning the patient's head may also reduce EKG artifact. One may need to change the pillow or bedsheet if it has become wet.

EMG artifacts may obscure the EEG. Neuromuscular blocking agents such as pancuronium or succinylcholine can be used to temporarily eliminate EMG artifacts. Since these drugs are paralytics, they should be used only with an order from a physician and administered by a nurse.

Respiration-related artifacts, by either the ventilator itself or head movement associated with respiration, may cause rhythmically recurring artifacts in association with the respiratory cycles. The waveforms are variable depending on the cases (see Fig. 15-21A–D and also Videos 15-7 and 15-8). Sometimes, movement of fluids accumulated in the ventilator circuit may produce artifacts. The technologist may need to monitor respirations by visually observing the chest movement or by using a transducer to record the respiratory movement. It may be necessary to temporarily disconnect the ventilator circuit to verify the disappearance of the events of concern. This has to be done by the ICU nurse, respiratory therapist, or ICU physician.

Other sources of artifacts include pacemakers, warming blankets, IV pumps, and dialysis units. Also, electrostatic artifacts can be caused by movements around the bed. As in any other EEG recording, low- and equal-electrode impedances minimize the introduction of artifacts. EEG is rarely ECI if any brainstem reflex remains, especially in adults. Conversely, as high as 20% of patients who meet the clinical criteria of brain death may still show some electrocerebral activity in their EEG for several hours to several days after clinical brain death was established.[37] However, the chance of long-lasting survival in clinically brain dead patients with minimal preservation of EEG activity is extremely unlikely.

Diffuse Encephalopathies Associated with Relatively Specific or Characteristic EEG Patterns

EEG is a sensitive and reliable test to evaluate the severity of cerebral dysfunction and to assess the progress of a disease process. However, most of the EEG abnormalities reflecting diffuse cerebral dysfunction are nonspecific and do not lead to a specific diagnosis. Nonetheless, there are several conditions in which the EEG shows a relatively specific or diagnostic pattern. Here, only those conditions as well as relatively common diseases in which EEG is requested are described in some detail. EEG findings in other remaining conditions are listed in Table 11-1 with reference citations.

HEPATIC ENCEPHALOPATHY

In the early stage of hepatic encephalopathy, EEG shows slowing of alpha rhythm, which is gradually replaced by theta and delta waves as the disease progresses. In the somnolent or mildly stuporous state, the EEG often shows triphasic waves (see Fig. 11-11).[124] This is characterized by a small negative wave followed by a prominent positive sharp wave and subsequent broad negative wave. It appears as a "blunt spike wave" in some cases and may be difficult to differentiate from the EEG of absence status or nonconvulsive status epilepticus (see Figs. 8-17, 13-1B, and 13-12B). Finding a well-defined spike among the sharp and wave complexes indicates epileptiform activity rather than triphasic waves of encephalopathy.

TABLE 11-1 Slowing and/or Paroxysmal Discharge in Different Cerebral Disorders

	Slowing	Paroxysmal Discharges	References
I. Metabolic Disorders			
Hypoglycemia	++ (D)	++ (D) Spk	38,39
Hyperglycemia (nonketotic)	+ (D)	+ (F) Spk	40,41
Hepatic encephalopathy	++ (D)	++ Triphasic	42,43
Uremic encephalopathy, acute	+ (D)	+ (D) Spk, triphasic waves	44,45
Uremic encephalopathy, chronic	+/− (D)	+ (D) Spk, photoparoxysmal response	46,47
Hypocalcemia (hypoparathyroidism)	++ (D)	++ (D) Spk	48
Hypercalcemia (hyperparathyroidism)	+ (D)	−	49
Hyponatremic (water intoxication)	++ (D)	+/−	50
II. Vitamin Deficiencies			
Vitamin B_6 (pyridoxine) deficiency	+/− (D)	++ (D) Spk	51
Vitamin B_1 (Wernicke's encephalopathy)	+ (D)	−	52
Vitamin B_{12} (pernicious anemia)	++ (D)	++ (D, F) Spk	53
III. Endocrine Diseases			
Adrenocortical insufficiency (Addison's disease)	+ (D)	−	54
Adrenocortical hyperfunction	Fast activity↑	−	55
Hypopituitarism (Sheehan's syndrome)	+ (D)	−	56
Hyperthyroidism	Fast activity↑	+	57
Thyrotoxicosis	Fast activity↑	+ (D) Triphasic wave	58
Hypothyroidism (myxedema)	+ (D)	+ (D) Spk	54,59
Acute porphyria	+ (D, F)	+ (D, F) Spk	60
IV. Degenerative Disorders			
Tay–Sachs disease	+ (D)	++ (D) Spk, myoclonus	61,62
Cherry red spot myoclonus syndrome	+/− (D)	++ (Positive spike at vertex), myoclonus	63
Gaucher's disease	+/− (D)	++ (D) Photoparoxysmal response	64
Globoid leukodystrophy (Krabbe's disease)	+ (D)	+ Hypsarrhythmia	65
Metachromatic leukodystrophy	+/− (D)	−	66
Adrenoleukodystrophy	+ (D)	−	67
Zellweger's syndrome	+ (D)	+ Spk	68
MELAS syndrome (mitochondrial myopathy, encephalopathy, lactic acidosis, and stroke)	+ (D)	+ (F) Spk, PLEDs	69
MERRF syndrome (myoclonus with epilepsy and ragged red fibers)	+/− (D)	+ (D)	70
PKU (phenylketonuria)	+ (D)	+ (D) Hypsarrhythmia	71,72
Batten's disease (neuronal ceroid lipofuscinosis)	++ (D)	++ (D) Spk by low-frequency photic stimulation (see Fig. 9-11)	73,74
Hallervorden–Spatz disease	+ (D)	+ (F, D) Delta/theta/Spk	75
Infantile neuroaxonal dystrophy (Seitelberger's disease)	Fast activity	+/− (D) Theta, delta	76,77
Wilson's disease (hepatolenticular degenerative disease)	+ (D)	+/− (D) Delta/theta/sharp waves	78
Menke's disease (kinky-hair disease)	+ (D)	+ (F) Spk, hypsarrhythmia	79

TABLE 11-1 Slowing and/or Paroxysmal Discharge in Different Cerebral Disorders (*Continued*)

	Slowing	Paroxysmal Discharges	References
Tourette syndrome	+/− (D)	+/− (D, F) Central Spk	80
Lafora disease	+ (D)	++ (D, F) Spk, photoparoxysmal response, myoclonus	81
Baltic myoclonic epilepsy (Unverricht–Lundborg type)	+ (D)	++ (D) Photoparoxysmal response	82
Alper's disease	+/−	++ (F, D)	83
Tuberous sclerosis	+ (D, F)	++ (F, D) Hypsarrhythmia	84,85
Sturge–Weber syndrome	+ (F)	+ (F) Spk, hypsarrhythmia	86
Down's syndrome	+/−	+/−	87
Hereditary optic nerve atrophy (Leber's disease)	+/−	−	88
Myotonic dystrophy	+ (D)	−	89
Congenital muscular dystrophy (Fukuyama type)	+ (D)	+ (D)	90
Angelman syndrome (happy puppet syndrome)	++ (D)	+ (D) Spk	91
Rett syndrome	+ (D)	++ (F) Spk, central Spk, Lennox–Gastaut syndrome (slows Spk wave)	92,93
V. Inflammatory/Infectious Disease			
Acute purulent meningitis	++ (D)	+ (D)	94
Infectious mononucleosis	+ (D)	+/− (D)	95
Aseptic meningitis	+/−	−	96
Encephalitis	++ (D)	+ (D)	94
Herpes encephalitis	++ (F)	++ (F) PLEDs (see Figs. 10-39 and 10-41A and B)	96
Rasmussen's encephalitis	+ (F)	++ (F)	97
Congenital rubella encephalitis	++ (D)	+ (D)	98
Progressive rubella panencephalitis	+ (D)	+ (D) Periodic discharges, myoclonus	99
Congenital cytomegalovirus disease	+ (D, F)	−	100
West Nile virus	+ (D)	−	101
Rabies	+ (D)	−	96
Rickettsial infections	+ (D, F)	+ (D, F)	96
Lyme disease	+ (D)	−	102
Fungal disease	+ (D, F)	−	96
AIDS (acquired immunodeficiency syndrome)	+ (D, F)	+ (D)	103
Cysticercosis	+ (D, F)	+ (F)	96
Echinococcosis	+ (D, F)	+ (D)	96
Toxoplasmosis	+ (D)	+ (D) Hypsarrhythmia	96,100
African trypanosomiasis (sleeping sickness)	+ (D)	+ (D)	96
Malaria	+ (D)	+/−	96
Sydenham's chorea	+ (D)	+/−	94
Neuro-Behçet's disease (uveomeningitis)	+ (D)	+ (D)	99
Neurosyphilis	+ (D, F)	+ (F)	94,96

(Continued)

TABLE 11-1 Slowing and/or Paroxysmal Discharge in Different Cerebral Disorders (*Continued*)

	Slowing	Paroxysmal Discharges	References
Hemiconvulsions, hemiplegia, and epilepsy (HHE syndrome)	+ (F)	+ (F) Spk, SW	104
Brain abscess	++ (F/D)	+ (F,D) PLEDs	105,106
VI. Dementia			
Alzheimer's disease	+ (D)	+/– Triphasic	107–109
Pick's disease (frontotemporal dementia)	–	–	110
Parkinson's disease	+ (D)	–	111
Progressive supranuclear palsy	+/– (D)	+ FIRDA (frontally predominant RDA*)	112
Dementia with Lewy bodies	+ (D)	+ FIRDA (frontally predominant RDA*)	113,114
Huntington's chorea	+/– low voltage	–	115,116
Normal pressure hydrocephalus	+/– (D)	+ (D) Slow-wave bursts	117
Depression	–	–	118
Creutzfeldt–Jakob disease	++ (D)	++ (D) Periodic triphasic waves (see Fig. 10-32A–D)	119,120
VII. Others			
Multiple sclerosis	+/– (D, F)	+/– (D, F)	94
Reye's syndrome	++ (D)	+14- and 6-Hz positive spikes (see Fig. 11-16)	121,122
Subacute sclerosing panencephalitis (SSPE)	+	++ (D) Periodic burst (see Fig. 10-31A and B)	96,123

++, prominent, frequent, high incidence; +, often present; +/–, may or may not be present or low incidence; –, most often not present or none; D, diffuse; F, focal; Spk, spike or spike wave; SW, spike and wave; FIRDA, frontal intermittent rhythmic delta activity; PLEDs, periodic lateralized epileptiform discharges; ↑, increase.

Triphasic waves in hepatic encephalopathy typically occur in a serial, rhythmic fashion at 2 to 4 Hz with bilaterally synchronous and symmetric distribution. They are usually frontally dominant and show a phase lag from anterior to posterior head regions.[124] While these *typical triphasic waves* are common in hepatic encephalopathy, atypical triphasic waves that have a more irregular waveform and more sporadic occurrence can be seen in other metabolic encephalopathies including uremia, hyperthyroidism, hypercalcemia, hyponatremia, hypoglycemia, lithium intoxication,[7,43] and postanoxic encephalopathy.[5] Triphasic waves usually disappear with deepening of the coma state. Despite the paroxysmal appearance of triphasic waves associated with hepatic coma, a complication of clinical seizures is not common. This is in contrast to triphasic waves of uremic encephalopathy in which seizure is a more common complication. No single biochemical abnormalities correlate well with the degree of encephalopathy or EEG alteration, although the role of hyperammonemia has been proposed.[125] In the state of profound coma when EEG is dominated by delta activity, there may be 14- and 6-Hz positive spike bursts presenting peculiar combinations of slow and fast activities.[126] Similar features have been reported in Reye's syndrome.[121]

REYE'S SYNDROME

This syndrome was a prevalent childhood encephalopathy in the early 1970s but has dramatically decreased since the avoidance of the use of aspirin for acute febrile illness in children.

Despite severe hepatic dysfunction, triphasic waves are not common. The degree of EEG abnormalities varies corresponding to the severity of the illness, ranging from minimal slowing of background activity to low-voltage nonreactive delta or burst suppression pattern. Poor prognosis is predicted when EEG shows low-voltage delta or burst suppression pattern.[121] Interestingly, a high incidence of 14- and 6-Hz positive spike bursts (Fig. 11-17A and B; see "14- and 6-Hz Positive Spike Bursts," Chapter 14; see also Figs. 14-1 to 14-5) was observed during coma associated with an EEG of dominant delta activity.[122] It is debatable if this represents preservation or precipitation of normal sleep pattern for children and adolescence during an acute illness. In some patients who showed abundant 14- and 6-Hz positive spikes during an acute coma state, the positive spikes were no longer present when the patients recovered from coma. This suggested that the positive spikes were precipitated during coma in Reye's syndrome.[127] The 14- and 6-Hz positive spikes have also been reported in coma with other childhood encephalopathies,[128] though not as prevalent as seen in Reye's syndrome.

UREMIC ENCEPHALOPATHY AND RELATED CONDITIONS

In the early stage of uremic encephalopathy, slowing of alpha rhythm and intermittent diffuse theta bursts appear. As the disease progresses, further slowing of background activity is associated with increased delta waves and occasionally with

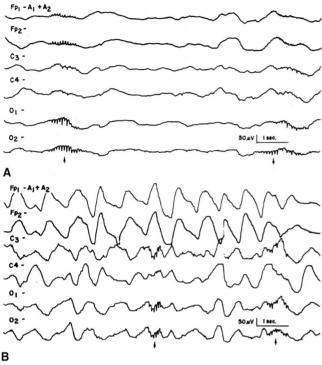

FIGURE 11-17 | EEG of a 10-year-old boy after diagnosis of Reye's syndrome. On the day of admission, when the patient was in deep coma, EEG showed diffuse slow (0.5- to 1-Hz) delta activity with occasional 14- and 6-Hz positive spike bursts **(A)**. On the 2nd day, EEG showed improvement with faster frequency and greater amplitude of delta activity, though the patient remained in coma. The 14- and 6-Hz positive spikes were still present **(B)**. (From Yamada T, Tucker RP, Kooi KA. Fourteen and six c/sec positive bursts in comatose patients. *Electroencephalogr Clin Neurophysiol* 1976;40:645–653, with permission.)

intermittent triphasic waves. The triphasic waves seen in uremic encephalopathy tend to be less rhythmic and more irregular (may be referred as "atypical triphasic waves") than typical triphasic waves as those seen in hepatic encephalopathy (see Fig. 11-12 and compare with Fig. 11-11; see also Fig. 8-17). Intermittent photic stimulation may induce photomyogenic or photoparoxysmal responses.[129] In some, bursts of spike wave or polyspike and wave may be seen with or without seizures. Seizures are seen in more than 30% of patients with acute renal failure,[130] while the incidence of seizure complication in chronic uremia is less than 10%.[46] *Dialysis disequilibrium syndrome* occurs during or immediately following dialysis. Despite improved blood chemistry, the patient may deteriorate clinically and may even have seizures. EEG also tends to be worsened with increased rhythmic or arrhythmic slow-wave bursts, occasionally including spikes or spike-wave discharges. The syndrome became rare when glucose was added to hemodialysis with modern dialysis methods.

Dialysis dementia is seen in patients receiving chronic hemodialysis for 3 to 4 years or longer and characterized by dementia, dysarthria, myoclonus, and seizures. EEG abnormalities may precede the clinical manifestation. EEG is characterized by prominent paroxysmal features with frontal dominant generalized delta bursts including FIRDA/frontally predominant RDA* or triphasic waves. Sharp and wave, spikes, and

spike and waves are also prominent.[131] These abnormalities may occur in association with normal or only minimally slowed background activity in the early stage. This condition also has become rare as a result of the use of aluminum-free dialysis.

HYPOXIC–ANOXIC CEREBRAL INSULT

EEG is extremely sensitive and prompt by reflecting the degree of cerebral ischemia. The changes start with slowing of the background activity followed by diffuse or frontally dominant high-amplitude rhythmic delta activity (FIRDA or frontally predominant RDA*), which rapidly progresses to a flattening of the EEG activity if the ischemia is severe. The whole sequence occurs within ½ to 1 minute if cerebral flow is not restored. These acute and possibly reversible EEG changes can be seen when performing intraoperative EEG recording during carotid endarterectomy surgery where the carotid artery must be clamped in order to surgically remove the plaque accumulated within the artery. Even if the blood flow is completely interrupted on the side of the surgery, in most patients, there is sufficient collateral blood flow from the opposite (nonsurgical side) carotid artery through the circle of Willis (see Fig. 5-11) to maintain blood flow on the side of occluded artery. In some patients, perhaps less than 15~20% of the patients, collateral blood flow is not sufficient to avoid ischemic damage to the brain unless a shunt is placed at the distal and proximal ends of occluded artery in order to maintain the blood flow on the side of occluded carotid artery. To decide if the shunt is needed, EEG is usually monitored to detect ischemic changes upon clamping of the artery. Depending on the degree of ischemia, various degrees of EEG changes are noted from slowing/depression of the background activity (the most sensitive EEG change is disappearance of fast and beta activity) to complete suppression on the side of surgery (Fig. 13-9A–G, Video 11-1A). Within a few to several minutes after the shunt is placed, EEG will return to its baseline pattern (see also Video 11-1B).

In hypoxic encephalopathy, various degrees of EEG abnormalities are found depending on the severity and length of the hypoxic–anoxic episode. The severity can be classified according to the grading of EEG abnormalities listed in "General Features of Diffuse EEG Abnormalities." Grade I or II suggests a favorable prognosis while burst suppression pattern or near ECS/ECI (grade V or VI) almost always results in a fatal outcome or neurovegetative state. Patients with grade III or IV show variable outcomes.

There are several characteristic EEG patterns associated with coma after severe hypoxia. One is a periodic pattern with bi- or triphasic sharp discharges appearing with intervals of 0.5 to 2 seconds with relatively quiet periods between the discharges (see Fig. 11-8A and B). The patient often exhibits myoclonus involving various body parts, but the jerks are not always time locked with the discharges (see Fig. 10-36; compare with Fig. 10-35A and B). The second is a burst suppression pattern with bursts consisting of various frequency activities including sharp waves or spikes (see "Burst Suppression Pattern" in this chapter; see Fig. 11-8A and B; see also Fig. 10-34A and B). The bursts usually recur with an interval of 4 to 8 seconds. Shorter bursts and longer suppression periods indicate greater severity of the cerebral insult. The burst suppression may be considered a subgroup of periodic patterns. The third is *BiPLEDs* or *BIPD** (see "Periodic Patterns" in this chapter; see also "Periodic Lateralized Epileptiform Discharges," Chapter 10; see also Fig. 10-42A and B). The fourth is *alpha-coma pattern* that presents with abundant alpha frequency activity and little or no delta waves and is associated with a clinical picture of coma (see "Alpha-Coma and Theta-Coma Pattern" in this chapter) (see Figs. 11-13 and 11-14).

HERPES SIMPLEX ENCEPHALITIS

Any focal or lateralized EEG abnormalities in the clinical setting of acute encephalitis raises a suspicion of herpes simplex encephalitis. In the early stage, focal or lateralized asymmetric delta activity appears with temporal or frontotemporal prominence. Within a few days to 2 weeks after the onset of illness, periodic or pseudoperiodic discharges consisting of sharp or sharp and slow-wave complexes appear with intervals of 1 to 5 seconds (PLEDs or LPD*) (see Figs. 10-39A and B and 10-40; see also "Periodic Discharges," Chapter 10). As the disease progresses, PLEDs may become bilateral, and they occur either synchronously or independently between the hemispheres (BiPLEDs or BIPD*) (see Fig. 10-42A and B).[132,133] Most of the PLEDs or LPD* represent interictal patterns. However, this could evolve to ictal patterns consisting of rhythmic sharp or spikes, either with (convulsive) or without (nonconvulsive) clinical seizure activity. It is, therefore, highly recommended to do continuous bed side EEG monitoring, once LPD* or BIPD is found in a routine EEG (see Figs. 10-38 through 10-43; see also Video 13-5). PLEDs/LPD may be more multifocal especially in infants with herpes simplex encephalitis.[134] The presence of PLEDs or BiPLEDs (BIPD) is not pathognomonic of the disease, but febrile illness and a rapid deterioration of neurological signs in association with this EEG pattern is highly suggestive of herpes simplex encephalitis. EEG may rapidly deteriorate to burst suppression pattern with a fatal outcome in some cases, while others may show progressive improvement, even to normalization of EEG.

SUBACUTE SCLEROSING PANENCEPHALITIS

SSPE is a progressive disease secondary to a chronic measles virus infection. It has become extremely rare since the introduction of measles immunization. The disease is manifested by abnormal movements and progressive intellectual deterioration. The EEG is characterized by periodic complexes consisting of bilaterally symmetric and synchronous, high-amplitude (may reach >1,000 μV) bursts of polyphasic delta mixed with sharp waves (GPD* or generalized periodic discharges). The bursts recur with intervals of 4 to 10 seconds (see Fig. 10-32A and B). The periodic bursts may be more prominent and distinct during the awake state. The myoclonic jerks, if present, are time locked with the bursts. Periodic complexes may be present at any stage of the disease, but they are usually seen during the intermediate stage. In the early stage of illness, the background activity may be well preserved and the bursts may occur infrequently every few minutes and may be present only in sleep.[135,136] As the disease progresses, the burst intervals become shorter.[135] In the later stages of the disease, polymorphic delta or FIRDA (frontally predominant GRDA*) may appear. Also, various types of epileptiform activity, including spikes, sharps, and spike-wave discharges, either in a focal or in a generalized form may occur.[135,136]

CREUTZFELDT–JAKOB DISEASE

This disease is a rapidly progressive dementia associated with various myoclonic jerks. In the early stage, EEG shows slowing of the background activity and increased theta–delta activity. The abnormalities may start with focal or unilateral prominence but eventually become bilaterally diffuse. As the disease progresses, the EEG is characterized by periodic diphasic or triphasic sharp discharges recurring with an interval of ½ to 1 second (GPD*) (see Fig. 10-33A–D; see also "Creutzfeldt–Jakob Disease," in the section of Diffuse Periodicity in Chapter 10). The periodic discharges may be subtle at first and unilaterally dominant, may only be present intermittently alternating with periods of no periodic pattern, and may be evident only in the awake EEG. In between the periodic discharges, background activity becomes increasingly slower until it is no longer discernible.

The configuration of triphasic waves in CJD is different from that of hepatic encephalopathy. The slow-wave components are more prominent in hepatic encephalopathy, while the sharp-wave components are more prominent in CJD. The periodic discharges in CJD are also different from those seen in SSPE. The paroxysmal discharges consist of complex bursts in SSPE rather than the simple transients seen in CJD. Also, periodic intervals are much longer (4 to 10 seconds) in SSPE than in CJD. The CJD patient exhibits random myoclonic jerks, but the jerks are not time locked with the sharp discharges, unlike SSPE in which the jerk tends to coincide with paroxysmal bursts. However, computerized back avenging technique ("jerk-locked" or "myoclonus triggered averaging") can reveal sharp/spike discharges that are time locked to the myoclonus.[137] (See Chapter 10, Myoclonic seizure.)

In the final stage of CJD, periodic discharges usually decrease or the interval between the discharges may lengthen,[138] but periodicity may remain until the terminal stage.[119]

Although the above described periodic patterns are characteristic of CJD and seen in more than 75% of proven cases,[119] some CJD patients, especially the atypical forms, ataxic, or amyotrophic variety of slow progression[139] or the familial type,[140] may not show a periodic EEG pattern. Less prominent and less periodic triphasic (or pseudoperiodic) patterns, which superficially resemble the periodic pattern of CJD, have been described in patients with rapidly progressive Alzheimer's dementia.[141] The triphasic periodic pattern can also occur with reversible toxic encephalopathy due to baclofen,[142] lithium,[143] levodopa,[144] anoxic encephalopathy,[145] and hepatic/uremic encephalitis.[146]

BATTEN'S DISEASE (CEREBROMACULAR DEGENERATION, NEURONAL CEROID LIPOFUSCINOSIS)

The onset of Batten's disease is usually during late infancy or childhood, characterized by loss of vision with macular degeneration, optic nerve atrophy, decline of mental function, and epileptic seizures. EEG abnormalities with marked slowing and paroxysmal discharges including spikes are present in the early stage of the illness. The most characteristic feature is large occipital spikes induced by slow flicker photic stimulation (see Fig. 9-11). These flicker-induced occipital spikes are seen only in the late infantile form (Bielschowsky–Jansky form) and not in the juvenile or adult forms.[147,148]

Dementing Illnesses

ALZHEIMER'S DISEASE

Alzheimer's disease is the most common dementing illness accounting for more than 50% of all dementia patients. Many studies have found a positive correlate between the severity of dementia and the degree of EEG abnormalities.[149–151] In the early stage of Alzheimer's disease, the EEG is usually normal. At this stage, quantitative EEG analysis using power spectrum has reported an increase in theta and decrease in beta activity without affecting alpha band frequency.[152,153] The routine EEG by visual inspection fails to reveal these early EEG changes.[151,152] Once dementia becomes moderate to severe, the EEG becomes abnormal in almost all patients; the alpha rhythm becomes slower and tends to lose reactivity to eyes opening/closing, and as the disease progresses, diffuse low to moderate amplitude irregular theta and delta activity appears[153] (Fig. 11-18). Epileptiform activity is rare, but sharp or triphasic waves may be seen in severely demented patients.[154] Triphasic waves tend to be more posteriorly dominant in contrast to the frontal dominant triphasic waves seen in metabolic encephalopathy.[108] Patients with abnormal EEGs in the early stage of illness or deteriorating EEGs tend to show a greater decline in coordinate motor functions and a higher frequency of extrapyramidal symptoms than patients with normal or stable EEG.[155] Also, patients with a greater degree of EEG abnormalities tend to have more delusions and hallucinations.[156] Biochemically, impaired cholinergic function appears to be responsible for loss of cognitive functions.[157]

HUNTINGTON'S DISEASE

The EEG of this autosomal-dominant disease is characterized by "flat" background activity.[158] Because of the low-voltage background activity, alpha rhythm is difficult to measure. Since low-voltage background pattern (<20 μV) is seen in about 10% of normal population, the "flat" EEG is not specific for the Huntington's disease. However, background activity of less than 10 μV is unusual in normal or other neurologic diseases and is found in one third of Huntington's patients (Fig. 11-19).[115] Hyperventilation often increases the amplitude of alpha rhythm in normal patients who otherwise have very-low-voltage background activity, but this does not occur in Huntington's patients. Sleep spindles, vertex sharp wave, and K complexes are also attenuated.[159] Of interest is that the amplitude of visual evoked potentials and median nerve somatosensory evoked potentials is also diminished.[160,161]

PARKINSON'S DISEASE AND DEMENTIA WITH LEWY BODIES

Approximately 30% to 50% of Parkinson's patients have abnormal EEGs consisting of slow background activity and increased theta–delta activity predominantly over the posterior head regions.[162,163] The incidence of dementia in idiopathic Parkinson's disease is estimated to be about 40%.[164] A significant number of nondemented Parkinson's patients also have abnormal EEGs (16%) though the abnormal incidence was statistically higher in dementia patients (44%).[165] In addition to dementia, increased motor disability correlates with increased

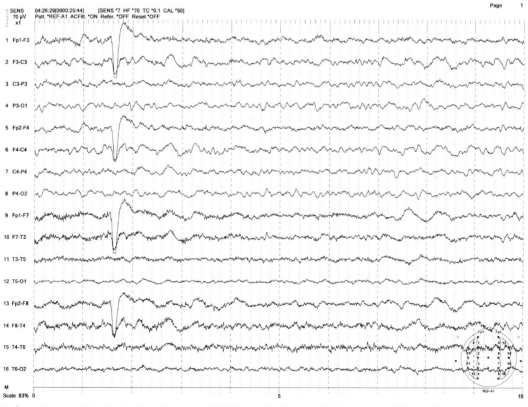

FIGURE 11-18 | A 60-year-old patient after diagnosis of Alzheimer's disease with the onset of illness about 2 years ago. Note irregular delta activity associated with variable mixed background activity consisting of alpha and theta rhythm. No paroxysmal activity was noted.

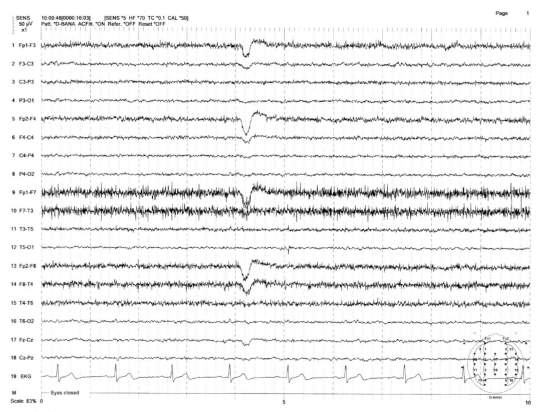

FIGURE 11-19 | A 43-year-old patient with diagnosis of Huntington's chorea. Note low-voltage EEG pattern without slow waves.

slowing of the EEG. The distinction has been made between Parkinson's disease with dementia and dementia with Lewy bodies, in which the latter shows an earlier onset of extrapyramidal and cognitive symptoms with the greater degree of EEG abnormalities than the former.[166] The frontally predominant RDA*/FIRDA is relatively common, seen ⅓ of the patients with Lewy bodies dementia.[113]

MULTI-INFARCT DEMENTIA

This dementia is a result of the cumulative effects of multiple ischemic cerebral infarcts.[167] EEG has limited value in differentiating vascular dementia from other types of dementia, though focal abnormalities such as spikes, sharp wave, and delta–theta slowing are more common in vascular dementia than in patients with Alzheimer's dementia.[150,168] One quantitative EEG study showed some spectral differences in Alzheimer's dementia patients having more delta and theta slow-wave power and less alpha power than in vascular dementia patients matched for severity of dementia.[169] However, distinction between Alzheimer's dementia and multi-infarct dementia is never certain because of considerable overlap in abnormal EEG patterns.

ANTI-NMDA RECEPTOR ENCEPHALITIS

The anti-NMDA (N-methyl-D-aspartate) receptor encephalitis was first introduced in 2005.[170] The disease is caused by an autoimmune reaction against NMDA receptors with paraneoplastic association.[170] The illness presents initially with flu-like symptoms followed by acute psychosis (agitation, paranoia,

etc.), altered cognition, and dyskinesia often affecting mouth and lips, and seizures (either convulsive or nonconvulsive, or both). The disease can be fatal but has a high probability of recovery with adequate treatment (steroid, immunoglobulin, and plasmapheresis). The EEG plays an important role for the diagnosis because EEG often shows a uniquely characteristic pattern, referred to "*extreme delta brush.*"[171,172] This consists of rhythmic or semirhythmic diffuse or lateralized 1- to 3-Hz delta activity mixed with intermittent 20- to 30-Hz beta or even faster than 30-Hz (gamma) activity superimposed over the delta wave (Fig. 11-20). The pattern usually disappears with spontaneous or induced arousal episodes. Because of extreme fast activity, it is at times difficult to differentiate from muscle artifacts, especially when associated with oral–buccal dyskinesia. Also, the effect of sedative drug (benzodiazepine, etc.) producing beta activity must be ruled out. The rhythmic delta pattern occurs continuously or intermittently, often with sharply contoured waveform, resembling electrographic ictal pattern (Fig. 11-21A). In fact, this could be considered status epilepticus (usually nonconvulsive)[173] if the pattern lasts longer than 5 minutes or BRD (brief rhythmic discharges; see also Chapter 10, section of Ictal vs. Interictal Epileptiform Discharges) for the shorter pattern (see also Fig. 10-43A).[174] In addition, the typical clinical seizures associated with clear ictal EEG changes are not uncommon[170] (Fig. 11-21B).

The Effect of Drugs on the EEG

Many patients who are examined in EEG laboratories are being treated with various medications. Especially in

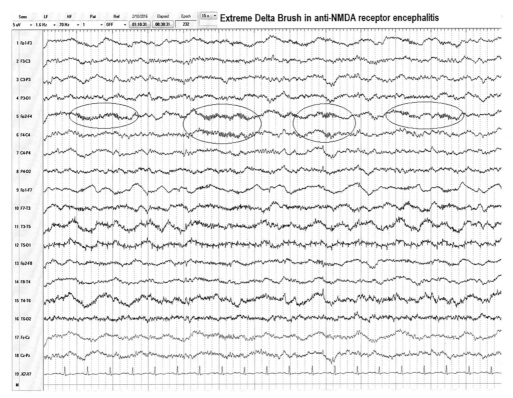

FIGURE 11-20 | A 33-year-old female with diagnosis of anti-NMDA receptor encephalitis associated with diagnosis of cystic teratoma. The initial presentation was focal seizure followed by psychotic behavior. The gamma range (>30 Hz) fast activity was noted over the decaling phase of delta waves over the frontal region (shown by *oval circles*), named as "extreme delta brush." Note the difference from the fast activity due to muscle artifacts over the temporal electrodes. The pattern was intermittently terminated by arousal episodes.

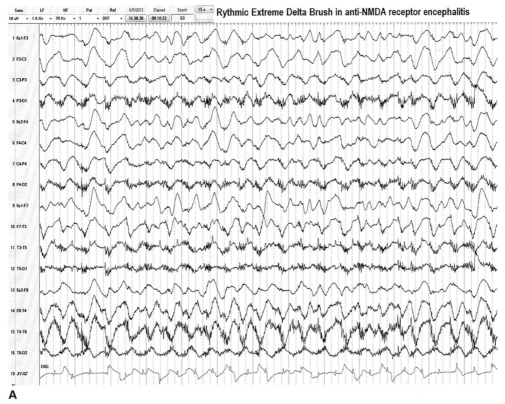

FIGURE 11-21 | A 27-year-old female with diagnosis of anti-NMDS receptor encephalitis, presented with somnolence, regression to child-like behavior and status epilepticus. The EEG showed rhythmic somewhat sharply contoured delta associated with rhythmic bursts of fast activity (probably partly contaminated by muscle artifacts from buccal movements) **(A)**. The patient also had intermittent episodes of non nonconvulsive status epilepticus with rhythmic right/left spike-wave bursts lasting more than 30 minutes **(B)**.

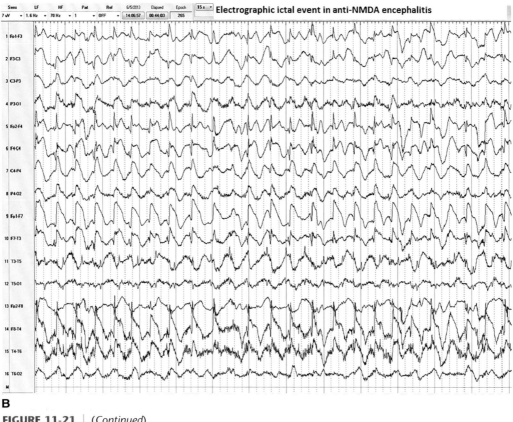

FIGURE 11-21 | (*Continued*)

psychiatric patients treated with therapeutic doses of neuroleptics or antidepressants, it is often difficult to distinguish if altered EEG patterns are due to a drug effect or intrinsic abnormalities. The drug effects on EEG are dependent on multiple factors. The effect may be different depending on the dose (therapeutic or toxic) or the duration of exposure. The effects also show considerable interindividual variability. Preexisting EEG abnormalities or neurological disorders can influence the impact of drug effects. In general, EEG abnormalities induced by drugs are expected to be bilaterally diffuse, but focal or lateralized abnormalities may also occur. EEG changes caused by medications mainly consist of (i) slowing of background alpha rhythm and/or increased theta and delta activity, (ii) increased beta activity, and/or (iii) appearance of paroxysmal activity with sharp waves, theta–delta waves, and at times including spike and spike-wave discharges. Because it is not possible to describe all the relevant medications in detail, only commonly used medications are described here. The remaining medications are listed in Table 11-2 with references.

ANTIPSYCHOTIC DRUGS

The *neuroleptics* (*phenothiazine*, *butyrophenone*, and *thioxanthene derivatives*) generally have more pronounced effects on the EEG compared to other drugs. The changes consist of slowing of alpha rhythm and increase of theta and delta activity and paroxysmal bursts of sharp and slow waves, occasionally spike and spike-wave complexes.[197,218] The bursts tend to be more prominent in the awake state than in sleep. These drugs may also increase preexisting epileptiform activity in epileptic patients. A new antipsychotic agent, *clozapine*, has a marked effect on EEG. As high as three fourths of patients receiving clozapine have a wide spectrum of EEG changes including generalized slowing and bilateral spike-wave discharges.[219,220] Abnormal EEGs are more common in patients receiving high dosage of clozapine.[221] In contrast to these antipsychotic agents, which have significant effects on EEG, another newer drug *risperidone* has no effect on EEG.[192]

ANTIDEPRESSANT DRUGS

Tricyclic antidepressants (*amitriptyline*, *desipramine*, *imipramine*, *nortriptyline*, and *protriptyline*) have similar but much less prominent effects as compared to the neuroleptics. The changes include slowing of alpha rhythm, increase of beta activity, and, in some cases, paroxysmal discharges including spikes and spike-wave discharges.[219,220] MAO (monoamine oxidase) inhibitors have a similar effect as tricyclic antidepressants. The effect of a therapeutic dose of lithium on the EEG varies from no or minimal EEG change to slowing of alpha rhythm.[222] FIRDA may be present and accentuated by hyperventilation.[223] Focal abnormalities may also occur.[222] The paroxysmal activity precipitated by a toxic level may include spikes or triphasic waves[223] (Fig. 11-22A and B) or periodic complexes resembling those of CJD.[143] It should be noted that one large retrospective study in patients receiving psychopharmaceutical agents found the highest incidence of abnormal EEGs in patients receiving clozapine (59%) and next highest in those receiving lithium (50%).[195]

TABLE 11-2 Drug Effects on EEG

	Therapeutic	Toxic	References
A. Anticonvulsants Anxiolytic Drugs			
Benzodiazepine	Increase fast (beta) activity (see Figs. 7-21 and 7-42)	Increase delta and spindle coma	175,176
Barbiturate	Increase fast (beta) activity	Increase delta, spindle coma, burst suppression, and ECS	177,178
Phenytoin	None or minimal	Slowing of alpha and increase delta and theta	179,180
Carbamazepine	None or mild slowing of alpha	Increase delta and theta	181,182
Valproic acid	None	Increase delta and theta	179,183
Lamotrigine	None	—	184,185
Tiagabine	None	—	186
Vigabatrin	None	—	187,188
Gabapentin	Minimally increase delta and theta and decrease alpha	—	189
Baclofen	—	Triphasic wave PLEDs/LPD*	190
B. Neuropsychiatric Drugs			
Neuroleptic drugs (phenothiazine, butyrophenone, and thioxanthene)	Decrease beta and increase theta and delta	Increase paroxysmal activity	191,192
Risperidone	None	—	193
Clozapine	Slow BA and spike wave	—	194,195
Lithium	Slow BA and FIRDA (frontally predominant RDA*)	Triphasic waves paroxysmal discharges	196,197
Tricyclic antidepressant (TCA)	Slow BA and decrease REM sleep	Increase slow waves and increase paroxysmal activity (spikes)	198,199
Selective serotonin reuptake inhibitor (SSRI)	Minimal or none	—	200
Cocaine	Increase beta	—	200
LSD (lysergic acid diethylamide)	Faster alpha and decrease slow wave	—	201
Marijuana (delta-9 tetrahydrocannabinol)	None	—	202
C. Immunosuppressive Agents			
Methotrexate	—	Focal delta, slow BA, and PLEDs (LPD*)	203,204
Ifosfamide	—	Increase delta, PLEDs/LPD*, and status epilepticus	205
L-Asparaginase	—	Increase delta	206
Cyclosporine	—	Focal slow and epileptiform activity	207
D. Toxic Agents			
Lead	—	Increased slow waves	208
Mercury	—	Increased slow waves and epileptiform activity	209
Manganese	—	Increase fast activity spike	210
Aluminum	—	Increase slow waves and spike	211
Carbon monoxide	—	Focal and diffuse epileptiform activity, and increase slow waves	212
Organophosphates pesticides	—	Increase slow waves, increase paroxysmal activity, and fast rhythmic activity	213

(Continued)

TABLE 11-2 Drug Effects on EEG (*Continued*)

	Therapeutic	Toxic	References
E. Others			
Morphine	Decrease REM sleep	Increase slow waves	214
Aminophylline	—	Increase paroxysmal discharges (PLEDs/LPD*)	215
Isoniazid	—	Increase slow waves, increase paroxysmal discharges, and status epilepticus	216
Penicillin	—	Status epilepticus	217

BA, background activity; ECS, electrocerebral silence; PLEDs, periodic lateralized epileptiform discharges; —, no data available.

ANXIOLYTIC OR HYPNOTIC DRUGS

Benzodiazepine derivatives are a potent activation of beta activity, which may persist as long as 2 to 3 weeks after the last oral administration. The degree of beta activation varies considerably from one subject to another. The alpha rhythm may become faster to the beta frequency range. In sleep, the amount of sleep spindles increases along with a paucity of vertex sharp waves and K complexes. Differentiating beta activity and sleep spindles may sometimes become difficult (see Figs. 8-3 and 8-4; and also Fig. 7-21). Instead of beta, gamma activity may be induced in some cases (see Fig. 7-22). Among the hypnotic or anxiolytic drugs that induce beta activity are *barbiturates, bromides, methaqualone, glutethimide,* and *meprobamate.* Focal depression of beta activity, especially when the patient is on these beta-inducing drugs, suggests focal cortical lesions (see Fig. 8-5, also Fig. 12-6).[224] Acute withdrawal of benzodiazepines[225] or barbiturates[226] may induce spike and spike-wave discharges and sometimes provoke clinical seizures. Photoparoxysmal and photomyogenic responses may occur in barbiturate withdrawal.[227] Despite the opposite effect to sedative drugs, cerebral stimulants such as D-amphetamine, methylphenidate, and cocaine and hallucinogens such as lysergic acid diethylamide (LSD) may also enhance beta activity.[228]

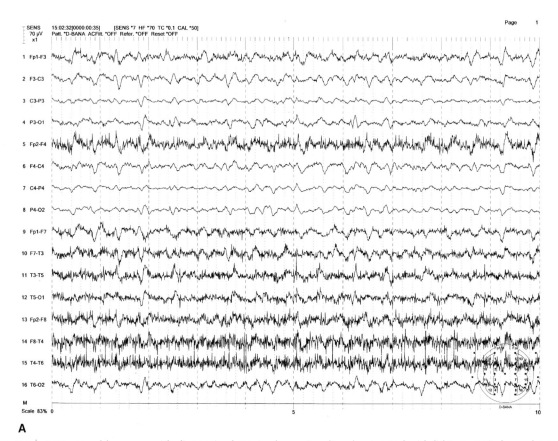

FIGURE 11-22 | A 55-year-old woman with diagnosis of manic–depressive disorder, treated with lithium. EEG showed nearly periodic triphasic sharp discharges **(A)**. Three weeks after discontinuing lithium, EEG showed disappearance of triphasic sharp discharges but background activity remained slow **(B)**.

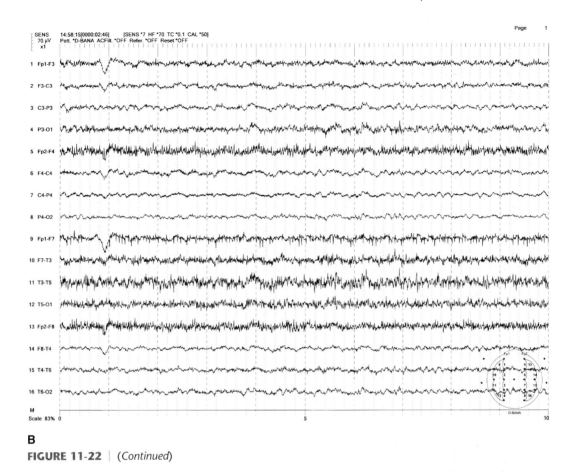

B

FIGURE 11-22 | (Continued)

ANTICONVULSANT DRUGS

In general, a visual inspection of the EEGs with an oral dose of antiepileptic drugs does not show significant EEG change at therapeutic drug levels. But slight slowing may be detected by quantitative EEG analysis even at the therapeutic drug level.[179,229] This applies to both phenytoin and carbamazepine, and the EEG changes are more pronounced with toxic drug levels. Valproic acid does not have much effect on background EEG activity but a toxic state will result in diffuse slowing.[230] The most significant effect of valproic acid is the reduction of generalized spikes and photoparoxysmal responses.[231] This effect contrasts to phenytoin[175] and carbamazepine,[232] which have little or no effect on interictal epileptiform discharges. For the effect of newer anticonvulsants, the reader may refer to the section "Paroxysmal Discharges and Seizure Diagnosis" in Chapter 10. Intravenous administration of benzodiazepine (diazepam, Alprazolam, lorazepam, midazolam, etc.), often used for treatment of status epilepticus, rapidly and effectively attenuates epileptiform activity.[233]

ETHANOL (ETHYL ALCOHOL)

During acute alcohol intoxication, mild slowing of the alpha rhythm may occur, but with severe intoxication, theta and delta slowing increases.[234] EEGs in chronic alcoholism are usually normal and show only slight slowing, if any.[235] Acute alcohol withdrawal may cause hallucinations, delirium, tremor, and epileptic seizures. EEG shows a desynchronized low-voltage pattern and may produce spikes.[236] In *Wernicke–Korsakoff encephalopathy* due to thiamine deficiency in chronic alcoholism, the EEG mainly shows diffuse slowing. Alcoholic encephalopathy may produce PLEDs (LPD) associated with focal seizure.[237] Alcohol withdrawal may also activate PLEDs (LPD*) in patients who have preexisting focal cerebral lesions.[238]

ANESTHETIC AGENTS

Most anesthetic agents produce similar EEG changes. However, some agents suppress the epileptiform activity, while others may accentuate or precipitate epileptiform discharges:

1. *Barbiturates* initially cause an increase of beta activity with reduction of alpha rhythm. As the dose increases, slow waves increase. At high doses, a burst suppression pattern appears. Barbiturate-induced coma for therapeutic purpose achieves and maintains a burst suppression pattern for a few to several days with the aid of EEG monitoring. The suppression period is dependent on the doses of barbiturate and can be as long as several hours. During a severe suppression period, the recording is electrically silent.
2. *Propofol* may act as a stimulant for epileptiform discharges at a low dose but suppress the epileptiform activity at high dose.[239] A high dose of propofol also has been used for inducing therapeutic burst suppression as a means to control refractory status epilepticus. Inducing a burst suppression pattern with Propofol is much quicker than barbiturate (Video 11-2).[240] Similar to barbiturates, abrupt withdrawal may precipitate seizures.

3. *Ketamine* at low doses causes a loss of alpha rhythm and a decrease of background amplitude. With a high dose, theta activity appears with an increase of beta activity.[240]
4. *Halogenated inhalation agents* (*desflurane, enflurane, halothane, isoflurane,* and *sevoflurane*) have EEG effects similar to those produced by barbiturates. At an induction dose, EEG may show sleep spindle-like activity in the frontal region. High concentrations produce reduction of amplitude and frequency of background activity.[240] All halogenated agents markedly suppress evoked potentials, especially motor evoked potentials; thus, they are not a suitable anesthesia for intraoperative surgical monitoring using somatosensory and/or motor evoked potentials.
5. *Nitrous oxide,* often used in combination with other halogenated agents, also increases very fast beta (gamma) activity (>30 Hz).[240] Pro and/or anticonvulsant properties of all the above inhalation agents have been inconclusive.
6. *Synthetic opiates* (*fentanyl, sufentanil,* and *alfentanil*) cause loss of alpha activity and increase of beta activity at low concentrations. With increased doses, theta and then delta activity increases. Burst suppression or ECS does not occur even with high doses of opioid agents. Instead, this may precipitate epileptiform activity.[241]

EEG in Head Injury

EEG shows various degrees of abnormalities depending on the severity of trauma, location of cerebral injury, and level of consciousness. The degrees of EEG abnormalities discussed in the first section of this chapter correlate well with the severity of posttraumatic coma, especially in the acute state.[242] EEG also assists in prognosticating the outcome after head injury.[243] Chronic stages of cerebral trauma show less correlation, though there is an overall correlation between EEG and clinical improvement, especially when evaluating serial EEGs.[244,245]

CEREBRAL CONCUSSION

Cerebral concussion is defined as brief and temporary cessation of brain functions secondary to blunt or closed head injury but without evidence of pathological damage to the brain. The patient loses consciousness briefly, which may accompany transient arrest of respiration, bradycardia, and a drop in blood pressure. These return to normal within a few seconds. The vast majority of patients with cerebral concussion with transient loss of consciousness have normal or borderline EEGs.[246] Some patients may become drowsy or sleepy after a concussion, with accompanying normal sleep EEG.[247] There may be some excess of slow waves during the awake state, but EEG normalization usually occurs quickly.

In contrast, some patients may show moderately abnormal EEGs with excessive theta–delta waves associated with normal neurological state and little or no complaints. These discrepancies between EEG abnormalities and clinical state may be found more often in children.[248] If the EEG is abnormal, the patient may have longer-lasting alteration of the mental state.[249]

CEREBRAL CONTUSION OR HEMORRHAGE

Cerebral contusion can be due to closed head injury or open and penetrating injury. It causes various degrees of brain tissue damage, hemorrhage, and/or brain edema. In contrast to concussion, contusions are associated with varieties and various degrees of EEG abnormalities. The abnormalities may be diffuse and/or focal. The degree of EEG abnormality correlates well with the patient's level of consciousness, ranging from minimal impairment of consciousness with minimal EEG abnormality to deep coma state associated with diffuse low-voltage delta activity or near ECI. A burst suppression pattern may occur in posttraumatic coma when complicated by cerebral anoxia.

The presence of sleep spindles is common, especially in the acute state (within 2 days after brain injury), which suggests a favorable prognosis.[26,27,29] The incidence of sleep spindles decreases in prolonged coma irrespective of outcome.[250,251]

In contrast to spindles, the presence of electrographic seizure activity during the acute stage carries a poor prognosis,[252] and the mortality is three times higher in patients with seizure than those without.[247] More than 50% of patients who have status epilepticus associated with motor manifestation will die within a few days.[252] Nonconvulsive (subclinical) status epilepticus also carries a grave prognosis.[252] The risk for developing epilepsy is significantly higher for patients with seizures in the acute stages than those without.[253] Early and late seizures are three times more common in patients with depressed skull fracture than those without.[247] Also, focal epileptiform activity associated with diffuse EEG abnormalities in the acute state carries a greater chance of subsequent chronic epilepsy than those with only a focal epileptiform pattern.[247]

References

1. Teasdale G, Jennett B. Assessment of coma and impaired consciousness. A practical scale. *Lancet* 1974;2:81–84.
2. Bickford RG, Butt HR. Hepatic coma: The electroencephalographic patterns. *J Clin Invest* 1955;34:790–799.
3. Cadilhac J. The EEG in renal insufficiency. In: Rmond A, ed-in-chief. *Handbook of Electroencephalography and Clinical Neurophysiology.* Vol. 15c. Amsterdam, The Netherlands: Elsevier, 1976:351–369.
4. Kuroiwa Y, Celesia GG. Clinical significance of periodic EEG pattern. *Arch Neurol (Chicago)* 1980;37:15–20.
5. Silverman D. The electroencephalogram in anoxic coma. In: Harner R, Naquet R, eds. *Altered States of Consciousness. Coma, Cerebral Death/Handbook of Electroencephalography and Clinical Neurophysiology.* Vol. 12. Amsterdam, The Netherlands: Elsevier, 1975:81–94.
6. Koufen H, Consbruch. Die Lithium-Intoxikation. Beobachtungen and 6 Fallen. *Nervenarzt* 1972;43:145–152.
7. Harner RN, Katz RI. Electroencephalography in metabolic coma. In: Harner R, Naquet R, eds. *Altered States of Consciousness, Coma, Cerebral Death. Handbook of Electroencephalography and Clinical Neurophysiology.* Vol. 12. Amsterdam, The Netherlands: Elsevier, 1975:47–62.
8. Hockaday JM, Potts F, Epstein E, et al. Electroencephalographic change in acute cerebral anoxia from cardiac or respiratory arrest. *Electroencephalogr Clin Neurophysiol* 1965;18:575–586.
9. Panpiglione G, Harden A. Resuscitation after cardiopulmonary arrest: Prognostic evaluation of early electroencephalographic findings. *Lancet* 1968;1:1261–1263.
10. Haider I, Matthew H, Oswald I. Electroencephalographic change in acute drug poisoning. *Electroencephalogr Clin Neurophysiol* 1971;30:23–31.
11. Weissenborn K, Wilkens H, Hawsmann E, et al. Burst suppression EEG with baclofen overdose. *Clin Neurol Neurosurg* 1991;93:77–80.
12. Pagni CA, Courjon J. Electroencephalographic modifications induced by moderate and deep hypothermia in man. *Acta Neurochir Suppl (Wien)* 1964;13:35–49.

13. Bird TD, Plum F. Recovery from barbiturate overdose coma with prolonged isoelectric electroencephalogram. *Neurology (Minneap)* 1968;18:456–460.

14. Jellish WS, Thalji Z, Fluter E, et al. Etomidate and thiopental-based anesthetic induction: Comparisons between different titrated levels of electrophysiologic cortical depression and response to laryngoscopy. *J Clin Anesth* 1977;1997:36–41.

15. Illievich UM, Petricek W, Schramm W, et al. Electroencephalographic burst suppression by propofol infusion in human: Hemodynamic consequence. *Anesth Analog* 1993;77:155–160.

16. Yli-Hankala A, Jantti V. EEG burst-suppression pattern correlates with the instantaneous heart rate under isoflurane anesthesia. *Acta Anaesthesiol Scand* 1990;34:665–668.

17. Chokroverty S. "Alpha-like" rhythm in electroencephalogram in coma after cardiac arrest. *Neurology (Minneap)* 1975;25:655–663.

18. Westmoreland BF, Klass DW, Sharbrough FW, et al. Alpha-coma. Electroencephalographic, clinical, pathologic and etiologic correlations. *Arch Neurol (Chicago)* 1975;32:713–718.

19. Young GB, Blume WT, Campbell VM, et al. Alpha, theta and alpha-theta coma: A clinical outcome utilizing serial recordings. *Electroencephalogr Clin Neurophysiol* 1994;91:93–99.

20. Chatrian GE, White LE, Shaw CM. EEG pattern resembling wakefulness in unresponsive decerebrate state following traumatic brainstem infarct. *Electroencephalogr Clin Neurophysiol* 1964;16:285–289.

21. Grindal AB, Suter C. "Alpha pattern coma" in high voltage electrical injury. *Electroencephalogr Clin Neurophysiol* 1975;38:521–526.

22. Yamada T, Steveland N, Kimura J. Alpha-pattern coma in a 2-year-old child. *Arch Neurol (Chicago)* 1979;36:225–227.

23. Synek VM, Synek BJL. Theta pattern coma, a variant of alpha pattern coma. *Clin Electroencephalogr* 1984;15:116–121.

24. Bergamasco B, Bergamini L, Doriguzzi T, et al. EEG sleep patterns as a prognostic criterion in post-traumatic coma. *Electroencephalogr Clin Neurophysiol* 1968;24:374–377.

25. Bricolo A, Turella G. Electroencephalographic pattern of acute traumatic coma: Diagnostic and prognostic value. *J Neurosurg Sci* 1973;17:278–285.

26. Chatrian GE, White LE, Daly D. Electroencephalographic pattern resembling those of sleep in certain comatose states after injuries to the head. *Electroencephalogr Clin Neurophysiol* 1963;15:272–280.

27. Rumpl E, Prugger M, Bauer G, et al. Incidence and prognostic values of spindles in post-traumatic coma. *Electroencephalogr Clin Neurophysiol* 1983;56:420–429.

28. Britt CW Jr. Non-traumatic "spindle-coma": Clinical, EEG and prognostic features. *Neurology (Minneap)* 1981;31:393–397.

29. Hansotia P, Gottschalk P, Green P, et al. Spindle coma: Incidence, clinico-pathologic correlates and prognostic value. *Neurology (Minneap)* 1981;31:83–87.

30. Dadmehr N, Pakalnis A, Drake ME. Spindle coma in viral encephalitis. *Clin Electroencephalogr* 1987;18:34–37.

31. Evans BM, Bartlett JR. Prediction of outcome in severe head injury based on recognition of sleep related activity in the polygraphic electroencephalogram. *J Neurol Neurosurg Psychiatry* 1995;59:17–25 (abstract).

32. Kaplan PW, Genoud D, Ho TW, et al. Clinical correlates and prognosis in early spindle coma. *Clin Neurophysiol* 2000;111:584–590.

33. Report of the Quality Standards Subcommittee of the American Academy of Neurology. Practice parameters for determining brain death in adults (Summary Statement). *Neurology (Minneap)* 1995;45:1012–1014.

34. Stecker MM, Sabau D, Sullivan L, et al. American Clinical Neurophysiology Society Guidelines. Guideline 3: Minimum technical standards for EEG recording in suspected cerebral death. *J Clin Neurophysiol* 2016;33(4):324–327.

35. The NINDS Collaborative Study of Brain-death. NINCDS Monograph No. 24, *NIH Publication No. 81-2286*. December 1980.

36. Guidelines for the determination of brain death in infants and children: An update for the 1987 task force recommendation. *Crit Care Med* 2011;39(9):2139–2155.

37. Grigg MM, Kelly MA, Celesia GG, et al. Electroencephalographic activity after brain death. *Arch Neurol* 1987;44:948–954.

38. Hoefer PFA, Guttmann SA, Sands IJ. Convulsive states and coma in cases of islet cell adenoma of the pancreas. *Am J Psychiatry* 1946;102:486–495.

39. Gibbs FA, Murray EL. Hypoglycemia convulsions. *Electroencephalogr Clin Neurophysiol* 1954;6:674.

40. Daniel JC, Chohroverty S, Barron KD. Anacidotic hyperglycemia and focal seizures. *Arch Intern Med* 1969;124:701–706.

41. Singh BM, Strobos RJ. Epilepsia partialis continua associated with nonketotic hyperglycemia: Clinical and biochemical profile of 21 patients. *Ann Neurol* 1980;8:155–160.

42. Karnaze DS, Bickford RG. Triphasic waves: A reassessment of their significance. *Electroencephalogr Clin Neurophysiol* 1984;57:193–198.

43. Fisch BJ, Klass DW. The diagnostic specificity of triphasic wave pattern. *Electroencephalogr Clin Neurophysiol* 1988;70:1–8.

44. Prill A, Quellhorst E, Scheler F. Epilepsy: Clinical and electrographic findings in patients with renal insufficiency. In: Gastaut H, Jasper HH, Bancaud J, eds. *The Physiopathogenesis of the Epilepsies*. Springfield, IL: Charles C Thomas, 1969:60–68.

45. Glaser GH. Brain dysfunction in uremia. In: Plum F, ed. *Brain Dysfunction in Metabolic Disorders*. New York: Raven Press, 1974:3173–3197.

46. Hughes JR. EEG in uremia. *Am J EEG Technol* 1984;24:1–10.

47. Tyler HR. Neurological complication of dialysis, transplantation and other form of treatment in chronic uremia. *Neurology (Minneap)* 1965;15:1081–1088.

48. Glaser GH, Levy LL. Seizures and idiopathic hypoparathyroidism: A clinical–electroencephalographic study. *Epilepsia (Amsterdam)* 1960;1:454–465.

49. Swash M, Rowan AJ. Electroencephalographic criteria of hypocalcemia and hypercalcemia. *Arch Neurol (Chicago)* 1972;26:218–228.

50. Saunders MG, Westmoreland BF. The EEG for evaluation of disorders affecting the brain diffusely. In: Klass DW, Daly DD, eds. *Current Practice of Clinical Electroencephalography*. New York: Raven Press, 1979:343–379.

51. Glaser GH. The EEG in certain metabolic disorders. In: Remond A, ed-in-chief. *Handbook of Electroencephalography and Clinical Neurophysiology*. Vol. 315C. Amsterdam, The Netherlands: Elsevier, 1976:316–325.

52. Dreifus PM, Victor M. Effects of thiamine deficiency on the cerebral nervous system. *Am J Clin Nutr* 1961;9:414–425.

53. Walton JN, Kiloh LG, Osselton JW, et al. The electroencephalogram in pernicious anemia and subacute combined degeneration of the cord. *Electroencephalogr Clin Neurophysiol* 1954;6:45–64.

54. Thiebaut F, Rohmer F, Wackenheim A. Contribution a l'etude electroencephalographique des syndromes endocriniens. *Electroencephalogr Clin Neurophysiol* 1958;10:1–30.

55. Glaser GH. Psychotic reactions induced by corticotropin (ACTH) and cortisone. *Psychosom Med* 1953;4:280–291.

56. Hughes R, Summers YK. Changes in electroencephalogram associated with hypopituitarism due to post-partum necrosis. *Electroencephalogr Clin Neurophysiol* 1956;8:87–96.

57. Jabbari B, Huott AD. Seizures in thyrotoxicosis. *Epilepsia* 1980;21:91–96.

58. Spatz R, Nagel J, Kollmannsberger A, et al. Das Elektroenzephalogramm bei der Hyperthyreose und im thyreotoxichen Koma. *Z EEG-EMG* 1975;6:14–18.

59. Harris R, Della-Rovere MD, Prior P. Electroencephalographic studies in infants and children with hypothyroidism. *Arch Dis Child* 1965;40:612–617.

60. Dow RS. The electroencephalographic finding in acute intermittent porphyria. *Electroencephalogr Clin Neurophysiol* 1961;13:425–437.

61. Schneck L. Clinical manifestation of Tay-Sachs disease. In: Volk BW, ed. *Tay-Sachs Disease*. New York: Grune & Stratton, 1964:16–30.

62. Pampiglione G, Lehovsky M. The evolution of EEG feature in Tay-Sach's disease and amaurotic family idiocy in 24 children. In: Kellaway P, Petersen I, eds. *Clinical Electroencephalography in Children*. New York: Grune & Stratton, 1968:287–306.

63. Engel J Jr, Rapin I, Giblin DR. Electrophysiological studies in two patients with cherry red spot-myoclonus syndrome. *Epilepsia* 1977;18:73–87.

64. Nishimura R, Omos-Lau N, Ajmone-Marson C, et al. Electroencephalographic findings in Gaucher's disease. *Neurology (Minneap)* 1980;30:152–159.

65. Andrews JM, Cancilla PA, Grippo J, et al. Globoid cell leukodystrophy (Krabbe's disease): Morphological and biochemical studies. *Neurology (Minneap)* 1971;21:337–352.

66. Pampiglione G. Some inborn metabolic disorders affecting cerebral electrogenesis. In: Holt KS, Coffey VP, eds. *Some Recent Advances in Inform Errors of Metabolism*. London, UK: Livingstone, 1968:80–100.

67. Mamoli B, Graf M, Toifl K. EEG pattern evoked potentials and nerve conduction velocity in a family with adrenoleukodystrophy. *Electroencephalogr Clin Neurophysiol* 1979;47:411–419.

68. Volpe JJ, Adams RD. Cerebro-hepato-renal syndrome of Zellweger: An inherited disorder of neuronal migration. *Acta Neuropath (Berlin)* 1972;20:175–198.

69. Bell AJ. MELAS syndrome: Overview and case study. *Am J EEG Technol* 1995;35:83–91.

70. Naibu S, Niedermeyer E. Degenerative disorder of the central nervous system. In: Niedermeyer E, Da Silva FL, eds. *Electroencephalography: Basic, Principles, Clinical Application and Related Fields*. 5th Ed. Philadelphia, PA: Lippincott Williams & Wilkins, 2005:379–401.

71. Metcalf DR. EEG in inborn errors of metabolism. In: Remond A, ed-in-chief. *Handbook of Electroencephalography and Clinical Neurophysiology*. Vol. 158. Amsterdam, The Netherlands: Elsevier, 1972:14–18.

72. Low NL, Bosma JF, Armstrong MD. Studies on phenylketonuria. VI EEG studies in phenylketonuria. *Arch Neurol Psychiatry (Chicago)* 1957;77:359–365.

73. Pampiglione G, Harden A. Neurophysiological identification of a late infantile form of neuronal lipidosis. *J Neurol Neurosurg Psychiatry* 1973;36:68–74.

74. Green JB. Neurophysiological studies in Batten's disease. *Dev Med Child Neurol* 1971;13:477–498.

75. Swaiman K, Smith SA, Trock GL, et al. Sea blue histocytes, lymphocytic cytosomes, movement disorders. 59 Fe uptake in basal ganglia in Hallervorden-Spatz disease or ceroid storage disease with abnormal isotope scan? *Neurology (Chicago)* 1983;33:301–305.

76. Ferriss GS, Happel LT, Duncan MC. Cerebral cortical isolation in infantile neuroaxonal dystrophy. *Electroencephalogr Clin Neurophysiol* 1977;43:168–182.

77. Radermecher FJ. Degenerative disease of the nervous system. In: Remond A, ed-in-chief. *Handbook of Electroencephalography and Clinical Neurophysiology*. Vol. 15A. Amsterdam, The Netherlands: Elsevier, 1977:162–191.

78. Heller GL, Kooi KA. The electroencephalogram in hepatolenticular degenerative (Wilson's disease). *Electroencephalogr Clin Neurophysiol* 1962;14:520–526.

79. White SR, Reese K, Sato S, et al. Spectrum of EEG findings in Menkes disease. *Electroencephalogr Clin Neurophysiol* 1993;87:57–61.

80. Krumholtz A, Singer HS, Niedermeyer E, et al. Electrophysiological studies in Tourette's syndrome. *Ann Neurol* 1983;14:638–641.

81. Roger J, Gastaut H, Toga M, et al. Epilepsie myoclonie progressive avec corps de Lafora (etude clinique, polygraphique et anatomique d' un cas). *Rev Neurol (Paris)* 1965;112:50–61.

82. Koskniemi M, Toivakka E, Donner M. Progressive myoclonus epilepsy. Electroencephalographic findings. *Acta Neurol Scand* 1974;50:333–359.

83. Walton A. A case study of Alpers' disease in siblings. *Am J EEG Technol* 1996;36:18–27.

84. Ganji S, Hellman CD. Tuberous sclerosis: Long-term follow-up and longitudinal electroencephalographic study. *Clin Electroencephalogr* 1985;16:219–224.

85. Lagos JC, Gomez MR. Tuberous sclerosis: Re-appraisal of a clinical entity. *Proc Mayo Clinic* 1967;42:26–49.

86. Jansen FE, van Huffelen AC, Witkamp ThD, et al. Diazepam-enhanced activity is Sturge-Weber syndrome: Its diagnostic significance in comparison with MRI. *Clin Neurophysiol* 2002; 113:1025–1029.

87. Ellingson RJ, Menolascino FJ, Eisen JD. Clinical-EEG relationship in mongoloids confirmed by karyotype. *Am J Ment Defic* 1970;74:645–650.

88. Rabache R, Francois P, Asselman R, et al. L'electroencephalographic dans 16 cas de maladie de Leber. *Rev Neurol (Paris)* 1960; 102:360–361.

89. Biejersbergen RSHM, Kemp A, Storm van Leeuwen W. EEG observation in dystrophia myotonia (Curschmann-Steinert). *Electroencephalogr Clin Neurophysiol* 1980;49:143–151.

90. Yoshioka M, Okuno T, Ito M, et al. Congenital muscular atrophy (Fukuyama type): Repeated CT studies in 19 children. *Comput Tomogr* 1981;5:81–88.

91. Guerrini R, DeLorey TM, Bonanni P, et al. Cortical myoclonus in Angelman syndrome. *Ann Neurol* 1996;40:39–48.

92. Niedermeyer E, Naidu S, Nogueira ed Melco A. The usefulness of electrocorticography in Rett syndrome. *Am J EEG Technol* 1991;31:27–37.

93. Robertson R, Langill L, Wong PKH, et al. Rett syndrome: EEG presentation. *Electroencephalogr Clin Neurophysiol* 1988;70:388–395.

94. Kooi KA, Tucker RP, Marshall RE. *Fundamentals of Electroencephalography*. 3rd Ed. Hagerstown, MD: Harper & Row, 1978.

95. Greenberg DA, Weinkle DJ, Aminoff MJ, et al. Complexes in infectious mononucleosis encephalitis. *J Neurol Neurosurg Psychiatry* 1982;45:648–651.

96. Radenmacker FJ. In: Remond A, ed-in-chief. *Infectious and Inflammatory Reaction, Allergy and Allergic Reaction: Degenerative Disease/Handbook of Electroencephalography and Clinical Neurophysiology*. Vol. 15, Part A. Amsterdam, The Netherlands: Elsevier, 1977.

97. Anderman F. *Chronic Encephalitis and Epilepsy. Rasumssen's Syndrome*. Toronto, Canada: Butterworth-Heinemann, 1991.

98. Desmond MM, Wilson GS, Melnick JL, et al. Congenital rubella encephalitis: Course and early sequelae. *J Pediatr* 1967;71:311–331.

99. Vinkin PJ, Bruyn GW, eds. *Infections of the Nervous System, Part 2. Neurology*. Vol. 34. Amsterdam, The Netherlands: North-Holland, 1978.

100. Dreyfus-Brisac C, Ellingson RJ. Hereditary, congenital and perinatal diseases. In: Remond A, ed-in-chief. *Handbook of Electroencephalography and Clinical Neurophysiology*. Vol. 15, Part B. Amsterdam, The Netherlands: Elsevier, 1972.

101. Klein C, Kimiagar I, Pollak L, et al. Neurological feature of West Nile virus infection during 2000 outbreak in a regional hospital in Israel. *J Neurol Sci* 2002;200:63–66.

102. Pachner AR, Steere AC. The triad of neurological manifestation of Lyme disease: Meningitis, cranial neuritis and radiculoneuritis. *Neurology (Minneap)* 1985;35:47–53.

103. Bernad PG. The neurological and electroencephalographic changes in AIDS. *Clin Electroencephalogr* 1991;22:65–70.

104. Gastaut H, Poirier F, Payan H, et al. HHE syndrome, hemiconvulsion, hemiplegia, epilepsy. *Epilepsia* 1959/1960;1:418–447.

105. Scott DF. *Understanding EEG: An Introduction to Electroencephalography*. London, UK: Gerald Duckworth, 1960.

106. LeBeau J, Dondey M. Importance diagnostique de certaines activites electroencephalographique lateralisees periodiques ou a tendance periodique au cours des abces du cerveau. *Electroencephalogr Clin Neurophysiol* 1959;11:43–58.

107. Brenner RP, Reynolds CF, Ulrich RF. Diagnostic efficacy of computerized spectral versus visual EEG analysis in elderly normal, demented and depressed subjects. *Electroencephalogr Clin Neurophysiol* 1988;169:110–117.

108. Primavera A, Traverso F. Triphasic waves in Alzheimer's disease. *Acta Neurol Belg* 1990;90:274–281.

109. Gordon EB, Sim M. The EEG in presenile dementia. *J Neuro Neurosurg Psychiatry* 1967;30:285–291.

110. Groen JJ, Endtz LJ. Hereditary Pick's disease: Second re-examination of the large family and discussion of other hereditary cases with particular reference to electroencephalography, a computerized tomography. *Brain* 1982;105:443–459.

111. Neufeld MY, Inzelberg R, Korczyn AD. EEG in demented and nondemented parkinsonian patients. *Acta Neurol Scand* 1988;78:1–5.

112. Su PC, Goldensohn ES. Progressive supranuclear palsy. Electroencephalographic studies. *Arch Neurol (Chicago)* 1973;29:183–186.

113. Calzetti S, Bortone E, Negrotti A, et al. Frontal intermittent rhythmic delta activity (FIRDA) in patients with dementia with Lewy bodies: A diagnostic tool? *Neurol Sci* 2002;23(Suppl.):S65–S66.

114. Crystal HA, Dickson DW, Lizardi JE, et al. Antemortem diagnosis of diffuse Lewy body disease. *Neurology (Minneap)* 1990;40:1523–1528.

115. Scott DF, Healthfield KWG, Toone B, et al. The EEG in Huntington's Chorea: A clinical and neuropathological study. *J Neurol Neurosurg Psychiatry* 1972;35:97–102.

116. Streletz LJ, Reyes PF, Zalewska M, et al. Computer analysis of EEG activity in dementia of the Alzheimer's type and Huntington's disease. *Neurobiol Aging* 1990;11:15–20.

117. Hashi K, Nishimura S, Kondo A, et al. The EEG in normal pressure hydrocephalus. *Acta Neurochir (Wien)* 1976;33:23–35.

118. Brenner RP, Reynolds CF, Ulrich RF. EEG findings in depressive pseudodementia and dementia with secondary depression. *Electroencephalogr Clin Neurophysiol* 1989;72:298–304.

119. Burger LJ, Rowan AJ, Goldensohn ES. Creutzfeldt–Jakob disease: An electroencephalographic study. *Arch Neurol (Chicago)* 1972;26:428–433.

120. Chiofano N, Fuentes A, Galvez S, et al. Serial EEG findings in 27 cases of Creutzfeldt–Jakob disease. *Arch Neurol (Chicago)* 1980;37:143–145.

121. Aoki Y, Lombroso CT. Prognostic value of electroencephalography in Reye's syndrome. *Neurology (Minneap)* 1973;23:333–343.

122. Yamada T, Tucker KP, Kooi KA. Fourteen and six c/sec positive bursts in comatose patients. *Electroencephalogr Clin Neurophysiol* 1976;40:645–653.

123. Westmoreland BF, Gomez MR, Blume WT. Activation of periodic complexes of subacute sclerosing panencephalitis by sleep. *Ann Neurol* 1977;1:185–187.

124. Silverman D. Some observations on the EEG in hepatic coma. *Electroencephalogr Clin Neurophysiol* 1962;14:53–59.

125. Gabuzda GJ. Ammonium metabolism and hepatic coma. *Gastroenterology* 1967;53:806–810.

126. Silverman D. Fourteen and six per second positive spike pattern in a patient with hepatic coma. *Electroencephalogr Clin Neurophysiol* 1964;16:395–398.

127. Yamada T, Young S, Kimura J. Significance of positive spike bursts in Reye's syndrome. *Arch Neurol* 1977;34:376–380.

128. Drury I. 14- and 6-positive bursts in childhood encephalopathies. *Electroencephalogr Clin Neurophysiol* 1989;72:479–485.

129. Jacob JC, Gloor P, Elawan OH, et al. Electroencephalographic changes in chronic renal failure. *Neurology (Minneap)* 1965;15:419–429.

130. Locke J, Merrill JP, Tyler HR. Neurologic complication of uremia. *Arch Intern Med* 1961;108:519–530.

131. Lederman RJ, Henry CE. Progressive dialysis encephalopathy. *Ann Neurol* 1978;4:199–204.

132. Gupta PC, Seth P. Periodic complexes in herpes simplex encephalitis: A clinical and experimental study. *Electroencephalogr Clin Neurophysiol* 1973;35:67–74.

133. Smith JB, Westmoreland BR, Reagan TJ, et al. A distinctive clinical EEG profile in herpes simplex encephalitis. *Mayo Clin Proc* 1975;50:469–474.

134. Mizrahi EM, Tharp BR. A characteristic EEG pattern in neonatal herpes simplex encephalitis. *Neurology (Minneap)* 1982;32:1215–1220.

135. Markand ON, Panzi JG. The electroencephalography in subacute sclerosing panencephalitis. *Arch Neurol (Chicago)* 1975;32:719–726.

136. Cobb W. The periodic events of subacute sclerosing leukoencephalitis. *Electroencephalogr Clin Neurophysiol* 1966;21:278–294.

137. Shibasaki H, Motomura S, Yamashita Y, Kuroiwa Y. Periodic synchronous discharges and myoclonus in Creutzfeldt–Jakob disease: Diagnostic application of jerk-locked averaging method. *Ann Neurol* 1981;9(2):150–156.

138. Lee RG, Blair RDG. Evolution of EEG and visual evoked response change in Jakob–Creutzfeldt disease. *Electroencephalogr Clin Neurophysiol* 1973;35:133–142.

139. Brown P, Cathala F, Castaigne P, et al. Creutzfeldt–Jakob disease: Clinical analysis of consecutive cases of 230 neuropathologically verified cases. *Ann Neurol* 1986;20:597–602.

140. Tietjen GE, Drury I. Familial Creutzfeldt–Jakob disease without periodic EEG activity. *Ann Neurol* 1990;28:585–588.

141. Watson CP. Clinical similarity of Alzheimer and Creutzfeldt–Jakob disease. *Ann Neurol* 1979;6:368–369.

142. Hormes JT, Benarroch EE, Rodriguez M, et al. Periodic sharp waves in baclofen-induced encephalopathy. *Arch Neurol (Chicago)* 1988;45:814–815.

143. Smith SJM, Kocen RS. A Creutzfeldt–Jakob like syndrome due to lithium toxicity. *J Neurol Neurosurg Psychiatry* 1988;51:120–123.

144. Neufeld MY. Periodic triphasic waves in levodopa-induced encephalopathy. *Neurology (Minneap)* 1992;42:444–446.

145. Nilsson BY, Olsson Y, Sourander P. Electroencephalographic and histopathological changes resembling Jakob–Creutzfeldt disease after transient cerebral ischemia due to cardiac arrest. *Acta Neurol Scand* 1972;48:416–426.

146. Brenner RP, Schaul N. Periodic EEG pattern: Classification clinical correlation and pathophysiology. *J Clin Neurophysiol* 1990;7:249–267.

147. Westmoreland BF, Sharbrough FW. The EEG in cerebromacular degeneration. *Electroencephalogr Clin Neurophysiol* 1978;45:28–29 (abstract).

148. Pinsard N, Livet MO, Saint-Jean M. A case of cerebral lipidosis with an atypical presentation. *Electroencephalogr Clin Neurophysiol* 1979;46:38 (abstract).

149. Liddell DW. Investigation of EEG findings in presenile dementia. *J Neurol Neurosurg Psychiatry* 1958;21:173–176.

150. Soininen H, Partanen VJ, Heilkala E-L, et al. EEG findings in senile dementia and normal aging. *Acta Neurol Scand* 1982;65:59–70.

151. Merskey H, Ball MJ, Blume WT, et al. Relationship between psychological measurements and cerebral organic changes in Alzheimer's disease. *Can J Neurol Sci* 1980;7:45–49.

152. Coben LA, Danziger WL, Berg L. Frequency analysis of the resting awake EEG in mild senile dementia of Alzheimer type. *Electroencephalogr Clin Neurophysiol* 1983;55:372–380.

153. Schreiter-Gasser U, Gasser T, Ziegler P. Quantitative EEG analysis in early onset Alzheimer's disease: Correlations with severity, clinical characteristics, visual EEG and CT. *Electroencephalogr Clin Neurophysiol* 1994;90:267–272.

154. Muller HF, Kral VA. The electroencephalogram in advanced senile dementia. *J Am Geriatr Soc* 1967;15:415–426.

155. Helkala E-L, Laulumaa V, Soininen H, et al. Different pattern of cognitive decline related to normal or deteriorating EEG in three year follow-up study with patients of Alzheimer's disease. *Neurology (Minneap)* 1991;41:528–532.

156. Lopez OL, Brenner RP, Becker JT, et al. EEG spectral abnormalities and psychosis as predictors of cognitive and functional decline in probable Alzheimer's disease. *Neurology* 1997;48:1521–1525.

157. Collerton D. Cholinergic function and intellectual decline in Alzheimer's disease. *Neuroscience* 1986;19:1–28.

158. Foster DB, Bagchi BK. Electroencephalographic observation in Huntington's chorea. *Electroencephalogr Clin Neurophysiol* 1949;1:247–248.

159. Sishta K, Troupe A, Marszalek KS, et al. Huntington's chorea: An electroencephalographic and psychometric study. *Electroencephalogr Clin Neurophysiol* 1973;36:387–393.

160. Oepen G, Doerr M, Thoden U. Visual (VEP) and somatosensory (SSEP) evoked potentials in Huntington's chorea. *Electroencephslogr Clin Neurophysiol* 1981;51:666–676.

161. Yamada T, Rodnitzky RL, Kameyama S, et al. Alteration of SEP topography in Huntington's patients and their relatives at risk. *Electroencephalogr Clin Neurophysiol* 1991;80:251–261.

162. England AC, Schwab RS, Peterson E. The electroencephalogram in Parkinson's syndrome. *Electroencephalogr Clin Neurophysiol* 1959;11:723–731.

163. Sirakov AA, Megan IS. EEG findings in Parkinsonism. *Electroencephalogr Clin Neurophysiol* 1963;15:321–322.

164. Goldenstein MA, Price BH. Non-Alzheimer dementias. In: Samuels MA, Feske SK, eds. *Office Practice on Neurology.* Philadelphia, PA: Churchill Livingston, 2003:873–886.

165. Green J, Haycool WM. Electroencephalographic changes in parkinsonian patients treated with levodopa and levodopa-amantadine in combination. *Clin Electroencephalogr* 1971;2:28–34.

166. Barber PA, Varma AR, Lloyd H, et al. The electroencephalogram in dementia with Lewy bodies. *Arch Neurol Scand* 2000;101:53–56.

167. Hachinski VC, Lassen NA, Marshall J. Multi-infarct dementia, a cause of mental deterioration in the elderly. *Lancet* 1974;2:207–210.

168. Bucht G, Adolfsson R, Winblad B. Dementia of the Alzheimer type and multi-infarct dementia. A clinical description and diagnostic problem. *J Am Geriatr Soc* 1984;32:491–498.

169. Sloan EP, Fenton GW. EEG power spectra and cognitive change in geriatric psychiatry: A longitudinal study. *Electroencephalogr Clin Neurophysiol* 1993;86:361–367.

170. Dalmau J, Gleichman AJ, Hughes EG, et al. Anti-NMDA-receptor encephalitis: Case series and analysis of the effects of antibodies. *Lancet Neurol* 2008;7:1091–1098.

171. Schmitt SE, Pargeon K, Frechette ES, et al. Extreme delta brush. A unique EEG pattern in adults with anti-NMDA receptor encephalitis. *Neurology* 2012;79(11):1094–1099.

172. Kirkpatrick MP, Clarke CD, Sonmezturk HH, et al. Rhythmic delta activity represents a form of nonconvulsive status epileptics in anti-NMDA receptor antibody encephalitis. *Epilepsy Behav* 2011;20:392–394.

173. Abbas A, Garg A, Jain R, et al. Extreme delta brushes and BIRDs in the EEG of anti-NMDA-receptor encephalitis. *Pract Neurol* 2016;16:326–327.

174. Abdullah S, Lim KS, Wong WF, et al. EEG is sensitive in early diagnosis of anti NMDAR encephalitis and useful in monitoring disease progress. *Neurology Asia* 2015;20(2):167–175.

175. Bazil CW, Pedley TA. General principles. Neurophysiological effects of anti-epileptic drugs. In: Levy RH, Mattson RH, Meldrum BS, et al., eds. *Antiepileptic Drugs.* 5th Ed. New York: Lippincott Williams & Wilkins, 2002:23–35.

176. Duncan JS. Antiepileptic drugs and the electroencephalogram. *Epilepsia* 1987;28:259–266.

177. Prichard JW. Barbiturates: Physiological effects I. In: Glasser GH, Perry JK, Woodbury DM, eds. *Antiepileptic Drugs: Mechanism of Action.* New York: Raven Press, 1980:505–522.

178. Sloan TB. Anesthetic effects on electrophysiologic recordings. *J Clin Neurophysiol* 1998;15:217–226.

179. Herkes GK, Lagerlund TD, Sharbrough FW, et al. Effects of antiepileptic drug treatment on the background frequency of EEG in epileptic patients. *J Clin Neurophysiol* 1993;10:210–216.

180. Roseman E. Dilantin toxicity: A clinical and electroencephalographic study. *Neurology (Minneap)* 1961;11:912–921.

181. Frost JD, Hrachovy RA, Glaze DG, et al. Alpha rhythm slowing during initiation of carbamazepine therapy. Implication for future cognitive performance. *J Clin Neurophysiol* 1995;12:57–63.

182. Rodin, EA, Rim CD, Rennick PM. The effects of carbamazepine in patients with psychomotor epilepsy: Results of double-blinded study. *Epilepsia* 1974;15:547–561.

183. Adam DJ, Luders H, Pippenger GH. Sodium valproate in the treatment of intractable seizure disorders: A clinical and electroencephalographic study. *Neurology (Minneap)* 1978;28:152–157.

184. Foletti G, Volanschi D. Influence of lamotrigine addition on computerized background EEG parameters in severe epileptogenic encephalopathies. *Eur Neurol* 1994;(Suppl. 1):S87–S89.

185. Mervaala E, Koivisto K, Hanninen T. Electrophysiological and neuropsychological profiles of lamotrigine in young and age-associated memory impairment (AAMI) subjects. *Neurology (Chicago)* 1995;46(Suppl. 4):S259.

186. Kalviainen R, Aikia M, Mervaala E, et al. Long-term cognitive and EEG effects of tiagabine in drug-resistant partial epilepsy. *Epilepsy Res* 1996;25:291–297.

187. Hammond EJ, Wilder BJ. Effects of gamma-vinyl-GABA on the human electroencephalogram. *Neuropharmacology* 1985;24:975–984.

188. Mervaala E, Partanen J, Nousiainen U, et al. Electrophysiologic effects of gamma-vinyl GABA and carbamazepine. *Epilepsy* 1989;30:189–193.

189. Saletu B, Grunberger J, Linzmayer L. Evaluation of encephalopathic and psychotropic properties of gabapentin in man by pharmaco-EEG and psychometry. *Int J Clin Pharmacol Toxicol* 1986;24:362–373.

190. Logothetis J. Spontaneous epileptic seizures and electroencephalographic changes in the course of phenothiazine therapy. *Neurology (Minneap)* 1967;17:869–877.

191. Itil TM. Convulsive and anticonvulsive properties of neuro-psycho-pharmaca. In: Niedermeyer E, ed. *Epilepsy. Modern Problem in Pharmacopsychiatry.* Vol. 4. Basel, Switzerland: Karger, 1970:270–305.

192. Cunningham Owens DG. Adverse effects of antipsychotic agents. *Drugs* 1996;51:895–930.

193. Neufeld MY, Rabey JM, Orlov E, et al. Electroencephalographic findings with low-dose clozapine treatment in psychotic Parkinsonian patients. *Clin Neuropharmacol* 1996;19:81–86.

194. Gunther W, Baghai T, Naber D, et al. EEG alterations and seizure during treatment with clozapine: A retrospective study of 283 patients. *Phamacopsychiatry* 1993;26:69–74.

195. Spatz R, Kugler J. Abnormal EEG activities induced by psychotropic drugs. *Electroencephalogr Clin Neurophysiol* 1982;36:549–558.

196. Small JG. EEG and lithium CNS toxicity. *Am J EEG Technol* 1986;26:225–239.

197. Fink M. EEG and human psychopharmacology. *Annu Rev Pharmacol* 1969;9:241–258.

198. Kurtz D. The EEG in acute and chronic drug intoxication. In: Glasser GH, ed. *Endocrine and Toxic Diseases/Handbook of Electroencephalography.* Vol. 15. Amsterdam, The Netherlands: Elsevier, 1976:88–104.

199. Bauer G, Bauer R. EEG, drug effects, and central nervous system poisoning. In: *Niedermeyer E*, Lopes da Silva FH, eds. *Electroencephalography: Basic Principle, Clinical Application and Related Fields.* 5th Ed. Baltimore, MD: Lippincott Williams & Wilkins, 2005:701–723.

200. Herning RI, Jones RT, Hooker WD, et al. Cocaine increases beta: A replication and extension of Hans Burger's historic experiments. *Electroencephalogr Clin Neurophysiol* 1985;69:470–477.

201. Brown BB. Subjective and EEG responses to LSD in visualizer and nonvisualizer subjects. *Electroencephalogr Clin Neurophysiol* 1968;25:372–379.

202. Volavka J, Dornbusch R, Feldstein S, et al. Effects of delta-9 tetrahydrocannabinol on EEG, heart rate, and mood. *Electroencephalogr Clin Neurophysiol* 1972;33:453 (abstract).

203. Fakhoury T, Abou-Khalil B, Blumenkopf B. EEG changes in intrathecal baclofen overdose: A case report and review of the literature. *EEG Clin Neurophysiol* 1998;107:339–342.

204. Kovnar E, Ward J. EEG manifestation of metabolic, toxic, degenerative and infectious disease. In: Holmes GL, Meske SL, eds. *Pediatric Clinical Neurophysiology.* Norwalk, CT: Appleton & Lange, 1992.

205. Pratt CB, Green AA, Horowitz ME, et al. Central nervous system toxicity following treatment of pediatric patients with ifosfamide mesna. *J Clin Oncol* 1986;4:1253–1261.

206. Land VL, Sutow WW, Fernbach DJ, et al. Toxicity of L-asparaginase in children with advanced leukemia. *Cancer* 1972;30:339–347.

207. Rubin AM, Kang H. Cerebral blindness and encephalopathy with cyclosporin A toxicity. *Neurology (Minneap)* 1987;37:1072–1076.

208. Audesirk G. Electrophysiology of lead intoxication: Effects on voltage sensitive ion channels. *Neurotoxicology* 1993;14:137–147.

209. Brenner RP, Snijder RD. Late EEG-findings and clinical status after organic mercury poisoning. *Arch Neurol* 1980;37:282–284.

210. Mellerio F, Kubicki S. Encephalopathy due to poisoning. In: Remond A, ed-in-chief. *Handbook of Electroencephalography and Clinical Neurophysiology.* Vol. 15A. Amsterdam, The Netherlands: Elsevier, 1977:108–135.

211. Alfrey AC, Le Gendre GR, Kachny WD. The dialysis encephalopathy syndrome. Possible aluminum intoxication. *N Engl J Med* 1976;294:184–188.

212. Leweke F, Damion MS, Kern A, et al. Zweizeitige Kohlen-monoxid-intoxication: Akinetisches Syndrom and Leukenzephalopathie. *Akt Neurol* 1999;26:86–90.

213. Okonek S, Rieger H. EEG Veranderungen bei Alkyl-phosphavegiftungen. *Z EEG–EMG* 1975;6:19–27, Elsevier 1963.

214. Young GB, Da Silva OP. Effect of morphine on the electroencephalograms of neonates: A prospective observational study. *Clin Neurophysiol* 2000;11:1955–1960.

215. Yarnell PR, Chu NS. Focal seizures and aminophylline. *Neurology (Minneap)* 1975;25:819–822.

216. Terman D, Teitebaum DT. Isoniazid self-poisoning. *Neurology (Minneap)* 1970;20:299–304.

217. Weinstein L. Penicillin and cephalosporins. In: Goodman LS, Gilman A, eds. *The Pharmacological Basis of Therapeutics.* New York: Macmillan, 1975:1130–1166.

218. Itil MT, Soldatos C. Epileptogenic effects of psychotropic drugs: Practical recommendation. *JAMA* 1980;244:1460–1463.

219. Gunther W, Baghai T, Naber D, et al. EEG alteration and seizures during treatment with clozapine: A retrospective study of 283 patients. *Pharmacopsychiatry* 1993;26:69–74.

220. Malow BA, Reese KB, Sato S, et al. Spectrum of EEG abnormalities during clozapine treatment. *Electroencephalogr Clin Neurophysiol* 1994;91:205–211.

221. Freudenreich O, Weinter RD, McEvoy JP. Clozapine-induced electroencephalogram changes as a function of clozapine serum levels. *Biol Psychiatry* 1997;42:132–137.

222. Helmchen H, Kanowshi S. EEG changes under lithium (Li) treatment. *Electroencephalogr Clin Neurophysiol* 1971;30:269 (abstract).

223. Smith JG. EEG and lithium CNS toxicity. *Am J EEG Technol* 1986;26:225–239.

224. Gotman J, Gloor P, Quesney LF, et al. Correlations between EEG changes induced by diazepam and localization of epileptic spikes and seizures. *Electroencephalogr Clin Neurophysiol* 1982;54:614–621.

225. Thomas P, Lebrun C, Chatel M. De novo absence status epilepticus as a benzodiazepine withdrawal syndrome. *Epilepsia* 1993;34:355–358.

226. Essig CF, Frasen HF. Electroencephalographic changes in man during use and withdrawal of barbiturates in moderate dose. *Electroencephalogr Clin Neurophysiol* 1958;10:649–656.

227. Wikler A, Essig CF. Withdrawal seizures following chronic intoxication with barbiturates and other sedative drugs. In: Niedermeyer E, ed. *Epilepsy, Modern Problems in Pharmacopsychiatry.* Vol. 4. Basel, Switzerland: Karger, 1970:185–199.

228. Fink M. EEG classification of psychoactive compounds in man: A review and theory of behavioral associations. In: Effron DH, ed. *Psychopharmacology: A Review of Progress 1957–1967. US Public Health Service Publication No. 1836.* Washington, DC: U.S. Government Printing Office, 1968:497–507.

229. Salinsky MC, Oken BS, Storzbach D, et al. Assessment of CNS effects of antiepileptic drugs by using quantitative EEG measures. *Epilepsia* 2003;44:1042–1050.

230. Adams DJ, Luders H, Pippenger CH. Sodium valproate in the treatment of intractable seizure disorders: A clinical and electroencephalographic study. *Neurology (Minneap)* 1978;28:152–157.

231. Harding GFA, Herrick CE, Jeavons PM. A controlled study of the effect of sodium valproate on photosensitive epilepsy and its prognosis. *Epilepsia* 1978;19:555–565.

232. Pyre-Phillips WEM, Jeavons PM. Effects of carbamazepine (Tegretol) on the electroencephalograph and ward behavior of patients with chronic epilepsy. *Epilepsia* 1970;11:236–273.

233. Sirven JI, Waterhouse E. Management of status epileptics. *Am Fam Physician* 2003;68(3):469–476.

234. Ehlers CL, Wall TL, Schuckit MA. EEG spectral characteristics following ethanol administration in young men. *Electroencephalogr Clin Neurophysiol* 1989;73:179–187.

235. Krauss GL, Niedermeyer E. Electroencephalogram and seizures in chronic alcoholism. *Electroencephalogr Clin Neurophysiol* 1991;78:97–104.

236. Niedermeyer E, Freund G, Krumholtz A. Subacute encephalopathy with seizures in alcoholics: A clinical electroencephalographic study. *Clin Electroencephalogr* 1981;12:113–129.

237. Mani J, Sitajayalakshmi S, Borgohain R, et al. Subacute encephalopathy with seizures in alcoholism. *Seizure* 2003;12:126–129.

238. Wang B, Bai Q, Jiao X, et al. Effect of sedative and hypnotic doses of propofol on the EEG activity of patients with or without history of seizure disorder. *J Neurosurg Anesthesiol* 1997;9:335–340.

239. Stecker MM, Kramer TH, Raps EC, et al. Treatment of refractory status epilepticus with propofol: Clinical and pharmacokinetic findings. *Epilepsia* 1998;39:18–26.

240. Mahla ME. Anesthetic effects on the electroencephalogram. *Neurol Sci Monitor* 1992;3:2–7.

241. Kearse LA Jr, Koski G, Husain MV, et al. Epileptiform activity during opioid anesthesia. *Electroencephalogr Clin Neurophysiol* 1993;87:374–379.

242. Stone JL, Ghaly RF, Hughes JR. Electroencephalography in acute head injury. *J Clin Neurophysiol* 1988;5:125–133.

243. Synek VM. Value of a revised EEG coma scale for prognosis after cerebral anoxia and diffuse head injury. *Clin Electroencephalogr* 1990;21:25–30.

244. Jabbari B, Vengrow MI, Salazar AM, et al. Clinical and radiological correlates of EEG in the late phase of head injury: A study of 515 Vietnam veterans. *Electroencephalogr Clin Neurophysiol* 1986;64:285–293.

245. Koufen H, Hagel KH. Systematic EEG follow-up study of traumatic psychosis. *Eur Arch Psychiatr Neurol Sci* 1987;237:2–7.

246. Scherzer E. Wert der Elektroenzephalographie beims Schadeltrauma. *Wien Klin Wschr* 1965;77:543–547.

247. Stockard JJ, Bickford RG, Aung MH. The electroencephalogram in traumatic brain injury. In: Vinken PJ, Bruyn GW, eds. *Handbook of Clinical Neurology.* Vol. 23. Amsterdam/Oxford: North-Holland, 1975:217–367.

248. Lenard HG. EEG-Veranderungen bee frischen Schadeltraumen im Kindesalter. *Med Wschr* 1965;107:1820–1827.

249. Kelly JP, Rosenberg JH. Diagnosis and management of concussion in sports. *Neurology (Minneap)* 1997;48:575–580.

250. Courjon J, Naquet R, Baurand C, et al. Valeur diagnostique de l'EEG dans les suites immediates des traumatismes craniens. *Rev EEG Neurophysiol* 1971;1:133–150.

251. Bricolo A, Turazzi S, Faccioli F, et al. Clinical application of compressed spectral array in long-term EEG monitoring of comatose patients. *Electroencephalogr Clin Neurophysiol* 1978;45:211–225.

252. Courjon J, Scherzer E. Traumatic disorders. In: Remmond A, Magnus O, Courjon J, eds. *Handbook of Electroencephalography and Clinical Neurophysiology.* Vol. 14. Amsterdam, The Netherlands: Elsevier, 1972:8–95.

253. Jennett WB. Early traumatic epilepsy. *Lancet* 1969;1:1023–1025.

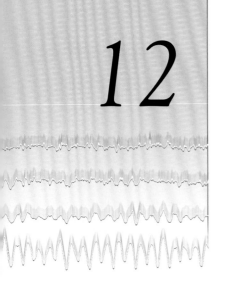

Focal EEG Abnormalities

THORU YAMADA and ELIZABETH MENG

General Characteristics of Focal EEG Abnormalities

Focal EEG abnormalities were first described in 1936 by Gray Walter in brain tumor patients.[1] The abnormalities were characterized by localized slow waves, which he termed "delta waves." Since then, EEG has served as an important, noninvasive diagnostic tool for localized cerebral lesions. However, this has changed with the advent of computerized tomography (CT) and magnetic resonance imaging (MRI) as these studies proved to be more accurate in the anatomical localization of lesions. However, EEG has remained an important tool for *functional assessment* of localized cerebral lesions. The potential for improved anatomical/spatial accuracy of EEG lies with the use of computerized quantitative methods. Although positron emission tomography (PET) scan and functional MRI can reveal functional alterations of the brain, EEG is superior in its temporal resolution. For example, focal cerebral dysfunction can be revealed almost instantaneously after the clamping of a carotid artery during endarterectomy surgery if the hemisphere on the side of clamped carotid artery encounters a risk of ischemia (see Video 11-1). Poor spatial resolution of scalp-recorded EEG is in part due to the distortion by volume conductors that lie between the cortex and scalp, that is, CSF (cerebrospinal fluid), dura, skull, and scalp. By the time the electrical activity reaches the scalp, the current is attenuated and distorted. Combining computerized EEG data and MRI will provide more accurate anatomical localization. The more accurate anatomical assessment of electrical source of interest from the brain can be made by MEG (magnetoencephalography). Focal EEGs are represented by the following findings:

1. Focal/unilateral amplitude depression or slowing of basic background activity (alpha, beta waves) without an increase in theta–delta slow waves (Fig. 12-1)
2. Focal/unilateral amplitude depression or slowing of basic background activity associated with an increase in theta–delta slow waves (Fig. 12-2)
3. Focal/unilateral theta–delta slow waves with preserved basic background activity (Fig. 12-3)
4. Focal/unilateral enhancement of basic background activity with or without associated slow waves (Fig. 12-4)
5. Focal/unilateral epileptiform activity with or without associated slow waves (Fig. 12-5)

ALTERATION OF BACKGROUND ACTIVITY

EEG recorded directly from the surface of a brain tumor shows no EEG activity. Slow waves appear some distance from the tumor location. Recorded from the scalp, depression, slowing, and disruption of the background rhythm are common findings near a lesion. In evaluating focal abnormalities, the EEG should be examined for symmetry of amplitude and frequency, continuity, and reactivity of the background activity between homologous areas. An amplitude asymmetry alone, without frequency asymmetry, should be treated cautiously as technical errors (i.e., unequal interelectrode distances between homologous electrode pairs or cancelation effect due to equipotential distribution between two electrodes) must be considered (see "Technical Pitfalls and Errors," Chapter 15; see also Figs. 15-47 and 15-48). The destructive lesions or lesions involving cortex and white matter tend to show attenuated background activity associated with delta activity (see Fig. 12-2). Slowed background rhythm with preservation of amplitude tends to occur in chronic lesions (see Fig. 12-3). Slowing of the alpha rhythm may occur in lesions not necessarily involving the occipital lobe. Slowing of background rhythm often accompanies theta–delta waves, disrupting normal continuity of background rhythm. Focal delta slow waves in a preserved background activity may be seen in subcortical lesions.

Focal or unilateral depression of beta rhythm, either intrinsic or drug induced, is also an important parameter in interpretation of a focal abnormality (Fig. 12-6). Beta depression is a sensitive indicator for cerebral ischemia. Beta depression may also be seen in the region of an epileptic focus. In sleep, unilateral depression of sleep spindles, vertex sharp waves, or other sleep patterns may be present on the side of a lesion (Figs. 12-7A and B and 12-8A and B). When EEG shows bilateral slowing, the side of slower frequency and/or decreased background activity is the worse hemisphere irrespective of amplitude asymmetry (Fig. 12-9).

Although amplitude depression and paucity of background activity are common findings of focal abnormality, higher-than-normal alpha rhythm amplitude on the side of a lesion may be seen in some cases, especially in slowly progressive or chronic lesions (Fig. 12-10A and B). Similarly, beta rhythm, mu rhythm, or sleep spindles may be augmented ipsilateral to the side of a lesion (Fig. 12-11).[2–6] Both ends of the spectrum, either depression or accentuation of sleep spindles, have been reported in

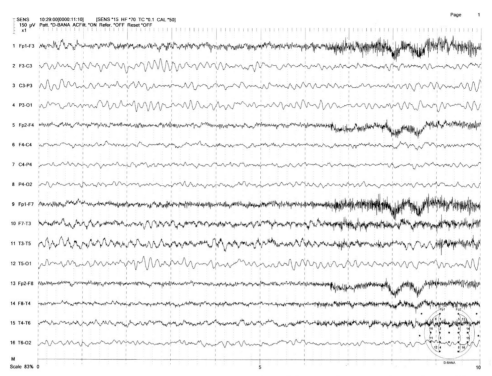

FIGURE 12-1 | A 6-year-old boy with a history of focal seizures involving left arm. There was depression and intermittent slowing of alpha rhythm over the right hemisphere but without significant focal delta–theta slow.

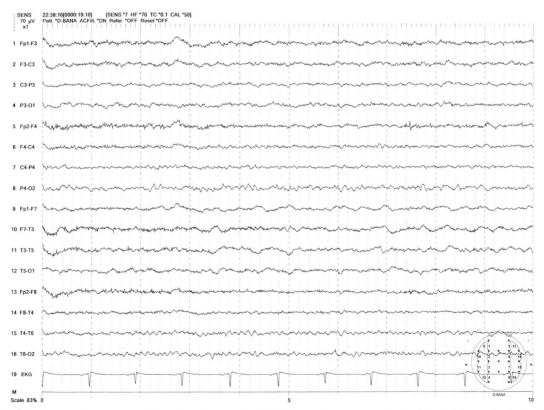

FIGURE 12-2 | A 62-year-old woman with acute aphasia and right-sided weakness secondary to left middle cerebral artery infarct. EEG showed decreased background activity along with more or less continuous polymorphic delta activity over the left hemisphere, while EEG on the right side is entirely normal.

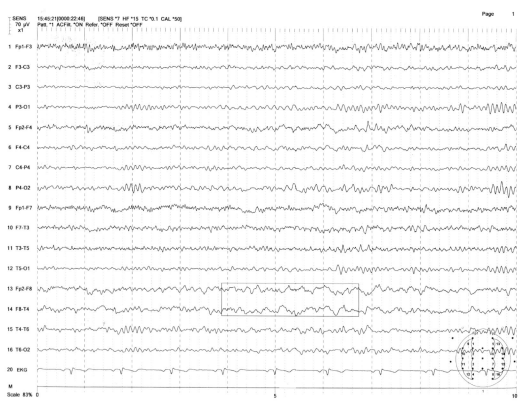

FIGURE 12-3 | A 27-year-old woman with a history of partial complex seizures secondary to arachnoid cystic lesion in right frontal lobe. Note polymorphic delta from right anterior temporal region, but with preserved symmetric background alpha rhythm. A portion of this example is shown in the *box*.

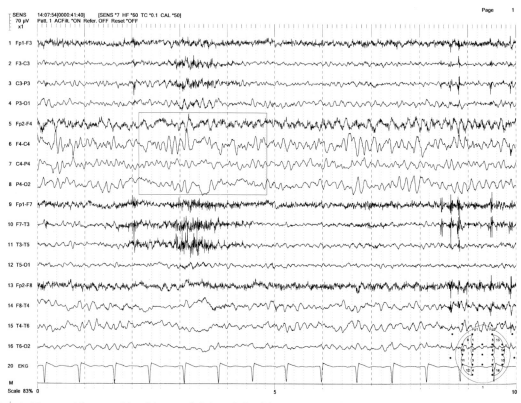

FIGURE 12-4 | A 49-year-old man with a history of right subdural hematoma and status post craniotomy on the right. EEG showed increased amplitude of background activity as well as underlying polymorphic delta slow waves over the right hemisphere. Increased background amplitude over the right is likely secondary to skull defect. A portion of this example is shown in the *box*.

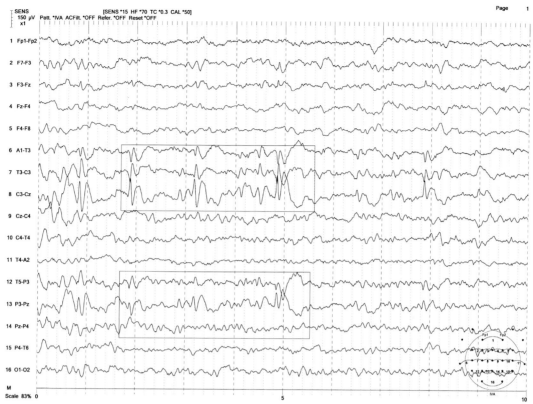

FIGURE 12-5 | A 6-year-old boy with a history of focal seizure with secondary generalization. Note spike maximum at C3 or P3 electrode along with irregular delta activity from left hemisphere (shown in *boxes*).

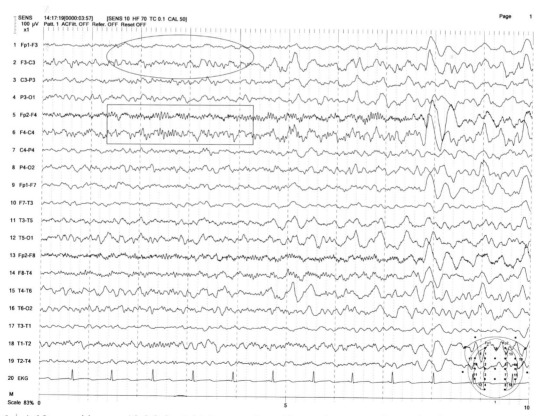

FIGURE 12-6 | A 19-year-old man with left frontal intraparenchymal hemorrhage secondary to head trauma. EEG showed bilaterally diffuse and bifrontal dominant delta–theta activity. There was consistent depression of beta activity over the left frontal region and this was the only lateralizing EEG finding (compare the channels shown by the *box* and *oval circle*).

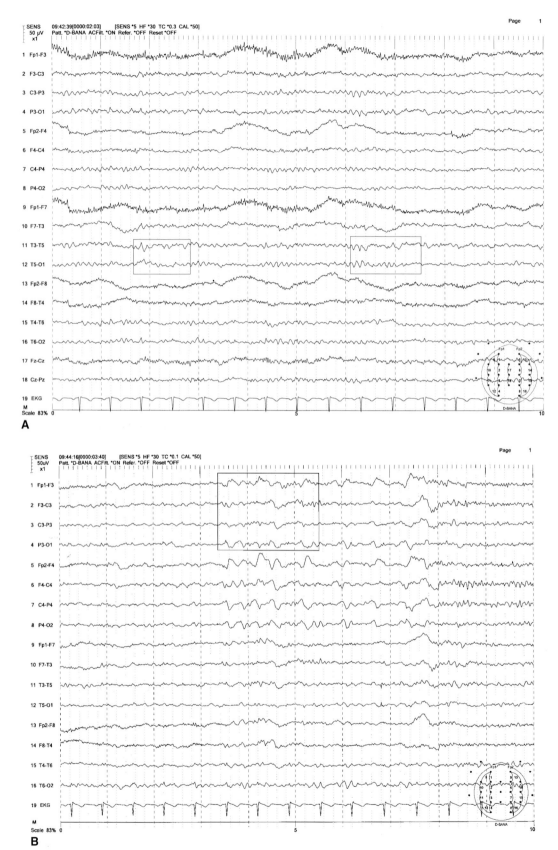

FIGURE 12-7 | A 47-year-old woman with a left chronic subdural hematoma. EEG showed only minimal slowing on left side (shown by *rectangular boxes*) **(A),** but sleep record showed consistent depression of V wave (shown by *rectangular box*) over the left hemisphere **(B).**

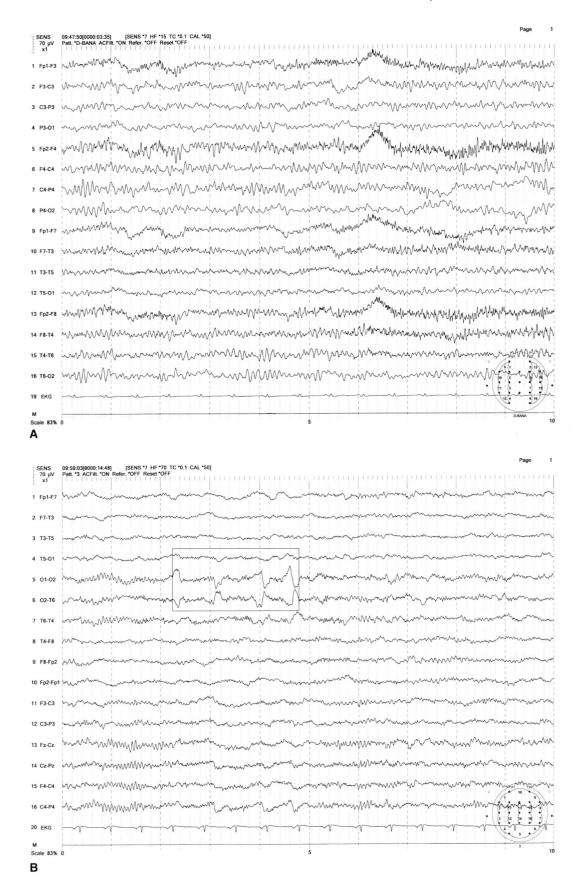

FIGURE 12-8 | A 46-year-old man with partial complex seizures secondary to left frontoparietal infarct 13 years ago. Awake EEG showed only decreased amplitude of background activity **(A)**. Sleep record showed consistent depression of sleep spindles and POSTs (shown by *rectangular box*) **(B)**.

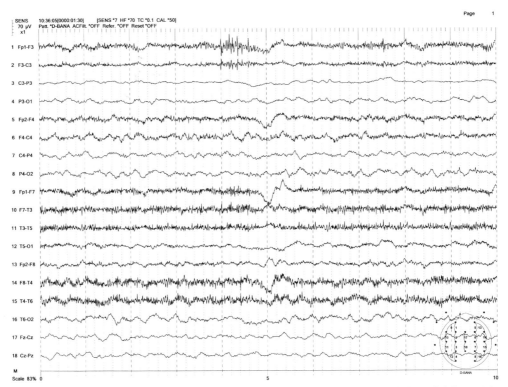

FIGURE 12-9 | A 6-year-old boy with developmental delay and right hemiparesis. EEG showed bilateral delta activity with slower and lower amplitude delta over the left hemisphere, indicating that left hemisphere is worse than right.

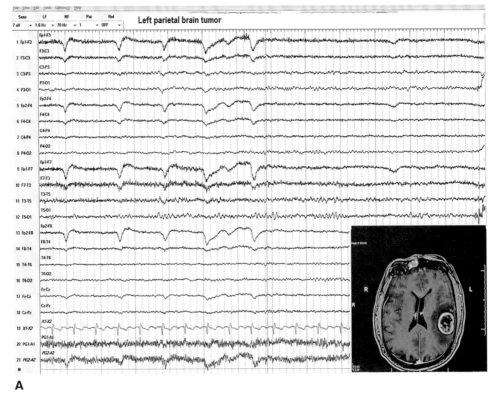

A

FIGURE 12-10 | Patient was a 60-year-old man presenting with sudden onset of slurred speech and right facial droop. MRI showed large parietal mass lesion with small hemorrhagic extending from posterior periventricular region **(A)**. EEG in awake showed left>right alpha rhythm without significant slow waves **(A)**. In sleep, there were irregular delta slow waves focused at left posterior head region **(B**, shown by *rectangular box*). This case illustrates very unusual EEG features showing enhanced alpha on the side of lesion (in common sense, right side should be considered abnormal side). Sleep record, however, showed delta slow waves in left posterior quadrant corresponding to the site of legion **(B).** This is also unusual since focal slow waves are usually more clear in awake than in sleep record (see Fig. 12-14). (This patient did not have skull defect or craniotomy at the time of this EEG recording.)

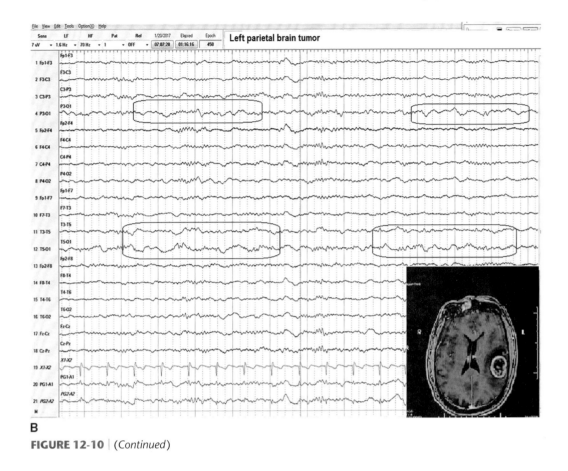

B

FIGURE 12-10 | (*Continued*)

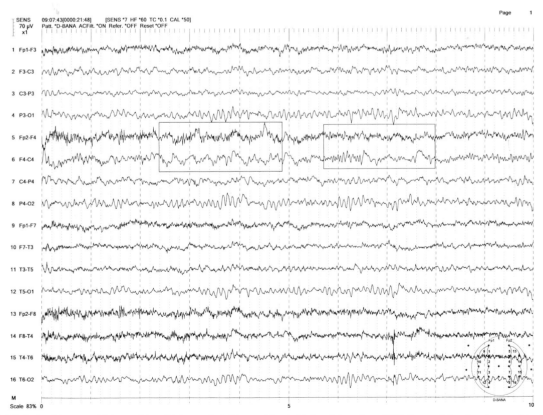

FIGURE 12-11 | An 11-year-old boy with a history of stable cyst in right frontal region. EEG showed focal polymorphic delta in right frontal region. Note increased beta activity in the same region (shown in *boxes*). There was no skull defect in this patient.

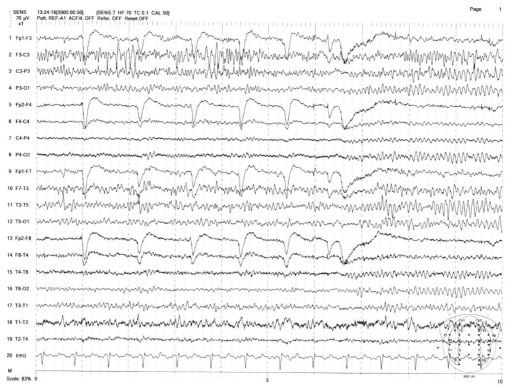

FIGURE 12-12 | A 26-year-old man with a history of closed head injury and left epidural hematoma, and status post craniotomy 6 months prior to the EEG. Note increased beta and "spiky" alpha and enhanced mu rhythm over the left central and midtemporal region (breach rhythm).

patients with Sturge–Weber syndrome (Fig. 12-12).[5] Similarly, marked attenuation or accentuation of beta rhythm has been reported on the side of a porencephalic cyst.[7]

Skull defect or burr hole secondary to craniotomy or head injury causes local enhancement of underlying EEG activity, especially beta rhythm. The focal amplitude accentuation secondary to skull defect is referred to as "breach rhythm" and is usually discreetly localized to one or two electrodes near the skull defect or burr hole site (Fig. 12-13; see also Fig. 7-20). This beta enhancement may result in a "spiky"-appearing activity, which includes "spike-like" or "sharp-like" transients. In fact, these are often difficult to differentiate from true spike or sharp discharges. If the "spiky" discharge is disproportionately larger or wider spread than the breach rhythm, it is likely true spike.

FOCAL DELTA ACTIVITY

Delta activity can be divided into two types by morphological characteristics, one is *arrhythmic* (*polymorphic*) and the other is *rhythmic* (*monomorphic or monorhythmic*). Arrhythmic delta activity (*ADA*) consists of serial waves of irregular shape with variable duration and amplitude, which occur continuously or intermittently. ADA reacts little to eye opening or alerting stimuli. Focal ADA is usually most evident in the awake state and becomes less distinct in non-REM sleep (Fig. 12-14A and B).

Focal ADA usually indicates a lesion involving subcortical white matter. Greater irregularity in waveforms, slower frequency, greater persistence, and less amount of superimposed or intermixed fast activity generally indicate a more severe and acute lesion. In determining the most affected area, the same rule applies. The region of slower frequency and lower amplitude

delta activity is more severely affected (see Fig. 12-9). Faster and higher amplitude delta, often mixed with alpha or theta, is more common at a distance further from the lesion.

Continuous ADA, especially when associated with loss of background activity, correlates highly with acute or rapidly progressive destructive lesions (see Fig. 12-2). Intermittent or less continuous ADA intermingled with theta or alpha background activity may be a sign of a chronic lesion or may occur during the recovery process of focal damage (see Fig. 12-3).

In contrast to the irregularly formed ADA, *intermittent rhythmic delta activity* (*IRDA*) or RDA* has a rhythmic sinusoidal waveform occurring as bursts or paroxysms. Classically, IRDA/RDA* was thought to represent a projected rhythm, thus correlating with deep midline lesions such as tumors in the thalamus, hypothalamus, or brainstem. IRDA/RDA* is now recognized to occur more commonly in toxic/metabolic encephalopathy than in focal intrinsic brain lesions. IRDA/RDA* has two characteristic distributions, one is frontally predominant RDA*/(*FIRDA*) and the other is occipitally predominant RDA (*OIRDA*). FIRDA/frontally predominant RDA* is usually seen in adult patients (see Fig. 6-3; see also Fig. 8-14), whereas OIRDA/ occipitally predominant RDA* occurs more commonly in children (see Fig. 8-15, see also Video 10-6).

Although IRDA is more common in metabolic, toxic, encephalopathy, it can occur in infratentorial lesions and is usually bilaterally symmetrical or shows shifting asymmetries. With supratentorial lesions, IRDA may be asymmetric, usually with greater amplitude on the side of the lesion.[8,9]

Unlike ADA which is resistant to reactivity, IRDA/RDA* tends to be augmented by eyes closing or hyperventilation and is attenuated by alerting stimuli.

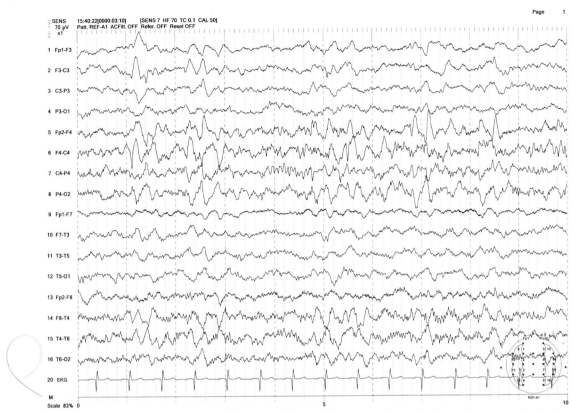

FIGURE 12-13 | A 5-year-old boy with diagnosis of Sturge–Weber syndrome and history of seizures. MRI showed atrophy of left frontal, parietal, and occipital lobes, enlarged left lateral ventricle, and left frontal calcification. This sleep EEG showed consistent depression of sleep spindles, V waves, and beta activity over the left hemisphere.

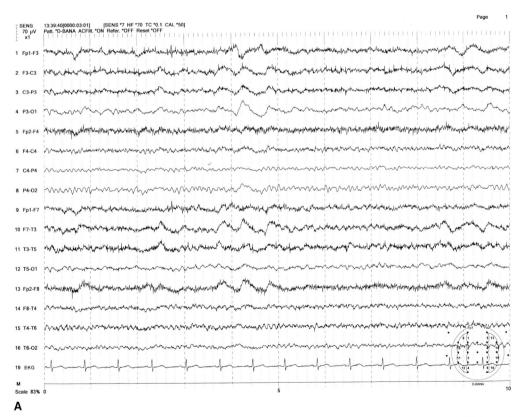

A

FIGURE 12-14 | A 44-year-old woman with right spastic hemiparesis secondary to head injury 11 years ago. MRI showed encephalomalacia on left temporal lobe and enlarged left lateral ventricle. EEG in awake state showed intermittent delta waves and decreased alpha rhythm over the left hemisphere **(A)**. In sleep, delta waves appear bilaterally and focal delta activity noted in awake state becomes unclear **(B)**.

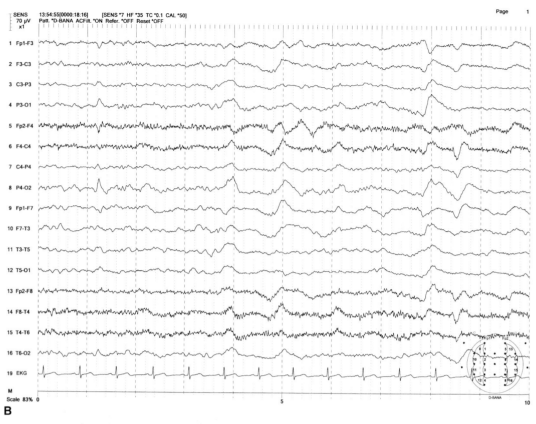

FIGURE 12-14 | (*Continued*)

FOCAL EPILEPTIFORM ACTIVITY

Focal or lateralized IRDA (LRDA*) implies potential seizure activity rather than focal structural lesion (see Chapter 10, section "Indication for CCEEG." See also Fig. 13-2A and B, Video 13-4).

FOCAL EPILEPTIFORM ACTIVITY

Cortical scarring following a cortical insult can give rise to epileptiform activity. Therefore, spike or spike-wave discharges occur more commonly in slowly progressive or static lesions than in rapidly destructive lesions. Epileptiform activity is seen in about 10% to 20% of patients with cerebral tumors. It is more common in low-grade tumors (i.e., astrocytoma) than in rapidly growing tumors (i.e., glioblastoma).[10] By the same token, the occurrence of focal spike activity is rare in acute and localized cerebrovascular accidents (CVAs), either infarction or hemorrhage. Focal spikes tend to appear in months or years after a CVA. When epileptiform activity appears in CVA, it commonly occurs in massive hemorrhage or infarction and EEG usually takes the form of PLEDs (*periodic lateralized epileptiform activity or LPD**) (see "Periodic Lateralized Epileptiform Discharges," Chapter 10; see also Figs. 10-38 to 10-41). PLEDs/LPD*'s are usually seen in patients with impaired consciousness, secondary to a massive and acute hemispheric lesion (infarction, anoxic cerebral insult, brain abscess, acute exacerbation of a glioblastoma, or herpes simplex encephalitis). These PLEDs/LPDs* could be asynchronous within the same hemisphere, either totally independent from each other (see Fig. 10-41A) or the discharges on one lobe could be time locked and lead the discharges on another lobe (see Fig. 10-41B, see also Video 13-2A and B). Of these, herpes encephalitis and

acute cerebral infarct are the most common etiologies. PLEDs / LPD* seen in an acute infarction are usually self-limited and tend to disappear within 1 to 2 weeks after the illness. LPD* in herpes encephalitis may evolve to BiPLEDs or BIPD* (bilateral independent periodic discharge) (see Fig. 10-42A and B).

LOCALIZATION VALUES

As stated earlier in this chapter, EEG is relatively poor in determining the accurate location of a lesion. The localization is at best left/right and anterior/posterior quadrant. False localization is not uncommon (Fig. 12-15). For example, lesions situated in the frontal lobe, parietal lobe, or even in the thalamus may show focal EEG abnormalities in the temporal region. Other false-positive findings commonly seen in the temporal lobes are focal EEG patterns without focal pathology, such as temporal slow waves of the elderly or wicket spikes. Conversely, EEG is highly sensitive for lesions in temporal lobe. EEG abnormalities may well precede CT or MRI findings in detecting brain tumors growing in the temporal lobe. Occipital lesions also show a high incidence of abnormalities with focal ADA and suppression or slowing of alpha rhythm.[11] In contrast, false-negative findings are relatively common for lesions involving the parietal lobe. EEG changes are often minimal, if any, in these lesions. However, focal abnormalities in the parietal lobe, especially with altered background activity, have a relatively high localizing value (Fig. 12-16). Frontal lobe lesions may show ADA over the frontal or temporal region. The frontally predominant RDA/FIRDA may be seen in frontal lobe lesions and may appear as bilateral, ipsilateral, or, less often, contralateral in its distribution.

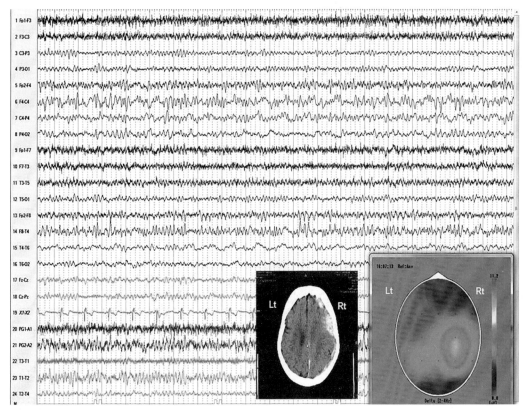

FIGURE 12-15 | A 35-year-old man with brain tumor at right frontal region extending to parietal region as shown in MRI scan (the left/right was intentionally reversed in order to match with EEG topography). There were delta slow waves in right hemisphere, maximum at parietal region, as shown by delta frequency topography. The localization was not quite accurate as shown by MRI localization.

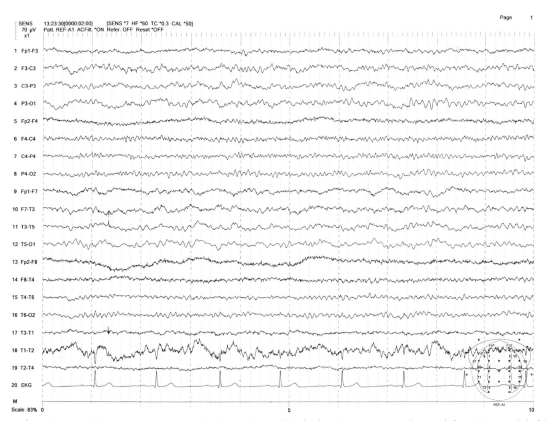

FIGURE 12-16 | A 74-year-old man presenting with dyscalculia and right hemiparesis secondary to left parieto-occipital infarct. EEG showed irregular delta activity from entire left hemisphere, maximum at parietal electrode indicated by phase reversal at P3 in parasagittal electrodes chain.

In deep, midline lesions such as tumors involving the basal forebrain or diencephalic structures, the incidence of EEG abnormality is less (at least 25% of patients have normal EEG) with less reliable localizing signs as compared to hemispheric lesions.[12,13] FIRDA/frontally predominant RDA* is the most frequent abnormality in these deep, midline lesions.

Subtentorial lesions involving the third ventricle or posterior fossa usually show a normal EEG. EEG becomes abnormal (characterized by frontally predominant or occipitally predominant RDA*, FIRDA, or OIRDA) only when increased intracranial pressure develops.[12,13] OIRDA, the occipitally predominant RDA* is more common in children.

DIAGNOSTIC SPECIFICITY OF FOCAL EEG ABNORMALITIES

Focal EEG abnormalities are rarely specific for diagnosing underlying focal pathologies. However, diagnostic probabilities are enhanced when clinical contexts are taken into account for interpreting EEG results. This applies even to normal EEG. For example, a normal EEG in awake patients with profound motor/sensory deficit rules out an extensive cortical lesion but points to a small deep or midline lesion such as a lacunar or capsular infarction. Similarly, disparity between extensive neurological deficits and minimal EEG changes may be seen in a brainstem lesion, for example, in a patient who is awake but mute and tetraplegic secondary to an infarction of bilateral ventral pons sparing the tegmentum (*locked-in syndrome*). The EEG in locked-in syndrome is usually normal with alpha rhythm that is reactive to various stimulations.[14] With bilateral

pontine lesions involving the tegmentum, the patient is in a deep comatose state, and EEG may show "alpha coma pattern" with posterior dominant normal alpha distribution,[15] in contrast to diffuse and anterior dominant alpha seen in postanoxic state (see Figs. 11-13 and 11-14A–D). It is usually not possible to differentiate between CVA and brain tumor based on focal EEG abnormalities. However, the presence of a well-defined focal spike lowers the possibility of acute stroke since focal spikes are more common in chronic lesions. If focal delta activity appears in the frontal or frontotemporal region, the probability of CVA is high since the middle cerebral artery (which is the most commonly affected artery in stroke) covers the frontal and temporal lobe territory (Fig. 12-17).

Focal EEG abnormalities associated with evidence of CSF pleocytosis suggest brain abscess or herpes simplex encephalitis. High-amplitude and exceedingly slow (<1 Hz) ADA often characterize brain abscess,[16] while PLEDs/LPD* are more characteristic for herpes simplex encephalitis.

Focal EEG with Focal Cerebral Disease

BRAIN TUMORS

The incidence and degree of abnormal EEG in detecting brain tumors varies depending on the size, location, and degree of malignancy of the tumor. Fast-growing and malignant tumors such as glioblastomas show greater and earlier EEG changes than slow-growing and benign tumors such as grade I

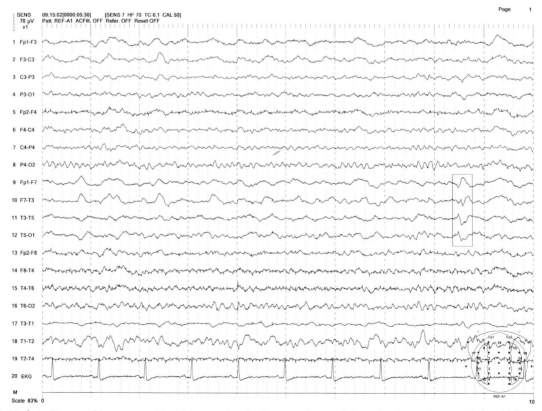

FIGURE 12-17 | A 67-year-old woman with a history of aphasia secondary to infarct in the territory of left middle cerebral artery 7 months prior to this EEG. Note polymorphic delta activity over the left hemisphere with emphasis to frontotemporal region and decreased alpha rhythm over the left occipital region. Also note a sharp transient at left temporal region (shown by *rectangular box*).

astrocytomas or meningiomas. Supratentorial tumors or tumors localized to the lateral convexity tend to show EEG abnormalities in the early stage, whereas EEG is relatively insensitive for deep-seated or midline tumors.

EEG is most sensitive in detecting abnormalities in temporal lobe tumors, especially anterior temporal lobe, showing polymorphic delta activity in the temporal electrodes. Frontal lobe tumors tend to cause high-amplitude delta activity in the corresponding frontal regions, often appearing as RDA*. Occipital tumors also show a high incidence of EEG abnormalities with focal slow waves at the occipital, parietal, and posterior temporal regions, often associated with decreased or slower alpha rhythms as compared to the intact side. EEG is least sensitive for parietal lobe tumors such as parasagittal meningiomas.[17] The abnormality may be focal depression of beta activity and/or focal spikes without polymorphic delta activity. Deep-seated tumors involving lateral and third ventricles, thalamus, hypothalamus, and basal ganglia tend to show bilateral abnormalities, often in the form of FIRDA or frontally predominant RDA/FIRDA or asymmetric LRDA. EEG is notoriously poor in detecting posterior fossa (infratentorial) tumors. If the EEG is abnormal, it may show bilateral delta activity as a form of OIRDA/occipitally predominant RDA, especially in children.[12]

The overall incidence of abnormal EEGs for supratentorial tumors is greater than 90%, but at least one fourth of EEGs are normal for deep midline, basal, and infratentorial tumors.[12,13]

Location of EEG abnormalities tends to be more widespread, perhaps reflecting functional disturbances rather than actual anatomical size. Further, it is well recognized that EEG abnormalities often localize to the temporal region irrespective of the tumor location.[18]

CEREBROVASCULAR ACCIDENTS

Subarachnoid Hemorrhage

EEG in acute subarachnoid hemorrhage is usually normal, especially if the patient's consciousness is not impaired. Along with clouding consciousness, EEG becomes abnormal with bilateral delta–theta activity. A focal abnormality suggests a complication such as a parenchymal hemorrhage or vasospasm causing ischemia.[19] Continuous EEG recording is usually requested in order to detect ischemic EEG changes so that appropriate treatment is initiated to prevent ischemic stroke (see "Indication of CCEEG" Chapter 13; see also Fig.13-8A–D).

Transient Ischemia Attacks

Most patients with transient ischemia attack (TIA) have normal EEGs. EEG recorded during or soon after a TIA may show relatively minor focal theta slowing.[20,21] Prominent ipsilateral focal delta activity is unlikely to be a sign of TIA.[22]

Ischemic Stroke

The degree of EEG abnormalities varies depending on the location and extent of ischemic lesions. Since ischemic stroke occurs most commonly in the territory of the internal carotid or the middle cerebral artery, EEG abnormality is often focused in the anterior and middle temporal regions and, to a less extent, in the frontal region. The EEG shows polymorphic delta activity with or without attenuation or slowing of background activity (see Figs. 12-16 and 12-17). Preservation of background activity is a favorable prognostic sign.[23] During the period of recovery, a progressive decrease of slow activity and recovery of background activity parallel the clinical improvement.

Large infarctions accompanied by cerebral edema and mass effect may lead to PLEDs /LPD* with or without clinical seizure. PLEDs/LPD* usually represent an acute cerebral insult and disappear in 2 to 3 weeks. Clinical seizures and epileptiform EEG activity (spikes and sharp discharges) appear to be higher in embolic than in thrombotic stroke.[24]

Stroke involving the anterior cerebral artery demonstrates polymorphic delta over the ipsilateral frontal area or RDA of unilateral dominance.[22]

Infarction within the territory of the posterior cerebral artery shows a loss or decrease of alpha rhythm on the side of the stroke along with focal slowing in the posterior temporal, parietal, and occipital regions.

Strokes in the brainstem usually do not give rise to abnormal EEG, especially when the patient is awake. Locked-in syndrome, which is characterized by quadriplegia and paralysis of all cranial nerve functions except for vertical eye movements, is secondary to an infarction in the ventral pons but sparing the posterior tegmentum. The EEG in locked-in syndrome usually shows normal awake and asleep patterns.[25] When infarction involves the reticular activating system (rostral pons, midbrain, or thalamus), the patients become comatose with EEG showing diffuse delta–theta activity and slow background rhythm.[26] EEG in lacunar infarction, which can produce hemiplegia and/or dense hemisensory loss,[27] is usually normal because the involved lesion is small and deeply seated. In fact, a focal EEG abnormality suggests a hemispheric lesion rather than a lacunar or capsular infarct.[27]

It is not certain if vascular etiology accounts for *transient global amnesia* (TGA). EEG of TGA is usually normal even during the attack.[28]

Cerebral Hemorrhage

Cerebral hemorrhage tends to occur in patients with hypertension. The cause might also be ruptured aneurysm or arteriovenous malformation (AVM) and bleeding from a neoplasm or with cerebral infarct. In general, patients with supratentorial hemorrhagic stroke are more acutely ill than patients with cerebral infarction, and consciousness is usually impaired. EEG shows focal frontotemporal dominant delta–theta activity on the affected hemisphere and becomes more bilaterally diffuse as the patients lapse into coma. Generally, EEG does not assist in differentiating hemorrhage from infarction.

Thalamic hemorrhage shows focal delta activity which may be associated with depressed sleep spindles.[29] Midbrain (mesencephalic) bleeding may cause diffuse theta range activity.[22] In patients with cerebellar infarct, EEG is usually normal if consciousness is impaired. In patients with cerebellar hemorrhage, it is of interest to note that the EEG may show delta activity in the contralateral hemisphere.[30]

BRAIN ABSCESS

EEG in brain abscess is characterized by large amplitude polymorphic slow delta activity (0.5 Hz) on the affected hemisphere,

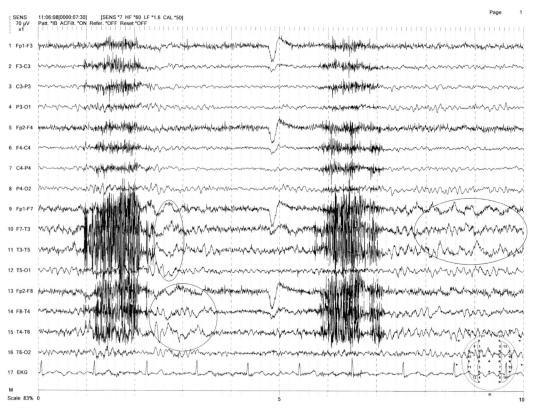

FIGURE 12-18 | A 78-year-old man with a history of diabetes and hypertension. MRI showed diffuse small-vessel disease with atherosclerotic change. EEG showed left/right shifting delta transients from temporal regions (shown by *oval circles*).

especially in the acute state.[31,32] Epileptiform discharges are common, and nearly one third of patients have clinical seizures during the acute illness.[33] LPD* may occur as a relatively rare complication.[31]

TEMPORAL SLOW WAVES IN THE ELDERLY

It is well recognized that there are increased delta–theta transients, at times including sharp components, from the temporal region, maximum at the midtemporal electrode, in subjects older than 60 to 70 (Fig. 12-18). These slow waves may be seen in 30% to 40% of normal volunteers over the age of 60.[34,35] For unknown reasons, the discharges are more common from the left than from the right temporal region. The discharges tend to increase during light drowsiness. Some investigators suggest that this is more common in patients with chronic cerebrovascular disease in the absence of major neurological deficit.[36,37] In fact, it is not uncommon to find a history of diabetes, hypertension, TIA, and/or hyperlipidemia in patients having excessive temporal slow wave patterns, especially in patients younger than 60.

Despite the normal functioning and lack of neurological deficit in these elderly individuals, some studies have found decreased performance on verbal fluency tests consistent with temporal lobe dysfunction.[37]

Nonetheless, focal slow waves from one or both temporal regions are common in elderly subjects without evidence of detectable pathology or neurological deficit. Therefore, the interpretation should be conservative and should not be considered to indicate focal pathology.

Sometimes, differentiation of these "normal" slow waves of elderly from pathological focal slow waves is difficult. Following are some helpful hints to aid in the differentiation:

1. The distribution of "normal" slow waves is limited to the temporal region and does not involve the parasagittal region.
2. "Normal" slow waves usually appear as a brief transient, lasting less than 1 second. Slow waves lasting longer than a few seconds are more likely pathological.
3. Most of the benign slow wave transients show a left/right shifting occurrence. Predominately unilateral slow waves are likely abnormal.

MIGRAINE HEADACHE

Many investigators have reported normal EEG when recorded during a headache-free period.[38–41] Others report a variety of abnormalities including hypersynchronous bursts and focal slowing,[41] prominent delta buildup to hyperventilation,[42] paroxysmal bursts, and slowing or sharp transients.[43] These varieties of EEG abnormalities may be attributed to the difference in types of migraines, age, gender, and timing of EEG recording in relation to the migraine attacks.

Some studies have reported that a photic driving response to a flash frequency above 20 Hz (called H-response) is thought to be characteristic for migraine.[43,44] However, this claim is not well-founded because there is great interindividual variability of photic driving responses among normal subjects.

EEG findings during migraine attacks also range from normal to abnormal. During a migraine attack, EEG may show focal abnormalities with slowing of background activity and/or

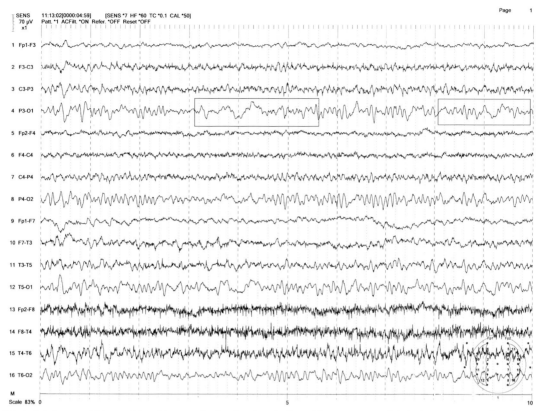

FIGURE 12-19 | A 16-year-old boy with a history of migraine headache with symptoms of right homonymous hemianopsia. EEG was recorded shortly after the migraine episode. EEG showed increased irregular delta over left occipital region (shown in *boxes*).

delta–theta activity corresponding to the side of the headache or contralateral to the side of neurological deficit (Fig. 12-19).[43] EEG is more likely to be abnormal during a hemiplegic migraine, which can show focal delta activity, at times associated with depression of beta activity.[42,43] During attacks of basilar migraine, EEG may show diffuse slow waves and monorhythmic high-amplitude delta waves (OIRDA/occipitally predominant RDA*) in the posterior head region, especially in children.[44–48] Abnormal brainstem auditory evoked potentials were reported during basilar migraine attack.[49] It should be noted that about one third of children with benign occipital spikes of childhood present with migraine-like headaches[50,51] (see "Childhood Epilepsy with Occipital Paroxysms and other Occipital Spikes," Chapter 10).

The relationship between migraine and epilepsy has been extensively debated but without convincing evidence of an etiological relationship. In fact, the coexistence of migraine and epileptic seizure disorder is uncommon. However, migraine may trigger an epileptic attack.[52,53] Conversely, there may be cases in which a seizure may trigger migraine.[54]

References

1. Walter WG. The localization of cerebral tumors by electroencephalography. *Lancet* 1936;2:305–308.
2. Kershman J, Conde A, Gibson WC. Electroencephalography in differential diagnosis of supratentorial tumors. *Arch Neurol Psychiatry* 1949;62:255–268.
3. Green RL, Wilson WP. Asymmetries of beta activity in epilepsy, brain tumor and cerebrovascular disease. *Electroencephalogr Clin Neurophysiol* 1961;13:75–78.
4. Daly DD. The effect of sleep upon the electroencephalogram in patients with brain tumors. *Electroencephalogr Clin Neurophysiol* 1968;25:521–529.
5. Jaffe R, Jacobs L. The beta focus: Its nature and significance. *Acta Neurol Scand* 1972;48:191–203.
6. Brenner RP, Sharbrough FW. Electroencephalographic evaluation in Sturge-Weber syndrome. *Neurology (Minneap)* 1976;26:629–632.
7. Yamada T, Kooi KA, Calhoun H. Relationship between high-voltage alpha or beta waves and obstructive hydrocephalus [abstract]. *Electroencephalogr Clin Neurophysiol* 1976;41:105.
8. Cordeau JP. Monorhythmic frontal delta activity in human electroencephalogram: A study of 100 cases. *Electroencephalogr Clin Neurophysiol* 1959;11:733–746.
9. Rowan AJ, Rudolf Nde M, Scott DF. EEG prediction of brain metastases. *J Neurol Neurosurg Psychiatry* 1974;37:888–893.
10. Kirstein L. The occurrence of sharp waves, spike and fast activity in supratentorial tumors. *Electroencephalogr Clin Neurophysiol* 1953;5:33–40.
11. Van der Drift JHA. *The Significance of Electroencephalography for the Diagnosis and Localization of Cerebral Tumors.* Leiden, the Netherlands: Stenfert Kroese NV, 1957.
12. Martinius J, Matthes A, Lombroso CT. Electroencephalographic features in posterior fossa tumor in children. *Electroencephalogr Clin Neurophysiol* 1968;25:128–139.
13. Daly D, Whelan JL, Bickford RG, Maccarty CS. The electroencephalogram in cases of tumors of the posterior fossa and third ventricle. *Electroencephalogr Clin Neurophysiol* 1953;5:203–216.
14. Bauer G, Gerstenbrand F, Rumpl E. Varieties of the lock-in syndrome. *J Neurol* 1979;221:77–92.
15. Westmoreland BF, Klass DW, Sharbrough FW, et al. Alpha-coma. Electrographic, clinical, pathologic and etiologic correlations. *Arch Neurol* 1975;32:713–718.

16. Vignadndra V, Ghee LT, Chawla J. EEG in brain abscess: Its value in localization compared to other diagnostic tests. *Electroencephalogr Clin Neurophysiol* 1975;38(6):611–622.

17. Klass DW, Daly DD, Electroencephalography in patients with brain tumor. *Med Clin North Am* 1960;44:1041–1051.

18. Strauss H, Ostrow M, Greenstein L, Lewyn S. Temporal slowing as a source of error in electroencephalographic localization. *Electroencephalogr Clin Neurophysiol Suppl* 1953;3:67.

19. Miller JHP. The electroencephalogram in cases of subarachnoid hemorrhage. *Electroencephalogr Clin Neurophysiol* 1953;5:165–168.

20. Madkour O, Elawan O, Hamdy H et al. Transient ischemic attack: Electrophysiological (conventional and topographic EEG) and radiological (CCT) evaluation. *J Neurol Sci* 1993;119:8–17.

21. Marshall DW, Brey BL, Morse MW. Focal and/or lateralized polymorphic delta activity: Association with either 'normal' or 'nonfocal' computerized tomographic scans. *Arch Neurol (Chicago)* 1988;45:33–35.

22. Van der Drift JHA, Kok NKD. The EEG in cerebrovascular disorders in relations to pathology. In: Remmond A, ed-in-chief. *Handbook of Electroencephalography and Clinical Neurophysiology*. Vol. 14A. Amsterdam, The Netherlands: Elsevier, 1972:12–30, 47–64.

23. Van der Drift JHA, Magnus O. The EEG in cerebral ischemic lesions. Correlation with clinical and pathological findings. In: Gastaut H, Meyer JS, eds. *Cerebral Anoxia and the Electroencephalogram*. Springfield, IL: Charles C. Thomas, 1961:180–196.

24. Rasheva M. Epileptic seizures in the acute stage of embolic stroke [abstract]. *Electroencephalogr Clin Neurophysiol* 1981;52:78.

25. Markand ON. EEG in the "locked-in" syndrome. *Electroencephalogr Clin Neurophysiol* 1976;40:529–534.

26. Schaul N, Gloor P, Gotman J. The EEG in deep midline lesion. *Neurology (Minneap)* 1981;31:157–167.

27. Petty GW, Labar DR, Fisch BJ, et al. Electroencephalography in lacunar infarction. *J Neurol Sci* 1995;134:47–50.

28. Mumenthaler M, Treig T. Anmestische Episoden. Analyse von 11 eigenen Beobachtungen. *Schweiz Med Wschr* 1984;114:1163–1170.

29. Hirose G, Saeki M, Kosoegawa H, et al. Delta waves in the EEGs of patients with intracerebral hemorrhage. *Arch Neurol (Chicago)* 1981;38:170–175.

30. Rasheva M, Stamenov E, Todorova P, et al. Dynamic of electrical activity of the brain in cerebellar hemorrhage [abstract]. *Electroencephalogr Clin Neurophysiol* 1981;52:78.

31. Michel B, Gastaut JL, Bianchi L. Electroencephalographic cranial computerized tomographic correlation in brain abscess. *Electroencephalogr Clin Neurophysiol* 1979;46:256–273.

32. Ziegler DK, Hoeffer PF. EEG and clinical findings in 28 verified brain abscess. *Electroencephalogr Clin Neurophysiol* 1952;2:41–44.

33. Legg NJ, Gupta PC, Scott DF. Epilepsy following cerebral abscess: A clinical and EEG study of 70 patients. *Brain* 1973;96:259–268.

34. Kooi KA, Guvener AM, Tupper CJ, Bagchi BK. Electroencephalographic patterns of the temporal region in normal adults. *Neurology (Minneap)* 1964;14:1029–1035.

35. Torres F, Faoro A, Loewenson R, et al. The electroencephalogram of elderly subjects revisited. *Electroencephalogr Clin Neurophysiol* 1983;56:397–398.

36. Niedermeyer E. The electroencephalogram and vertebrobasilar artery insufficiency. *Neurology (Minneap)* 1963;13:412–422.

37. Visser SL, Hooijer C, Jonker C, et al. Anterior temporal focal abnormalities in normal aged subjects, correlations with psychological and CT brain scan findings. *Electroencephalogr Clin Neurophysiol* 1987;66:1–7.

38. Ulett GA, Evans D, O'Leary JL. Survey of EEG findings in 1,000 patients with chief complaint of headache. *Electroencephalogr Clin Neurophysiol* 1952;4:463–470.

39. Bille B. Migraine in school children. *Acta Paediatr Suppl (Uppsala)* 1962;51:136.

40. Gibbs FA, Gibbs EL. *Atlas of Electroencephalography*. Vol. 3. Reading, MA: Addison-Wesley, 1964.

41. Heyck H. *Neue Beitrage zur Klinik und Pathogenese der Migraine*. Stuttgart, Germany: Thieme, 1956.

42. Weil AA. EEG findings in a certain type of psychosomatic headache: Dysrhythmic migraine. *Electroencephalogr Clin Neurophysiol* 1952;4:181–186.

43. Golla FL, Winter AL. Analysis of cerebral responses to flicker in patients complaining of episodic headache. *Electroencephalogr Clin Neurophysiol* 1959;11:539–549.

44. Smyth VOG, Winter AL. The EEG in migraine. *Electroencephalogr Clin Neurophysiol* 1964;16:194–202.

45. Schoenen J, Jamart B, De Pasqua V, et al. Mapping of EEG and auditory event-potentials in migraine [abstract]. *Electroencephalogr Clin Neurophysiol* 1990;75:S134.

46. Heyck H. Varieties of hemiplegic migraine. *Headache* 1973;12:135–142.

47. Gastaut JL, Yermenos F, Bonnefoy M, et al. Familial hemiplegic migraine. EEG and CT scan study of two cases. *Ann Neurol* 1981;10:392–395.

48. Lapkin MS, French JH, Golden GS, et al. The electroencephalogram in childhood basilar migraine. *Neurology (Minneap)* 1977;27:580–583.

49. Yamada T, Dickins QS, Arensdorf K, et al. Basilar migraine: Polarity dependent alteration of brainstem auditory evoked potentials. *Neurology (Minneap)* 1986;36:1256–1260.

50. Panayiotopoulos CP. Basilar migraine? Seizures and severe epileptic EEG abnormalities. *Neurology (Minneap)* 1980;30:1122–1125.

51. Gastaut H, Zifkin BG. Benign epilepsy of childhood with occipital spike and wave complexes. In: Andermann F, Lugaresi E, eds. *Migraine and Epilepsy*. Boston, MA: Butterworth, 1987:47–81.

52. Camfield PR, Metrakos K, Andermann F. Basilar migraine, seizures and severe epileptiform EEG abnormalities. *Neurology (Minneap)* 1978;28:584–588.

53. Niedermeyer E. Migraine-triggered epilepsy. *Clin Electroencephalogr* 1993;24:37–43.

54. Jacob J, Goadsby PJ, Duncan JS. Use of sumatriptan in post-ictal migraine headache [abstract]. *Neurology (Minneap)* 1996;47:1104.

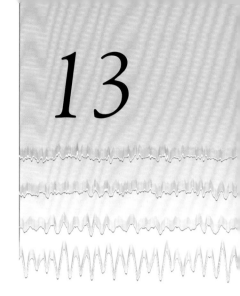

Continuous EEG Monitoring for Critically Ill Patients (CCEEG)

THORU YAMADA and ELIZABETH MENG

Introduction

The recent advancement in computer technology has allowed continuous EEG recording at the patient's bedside. This has become possible because of increased memory size, fast processing speed, and also improved video screen resolution. Continuous and long-term monitoring of EEG allows the evaluation of dynamic changes of brain function that may not be visible by clinical examination alone. With accumulation of continuous EEG data in the intensive care unit (ICU), it has become apparent that nonconvulsive seizures (NCS) or nonconvulsive status epilepticus (NCSE) are relatively common in acutely ill, comatose or stuporous patients. Because of the lack of motor manifestation, NCS can easily be overlooked without continuous EEG recording. In this context, we adopt the term CCEEG (continuous critical care EEG) to distinguish it from LTM EEG (long-term monitoring of EEG) used primarily for evaluation of epilepsy patients. Because of the intermittent and unpredictable occurrence of NCS, a single 20- to 30-minute EEG recording would likely miss capturing these seizures. The value of CCEEG has been further strengthened by concomitant video recording, networking capability, ability of storing large amounts of data for many hours (>24 hours), and also the automatic computer analyses of seizure/spike detection and various quantitative EEG analyses by power spectrum measurement.

Indication for CCEEG

The most common reason for CCEEG is to find out if the patient is having NCSE or intermittent episodes of NCS in the acutely ill comatose or obtunded patients. The following clinical conditions raise the question of NCSE or NSC.
- The expected recovery does not occur after brain surgery.
- The patient does not gain consciousness after head trauma.
- Consciousness remains impaired with paucity of positive physical finding or lack of radiological examination.
- There is fluctuating mental status without explainable cause.
- Unexplainable comatose or obtunded state.
- There is no recovery after convulsive status epilepticus or single seizure.

Other justifiable reasons for performing CCEEG include episodes of seizure-like symptoms such as muscle twitching, body posturing, eye deviation, chewing, pupillary abnormalities, or autonomic symptoms, but without overt convulsion.[1-4] The CCEEG may also be indicated for evaluation of vasospasms or cerebral ischemia, especially after subarachnoid hemorrhage (SAH) or interventional neuroradiological procedures.[5,6] CCEEG may also be used for the evaluation of progressively changing brain function, either worsening or improving, for the purpose of prognostication.[7,8] CCEEG is also indicated for guidance in maintaining a therapeutic burst suppression pattern with barbiturates or other anesthetic/sedative drugs[9,10] and for assessment of the treatment efficacy for NCS and NCSE. CCEEG is now a routine protocol for detection of NCS or NCSE in patients undergoing therapeutic hypothermia after anoxic brain insult secondary to cardiac arrest.[11,12]

The decision to switch to CCEEG may also be based on the finding of certain abnormal EEG patterns on the routine or initial recording. They include generalized (GPD*) (Video 13-1, see Figs. 10-33D and 10-35) or lateralized periodic discharges (PLEDs/LPD*) (see Figs. 10-39 and 10-40) (Video 13-2A and B), SIRPID (Fig. 13-1A–C, see also Fig. 10-38A and B) (Video 13-3A and B), lateralized rhythmic delta activity (LRDA) (Fig. 13-2A and B) (Video 13-4), or brief (potentially) ictal rhythmic discharges (B(I)RD) (Fig. 13-3A and B) (Video 13-5), because these patterns are more likely to develop NCS or NCSE[13-15] (see section of "Evaluation of CCEEG for NSC and NCSE" in this chapter). As shown in Video 13-2A and B, PLEDs/LPD between two regions may show synchronous (Video 13-2A) or asynchronous discharges (Video 13-2B, see also Fig. 10-41) within the same hemisphere. SIRPIDs may consist of variable waveforms, ranging from blunt sharp-wave triphasic form (Video 13-3A, see Fig. 13-1B) to frank spike-wave discharges (Video 13-3B, see Fig. 10-38B). This often makes it difficult to decide if the patient should be treated as having seizure.

---

*Some of EEG terminology is adopted from recent ACNS standard; Hirsch LJ, LaRoche SM, Gaspard N, et al. American Clinical Neurophysiology Society's standardized critical care EEG terminology: 2012 version. *J Clin Neurophysiol* 2013;301:1–27. They are labeled with * marks (see Table 13-1).

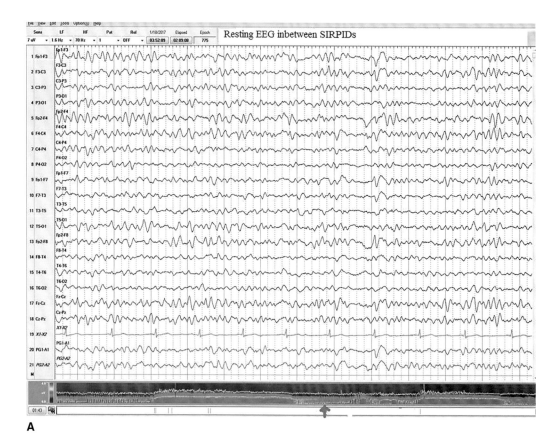

A

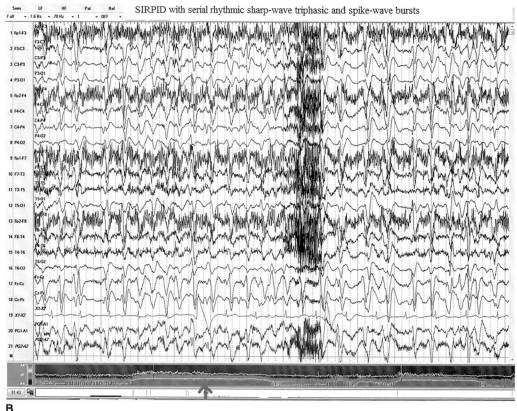

B

FIGURE 13-1 | An 89-year-old female presented with intraparenchymal hemorrhage. She was obtunded when EEG monitoring started. There were three different EEG patterns; one was diffuse theta and delta slow waves without paroxysmal discharges. This occurred when there were no muscle artifacts **(A)** EEG sample was taken at *arrow* in DSA). When muscle artifacts increased, sporadic generalized triphasic waves were induced, and this was short-lasting SIRPID **(B)**. With prolonged and greater degree of muscle artifact increase, EEG showed continuous and rhythmic generalized sharp-wave triphasic waves, which were much more "spikey" than the short-lasting SIRPID **(C)**. DSA represents 4 hours of EEG segment and this indicated two prolonged episodes of SIRPID and multiple short-lasting SIRPID **(C)** within 4 hours recording.

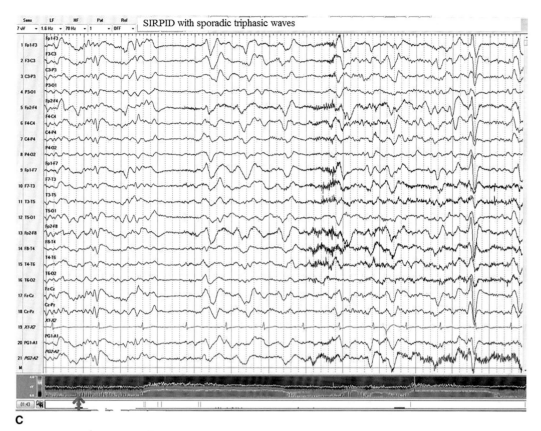

C

FIGURE 13-1 | (Continued)

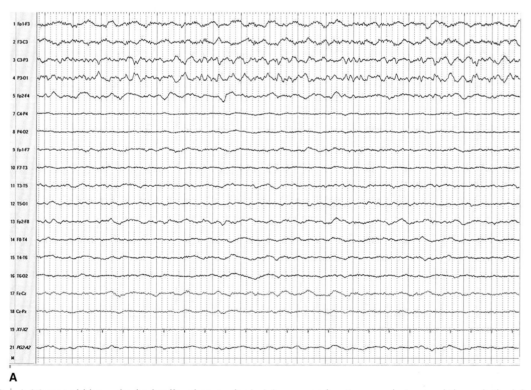

A

FIGURE 13-2 | A 16-year-old boy who had suffered severe brain injury secondary to a gunshot wound through the left orbit passing through the entire left hemisphere. EEG showed depressed electrical activity over the right hemisphere and semirhythmic delta from left frontal region (LRAD*) **(A)**. Nonconvulsive electrographic ictal discharges occurred intermittently with repetitive spikes involving left frontal region (same region as of delta activity), which progressed from 2 to 1 Hz **(B)**.

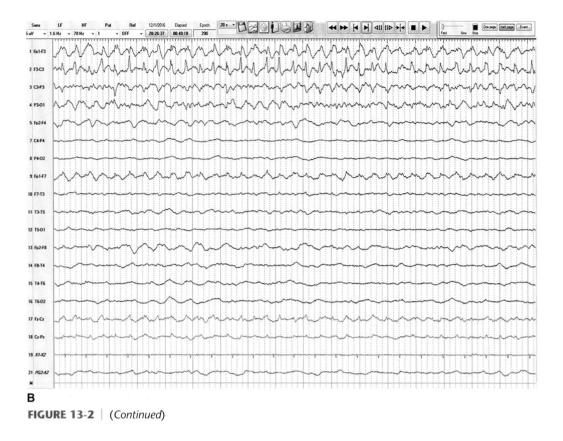

B

FIGURE 13-2 | (Continued)

Incidence of NCSE or NCS in the ICU

NCS is defined as an electrographic seizure without overt clinical signs of seizures, though patients may have subtle face or limb twitching, eye deviation, eyelid twitching, chewing, muscle tone increase, nystagmus, pupillary changes, or other autonomic signs (blood pressure change, respiration change, tachycardia or bradycardia, sweating, etc.). These clinical changes are diagnosed as seizures only by observing repeatedly the same subtle clinical sign correlating with consistent EEG changes (Video 13-6A and B). NCSE was traditionally defined when NCSs occur continuously or near continuously lasting more than 30 minutes.[16,17] But recent guidelines proposed in 2016 by the American Epilepsy Society define status epilepticus as when a seizure lasts longer than 5 minutes.[18] This applies for both convulsive seizures and NCSs.[18] Yet another consensus proposed by American Clinical Neurophysiology Society for use with neonates is "*summated duration of a seizure comprised of greater than or equal to 50% of an arbitrarily defined one hour epoch.*"[19]

The overall incidence of NCS or NCSE in patients who are in coma or unexplained altered mental status in ICU settings (inclusive of pediatric patients) varies from about 10% to 50%.[20–23] Of various etiologies, the postconvulsive status epilepticus patients have the highest incidence of NCS or NCSE; one study showed close to half the patients who had convulsive status epilepticus developed NCS (14% of these were NCSE) after the convulsions had stopped clinically.[24]

Another common cause for NCS is postanoxic cerebral insult following cardiac or respiratory arrest, ranging from 10% to 60% (see Fig. 10-36), although myoclonic convulsive seizures are not uncommon (Video 13-7).[25–27] NCS or NCSE may also occur during therapeutic hypothermia after anoxic cerebral insult secondary to cardiac arrest and could occur during the rewarming period.[10,11,26] The NCS or NCSE associated with ischemic brain injury carries a grave prognosis.[27]

NCS and NCSE are also common in toxic metabolic encephalopathy (uremia, hypertensive encephalopathy, drug intoxication or withdrawal, hepatic failure, hypo- and hyperglycemia)[28] and patients with postoperative brain surgery,[29–31] traumatic brain injury,[32–34] intracerebral hemorrhage,[34–36] ischemic stroke,[35–38] and SAH.[39,40] The incidence of NCS in these conditions varies, ranging from 10% to 30%. The incidences of NCS and NCSE are generally higher in neonates, infants, and children in NICU (neonatal ICU) or PICU (pediatric ICU)[41–44] than in adults. One study showed 44% of patients in PICU or NICU who underwent CCEEG monitoring had NCS and 75% of these were NCSE.[21] It is expected that the probability of capturing seizures (either clinical or nonconvulsive) would be higher with CCEEG than with a routine 30-minute recording in the ICU setting. EEGs of 30 to 60 minutes will likely miss more than half of the seizures captured in CCEEG.[22,43,45] With CCEEG, about 80% to 95% of NCS was captured within 24 to 48 hours.[23,45–47] It is therefore reasonable to stop monitoring if there are no seizures for 2 days after the last seizure.

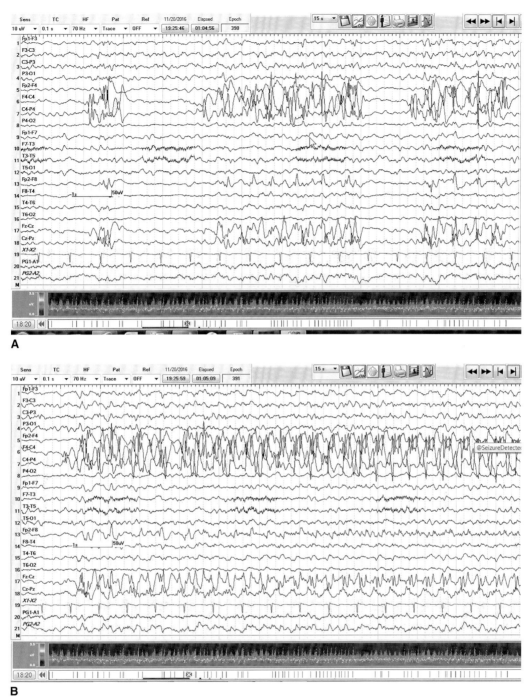

FIGURE 13-3 | A 64-year-old woman with right frontal hemorrhage with SAH after fall. EEG recording started after surgical evacuation of hematoma. EEG showed recurrent, mostly brief (<10 seconds) irregular spike-wave bursts from frontal region **(A)**. These are consistent with B(I)RD. DSA showed brief, repetitive, almost regularly recurring numerous episodes of power increase reflecting B(I)RD. Intermittently, there were longer episodes of spike-wave burst with more rhythmic configuration, which was consistent with NCS **(B)**.

However, more than 2 days of monitoring may be required for a patient who has frequent interictal epileptiform activity and periodic discharges or those withdrawing from pharmacological sedation. On the other hand, the chance of capturing a seizure in CCEEG (72 hours) without any epileptiform activity during the first 2 hours is less than 5%.[48] Although the study cohort was biased because CCEEG was ordered primarily for a question of NCS, one study disclosed 83% (49 out of 59 patients) had NSC and almost half (47% or 23 of 49) of these had NSCE.[16] Similarly, NSC was found in 18% to 35%,[23,24] and up to 75% of these patients had NCSE.[48] Also in postcardiac arrest patients undergoing hypothermia, similar results have been reported even with a 30-minute recording.[50]

Recording Technology of CCEEG

The electrodes used for CCEEG are the same as used in routine EEG (silver–silver chloride or gold). Because the EEG is recorded without the attendance of a technologist most of the time, it is important that the electrodes are attached securely enough for many hours of recording. In some cases, extra or redundant electrodes may be placed. This is especially true for the "system" or "common" reference; if the system reference is removed, the entire recording will be lost. In addition to EEG electrodes, EKG electrodes should always be placed because EKG contamination, especially abnormal EKG, can mimic epileptiform activity (Chapter 15, see Fig. 15-15). EKG can also sometimes provide important clues for cardiac-related spells such as vasovagal syncope (see Fig. 10-46A–D) or seizure causing cardiac abnormality (see Video 10-14). Other important electrodes are eye monitors to record the electrooculogram. This is necessary for the differentiation of frontal delta activity from eye movement artifacts (see Chapter 15, Eye Movement Artifacts, see also Figs. 8-16A and B, 15-3, 15-4, and 15-5). All electrodes are best secured with collodion. The use of paste is not recommended for long-term recording. Electrodes for recording EMG (electromyograph) may be applied over appropriate muscles, especially when the patient shows muscle twitches or involuntary movements.

Because ICU patients often undergo MRI or CT scan during the monitoring session, the electrodes must be removed before and replaced after the examination is done. This is a nuisance and is time consuming for technologists. MRI- or CT scan-compatible electrodes have now become commercially available. Subdermal needle electrodes (disposable stainless steel) can be used for rapid application and may be preferentially used for patients with skin problems or for patients who have fresh surgical wounds on the scalp. However, needle electrodes attenuate low-frequency signals. Also, they are not suitable for long-term recording. Other recently introduced electrodes are subdermal wire electrodes, which are made of Teflon-coated wire with a silver–chloride tip. These are suitable for long-term recording[51] and can be made compatible for CT or MRI scan. An electrode cap may be used for quick application when an EEG technologist is not available but is not suitable for long-term recording, so it should be replaced when the EEG technologist becomes available.

In some cases, polygraphic recording with respiratory airflow, a pulse oximetry (oxygen saturation), or intracranial pressure monitoring can be monitored by adding DC amplifiers.[52] Additionally, the output from an ICU monitoring device, which includes blood pressure, body temperature, EKG, SaO_2 saturation, etc., can be incorporated into the EEG recording.

Since the ICU is usually considered to be an electrically "hostile/noisy" environment because of the number of electrical devices attached to or working around the patient, it is important to mitigate the electrical interference emanating from these devices which will affect the EEG recording. The most important technical issue is to have well-secured and low-impedance electrodes. If high-frequency noise cannot be eliminated, a lower high-frequency filter may be used, but one should be cautious in EEG interpretation since lowering the high-frequency filter, for example, from 70 to 15 Hz may change the muscle or movement artifacts to look like spike discharges

or beta activity (see Chapter 15, Figs. 15-38 and 15-39A and B, see also Fig. 2-13).

Using a covering or wrapping over the entire set of electrodes helps to minimize accidental dislodging of the electrodes. The electrode wires should be bundled together and placed away from other instruments and at a distance from the patient's reach. Even if the patient is immobile, physicians or other ICU personnel may move the head or body without consideration of the attached EEG wires.

In addition to the EEG, video recording with audio helps to identify seizure versus artifacts from various activities in the ICU. EEG activity mimicking seizure patterns can be created by chewing, rhythmic massage, patting, rhythmic chest percussion, shaking, rubbing, tremors, etc. (see Chapter 15). Since EEG is recorded most of the time without bedside attendance of an EEG technologist, video recording is essential in order to review the patient's behavior, seizure activity, and also any activities surrounding the patient's bedside to differentiate artifacts from genuine EEG activity. Also, audio with video often provides additional useful information to evaluate the patient's behavior or surrounding environment (see Video 7-2; see also Video 15-15). The video screen is usually set up at the patient's bedside and should also be remotely transmitted to the reading/control room and/or nursing station. The video camera ideally can be controlled remotely for zooming, focusing, and pan/tilt motion.

With the start of EEG monitoring, the technologist should test the patient's responsiveness by calling his name or asking questions. Glasgow Coma Scale can be used to quantify the level of consciousness (see Chapter 11, section "General Features of Diffuse EEG Abnormalities"). If there is no response, the technologist delivers stronger stimulation by touch or shaking. If there is no response to that, the stimulus intensity is increased to painful stimulus (nail bed pressure or sternum rub).

The technologist should check the integrity of the recording at least twice daily or as frequently as needed depending on the case. The initial recording of 30 to 60 minutes should be reviewed by the electroencephalographer (EEGer) and the result should be reported to the referring physician in a timely manner. EEG should be reviewed at least every 12 hours or as often as possible depending on the progress of the disease condition. If the patient has some type of spell, the technologist should ask the nurse, medical staff, or family member to mark the events, with a push button marker that registers on the EEG recording. ICU nursing staff may be able to write the time of the event and describe the clinical features of the event in the medical record. When an event button is pushed, it can generate an "alert" signal to the nursing station and to the remote reading room and/or EEG staff. The technologist also needs to pay attention to medication changes, especially anticonvulsants, anesthetics, and sedative drugs or muscle relaxants.

If the recording continues more than several days, the skin/scalp should be checked for the presence of irritation or "breakdown." If present, the primary physician and/or EEGer should be alerted and appropriate measures should be taken. It is possible to continue the EEG recording by slightly displacing the electrode locations, but this should be clearly documented. The disc electrodes may be switched to needle or subdermal wire electrodes.

Commercially available EEG instruments are now capable of transmitting EEG data with video online to remote sites through the Internet. Thus, EEG information can be accessed anytime and anywhere. As long as the patient's confidentiality is kept secure (according to HIPAA regulations), this is an extremely convenient and important advancement for the EEG technologist, EEGer, and referring physician. The electroencephalographer can periodically check the evolution of EEG change, if any, and the technologist can check the integrity of the EEG recording throughout the day as needed at a remote site. Remote access also allows sending EEG data with video from a local community hospital to major medical centers where expert EEGers or epileptologists are available for consultation to provide prompt and appropriate evaluation and treatment for the patient. Successful CCEEG and appropriate management for the patient are based on close communication between the referring physician, nursing staff, EEGer, and technologist.

Evaluation of CCEEG for NCS or NCSE

The evaluation of interictal and ictal patterns is essentially the same as with routine EEG, but distinction between ictal, interictal, and nonictal patterns is not always clear. When frequent spike or spike-wave discharges occur in a random sequence, they are likely of the interictal pattern. Episodes of progressively changing patterns in frequency and amplitude or rhythmic wave forms are likely ictal events. The most difficult case is deciding between NCSE/NCS and metabolic encephalopathy such as hepatic encephalopathy when a more or less continuous rhythmic or periodic sharp–delta triphasic wave occurs (see Fig. 8-17, see also Fig. 10-37B, compare Fig. 13-1B and C). It was once thought triphasic waves that were abolished by short-acting benzodiazepines were ictal discharges, but it is now known that the triphasic waves associated with metabolic encephalopathy can also be abolished by benzodiazepine[53]; thus, this does not help to distinguish between the two. If, however, the patient shows clinical improvement promptly, it is likely NCSE. In general, the triphasic waves of ictal patterns show a more "spiky" configuration than the triphasic waves of metabolic origin; therefore, finding the "spike" is important to distinguish them (see Fig. 8-17, see also Fig. 13-1B).

Periodic discharges, either generalized (GPD*) or lateralized (PLED/LPD*) are fairly common EEG patterns seen in CCEEG in an ICU setting. GPD*s can take a variety of waveforms from rhythmic delta, triphasic waves to frank spike-wave discharges. It is difficult to determine if the GPD* represent a metabolic origin or an interictal or ictal pattern. Generally speaking, triphasic waves with a frequency less than 2 Hz are likely metabolic in origin and those faster than 3-Hz GPD represents an ictal pattern.[20,54] Another situation where it is difficult to distinguish ictal versus interictal patterns is periodic lateralized epileptiform discharges (PLEDs/LPD*). Most PLEDs/LPD* are interictal or postictal patterns. Once PLEDs/LPDs are found, CCEEG at least a few to several days should be in order, to look for the electrographic ictal events in between interictal PLEDs/LPD* (see Chapter 10, Fig. 10-39A and B, see also Fig. 13-10). Some PLEDs/LPD* are clearly ictal when associated with focal limb jerking, which is time locked to the discharges (epilepsia partialis continua) (Video 13-8). One study proposed two types of PLEDs; "PLEDs plus" are associated with rhythmic fast activity and "PLEDs proper" are without rhythmic fast activity. PLEDs plus had higher chance of seizure than PLEDs proper.[55]

Other patterns that are difficult and/or controversial are SIRPID (stimulus-induced rhythmic periodic or ictal discharges) and B(I)RD (brief potentially ictal rhythmic discharges or brief ictal/interictal rhythmic/repetitive discharges). It is controversial if SIRPID with a triphasic pattern should be treated as a seizure event. One study recommended conventional antiepileptic treatment,[56] while another study advocated against aggressive treatment because there was no increased cerebral blood flow with SIRPID.[57] It seems to be reasonable to treat SIRPID as a seizure event if it consists of unequivocal spike-wave bursts (see Fig. 10-38B, see also Fig. 13-1B). It is also not uncommon that the same patient will show SIRPID with clear spike wave at one time and also blunt triphasic pattern at another time (see Fig. 13-1B and C).

B(I)RD is defined as an evolving rhythmic pattern resembling an ictal pattern but lasting less than 10 seconds. BIRD was initially described in neonates[58] and was reported to be associated with hypoxic ischemic encephalopathy and neurodevelopmental sequelae.[59,60] B(I)RDs often coexist with otherwise clear ictal patterns (see Fig. 13-3A and B, see also Video 13-5). More than 90% of adult patients who had B(I)RD subsequently developed NCS or NCSE and more than half of them also showed PLEDs or LPD independently.[61] It is, therefore, reasonable to switch to CCEEG once B(I)RD is found in an initial EEG and the patient should be treated as if he had seizures.

The Assessment of Progress for Acute Cerebral Dysfunction

The CCEEG can be utilized not only for finding episodic events such as seizure but also for assessing the progress of acutely injured brain function and its prognostication during the course of illness. CCEEG showing reactivity to external stimulation, spontaneous change, episodic sleep patterns, or a progressive decrease of slow waves replaced by faster frequency activity suggests a favorable prognosis. The prognosis is unfavorable if CCEEG shows relentless and monotonous patterns without reactivity or variability.[61-63] EEG is especially sensitive to cerebral ischemia, which shows initially a decrease of fast (beta) activity followed by an increase of delta slow waves as ischemia progresses. This occurs when cerebral blood flow is below 18 to 25 mL/100 g/min.[64,65] CCEEG is often used during the acute phase of SAH because vasospasm occurs in 50% to 70% of patients after SAH.[66] The vasospasms tend to occur within 3 to 14 days after the onset of SAH and cause cerebral ischemia or infarction in close to 50% of the patients.[67] Because prompt treatment can prevent cerebral infarction or ischemia, early detection of these events is important. The vasospasms can be detected by transcranial Doppler or angiography, but these tests evaluate the vascular state only at the time of examination. CCEEG reflects brain function continuously and is useful for the timely detection of EEG changes when vasospasm occurs. The EEG worsening can be reflected by increased slow waves, with either diffuse or focal pattern.[4,68] EEG also helps to evaluate the effectiveness of treatment. Using quantitative EEG (qEEG) analyses, various algorithms have been introduced to automatically detect the deterioration or improvement of EEG activity after SAH. EEG deterioration due to vasospasms was detected by the reduction of total spectral power,[69] decrease in alpha frequency power[68] or reduction of alpha/delta frequency power ratio after stimulation[4] (see Fig. 13-9A–G). Ischemic infarction can be detected by brain symmetry index based on the difference of mean spectral power of 1 to 25 Hz between the left and right hemispheres.[70]

Seizure and Spike Detection Algorithms

Page-by-page review of CCEEG is time consuming for the EEG technologist and for the EEGer. In order to reduce the vast amounts of EEG data to be reviewed, automatic seizure or spike detection computer programs are commercially available. Despite much improvement and sophistication in computer technology in recent years, spike or seizure detection programs are far from perfect (Fig. 13-4). The computer detects muscle activity or various sharply formed artifacts as spikes and any rhythmic activity or any rhythmic artifact could be detected as a seizure (ictal) event. In reality, more than 90% of the computer-detected spikes or ictal events are false-positive detections. The computer is still not capable of complex analyses of waveforms, spatial distribution, and temporal factors of a given wave or pattern that experienced EEGer can instantaneously recognize and differentiate seizure/spike versus artifacts. The seizure detections are based on sudden amplitude, frequency, and waveform change

with rhythmic characters. Again, computers could falsely detect artifacts created by rhythmic movements as seizures (Fig. 13-4B, Video 13-9). Despite significant deficits, the seizure and spike detection programs are still useful by allowing the computer to detect abundant false-positive data, which reduces the amount of EEG data to be reviewed using page-by-page mode. One should also be aware of false-negative results; the computer will likely fail to detect electrodecremental seizures or short-lasting or less rhythmic ictal discharges.

The Use of Quantitative EEG Analyses for CCEEG

The standard visual analysis requires considerable amount of time even by skilled EEGer to review the entire 24-hour EEG. In addition to the spike or electrographic seizure detection program, quantitative analyses using spectral power by Fourier transformation helps to identify transient or gradual changes of the power spectrum during CCEEG. If qEEG is performed appropriately, the data and figures created by qEEG can be screened by personnel who are not familiar with EEG. However, because qEEG cannot differentiate various artifacts from genuine EEG activity and also is unable to differentiate various waveforms, one should never rely solely on the qEEG without correlating original EEG data. Therefore, it is important to use dual monitors to view the ongoing EEG on one and accumulating qEEG data on the other monitor. The final interpretation of the CCEEG still relies on the skilled EEGer.

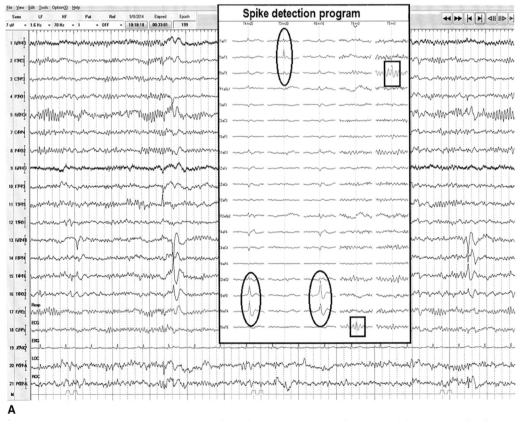

A

FIGURE 13-4 | **(A)** An example of computer-detected spikes. The program correctly detected three types of spikes, maximum at T4, T3, and F8. But "spiky" beta activities were falsely detected also as spikes (left two columns). **(B)** An example of falsely detected ical event (top figure on left column) by left > right rhythmic theta bursts (right column). This was caused by rhythmic head shaking (see Video 13-9). The proof of artifacts is shown by triple phase reversal at F3, C3 and P3 electrodes (example are shown by vertical lines).

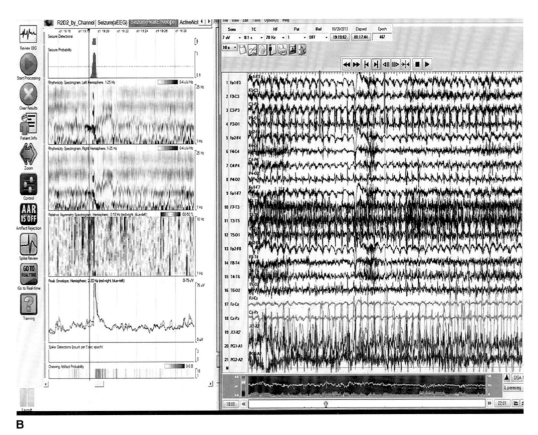

B

FIGURE 13-4 | (*Continued*)

The commonly used qEEGs are compressed spectral array (CSA) or density spectral array (DSA). CSA is created by plotting the frequency values along the *x*-axis and successive epochs (time) along the *y*-axis. The amplitude of spectral power, calculated from fast Fourier transforms, is then expressed by the height of vertical deflection, which gives three-dimensional effects with *x*-axis for frequency and *y*-axis for time and height of wave for power values (Fig. 13-5). DSA is expressed by

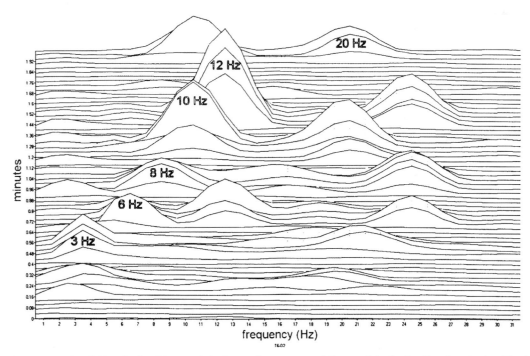

FIGURE 13-5 | An example of CSA display. The *x*-axis indicates frequency and the *y*-axis indicates time in minutes. The height of each tracing represents the amount of EEG power. This CSA was created by intermittent photic stimulation at 3, 6, 8, 19, 12, and 20 Hz stimulus rates. (From Scheuer MK, Wilson SB. Data analysis for continuous EEG monitoring in the ICU: seeing the forest and the trees. *J Clin Neurophysiol* 2004;21:353–378, with permission.)

DSA

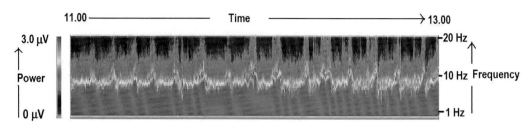

FIGURE 13-6 | An example of DSA display. The *x*-axis indicates time and the *y*-axis indicates frequency. The amount of EEG power is expressed by different colors with the highest power in *red* and the weakest power in *blue*. This shows power spectrum changes for 2 hours, revealing cyclic power alteration with increased power and frequency changes. The *yellow zigzag line* in this and subsequent figures represent SEF of 85% reflecting frequency shift. The *rising line* indicates increase of faster frequency activity.

depicting the spectral power amplitude by a gray scale or color differences with time on the *x*-axis and frequency values on the *y*-axis (Fig. 13-6). In creating CSA or DSA, it is possible to select any single electrode or multiple electrodes or combinations of all electrodes from the left and/or right hemisphere in order to maximize or enhance the frequency change against time. The DSA is often combined with *spectral edge frequency (SEF)*, which is for the frequency below a certain percentage (usually 85% to 95%) of the total power of a given signal location. For example, 85% SEF is the frequency in which 85% of the EEG spectrum power resides. The SEF is useful to see the shift of frequency in time, especially because ictal events are often expressed by increased fast activity, thus raising the SEF line (Fig. 13-7A and B).

The time scale of DSA can also be changed; a shorter time scale allows more detailed analyses of short-lasting epochs, but this may make it more difficult to recognize the gradual changes of the EEG pattern. A longer time scale reveals the event of gradually changing EEG patterns more clearly (Fig. 13-8A–D). Also, DSA with time scale of 4 to 6 hours is useful to recognize by one glance if the event is a long- or short-lasting one or severe or a less severe one (see Fig. 13-1A–C).

Other methods of qEEG include very simplified techniques such as amplitude-integrated EEG in which a simple calculation of rectified EEG amplitudes[71] to the highly sophisticated method using EEG bispectrum analysis, which is a signal-processing technique that determines both EEG linear (frequency and power) and nonlinear (phase and harmonic) components and quantitates the interfrequency phase coupling of EEG signals.[72–74] For example, quantitative EEG trends is useful for detecting cerebral ischemia by demonstrating left/right FFT power spectrogram, left/right asymmetric index, left/right alpha to delta ratio values, suppression ratio, etc. (Fig. 13-9A–G). This is especially true when evaluating the quantitative difference of hemispheric power of slowly or progressively changing frequency.

The reader can obtain more detailed information about CCEEG from recent consensus statement issued by the ACNS (American Clinical Neurophysiologic Society).[75,76] ACNS also proposed new terminology for CCEEG.

Here, we present several cases of CCEEG in which DSA provided valuable information (Cases 1 to 6).

Case No. 1: Patient was an 85-year-old man with multiple medical histories that included hypertension, type II diabetes mellitus, COPD, and obstructive sleep apnea. He was found unresponsive and was observed to show intermittent episodes of head turning with rightward gaze preference and rigidity of the left arm. The EEG on admission, when the patient was comatose, showed PLEDs/LPD* from the right hemisphere with frontal dominance (Fig. 13-10A, upward arrow indicates the time this EEG sample was depicted). The DSA depicted from the right parasagittal electrodes showed rhythmic and cyclic changes of spectral power with approximately 5- to 10-minute intervals; the trough of the spectral power corresponded with the PLEDs/LPD* and its peak corresponded to the ictal discharges with increased fast activity in the right frontal region (Fig. 13-10B). The examination of the video showed that no apparent clinical seizure activity was associated with the ictal discharges. By counting the number of peaks shown by DSA, close to 40 seizures was recorded within the first 5 hours of the recording. Further detailed evaluation of power spectrum changes showed that the power increased gradually, ultimately evolving to the ictal event, which was almost predictable (Fig. 13-10B). The trough of each cyclic event corresponded with the return of PLEDs/LPDs pattern The DSA became a stable pattern at 9 hours after the start of monitoring, implying no further ictal event, but PLEDs/LPDs continued (Fig. 10-10C).

Case No. 2: Patient was an 80-year-old woman, with past histories of cardiomyopathy and hypothyroidism, and was found unconscious apparently after cardiac arrest. The patient was comatose when the initial EEG was obtained. The EEG showed bilaterally diffuse, nearly periodic sharp-/spike-wave discharges (GPD*) with intervals of 1 to 1½ seconds (Fig. 13-11A, upward arrow indicates the time of this EEG sample was depicted). These periodic discharges were not continuous but intermittently faded away, replaced by burst suppression pattern, which corresponded to a decrease of spectral power (Fig. 13-11B). After about 2 hours of recording, DSA started to show an episode of different power spectrum from the earlier recording exhibiting four discrete band paths with abrupt onset. These DSA changes corresponded with a sudden emergence of 6-Hz spike discharges involving primarily the right temporal region and their harmonic frequencies

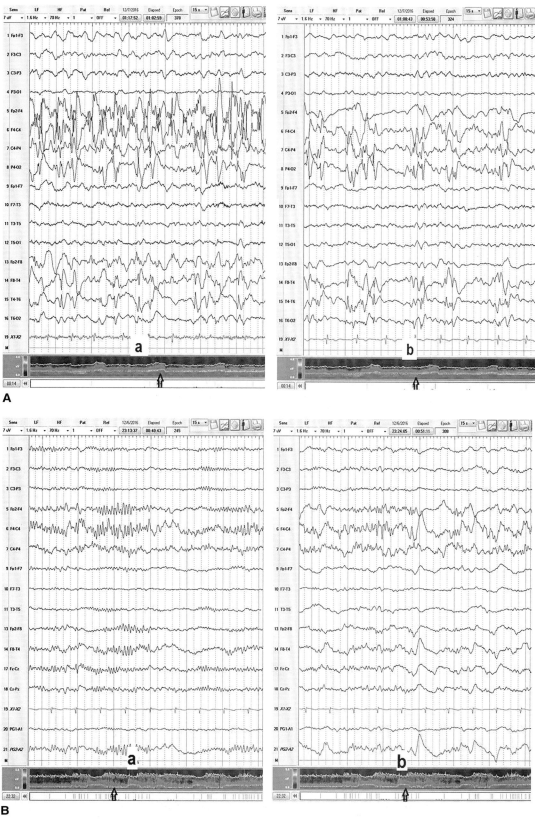

FIGURE 13-7 | Example of SEF **(A)** changes in relationship with changes of frequency powers. With increased beta activity associated with ictal events, DSA shows increased fast activity. This increase of fast activity relative to slow waves shifts the SEF to higher-frequency range (*a*), which contrasts to the SEF shift to the slower-frequency range during interictal period when fast activity was less relative to the slow waves (*upward arrow* indicates the time when this EEG sample is depicted). In contrast to the example, **A B** shows opposite SEF deflection; when fast activity is more dominant than slow waves, SEF shifts to higher-frequency range (*a*). When slow waves become more dominant than the fast activity, SEF shifts to lower-frequency range (*b*).

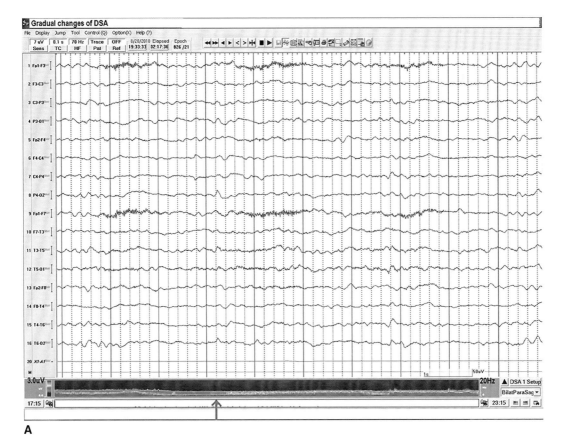

A

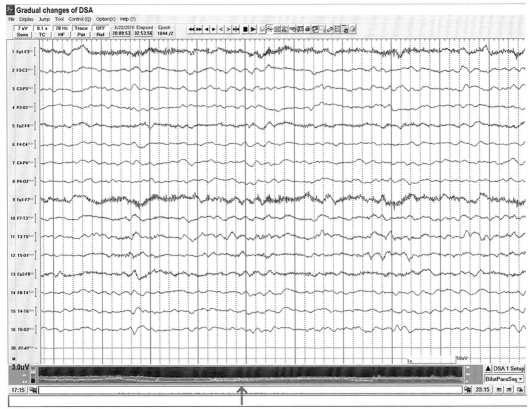

B

FIGURE 13-8 | The patient was a 75-year-old woman who was diagnosed with SAH (subarachnoid hemorrhage) after acute onset of headache and seizure. The EEG showed diffuse 5- to 6-Hz theta and low-voltage delta waves **(A)**. (The *upward arrow* indicates the time of the EEG sample obtained). The DSA revealed gradual increase of spectral power **(B)** and **(C)**. These changes were reflected by the gradual increase of delta–theta amplitude and finally emergence of broad triphasic waves **(D)**. Because these EEG changes were gradual and relatively subtle, their detection might have been missed using page-by-page mode of EEG without the help of DSA.

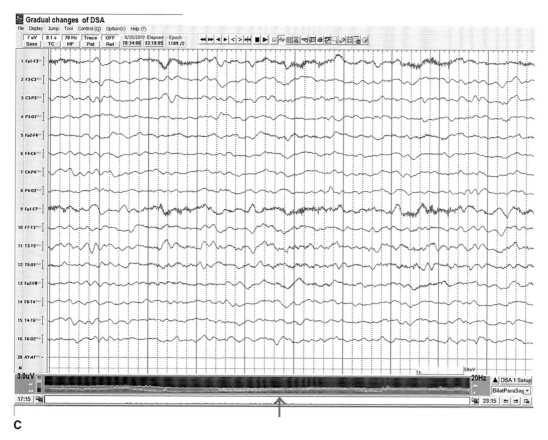

C

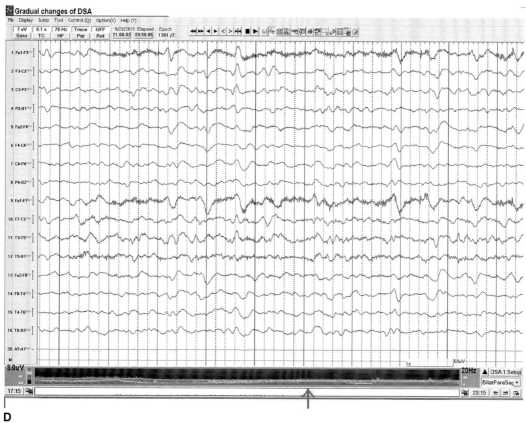

D

FIGURE 13-8 | (*Continued*)

(12 and 18 Hz) in addition to the underlying delta frequency activity (Fig. 13-11C). These discharges occurred independently from diffuse and recurrent sharp/spike discharges. With some of these 6-Hz spike episodes, the video showed left arm twitching synchronous to the spike discharges, indicating that these were clinical as well as electrographic ictal events. This unusually fixed frequency of 6-Hz spikes (without evolution) created two harmonic frequency activities at 12 and 18 Hz. DSA showed recurrent episodes of these 6-Hz spike discharges.

Case No. 3: Patient was a 48-year-old man who suffered from ventricular tachycardia in the emergency room while he was being evaluated for his chest pain. At the time of the EEG recording, the patient was comatose. The EEG showed diffuse and low-voltage delta with superimposed beta and alpha activities (Fig. 13-12A). The DSA showed fluctuating spectral power with intermittent increase of

power lasting variable durations (Fig. 13-12B). These episodes of power increase were reflected by increased diffuse triphasic sharp/delta waves that were always associated with increased muscle tone (SIRPID). These changes occurred with spontaneous arousal or when the nurses were working with the patient. At a glance of the DSA, it was possible to find 4 prolonged episodes of SIRPID within 2 hours of recording.

Case No. 4: A 93-year-old man was found unconscious on the street. He was found to have left subdural hematoma and SAH. He underwent left hemicraniotomy. Postsurgery EEG showed diffusely depressed activity with slightly higher background amplitude on the left hemisphere. There were interictal sharp and polyspikes from left hemisphere, maximum at left parietal electrode (Fig. 13-13A, Video 13-10A). The ictal events were associated with rhythmic spikes mixed with beta activity focused at the left parietal region without associated

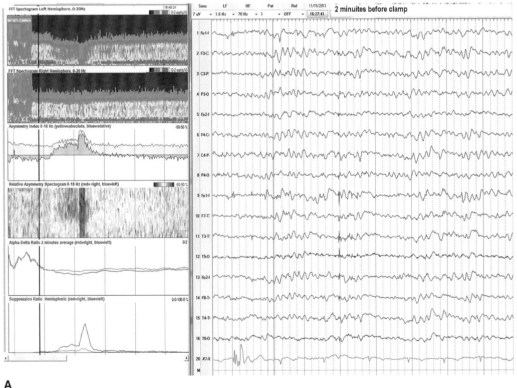

A

FIGURE 13-9 | More detailed quantitative EEG analysis is shown by an example recorded during left carotid endarterectomy. Preclamp EEG showed diffuse and symmetric alpha–theta with underlying delta and interspersed brief suppression periods **(A)**. The left graphic figures show (from *top* to *bottom*) left/right FFT spectrogram, left/right asymmetric index (with left > right higher power, *green* area becomes higher than horizontal line), relative asymmetry spectrogram with red color indicating greater power on the right, alpha–delta ratio (*red for right, blue for left*), and suppression index (*red for right, blue for left*). (*Thick vertical line* matches with the time of EEG.) Before the carotid was clamped as baseline EEG **(B)**, there was slight increase of power on the right hemisphere indicated by *blue color* in relative asymmetry spectrogram and by green downward trend in left/right asymmetric index. Two minutes after the clamp **(C)**, left spectrogram started to show decrease of fast and also delta frequency activity and asymmetric index (*green*) started to rise above the horizontal line with relative asymmetry spectrogram changing to red, indicating decrease of power on the left. At this time, EEG change was not convincing or at best questionable. Four minutes after the clamp **(D)**, further decrease of FFT spectrum power along with increase asymmetric index. EEG started to show slight depression of activity on the left, especially on the temporal region. Five and half minutes after the clamp **(E)**, the asymmetry with depressed power on the left reached the peak with the clear and much greater suppression ratio on the left than on the right. By then, EEG suppression on the left became quite obvious. Immediately after the shunt placement **(F)**, all parameters started to show reverse directions, and 4 minutes after the shunt placement, EEG became symmetric pattern **(G)**. This case illustrates that qEEG helps to recognize subtle and/or slow/progressive EEG changes and to objectify the visual impression even for seasoned EEGer.

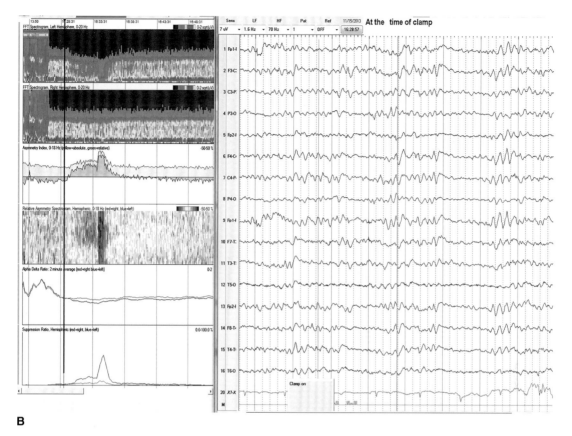

B

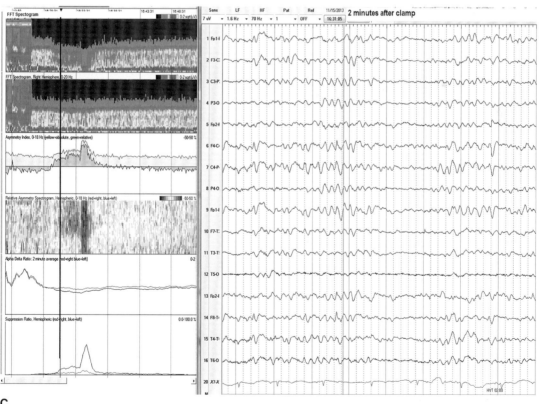

C

FIGURE 13-9 | (Continued)

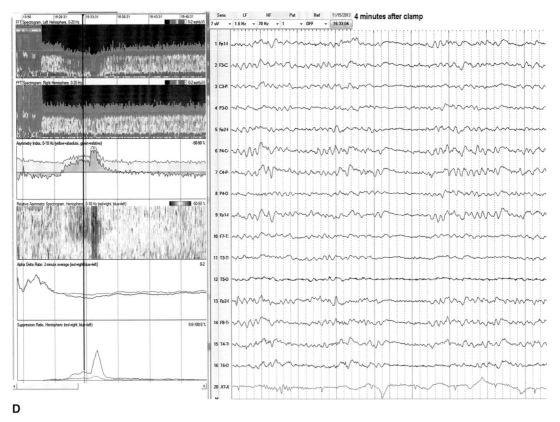

D

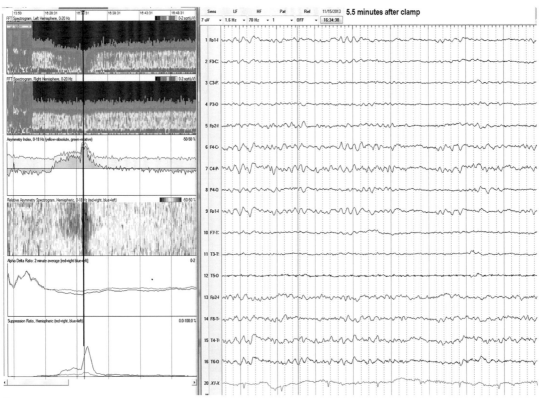

E

FIGURE 13-9 | (*Continued*)

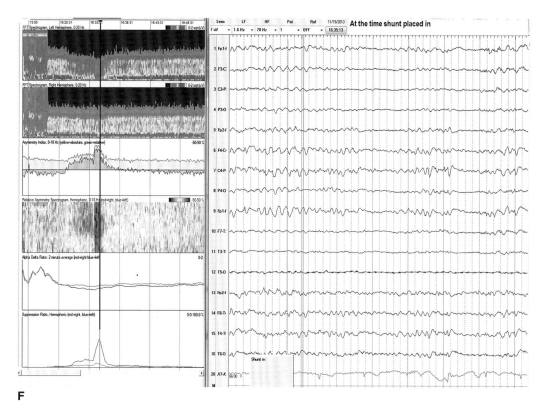

F

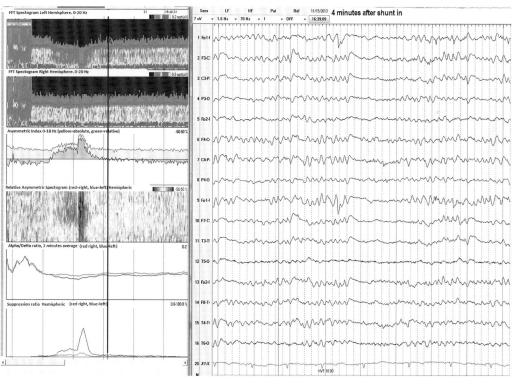

G

FIGURE 13-9 | (Continued)

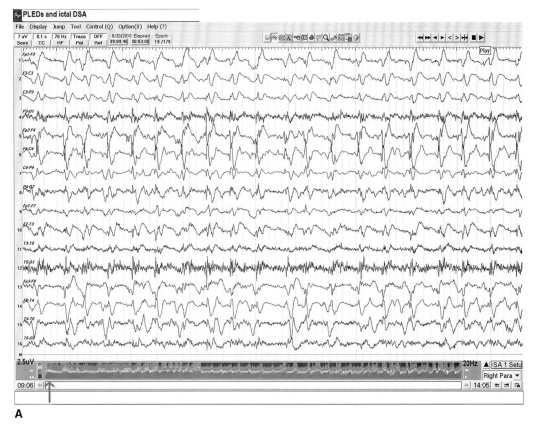

A

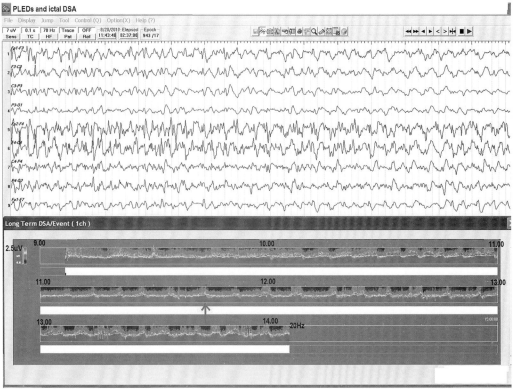

B

FIGURE 13-10 | This is Case 1 patient. With the start of the monitoring (time for this EEG sample is indicated by *arrow*), EEG showed right > left periodically recurring spike discharges (PLEDs/LPD) **(A)**. The DSA of 5 hours' time span later showed cyclic power changes. The details of these cyclic changes are better viewed by expanding time scale to 2 hours per line **(B)**, which revealed there was gradual increase of power and at the peak (indicated by *arrow*), EEG showed electrographic ictal discharges with recurrent polyspike wave involving right frontal region. Subsequent DSA showed stable pattern corresponding to PLED/LPD* as an interictal pattern and no ictal event was recorded for this 2-hour segment **(C)**. DSA was helpful to real that the cyclic ictal events varied in the intensity and duration and also occurred not exactly the same intervals. Also, DSA revealed the overall sequences of EEG changes against time.

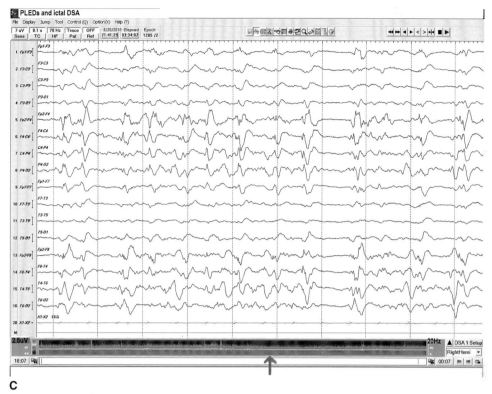

C

FIGURE 13-10 | (Continued)

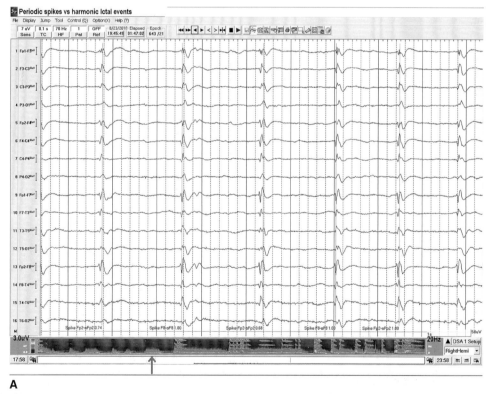

A

FIGURE 13-11 | This is Case 2 patient. During early phase of monitoring, EEG at the time indicated by *arrow* showed episode of diffuse periodic sharp discharges (GPD*) coinciding with some increase of delta slow-wave power shown in DSA. (**A:** this and subsequent figures represent DSAs of 6 hours' time span.) This was followed by the decreased power when EEG showed burst suppression pattern with 1 to 2 seconds theta bursts followed by suppression periods of 1 to 3 seconds (**B**). About 2 hours after the start of monitoring, there were sudden changes in DSA profile showing three distinct frequency bands in addition to the delta band frequency. These three bands corresponded to sudden occurrence of 6-Hz spikes in the right temporal region spreading to the parasagittal electrodes that appeared independently from diffuse frontal dominant sharp and spike waves (**C**). Apparently, 6-Hz fixed frequency spikes created additional harmonic responses at 12 and 18 Hz due to their consistent and fixed frequency throughout the event. Some of these are 6-Hz spikes. This DSA clarified the presence of three different types EEG changes.

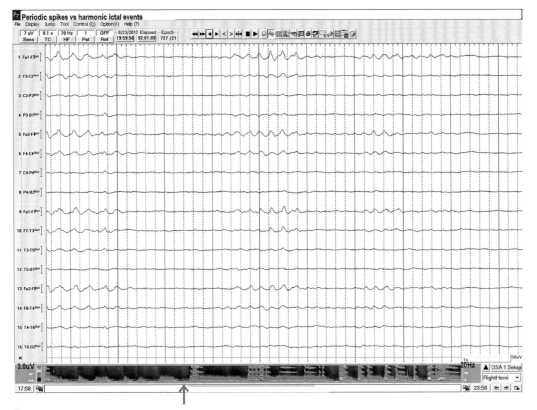

B

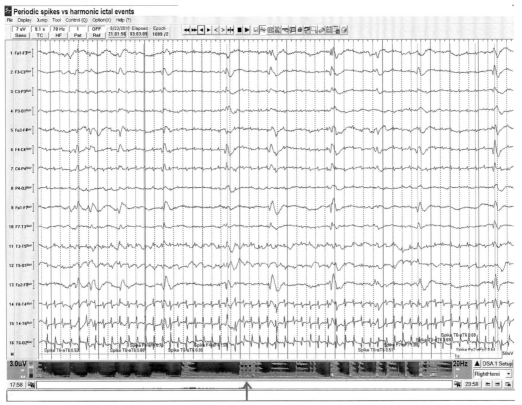

C

FIGURE 13-11 | (Continued)

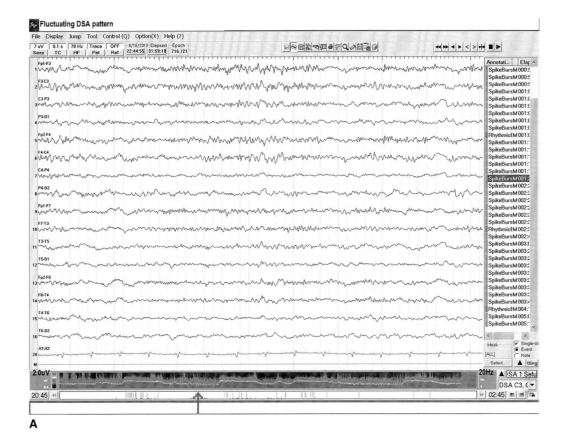

A

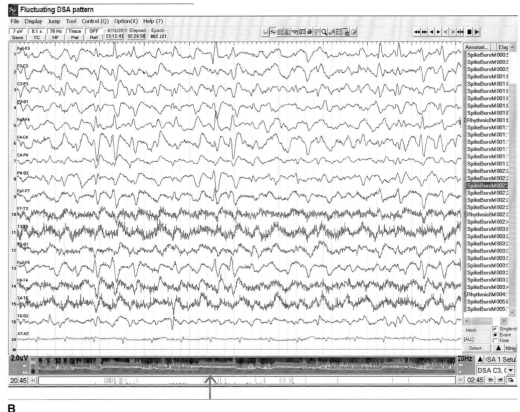

B

FIGURE 13-12 | **(A)** This is a Case 3 patient. When the patient was quiet without muscle tone artifacts, EEG showed diffuse delta with superimposed beta/alpha activities without any paroxysmal activity. **(B)** The *arrow* indicates at the time of this EEG sample was depicted). Whenever the patient was aroused spontaneously or by others, EEG started to show generalized semirhythmic triphasic bursts along with increased muscle artifacts (SIRPID). DSA showed increased power with each SIRPID episodes. Within 2 hours epoch, DSA showed 4 SIRPID episodes.

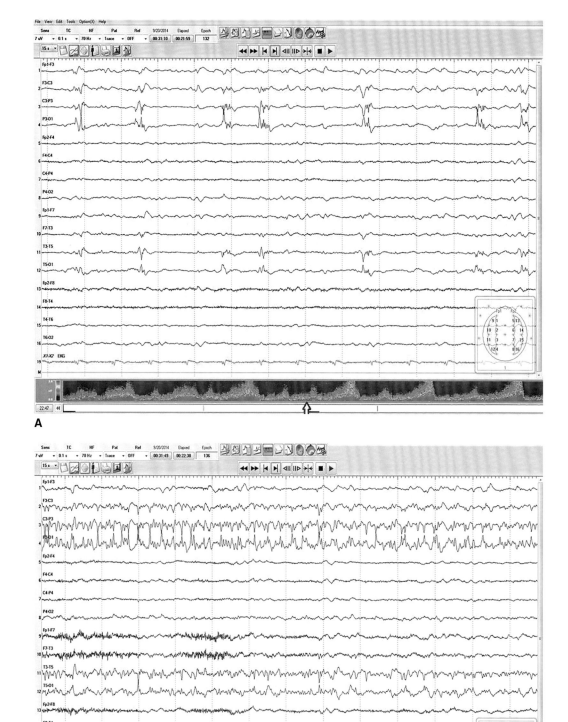

FIGURE 13-13 | This is a Case 4 patient. This EEG showed repetitive nonperiodic spikes followed by small beta activity arising from left posterior head region **(A)**. (This EEG sample was taken at the time indicated by *arrow* in DSA.) When DSA showed increased power including fast-frequency activity **(B)**, this corresponded with repetitive spikes mixed with beta activity from the left parietal region, the same location as of interictal discharges. This was nonconvulsive ictal event. In another occasion, there was greater and longer-lasting power increase than the event shown in **B**. This corresponded with convulsive seizure **(C)**; rhythmic muscle twitch artifacts occurred in synchronous with spike-wave bursts (Video 13-10A and B). By glance at DSA, it becomes evident that the smaller power (shown by *circle*) and larger power (shown by *rectangular box*) increases correspond with nonconvulsive and convulsive seizures, respectively.

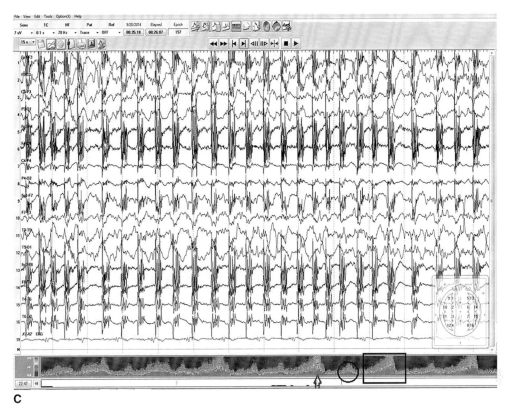

C

FIGURE 13-13 | (*Continued*)

clinical change (Fig. 13-13B). When this nonconvulsive ictal pattern prolonged, the discharges became more widely spread and the patient showed mouth/face twitching (Fig. 13-13C, Video 13-10B). DSA (4 hours) showed intermittent episodes of increased power (greater increase of slower frequency activity). There were small and larger peaks, which corresponded with nonconvulsive and convulsive seizures, respectively. Also, DSA showed each seizure occurred with gradual increase of power (spikes and slow waves) before ictal event. A total of 7 "large" and 6 "small" seizures were evident by DSA.

Case No. 5: A 68-year-old female underwent aortic valve replacement surgery and the procedure was complicated by circulatory arrest. EEG on the first day after surgery showed diffuse delta–theta slowing with slightly higher amplitude on the left hemisphere. Day 2 EEG started to show recurrent electrographic ictal events (Fig. 13-14A). These events occurred periodically with remarkably regular intervals with every 6 to 7 minutes as shown in DSA. In between ictal events, EEG showed diffuse delta–theta slowing and

some sharp transients from left hemisphere (Fig. 13-14B). All seizures were alike with stereotyped evolution. A total of 37 seizures were recorded during this 4-hour segment. Detailed evolution of the ictal event is shown in Video 13-11.

Case No. 6: Patient was a 61-year-old female with a past medical history of end-stage liver disease with cirrhosis secondary to hepatitis C. She presented with acute mental status change and generalized tonic–clonic convulsions. By the time CCEEG started, she was in comatose state. CCEEG showed recurrent episodes of electrographic ictal events arising from either left or right hemisphere independently. Most of the ictal events from left and right hemispheres occurred alternately or partially overlapped each other. Each ictal event lasted 4 to 5 minutes. The sequence of ictal events represented by beta activity from each hemisphere is well demonstrated by qEEG application. Detailed evolution of ictal events are shown in Video 13-12.

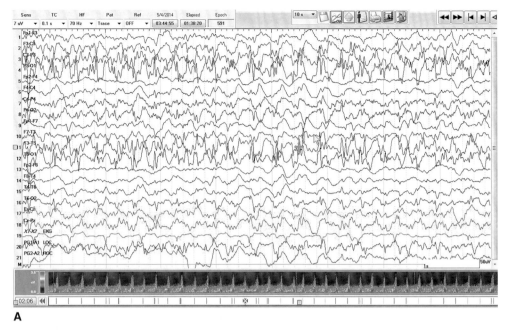

A

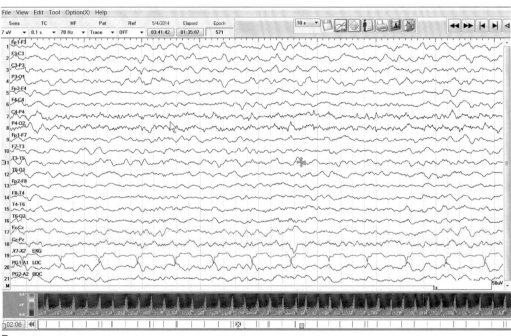

B

FIGURE 13-14 │ This is Case 5 patient. The EEG **(A)** is depicted at the middle of ictal event showing rhythmic bursts of polyspike waves from left hemisphere, maximum at parietal and posterior–temporal region. This EEG sample was taken at the peak of highest power in DSA (shown at *red star* mark) **(A)**. In between the ictal events **(B)**, EEG showed diffuse theta–delta slowing with slightly greater amplitude in the left hemisphere and some interspersed broad sharp transients from left parasagittal or temporal region. This EEG sample was taken at the time of lower power in DSA (shown by *red star* mark). A total of 37 ictal events were recorded within this 4 hours' segment. Video 13-11 shows detailed evolution of seizure event.

ACNS Standardized Critical Care EEG Terminology: 2012 version
Reference Chart

Main term 1	Main term 2	Plus (+) Modifier
G Generalized - Optional: Specify frontally, midline or occipitally predominant **L** Lateralized - Optional: Specify unilateral or bilateral asymmetric - Optional: Specify lobe(s) most involved or hemispheric **BI** Bilateral Independent - Optional: Specify symmetric or asymmetric - Optional: Specify lobe(s) most involved or hemispheric **Mf** Multifocal - Optional: Specify symmetric or asymmetric - Optional: Specify lobe(s) most involved or hemispheric	**PD** Periodic Discharges **RDA** Rhythmic Delta Activity **SW** Rhythmic Spike and Wave OR Rhythmic Sharp and Slow Wave OR Rhythmic Polyspike and Wave	**No +** **+F** Superimposed fast activity–applies to PD or RDA only **+R** Superimposed rhythmic activity–applies to PD only **+S** Superimposed sharp waves or spikes, or sharply contoured–applies to RDA only **+FR** If both subtypes apply–applies to PD only **+FS** If both subtypes apply–applies to RDA only

Major modifiers

Prevalence	Duration	Frequency	Phases[1]	Sharpness[2]	Absolute Amplitude	Relative Amplitude[3]	Polarity[2]	Stimulus Induced	Evolution[4]
Continuous ≥90%	Very long ≥1 h	≥4/s	>3	Spiky <70 ms	High ≥200 µV	>2	Negative	SI *Stimulus Induced*	Evolving
		3.5/s	3					Sp *Spontaneous only*	Fluctuating
Abundant 50%–89%	Long 5–59 min	3/s		Sharp 70–200 ms	Medium 50–199 µV	≤2	Positive		
		2.5/s	2						Static
Frequent 10%–49%	Intermediate duration 1–4.9 min	2/s	1	Sharply contoured >200 ms	Low 20–49 µV		Dipole	Unk *Unknown*	
		1.5/s							
Occasional 1%–9%	Brief 10–59 s	1/s			Very low <20 µV		Unclear		
		0.5/s		Blunt >200 ms					
Rare <1%	Very brief <10 s	<0.5/s							

Minor modifiers

Onset	Triphasic[5]	Lag
Sudden ≤3 s	Yes	A-P Anterior-Posterior
Gradual >3 s	No	P-A Posterior-Anterior
		No

NOTE 1: Applies to PD and and SW only, including the slow wave of the SW complex
NOTE 2: Applies to the predominant phase of PD and the spike or sharp component of SW only
NOTE 3: Applies to PD only
NOTE 4: Refers to frequency, location or morphology
NOTE 5: Applies to PD or SW only

Sporadic Epileptiform Discharges

Prevalence
Abundant ≥1/10 s
Frequent 1/min–1/10 s
Occasional 1/h–1/min
Rare <1/h

Background

Symmetry	Breach effect	PDR	Background EEG frequency	AP Gradient	Variability	Reactivity	Voltage	Stage II Sleep Transients	Continuity
Symmetric	Present	Present Specify frequency	Delta	Present	Present	Present	Normal ≥20 µV	Present and normal	Continuous
Mild asymmetry ≤50% Amp. 0.5–1/s Freq.	Absent	Absent	Theta	Absent	Absent	SIRPIDs only	Low 10–20 µV	Present but abnormal	Nearly continuous: ≤10% periods of suppression (<10 µV) or attenuation (≥10 µV but <50% of background voltage)
Marked asymmetry >50% Amp. >1/s Freq.	Unclear		≥Alpha	Reverse	Unclear	Absent	Suppressed <10 µV	Absent	Discontinuous: 10–49% periods of suppression or attenuation
						Unclear			Burst-suppression or Burst-attenuation: 50–99% periods of suppression or attenuation
									Suppression

(Hirsch LJ, Roche SM, Gaspard N, et al. American Clinical Neurophysiology Society's Standardized Critical Care EEG Terminology: 2012 version. *J Clin Neurophysiol* 2013;30:1–27 Wolters Kluwer/Lippincott Williams & Wilkins with permission)

References

1. Hirsch LJ, LaRoche SM, Gaspard N, et al. American Clinical Neurophysiology Society's standardized critical care EEG terminology: 2012 version. *J Clin Neurophysiol* 2013;30(1):1–27.

2. Jirsch J, Hirsch LJ. Nonconvulsive seizures: Developing a rational approach to the diagnosis and management in the critically ill population. *Clin Neurophysiol* 2007;180:1660–1670.

3. Lowenstein DH, Aminoff MJ. Clinical and EEG features of status epilepticus in comatose patients. *Neurology* 1992;42:100–104.

4. Kaplan PW. Behavioral manifestations of nonconvulsive status epilepticus. *Epilepsy Behav* 2002;3:122–139.

5. Claassen J, Hirsch LJ, Kreiter KT, et al. Quantitative continuous EEG for detecting delayed cerebral ischemia in patients with poor-grade subarachnoid hemorrhage. *Clin Neurophysiol* 2004;115(12):2699–2710.

6. Vaspa PM, Nuwer MR, Juhasz C, et al. Early detection of vasospasms after acute subarachnoid hemorrhage using continuous EEG ICU monitoring. *Electroencephalogr Clin Neurophysiol* 1997;103:607–615.

7. Young GB, Wang JT, Connolly JF. Prognostic determination in anoxic-ischemic and traumatic encephalopathies. *J Clin Neurophysiol* 2004;21:379–390.

8. Stevens RD, Sutter R. Prognosis in severe brain injury. *Crit Care Med* 2013;41:1104–1123.

9. Doenicke AW, Kugler J, Kochs E, et al. Narcotrend monitor and the electroencephalogram in propofol-induced sedation. *Anesth Analg* 2007;105:982–992.

10. Mirski MA, Hemstreet MK. Critical care sedation for neuroscience patients. *J Neurol Sci* 2007;261:16–34.

11. Sandroni C, Cavallaro F, Callaway CW, et al. Predictors of poor neurological outcome in adult comatose survivors of cardiac arrest: A systematic review and meta-analysis. Part 1: Patients not treated with therapeutic hypothermia. *Resuscitation* 2013;85:1310–1323.

12. Sandroni C, Cavallaro F, Callaway CW, et al. Predictors of poor neurological outcome in adult comatose survivors of cardiac arrest: A systematic review and meta-analysis. Part 2: Patients treated with therapeutic hypothermia. *Resuscitation* 2013;85:1324–1338.

13. Foreman B, Claassen J, Abou Khaled KJ, et al. Generalized periodic discharges in the critically ill: A case–control study of 200 patients. *Neurology* 2012;79:1951–1960.

14. Ong C, Gilmore E, Claassen J, et al. Impact of prolonged periodic epileptiform discharges on coma prognosis. *Neurocrit Care* 2012;17:39–44.

15. Gaspard N, Manganas L, Rampal N, et al. Similarity of lateralized rhythmic delta activity to periodic lateralized epileptiform discharges in critically ill patients. *JAMA Neurol* 2013;70:343–349.

16. Jordan K. Nonconvulsive status epilepticus in acute brain injury. *J Clin Neurophysiol* 1999;16:332–340.

17. Young GB, Jordan KG, Doig GS. An assessment of nonconvulsive seizures in the intensive care unit using continuous EEG monitoring: An investigation of variables associated with mortality. *Neurology* 1996;47:83–89.

18. Trinka E, Cook H, Hesdorffer D, et al. A definition and classification of status epileptics-report of ILAE task force of status epileptics. *Epilepsia* 2015;56(10):15–23.

19. Tsuchida TN, Wusthoff CJ, Shellhaas RA, et al. American Clinical Neurophysiology Society standardized EEG terminology categorization for the description of continuous EEG monitoring in neonates: Report for the American Clinical Neurophysiology Society Critical Care Monitoring Committee. *J Clin Neurophysiol* 2013;30:161–173.

20. Towne AR, Waterhouse EJ, Boggs JC, et al. Prevalence of nonconvulsive status epilepticus in comatose patients. *Neurology* 2000;54:340–345.

21. Jette N, Claassen J, Emerson RG, et al. Frequency and predictors of nonconvulsive seizures during continuous electroencephalographic monitoring in critically ill children. *Arch Neurol* 2006;63:1750–1755.

22. Claassen J, Mayer SA, Kowalski RG, et al. Detection of electrographic seizures with continuous EEG monitoring in critically ill patients. *Neurology* 2004;62:1743–1748.

23. Privitera M, Hoffman M, Moore JL, Jester D. EEG detection of nontonic-clonic status epilepticus in patients with altered consciousness. *Epilepsy Res* 1994;18:155–166.

24. DeLorenzo RJ, Waterhouse EJ, Towne AR, et al. Persistent nonconvulsive status epilepticus after the control of convulsive status epilepticus. *Epilepsia* 1998;39:833–840.

25. Krumholz A, Stern BJ, Weiss HD. Outcome from coma after cardiopulmonary resuscitation: Relation to seizures and myoclonus. *Neurology* 1988;38:401–405.

26. Wright WL, Geocadin RC. Postresuscitative intensive care: Neuroprotective strategies after cardiac arrest. *Semin Neurol* 2006;26:396–402.

27. Rossetti AO, Logroscino G, Liaudet L, et al. Status epilepticus: An independent outcome predictor after cerebral anoxia. *Neurology* 2007;69:255–260.

28. Oddo M, Carrera E, Claassen J, et al. Continuous electroencephalography in the medical intensive care unit. *Crit Care Med* 2009;35:2051–2056.

29. Foy PM, Copeland GP, Shaw MD. The incidence of postoperative seizures. *Acta Neurochir (Wien)* 1981;55:253–264.

30. Kvam DA, Loftus CM, Copeland B, Quest DO. Seizures during the immediate postoperative period. *Neurosurgery* 1983;12:14–17.

31. Baker CJ, Prestigiacomo CJ, Solomon RA. Short-term perioperative anticonvulsant prophylaxis for the surgical treatment of low-risk patients with intracranial aneurysms. *Neurosurgery* 1995;37:863–870.

32. Annegers JF, Grabow JD, Groover RV, et al. Seizures after head trauma: A population study. *Neurology* 1980;30:683–689.

33. Temkin NR, Dikmen SS, Wilensky AJ, et al. A randomized, double-blind study of phenytoin for the prevention of post-traumatic seizures. *N Engl J Med* 1990;323:497–502.

34. Lee S, Lui T, Wong C, et al. Early seizures after moderate closed head injury. *Acta Neurochir* 1995;137:151–154.

35. Bladin CF, Alexandrov AV, Bellavance A, et al. Seizures after stroke: A prospective multicenter study. *Arch Neurol* 2000;57:1617–1622.

36. Claassen J, Jette N, Chum F, et al. Electrographic seizures and periodic discharges after intracerebral hemorrhage. *Neurology* 2007;69:1356–1365.

37. Szaflarski JP, Rackley AY, Kleindorfer DO, et al. Incidence of seizures in the acute phase of stroke: A population-based study. *Epilepsia* 2008;49:974–981.

38. Camilo O, Goldstein LB. Seizures and epilepsy after ischemic stroke. *Stroke* 2004;35:1769–1775.

39. Butzkueven H, Evans AH, Pitman A, et al. Onset seizures independently predict poor outcome after subarachnoid hemorrhage. *Neurology* 2000;55:1315–1320.

40. Rhoney DH, Tipps LB, Murry KR, et al. Anticonvulsant prophylaxis and timing of seizures after aneurysmal subarachnoid hemorrhage. *Neurology* 2000;55:258–265.

41. Hosain SA, Solomon GE, Kobylarzx EJ. Electroencephalographic patterns in unresponsive pediatric patients. *Pediatr Neurol* 2005;32:162–165.

42. Tay SK, Hirsch LJ, Leary L, et al. Nonconvulsive status epilepticus in children: Clinical and EEG characteristics. *Epilepsia* 2006;47:1504–1509.

43. Abend NS, Gutierrez-Colina AM, Topjian AA, et al. Nonconvulsive seizures are common in critically ill children. *Neurology* 2011;76:1071–1077.

44. Abend NS, Amdt DH, Carpenter JL, et al. Electrographic seizures in pediatric ICU patients: Cohort study of risk factors and mortality. *Neurology* 2013;81:383–391.

45. Pandian JD, Cascino GD, So EL, et al. Digital video-electroencephalographic monitoring in the neurological-neurosurgical intensive care unit: Clinical features and outcome. *Arch Neurol* 2004;61:1090–1094.

46. Abend NS, Douglas DJ, Hahn CD, et al. Use of EEG monitoring and management of non-convulsive seizures in critically ill patients: A survey of neurologists. *Neurocrit Care* 2010;12:382–389.

47. Shahwan A, Bailey C, Shekerdemian L, Harvey AS. The prevalence of seizures in comatose children in the pediatric intensive care unit: A prospective video EEG study. *Epilepsia* 2010;51:1198–1204.

48. Westover MB, Shasi MM, Bianchi MT, et al. The probability of seizures during EEG monitoring in critically ill adults. *Clin Neurophysiol* 2014;126:463–471.

49. Jordan KG. Nonconvulsive seizures (NCS) and nonconvulsive status epilepticus (NCSE) detected by continuous EEG monitoring in neuro ICU. *Neurology* 1992;42:194–195.

50. Crepeau AZ, Fugate JE, Mandrekar J, et al. Value analysis of continuous EEG in patients during therapeutic hypothermia after cardiac arrest. *Resuscitation* 2014;85:785–789

51. Martz GU, Hucek C, Quigg M. Sixty day continuous use of subdermal wire electrodes for EEG monitoring during treatment of status epilepticus. *Neurocrit Care* 2009;11:223–227.

52. Kull II, Emerson RG. Continuous EEG monitoring in the intensive care unit: Technical and staffing considerations. *J Clin Neurophysiol* 2005;22:107–118.

53. Fountain NB, Waldman WA. Effects of benzodiazepines on triphasic waves: Implications for nonconvulsive status epilepticus. *J Clin Neurophysiol* 2001;18:345–352.

54. Kaplan PW. EEG criteria for nonconvulsive status epileptics. *Epilepsia* 2007;48(Suppl 8):39–41.

55. Reiher J, Rivest J, Grand Maison F, Leduc CP. Periodic lateralized epileptiform discharges with transitional rhythmic discharges: Association with seizures. *Electroencephalogr Clin Neurophysiol* 1991;78:12–17

56. Lee JW. EEG in the ICU: What should one treat, what not? *Epilptologie* 2012;29:210–217.

57. Zeiter SR, Turtzo LC, Kaplan PW. SPECT-negative SIRPID argues against treatment as seizure. *J Clin Neurophysiol* 2011;28:493–496.

58. Shewmom DA. What is a neonatal seizure? Problems in definition and quantification for investigative and clinical purposes. *J Clin Neurophysiol* 1990;7:315–368.

59. Oliveira AJ, Nunes ML, Haertel LM, et al. Duration of rhythmic EEG patterns in neonates; new evidence for clinical and prognostic significance of brief rhythmic discharges. *Clin Neurophysiol* 2000;111:1646–1653.

60. Nagarajan L, Palumbo L, Ghosh S. Brief electroencephalography rhythmic discharges (BERDs) in the neonate with seizures: Their significance and prognostic implications. *J Child Neurol* 2011;26(12):1529–1533.

61. Yoo JY, Rampal N, Petroff OA, et al. Brief potentially ictal rhythmic discharges in critically ill adults. *JAMA Neurol* 2014;71(4):454–462.

62. Bergamasco B, Bergamini L, Doriguzzi T, et al. EEG sleep patterns as a prognostic criterion in post-traumatic coma. *Electroencephalogr Clin Neurophysiol* 1968;24:374–377.

63. Bricolo A, Turella G, Ore GD, et al. A proposal for the EEG evaluation of acute traumatic coma in neurosurgical practice. *Electroencephalogr Clin Neurophysiol* 1973;34:789.

64. Bricolo A, Turazzi S, Faccioli F. Combined clinical and EEG examinations for assessment of severity of acute head injuries: Electrophysiological methods. *Acta Neurochir Suppl* 1979;28:35–39.

65. Astrup J, Siesjö BK, Symon L. Thresholds in cerebral ischemia—The ischemic penumbra. *Stroke* 1981;12:723–725.

66. Baron JC. Perfusion thresholds in human cerebral ischemia: Historical perspective and therapeutic implications. *Cerebrovasc Dis* 2001;11:2–8.

67. Weir B, Grace M, Hansen J, Rothberg C. Time course of vasospasm in man. *J Neurosurg* 1978;48:173–178.

68. Kirmani JF, Qureshi AI, Hanel RA, et al. Silent cerebral infarction in poor-grade patients with subarachnoid hemorrhage. *Neurology* 2002;58:159.

69. Vespa PM, Nuwer MR, Juhasz C, et al. Early detection of vasospasm after acute subarachnoid hemorrhage using continuous EEG ICU monitoring. *Electroencephalogr Clin Neurophysiol* 1997;103:607–615.

70. Labar DR, Fisch BJ, Pedley TA, et al. Quantitative EEG monitoring for patients with subarachnoid hemorrhage. *Electroencephalogr Clin Neurophysiol* 1991;78:325–332.

71. de Vos CC, van Maarseveen SM, Brouwers PJ, van Putten MJ. Continuous EEG monitoring during thrombolysis in acute hemispheric stroke patients using the brain symmetry index. *J Clin Neurophysiol* 2008;25:77–82.

72. Maynard DE, Jenkinson JL. The cerebral function analyzing monitor. Initial clinical experience, application and further development. *Anesthesia* 1984;39:678–690.

73. Simmons LE, Riker RR, Prato BS, Fraser GL. Assessing sedation during intensive care unit mechanical ventilation with the bispectral index and the sedation-agitation scale. *Crit Care Med* 1999;27:1499–1504.

74. Scheuer MK, Wilson SB. Data analysis for continuous EEG monitoring in the ICU: Seeing the forest and the trees. *J Clin Neurophysiol* 2004;21:353–378.

75. Herman ST, Abend NS, Bleck TP, et al. Consensus statement on continuous EEG in critically ill adults and children, part I: Indication. *J Clin Neurophysiol* 2015;32(2):87–95.

76. Herman ST, Abend NS, Bleck TP, et al. Consensus statement on continuous EEG in critically ill adults and children, part II: Technical specification, and clinical practice. *J Clin Neurophysiol* 2015;32(2):96–108.

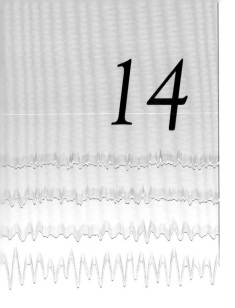

14

Benign EEG Patterns

THORU YAMADA and ELIZABETH MENG

This chapter is devoted to several EEG patterns that are seemingly abnormal because the waveform resembles epileptiform activity, the discharge has an asymmetric distribution, or the rhythmic pattern mimics an ictal (seizure) discharge. Correctly recognizing these variants is important in order to avoid overinterpreting their clinical significance. There may be some controversy and difference of opinion about these patterns, but most are in agreement that they are patterns of normal variants.

14- and 6-Hz Positive Spike Bursts

Historically, *14- and 6-Hz positive spikes* have been the most extensively discussed by many investigators and have created much controversy in regard to their clinical significance. The pattern has a characteristic waveform, frequency, and distribution—comb-shaped positive spikes maximum at the posterior temporal/occipital electrodes with a frequency of 13 to 17 Hz and/or 5 to 7 Hz, mostly consisting of 14 Hz and/or 6 Hz. They occur predominately in light sleep. The pattern may appear as a 14- and 6-Hz positive spike complex (Fig. 14-1), 14-Hz positive spikes alone (Fig. 14-2), or 6-Hz positive spikes alone (Fig. 14-3). The 6-Hz positive spikes tend to appear in early childhood and in adults, while 14-Hz positive spikes are more common in older children and adolescents.[1] The pattern is well visualized with a circumferential montage which includes occipital and posterior temporal electrodes. The pattern is also well demonstrated with an ear reference recording. However, ear reference ipsilateral to the side of the spikes is often active and contamination of the spike discharge results in seemingly "negative" spikes at the frontal region (Fig. 14-4A). An alternative montage is to use the contralateral ear reference, which increases the interelectrode distance and eliminates the contamination (Fig. 14-4B).

Since the discovery of this pattern by Gibbs and Gibbs,[2] who regarded it as the evidence of thalamic and hypothalamic epilepsy, there have been numerous studies correlating 14- and 6-Hz positive spikes with autonomic nervous system dysfunctions and psychiatric and/or behavioral disorders.[3–7] However, the enthusiasm for these clinical correlates faded when it became evident that the pattern was often seen in normal individuals, especially in adolescents.[8,9] One study showed that the incidence of 14- and 6-Hz positive spikes was 40% to 60% in 14- to 16-year-old adolescents.[8] The pattern is rarely seen in individuals before the age of 5 or after the age of 25.

The 14- and 6-Hz positive spike burst can be readily identified because of its characteristic waveform, distribution, and polarity. In some cases, 14- and 6-Hz positive spike bursts precede generalized slow waves, making the complex look abnormal (Fig. 14-5). A more difficult situation may be when the 14- and 6-Hz positive spike bursts precede a negative spike and wave burst. It is debatable if this should be regarded as abnormal.

One interesting clinical correlation of 14- and 6-Hz positive spikes is a high incidence of the discharge in patients with Reye's syndrome[10] (see Fig. 11-17A and B). The discharges appear during the acute coma state and disappear after recovery from coma.[11] Also, 14- and 6-Hz positive bursts have been reported in an adult patient with hepatic coma[12] and children with diverse encephalopathies including Reye's syndrome.[13]

Small Sharp Spikes

Small sharp spikes (SSS) are also known as *benign epileptiform transients of sleep* (BETS). The pattern is characterized by a small, usually less than 50 µV, mono- or diphasic spike of short duration (<50 ms). In a bipolar derivation, it often appears as a small "needle-like" spike (Fig. 14-6A). Recording with an ear reference montage (Fig. 14-6B) will show more widely distributed, often larger amplitude spikes than those recorded with it a bipolar montage. Because of the wide spread and fairly even distribution of the spike, bipolar recording tends to be canceled out, often making it appear to be more focal than if seen in a referential recording. The morphology of SSS may vary from predominantly negative to diphasic or to predominantly positive polarity within the same individual. SSS also tends to shift from side to side (Fig. 14-7A and B). This is essentially a pattern in adulthood with a peak age between 20 and 25 years,[14] and it is extremely rare before the age of 10.

SSS are regarded as a normal pattern, but the differentiation from a genuine epileptiform spike is sometimes difficult. The following points aid in differentiating between the two:

1. Because SSS tends to show a variable morphology and a side-to-side shift, a consistent localization and morphology are likely to indicate epileptiform activity.
2. Since SSS appears only in stage I or II sleep, spikes appearing in the awake state or in deep sleep are more likely to be epileptiform activity.

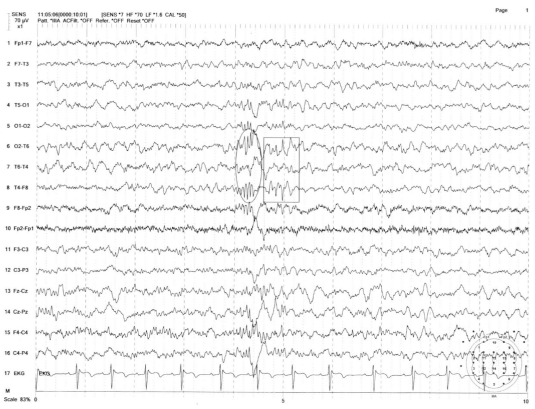

FIGURE 14-1 | An example of 14- and 6-Hz positive spike bursts in an 8-year-old boy. Note positive phase reversal at T6 and T4 electrodes (shown in *oval circle*) and 6-Hz positive spikes (shown in *rectangular box*) with equipotential at T6 and T4.

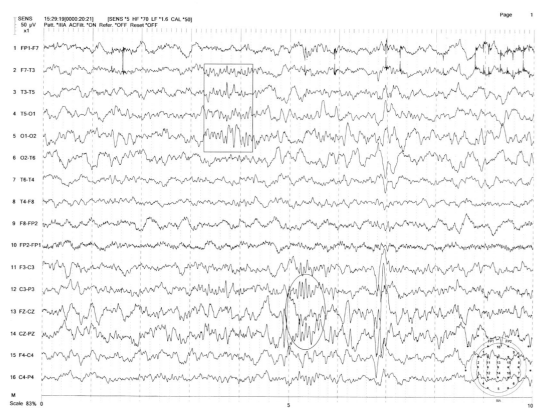

FIGURE 14-2 | An example of 14-Hz positive spikes in a 10-year-old girl. Note the difference of waveform and distribution between positive spikes (shown in *rectangular box*) and sleep spindles (shown in *oval circle*).

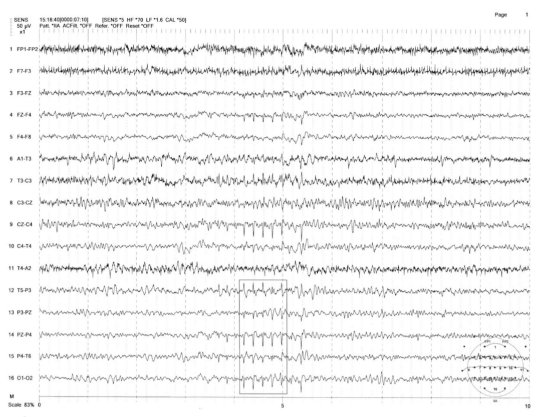

FIGURE 14-3 | An example of 6-Hz positive spikes in a 4-year-old boy (shown in *box*). Note positive phase reversal at P3 electrode.

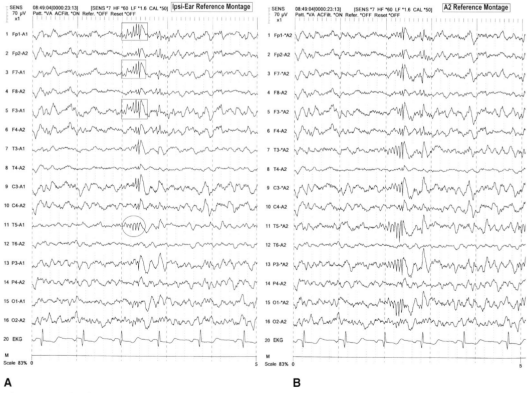

A   **B**

FIGURE 14-4 | An example of 14-Hz positive spikes in a 16-year-old girl, comparing ipsi- and contra-ear (mastoid) referential recordings. The ipsi-ear referential recording shows "up-going" ("negative") spikes at Fp1, F7, and F3 electrodes (shown by *boxes*) and "down-going" (positive) spikes at T5 electrode (shown by *oval circle*) **(A)**. This relationship is not due to dipole distribution of the spike, but instead it is due to ear (A1) reference electrode, which is active (contaminated) with positive polarity, resulting in up-going deflection in anterior electrodes. When all electrodes are referenced to A2 avoiding A1 contamination, this results in true distribution and polarity of positive spikes **(B)**. (**A** and **B** are the same EEG samples.)

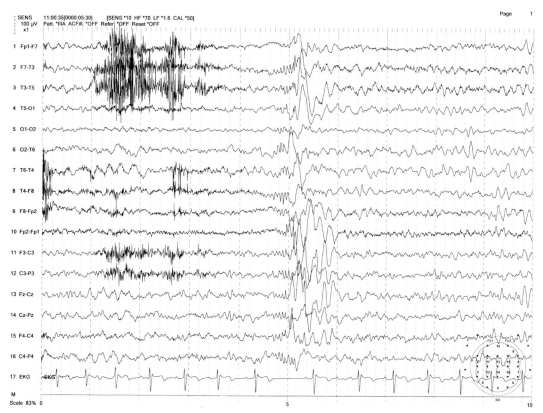

FIGURE 14-5 | An example of 14- and 6-Hz positive spike bursts preceding theta–delta burst in a 15-year-old boy. This resembles a polyspike burst preceding theta–delta activity. One should be cautious not to overinterpret this as an abnormal discharge.

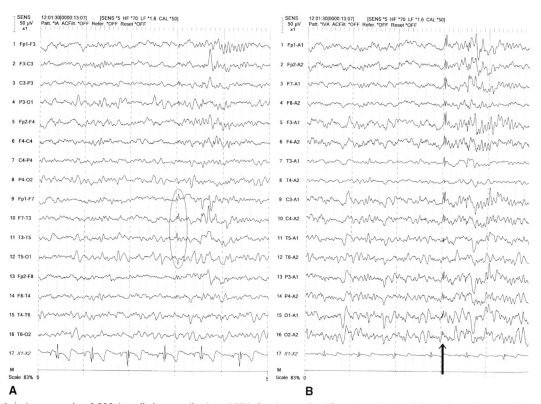

FIGURE 14-6 | An example of SSS (small sharp spikes) or BETS (benign epileptiform transients of sleep) in a 55-year-old man, comparing bipolar and referential recording. The small spike of short duration is localized at the left temporal region in bipolar derivation (shown in *oval circle in* **A**), while the same spike has a much wider distribution in referential recording (shown by *arrow in* **B**). (**A** and **B** are the same EEG samples.)

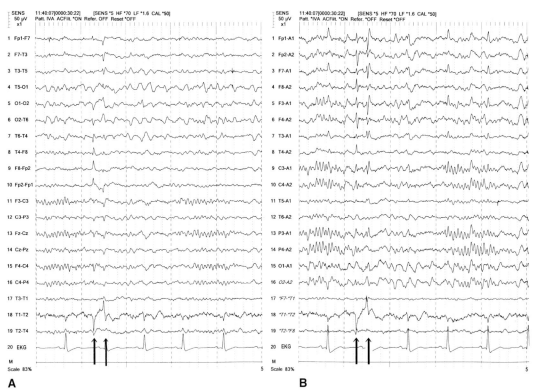

FIGURE 14-7 | Another example of SSS or BETS in a 63-year-old woman showing two small spikes in close sequence, maximum at temporal regions in bipolar recording. Left arrow for left and right for right temporal dominant spikes **(A)**. With referential recording, these two spikes are more widely distributed. Note the difference in morphology between the two spikes with the first one being predominantly negative-positive configuration (*left arrow*) and the second one (*right arrow*) being predominantly positive-negative configuration **(B)**. (**A** and **B** are the same EEG samples.)

3. SSS usually appears as a single transient and does not occur in rhythmic trains; thus, rhythmically recurring spikes are likely abnormal discharges.
4. SSS are not usually followed by a prominent wave. Therefore, a spike associated with a spike-wave complex is likely epileptiform activity.
5. SSS does not disturb the background activity.

It is generally agreed that SSS has no correlation with epilepsy and is a normal pattern,[14–17] though some investigators regard the pattern with a "moderate epileptogenic property."[18,19]

6-Hz Spike and Wave Bursts (Phantom Spike and Wave)

The *6-Hz spike and wave bursts*, also termed "*phantom spike and wave*,"[20] consist of rhythmic spike-wave bursts with a frequency of 5 to 7 Hz, most commonly at 6 Hz, occurring in the parasagittal regions, often maximum at the parietal and occipital electrodes (Fig. 14-8). The morphology of the spike consists of a very sharp deflection of small amplitude and short duration, often resembling a muscle twitch artifact. The bursts usually last 1 to 2 seconds and appear most commonly in awake, drowsiness, and light sleep. The incidence of this pattern is relatively rare and estimated to be seen in 2% of the population, both adolescents and adults. In some occasions, 6-Hz spike-wave bursts resemble 6-Hz positive spikes, and the differentiation between the two can be difficult.[21] The clinical significance of this pattern is still disputed. Some studies found a relatively high (50% to 60%) correlation with a seizure

history,[1,22] while others did not.[23,24] The general consensus is that this pattern is a normal variant and not a reliable indicator of seizure.

Two types of 6-Hz spike-wave bursts have been proposed by Hughes[25] as an aid in determining clinical correlates. He used the acronyms of *FOLD* and *WHAM*. FOLD stands for **F**emale, **O**ccipital dominant, **L**ow amplitude, and **D**rowsiness. WHAM stands for **W**ake, **H**igh amplitude, and **A**nterior dominant in **M**ale (Fig. 14-9). FOLD is considered to be a nonspecific and benign variant, while WHAM is more likely associated with a seizure history.

Wicket Spikes

Wicket spikes resemble mu or wicket rhythm seen in the central region, but they occur in the temporal electrodes. Wicket spikes usually appear as brief (<1 second) bursts at 6 to 11 Hz in a crescendo–decrescendo form of sharply contoured alpha or sharp activity.[26] The discharges occur bilaterally independently, arising from the left or right temporal region, usually maximum at the midtemporal electrode (Figs. 14-10 and 14-11). They are predominantly seen in adults older than 50 years. The clinical significance is minor or at best uncertain and is generally regarded as a normal variant. Like temporal slow waves of the elderly (see "Temporal Slow Waves in the Elderly," Chapter 12; see also Fig. 12-18), a possible relationship with cerebrovascular disease has been proposed.[27]

When a wicket spike appears as a single transient instead of a train of discharges, it may be difficult to differentiate wicket spikes from epileptiform spikes. The absence of slow waves

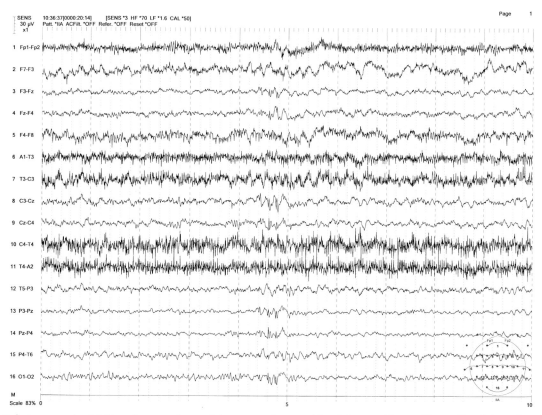

FIGURE 14-8 | An example of 6-Hz spike-wave bursts (phantom spike wave) in a 32-year-old man. Note spike of short duration followed by small wave with frequency close to 6 Hz distributed diffusely but with parietal dominance.

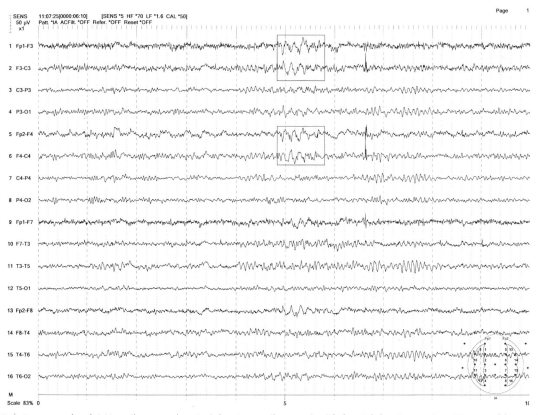

FIGURE 14-9 | An example of 6-Hz spike-wave bursts (phantom spike wave) with frontal dominance in a 45-year-old man. Note frontal dominant small spike-wave with frequency close to 6 Hz (shown in *boxes*).

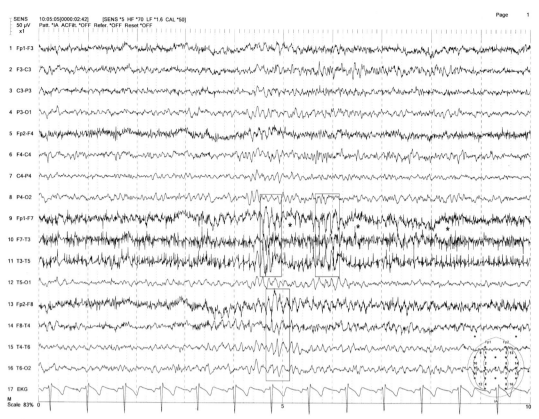

FIGURE 14-10 | An example of wicket spikes in a 76-year-old man. The spikes occur independently from both temporal regions, maximum at the mid or anterior temporal electrodes (shown by *boxes*). Also note delta transients from the left temporal region (marked by ***), which are temporal slow of elderly, a nonspecific finding.

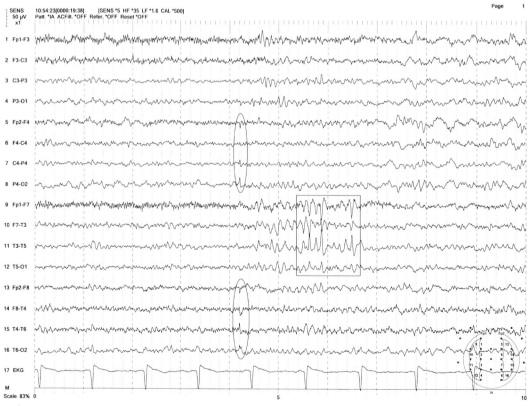

FIGURE 14-11 | An example of wicket spikes in a 65-year-old man. This EEG sample shows wicket spikes (shown in *box*) and also SSS (shown in *ovals*). Note the difference in distribution. Wicket spikes are restricted to temporal region, while SSS are more widely distributed.

following and a preserved background favor wicket spikes. An equal rise and decay of the sharp waveform also favors a wicket spike (epileptiform sharp activity often shows a steep rise or decay; see "Transients and Bursts," Chapter 6; Fig. 6-5C; see also Fig. 8-21).

Rhythmic Midtemporal Theta of Drowsiness

Rhythmic midtemporal theta of drowsiness (RMTD) was earlier termed "*psychomotor variant*"[1,2] because it resembles the rhythmic ictal activity of a "psychomotor" seizure (temporal lobe seizure), but the use of this term has been discouraged because the pattern has no relation with the temporal lobe or psychomotor seizures.[28] The preferred term is now *rhythmic midtemporal theta of drowsiness* or *RMTD*. The pattern consists of rhythmic 5- to 7-Hz theta bursts, usually maximum at midtemporal electrodes, which sometimes spread widely to the parasagittal region (Fig. 14-12). The waveform often has a notched peak on the rising phase (Fig. 14-13). The rhythmic train lasts from 1 to 2 seconds to as long as 1 min. Prolonged runs of RMTD resemble ictal discharges, but characteristic monorhythmic patterns without progressively changing frequency and/or amplitude often seen in true ictal events can distinguish them.

Although some authors have related RMTD to personality disorder and autonomic nervous system dysfunction,[1,29,30] it is now generally accepted that this is a pattern of normal variants and, at best, a nonspecific finding having no clinical significance with seizure or other neurological symptoms.[23]

Midline Theta Rhythm

Midline theta rhythm was originally described by Ciganek[31] who thought it was related to temporal lobe epilepsy. The discharge consists of a focal theta rhythm at 5 to 7 Hz, maximum in the midline region at Cz or Fz (Fig. 14-14). It appears during wakefulness and drowsiness. The pattern is now considered to be a nonspecific variant of normal rhythm.[32]

Subclinical Rhythmic Electrographic Discharge in Adults

Subclinical rhythmic electrographic discharge in adults (SREDA) is an exceedingly rare pattern with an incidence of only 0.02% to 0.045% of routine EEG studies[33] and is mainly seen in people older than 50 years. This pattern was originally described by Naquet et al.,[34] and the discharge was thought to be facilitated by temporary hypoxic conditions. However, later studies from the Mayo group have indicated that SREDA represents a benign EEG pattern that has little or no diagnostic significance,[35–37] despite its resemblance to a progressively changing ictal discharge. The pattern occurs mainly in the waking state or in light drowsiness and is sometimes precipitated by hyperventilation. There are two types of onset; one is an abrupt onset of widespread repetitive monorhythmic sharp discharges, and the other is a gradual onset starting with a few single sharp discharges (Fig. 14-15A–D). This is followed by rhythmic delta and then by sharply contoured theta activity. The sequence of progressive change tends to be slow to fast

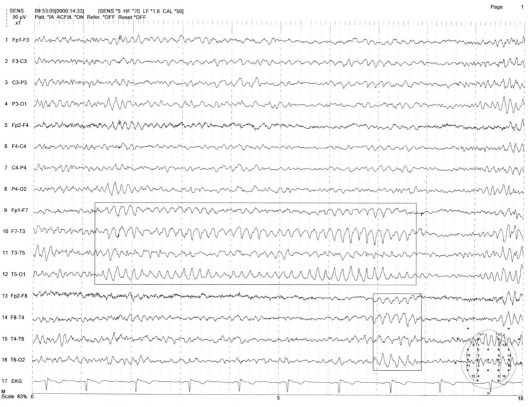

FIGURE 14-12 | An example of RMTD (rhythmic temporal theta of drowsiness) in a 32-year-old woman. Note rhythmic, sharply contoured theta activity arising independently from the left and right temporal regions seen during drowsiness (shown in *boxes*).

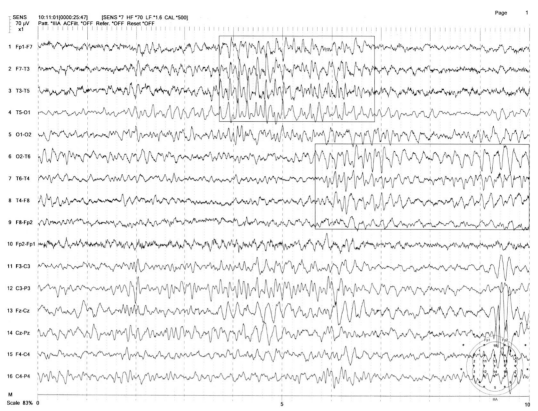

FIGURE 14-13 | An example of RMTD in a 45-year-old woman. Note rhythmic sharp theta with notched wave configuration arising from left and right temporal region independently seen during sleep (shown in *boxes*).

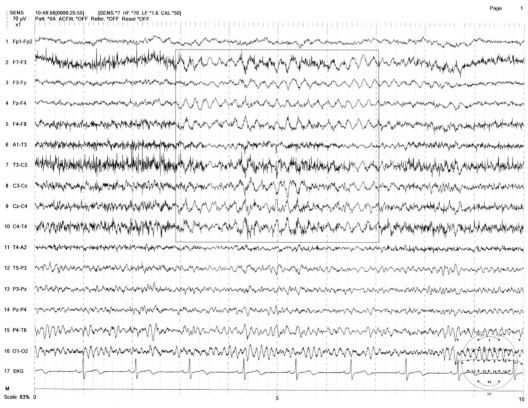

FIGURE 14-14 | An example of midline theta in a 36-year-old man. Note 4.5-Hz rhythmic theta bursts maximum at midline electrodes seen in awake state (shown in *box*).

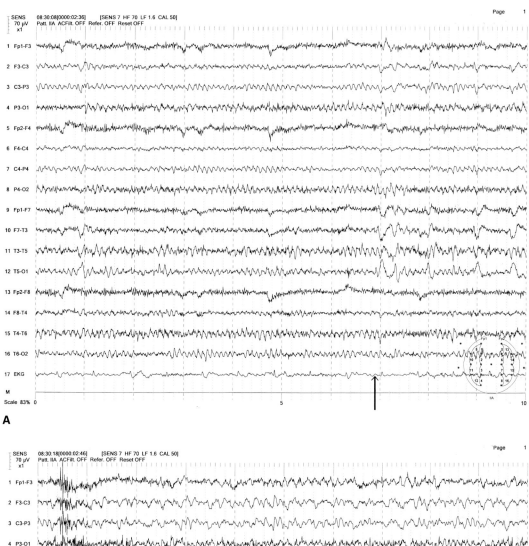

A

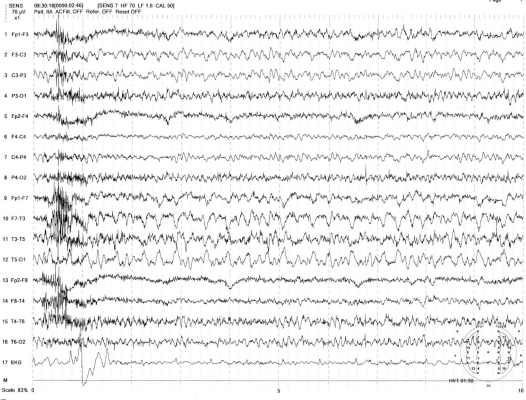

B

FIGURE 14-15 | An example of SREDA (subclinical rhythmic electrographic discharges in adult) in a 45-year-old woman. The episode started shortly after hyperventilation, with the onset of repetitive, broad, and sharp discharges from left temporal region. The *arrow* indicates the onset of the discharges **(A)**. This was followed by semirhythmic sharply contoured theta **(B)** progressively changing to faster frequency **(C)**. The episode abruptly ended without any postictal slowing **(D)**. The patient was asymptomatic throughout.

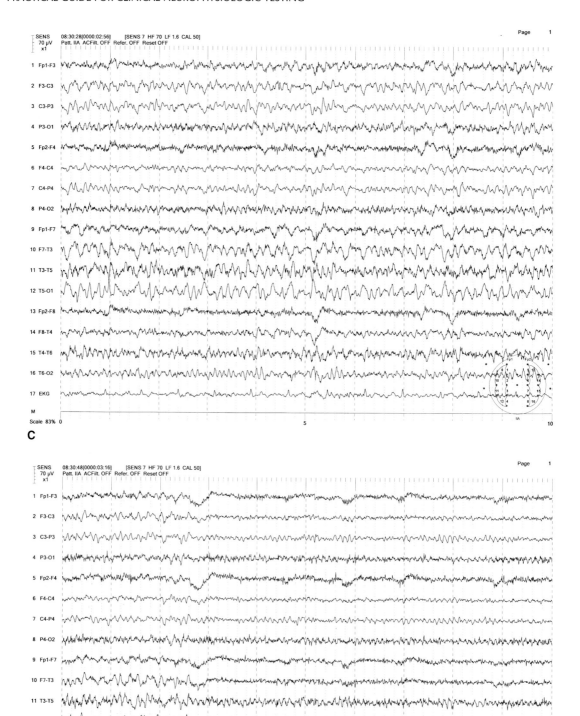

FIGURE 14-15 | (*Continued*)

activity, which is in contrast to a typical ictal event in which the waveform tends to change progressively from fast to slow activity. The duration of the event may range from 20 seconds to a few minutes.

Others

Other patterns that look "abnormal" but are considered to be normal variants are *slow alpha variant* (see "Alpha Variants," Chapter 7; see Fig. 7-16), *breach rhythm* (see "Beta rhythm/activity," Chapter 7; see Fig. 7-20), and *temporal slow of the elderly* ("Temporal Slow Waves in the Elderly," Chapter 12; see Fig. 12-18). These patterns are described elsewhere.

References

1. Gibbs FA, Gibbs EL. *Atlas of Electroencephalography*. Vol. 3. Reading, MA: Addison-Wesley, 1964.
2. Gibbs EL, Gibbs FA. Electrographic evidence of thalamic and hypothalamic epilepsy. *Neurology (Minneap)* 1951;1:136–144.
3. Gibbs FA, Gibbs EL. Fourteen and six per second positive spikes. *Electroencephalogr Clin Neurophysiol* 1963;15:353–358.
4. Henry CE. Positive spike discharges in the EEG and behavior abnormality. In: Glaser GE, ed. *EEG and Behavior*. New York: Basic Books, 1963:315–344.
5. Hughes JR. A review of the positive spike phenomenon: Recent study. In: Hughes JR, Wilson WP, eds. *EEG and Evoked Potentials in Psychiatry and Behavioral Neurology*. Boston, MA: Butterworth-Heinemann, 1983:295–324.
6. Schwade ED, Geiger SG. Matricide with electroencephalographic evidence of thalamic and hypothalamic disorder. *Dis Nerv Syst* 1953;14:18–20.
7. Shimoda Y. The clinical and electroencephalographic study of the primary diencephalic epilepsy or epilepsy of brainstem. *Acta Neuroveg (Wien)* 1961;23:181–191.
8. Lombroso CT, Schwartz IH, Clark DM, et al. Ctenoids in healthy youth. Controlled study of 14 and 6-per-second positive spiking. *Neurology (Minneap)* 1966;16:1152–1158.
9. Little SC. A general analysis of the fourteen and six per second dysrhythmia. In: *Proceedings of the 6th International Congress Electroencephalography and Clinical Neurophysiology*. Vienna, Austria: Wiener Med Akad, 1965:313–315.
10. Yamada T, Tucker RP, Kooi KA. Fourteen and six c/sec positive bursts in comatose patients. *Electroencephalogr Clin Neurophysiol* 1976;40:645–653.
11. Yamada T, Young S, Kimura J. Significant of positive spike bursts in Reye's syndrome. *Arch Neurol (Chicago)* 1977;34:246–249.
12. Silverman D. Fourteen and six-per second positive spike pattern in a patient with hepatic coma. *Electroencephalogr Clin Neurophysiol* 1964;16:395–398.
13. Drury I. 14- and 6-Hz positive bursts in diverse encephalopathies of childhood. *Electroencephlogr Clin Neurophysiol* 1989;72:12 (abst.).
14. Klass DW, Westmoreland BF. Nonepileptogenic epileptiform electroencephalographic activity. *Ann Neurol (Chicago)* 1985;18:627–635.
15. Reiher J, Klass DW. Two common EEG patterns of doubtful clinical significance. *Med Clin North Am* 1968;52:933–940.
16. White JC, Langston JW, Pedley TA. Benign epileptiform transients of sleep: Clarification of the small spike controversy. *Neurology (Minneap)* 1977;27:1061–1068.
17. Gutrecht JA. Clinical implications of benign epileptiform transients of sleep. *Electroencephagr Clin Neurophysiol* 1989;72:486–490.
18. Hughes JR, Gruener GT. Small sharp spike revisited: Further data on this controversial pattern. *Electroencephalogr Clin Neurophysiol* 1984;15:208–213.
19. Saito F, Fukushima Y, Kubota S. Small sharp spikes: Possible relationship to epilepsy. *Clin Electroencephalogr* 1987;18:114–119.
20. Marshall C. Some clinical correlates of the wave and spike phantom. *Electroencephalogr Clin Neurophysiol* 1955;7:633–636.
21. Silverman D. Phantom spike-waves and fourteen and six per second positive spike pattern: A consideration of their relationship. *Electroencephalogr Clin Neurophysiol* 1967;23:203–217.
22. Hughes JR. A review of the 6/sec spike and wave complex. In: Hughes JR, Wilson WP, eds. *EEG and Evoked Potential in Psychiatry and Behavioral Neurology*. Boston, MA: Butterworth–Heinemann, 1983:325–346.
23. Klass DW, Westmoreland BF. Nonepileptogenic epileptiform electroencephalographic activity. *Ann Neurol* 1985;18:627–635.
24. Thomas JE, Klass DW. Six-per-second spike-and-wave pattern in electroencephalogram: Reappraisal of its clinical significance. *Neurology (Minneap)* 1968;18:587–593.
25. Hughes JR. Two forms of the 6/sec spike and wave complex. *Electroencephalogr Clin Neurophysiol* 1980;48:535–550.
26. Reiher J, Lebell M. Wicket spikes: Clinical correlates of a previously undescribed EEG pattern. *Can J Neurol Sci* 1977;4:39–47.
27. Asokan G, Pareja J, Niedermeyer E. Temporal minor slow and sharp EEG activity and cerebrovascular disease. *Clin Electroencephalogr* 1987;18:201–210.
28. Chatrian GE, Bergamini L, Dondey M, et al. A glossary of terms most commonly used by clinical electroencephalographers. *Electroencephalogr Clin Neurophysiol* 1974;37:538–548.
29. Garvin JS. Psychomotor variant pattern. *Dis Nerv Syst* 1968;29:307–309.
30. Lipman IL, Hughes JR. Rhythmic mid-temporal discharges: An electro-clinical study. *Electroencephalogr Clin Neurophysiol* 1969;27:43–47.
31. Ciganek L. Theta-discharge in middle-line-EEG symptoms of temporal lobe epilepsy. *Electroencephalogr Clin Neurophysiol* 1961;13:669–673.
32. Westmoreland BF, Klass DW. Midline theta rhythm. *Arch Neurol (Minneap)* 1986;43:139–141.
33. Herranz F, Lopez S. Subclinical paroxysmal rhythmic activity. *Electroencephalogr Clin Neurophysiol* 1984;4:419–442.
34. Naquet R, Louard C, Rhodes J, et al. A propos de certaines decharges paroxystiques du carrefour temporo-parieto-occipital: Leur activation par l'hypoxie. *Rev Neurol (Paris)* 1961;105:203–207.
35. Miller CR, Westmoreland BF, Klass DW. Subclinical rhythmic EEG discharge of adults (SREDA): Further observations. *Am J EEG Technol* 1985;25:217–224.
36. O'Brien TJ, Sharbrough FW, Westmoreland BF, et al. Subclinical rhythmic electrographic discharge of adults (SREDA) revisited: A study using digital EEG analysis. *J Clin Neurophysiol* 1998;15:493–501.
37. Westmoreland BF, Klass DW. Unusual variants of subclinical rhythmic electrographic discharge of adult (SREDA). *Electroencephalogr Clin Neurophysiol* 1997;102:1–4.

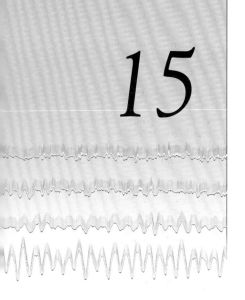

15

Artifact Recognition and Technical Pitfalls

THORU YAMADA and ELIZABETH MENG

Artifact Recognition

Artifacts are recorded activities that originate somewhere other than the area of interest. When recording an ECG (electrocardiogram), anything recorded which does not originate in the heart is considered an artifact. When recording EEG, anything recorded that is not cerebral in origin is considered an artifact. No EEG is free of artifacts. Identifying artifacts correctly is an essential role of an expert in EEG. This applies to both EEG technologists and electroencephalographers. Identifying, documenting, and eliminating artifacts are major roles of an EEG technologist. Some high-amplitude artifacts can totally obscure EEG activity. Some are of low amplitude and can subtly minimize or distort the cerebral activity. The artifacts are, however, not always useless. Some artifacts provide crucial information for an appropriate interpretation. Correlating artifacts with an ongoing EEG is an integral part of a skilled EEG interpretation. Artifacts can be grouped by origin such as:

1. Artifacts of physiological origins
2. Artifacts associated with body or head movements
3. Artifacts of nonphysiological (electrical) origins

PHYSIOLOGICAL ARTIFACTS

Physiological artifacts originate from the body itself. The contamination of physiological artifacts is inevitable in any EEG, though artifacts can be modified or minimized by appropriate technical adjustments.

Myogenic Artifacts (EMG; Electromyography)

EMG artifacts arise from nearby muscles introducing "muscle artifacts" mostly in the temporal and frontal electrodes. In spite of the technologist's efforts to relax the patient and reduce muscle artifacts, some patients, especially the elderly or uncooperative ones, may continue to show tonic muscle artifacts. The frequency of EMG artifacts varies from patient to patient.

When EMG is excessive and unrelenting, it can be minimized by lowering the high filter from 70 to 35 or 15 Hz. When this is necessary, caution should be exercised because filtered muscle can resemble beta activity (see Fig. 15-39A and B). Also, filtered muscle artifacts could mimic "spike" discharges (see Fig. 15-40A and B). EMG artifacts are usually prominent

in the ear or mastoid electrodes because of the proximity to the temporalis muscles. If the contamination of artifacts is excessive, the reference can be switched to the vertex (Cz) where muscle artifacts are minimal (Fig. 15-1A and B).

Tonic muscle artifacts, on the other hand, provide a useful clue to determine the patient's level of consciousness. Tonic muscle artifacts usually diminish during drowsiness. An awake or drowsy-appearing EEG coupled with an absence of tonic muscle artifact raises the possibility of rapid eye movements (REMs) sleep (see Fig. 7-45F). REM, scanning eye movement while eyes are open, or nystagmus causes a lateral rectus muscle twitch artifact (this is caused by activation of cranial nerve VI), which is recorded at F7 or F8 electrodes (see Figs. 15-9 and 15-10).

Muscle artifact may appear as a single muscle "twitch." This discharge is usually of a much shorter duration than an epileptiform spike. When they occur in sleep, however, "muscle spikes" tend to have a longer duration, and sometimes resemble the spikes of cerebral origin. Unusually, narrow and closed field distribution or random and scattered occurrence of these muscle spikes aids to distinguish them from epileptiform spikes (Fig. 15-2A). Repetitive muscle twitch artifacts resemble repetitive spikes or ictal (seizure) discharges or may obscure the background activity (Fig. 15-2B).

In comatose patients with decerebrate rigidity, shivering, or myoclonic twitches, pharmacologic paralysis may be necessary to distinguish the cerebral activity from artifacts (see Fig. 10-35A and B). Drugs like rocuronium, pancuronium, or succinylcholine can be used only when the patient is intubated, mechanically ventilated, and with an order from a physician (see Video 13-7). Swallowing or chewing results in a distinctive and diffuse crescendo–decrescendo type of muscle artifacts (see Fig. 15-18A and B).

Eye Movement Artifact

The eyeball can be regarded as a dipole with positivity toward the cornea and negativity toward the retina. When the eyeballs are in a fixed position, the dipole does not yield any potential change in the EEG. But, when the eyeball moves, this moving dipole generates a large and slow AC potential, detected by electrodes near the eyeballs. When the eyes close or blink, both eyeballs move in a conjugate upward direction (the Bell phenomena). This results in a positive deflection, which is maximal at Fp1 and Fp2 (Fig. 15-3, Video 15-1A, see also Fig. 8-16A

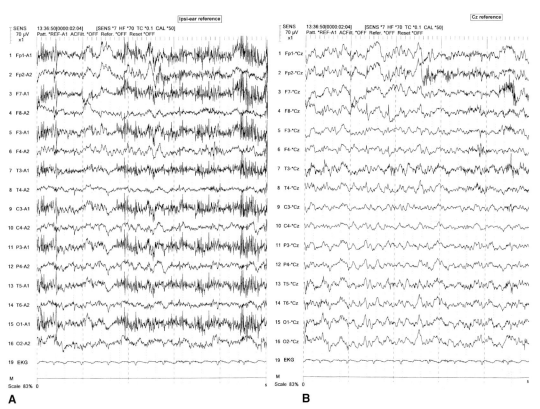

FIGURE 15-1 | EMG artifact arising from the left ear (A1) **(A)**. Because of close proximity of the ear to the temporalis muscle, ear reference recording is often contaminated by EMG artifact. This can be minimized with the use of Cz reference **(B)**. (**A** and **B** are the same EEG samples.)

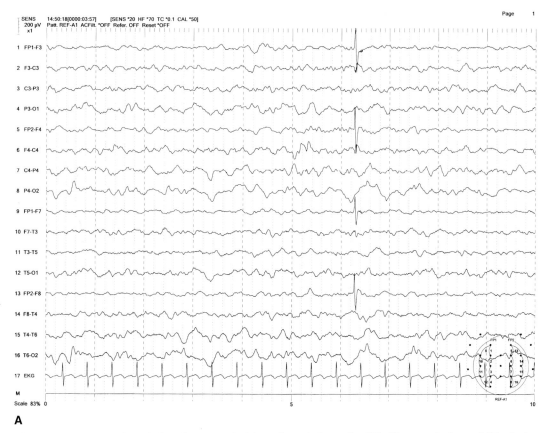

FIGURE 15-2 | Examples of "muscle spike" artifact recorded from frontal electrodes **(A)**. The morphology of this discharge resembles a real "spike," but the narrow field distribution of this discharge (restricted to Fp1 and Fp2) revealed on a double banana montage supports this as an artifact, not a cerebral potential. Another example is repetitive "muscle spikes" resembling ictal (seizure) discharges **(B)**.

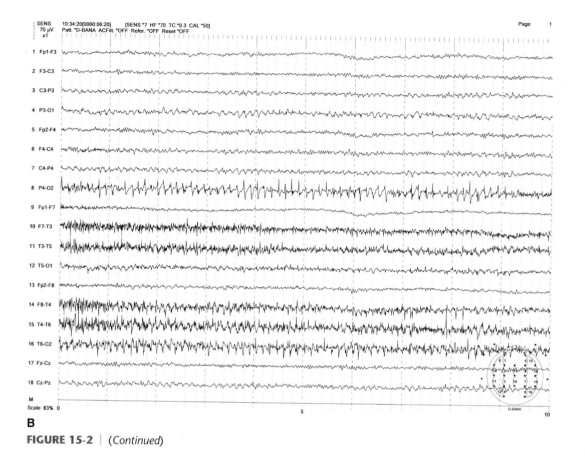

B

FIGURE 15-2 | *(Continued)*

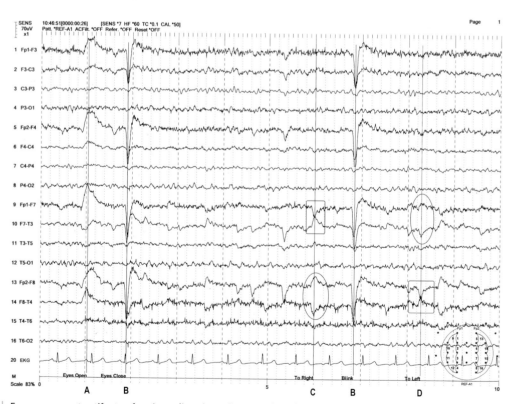

FIGURE 15-3 | Eye movement artifacts of various directions. Eye opening shows a negative deflection at Fp1 and Fp2 **(A)**. Eye closing or blink shows a positive deflection at Fp1 and Fp2 **(B)**. Horizontal eye movements show opposite polarity between F7 and F8; with right horizontal movement, F8 becomes positive (shown by *circles*) and F7 becomes negative (shown by *rectangular box*) **(C)**. The deflections are reversed for left horizontal eye movements **(D)**.

and B). Conversely, when the eyes open, a downward eye movement causes a negative potential at Fp1 and Fp2. Horizontal eye movements are reflected maximally at F7 and F8 with these two electrodes being charged in opposite polarities. Looking to the left causes positivity at F7 and negativity at F8; the reverse is true when looking to the right (Video 15-1B, see also Fig. 15-3).

In order to determine with certainty if a discharge represents eye movement or real cerebral activity, it may be necessary to use additional electrodes called eye monitors. In monitoring eye movements using two channels on each side, one electrode is placed just above the eye (Fp1 and Fp2 can be used), and one just below the eye (infraorbital: IO) on each side. Each is referred to the ipsilateral ear reference. Using this montage, the relationship between Fp and IO is out of phase for vertical eye movement and in phase for cerebral activity (see Fig. 15-4A and B, see also Fig. 8-16A).

An alternative derivation utilizes electrodes placed above the outer canthus of the left eye (LOCa) and below the outer canthus of the right eye (ROCb) or vice versa. Recording between LOCa-A1 and ROCb-A2, both vertical and horizontal eye movements, will show an out-of-phase deflection (see Fig. 15-4A and B, see also Fig. 8-16B) (see also Video 15-1A and B).

Without eye monitors, it can be difficult to differentiate bifrontal delta activity from vertical eye movement artifact. In general, the potential gradient of an eye movement from frontal to posterior electrodes is steep and rapidly dissipates in the posterior electrodes. This gradient is more gradual for frontal delta activity of cerebral origin (Fig. 15-5).

Some subjects have subtle and rapid eyelid fluttering accompanying rhythmic artifacts. This causes rhythmic theta or alpha range activity at Fp1 and Fp2 electrodes called *eye flutter artifacts* (Fig. 15-6A) (Video 15-2A). Some can even control the frequency of eye flutter (Video 15-2B). Eye flutter artifacts may also be induced by repetitive photic stimulation (Fig. 15-6B).

Asymmetric eye movement artifacts can mimic focal delta activity. This can occur when the patient has a prosthetic eye or diseased eye ball (Fig. 15-7). A severely diseased eyeball with a loss of normal ocular potential could also result in asymmetric eye movement artifacts despite the eyes moving in a normal and conjugate manner. Of course, asymmetric eye movement artifacts can be expected if there is asymmetrical electrode placement between homologous electrodes. An astute technologist should notice the asymmetries and clarify the reason for asymmetric eye movement potentials.

Another important artifact to be recognized is slow-drifting (horizontal) eye movements. This signifies that the patient is becoming drowsy and should not be disturbed if a sleep recording is desired (Fig. 15-8). Rapid horizontal eye movements are often accompanied by lateral rectus muscle twitch artifact, which can be detected at F7 or F8 electrodes. Because a lateral rectus muscle twitch causes the eye to move toward the contracted muscle, the twitch artifact is always followed by a deflection of positive polarity. This is best seen in REM sleep (see Fig. 7-45F) or in a patient who has nystagmus (Fig. 15-9).

Horizontal eye movements can be recognized because of the opposite polarities between F7 and F8 electrodes. Figure 15-10 shows unusual horizontal eye movement of rhythmic character (opsoclonus) resembling frontal delta activity (compare with Figs. 15-8 and 15-9).

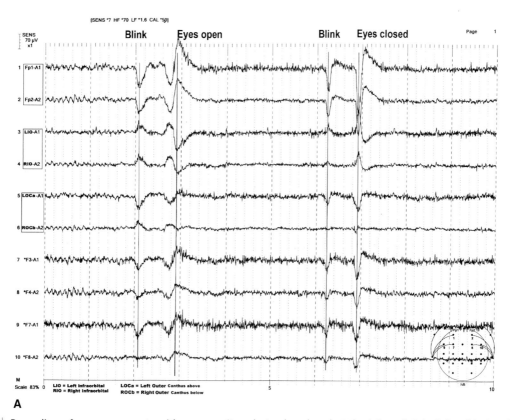

FIGURE 15-4 | Recording of eye movements with eye monitor electrodes placed at the left and right infraorbital region (LIO/RIO at channels 3/4), just above the left outer canthus, and just below the right outer canthus (LOCa/ROCb at channels 5/6). Vertical eye movements recorded from infraorbital electrodes are out of phase with the frontopolar electrodes. Lateral canthus electrodes are out of phase with each other for either eye-opening or eye-closing movements **(A)** and also for horizontal eye movement **(B)**. Note that the diffuse but bifrontal dominant inphase delta activities at all electrodes are consistent either with glossokinetic or frontal dominant delta activity potential (shown by *box*); compare with Figure 15-11.

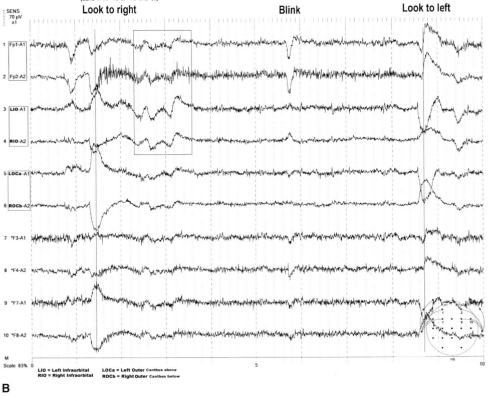

B

FIGURE 15-4 | (*Continued*)

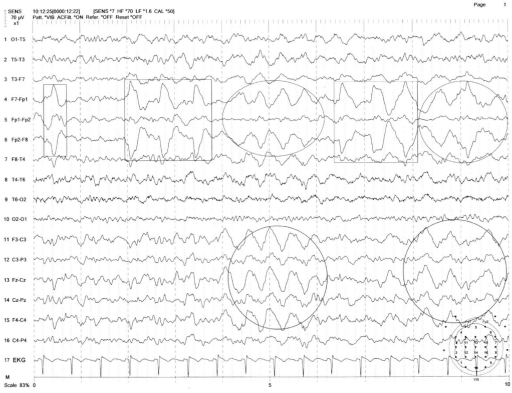

FIGURE 15-5 | Different field distribution between eye movement and frontal dominant delta activity. The potential fields of eye movement (blink artifacts) are relatively restricted to Fp1 and Fp2 electrodes (shown by *rectangular boxes*), whereas frontal delta activity (FIRDA/frontally dominant GPD* in this case) shows much wider distribution spreading posteriorly (shown by *circles*).

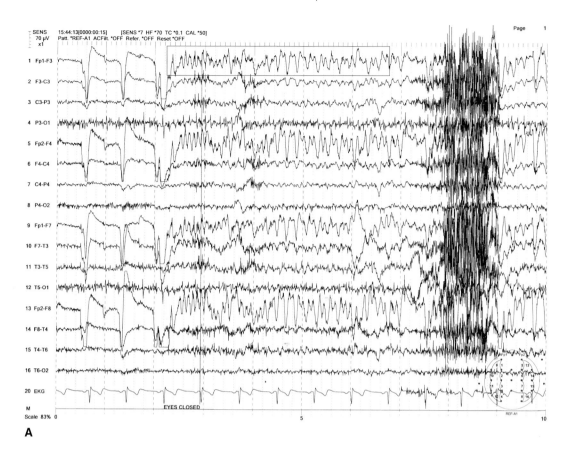

A

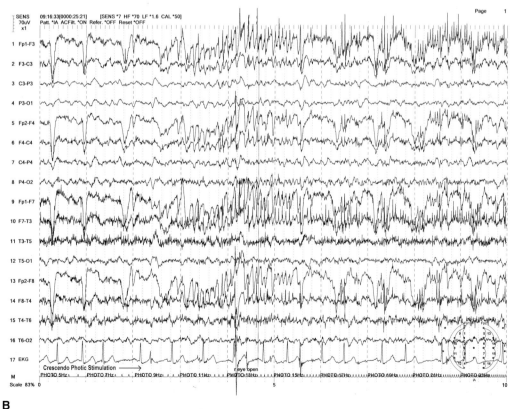

B

FIGURE 15-6 | An example of eye flutter artifact. Rapid eyelid movements associated with fast blinking called "eye flutter" show rhythmic alpha or theta range activity localized to Fp1 and Fp2 electrodes (shown by *rectangular box*) while eyes are closed **(A)**. Eye flutter artifacts can be differentiated from cerebral activity by their restricted distribution limited to Fp1 and Fp2 electrodes. In order to verify this, eye monitor electrodes would be helpful (see Fig. 15-4A). The same patient had similar eye movements induced by photic stimulation with the frequency time locked with photic flashes **(B)**.

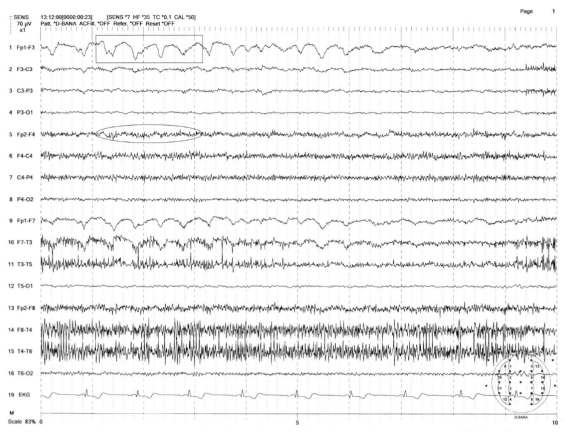

FIGURE 15-7 | A patient with prosthetic eye on the right is shown by the absence of eye movement (blink) artifacts at Fp2 (compare the patterns, shown in *rectangular box* and in *oval circle*).

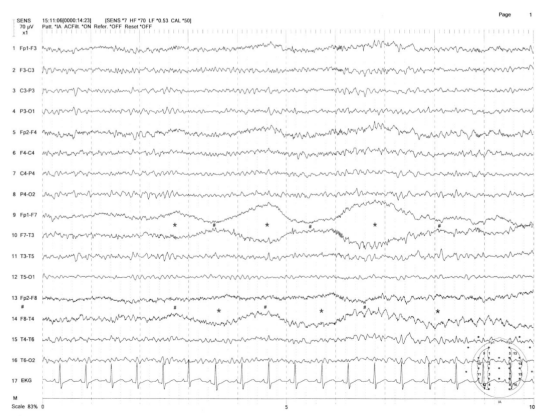

FIGURE 15-8 | Slow-drifting eye movements during approaching drowsiness. Note opposite polarities between F7 and F8 electrodes concomitantly (positivity is marked by *asterisk* and negativity is marked by #).

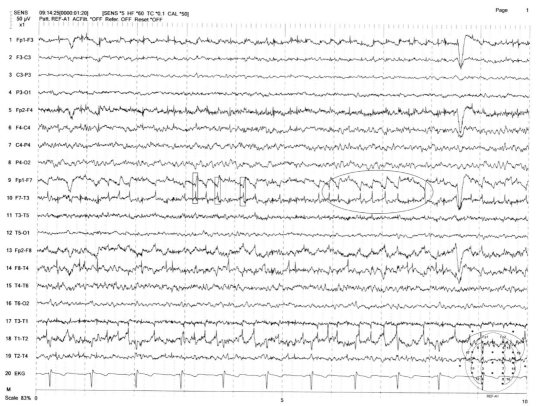

FIGURE 15-9 | An example of rapid horizontal eye movements (nystagmus). Note repetitive lateral rectus muscle twitches mostly at F7 electrodes (examples are indicated by *rectangular boxes*), followed by positive deflection (shown by *oval circle*) with concomitant negative deflection at F8 electrode.

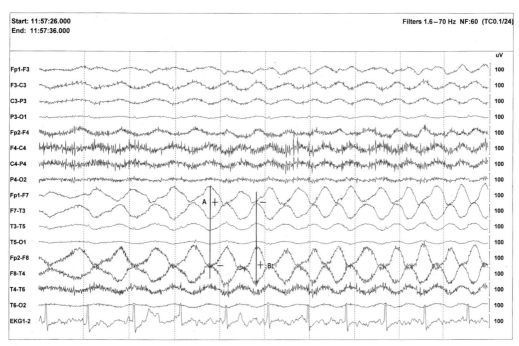

FIGURE 15-10 | Unusually rhythmic eye movements (opsoclonus) artifacts seen in a patient with acute hemorrhagic stroke in the thalamus extending to the brainstem. This is not frontal delta activity but horizontal eye movements. The eye movements are verified by opposite polarity between F7 and F8 electrodes. Note positive deflection F7 (*A*) and F8 (*B*) indicating eye movement to the left and to the right, respectively.

Glossokinetic Artifact

Another artifact which resembles frontal delta activity or eye movement artifacts is *glossokinetic potential* associated with tongue movement. The tongue, like the eye, is electrically charged with negativity at the tip and positivity at the root. When the tongue moves, especially when touching the roof of the pharynx, the change in the electrical field spreads to the scalp. This causes single or rhythmic diffuse delta waves, especially prominent in the frontal region resembling vertical eye movement artifact (Fig. 15-11). This glossokinetic potential can be reproduced by asking the patient to say words including an "L" sound such as "lilt" (Video 15-3). Unlike the eye movement potentials, the contamination of the glossokinetic potential to the scalp electrodes varies considerably from one person to another; the same tongue movement brings out large artifacts in some but not in others.

The more difficult differentiation is between glossokinetic potential and frontal delta activity. The infraorbital electrode helps in the differentiation. Both *glossokinetic potential* and frontal delta activity show an inphase deflection between Fp (frontopolar) and IO (infraorbital) electrodes, but the amplitude of a glossokinetic potential is larger at the IO than the Fp electrode, while frontal activity is larger at the Fp than the IO electrode (Fig. 15-12, see also Fig. 8-16) (Video 15-4). Without eye monitor electrodes, vertical eye movements and glossokinetic potentials can be differentiated by the wider distribution of the latter than the former (Fig. 15-13).

Electroretinogram

Electroretinogram (ERG) is seen as a response to photic stimulation and is conventionally recorded from a contact lens electrode placed directly over the eyeball. In some subjects, however, the ERG can be recorded from Fp1 and Fp2 electrodes. The potential consists of two major components, "a" and "b" waves appearing as a small sharp and wave complex (Fig. 15-14A). The response is time locked to the flicker frequency. ERG is often seen in electrocerebral silence (ECS) recordings because of the high-amplification recording with absence of interfering EEG activity and still remaining function of the retina. These normal physiological responses from the retina must be distinguished from the nonphysiological artifact in which the electrode reacts to a light source. This can be differentiated by delivering high-frequency flashes (>30 Hz). The ERG cannot react to high-frequency flashes (Fig. 15-14B), but electrode artifact continues without diminishing amplitude. Alternatively, the electrode in question may be covered by an opaque material. ERG persists but electrode artifact disappears.

Cardiac Artifacts

ELECTROCARDIOGRAM ARTIFACT. The artifacts from electrocardiogram (ECG) can usually be identified easily because of their regular form and repetition. If, however,

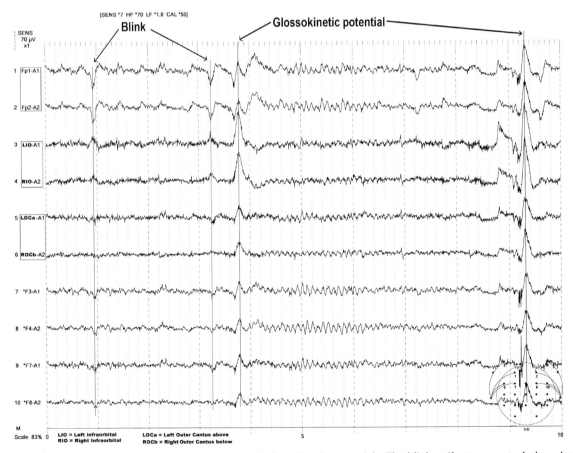

FIGURE 15-11 | The relationship between blink artifacts and glossokinetic potentials. The blink artifacts are out of phase between Fp and infraorbital (IO) electrodes, whereas the glossokinetic potentials show inphase between the two with the greater amplitude at the IO electrodes than Fp electrodes. (This distinguishes between glossokinetic potential and frontal delta slow waves; see also Fig. 15-12A and B, also Video 15-3.)

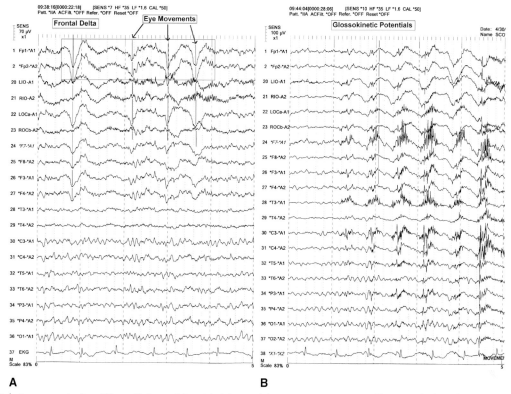

FIGURE 15-12 | An example for differentiation of frontal delta activity, eye movement artifacts, and glossokinetic potential using eye monitor derivations. The eye movement (*vertical*) artifacts show out-of-phase relationship between Fp and IO, but frontal delta activity shows inphase relationship between Fp and IO electrodes and also between LOCa and ROCb electrodes **(A)**. The glossokinetic potential shows inphase relationship between IO and Fp electrodes **(B)** but differs from frontal delta by greater amplitude of activity at IO than Fp electrode. It is not possible to differentiate frontal delta activity from eye movement or glossokinetic artifacts if examining only Fp electrodes because of similarity of these three activities.

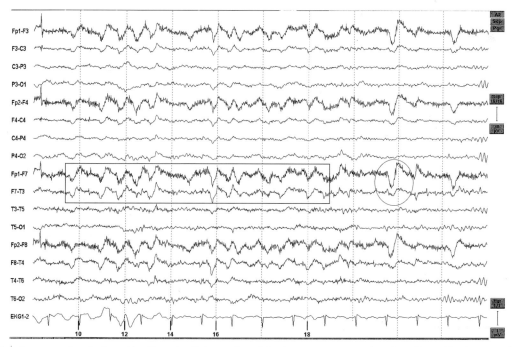

FIGURE 15-13 | An example of glossokinetic potentials produced by tongue movements when the patient was verbally counting. Note the difference in distribution between glossokinetic potentials and eye movement (blink) artifacts; glossokinetic potentials are more widely distributed with a slower potential gradient from the anterior to posterior head region (shown in *rectangular box*) as compared to the eye movement artifacts, which are more restricted to Fp1/Fp2 with a steep gradient from the anterior to posterior (shown in *circle*).

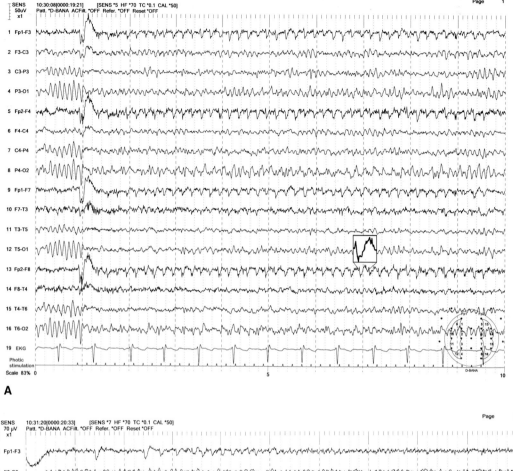

A

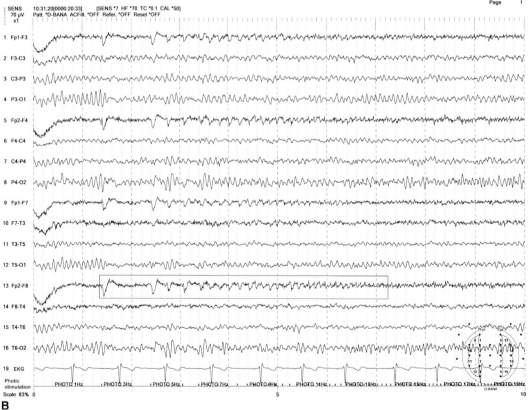

B

FIGURE 15-14 | An example of ERG (electroretinogram) seen in Fp1 and Fp2, produced by repetitive photic flashes **(A)**. Each ERG, time locked with each flash, consists of a small spike-wave complex referred to as "a" and "b" waves (one ERG is enlarged shown by the *box*). ERG responds to the progressively changing flash frequency but becomes smaller with faster frequencies and fades out at around 18 Hz **(B)** (shown by *rectangular box*).

ECG rhythm is irregular or has an abnormal waveform, the contamination of ECG artifact onto the EEG could mimic sharp or spike discharges. For this reason, ECG monitoring should be done routinely.

ECG artifacts most commonly appear in ear reference montages. Because of the vector direction of the QRS complex, A1 and A2 are charged with opposite polarities (see Fig. 2-23A). Electronically connecting A1 and A2 (linked ear reference), therefore, will reduce the ECG artifacts (see Fig. 2-23B). ECG artifacts are usually large in a stout person with a short neck. ECG contamination is usually minimal in bipolar recordings. If one channel shows disproportionately large ECG artifact in a bipolar montage, high impedance in one electrode should be suspected (see Fig. 15-34). Some ECG abnormalities such as PVC (premature ventricular contraction) occur irregularly and, when transmitted to the scalp electrodes, mimic abnormal EEG discharges (Fig. 15-15A). On some occasions, a part of the ECG complex such as T wave can contaminate onto the EEG (Fig. 15-15B).

ECG contamination is unavoidable in most ECS recordings because of the high sensitivity (S = 2μV) used for ECS recording and the absence of cerebral activity. Increased conductivity by sweat or a wet pillow or bedsheet may potentiate ECG transmission to the scalp electrodes. Changing the head position may attenuate ECG artifacts. At the increased sensitivity used in ECS recording, a systolic pulse wave may cause minute vibrations of the body on the bed, thereby inducing capacitive changes and movement of the electrodes (ballistocardiographic artifact) producing low-voltage rhythmic waves resembling cerebral activity.

PULSE ARTIFACT. Another artifact with cardiac origin is pulse artifact. If an electrode lies near a small scalp artery, rhythmic waves related to ECG rhythm may be recorded. Because of the time required for a pulse wave to travel from the left ventricle to the scalp, the pulse artifact lags the QRS complex by 200 to 300 ms. Usually, pulse artifacts are recognized by rhythmic delta activity time locked with the ECG rate. But the artifacts could resemble focal delta activity, especially when the ECG rhythm is irregular (Fig. 15-16B). Also, the artifact can appear in a variety of waveforms (Fig. 15-16B–D). In some occasions, ECG artifacts appear as repetitive sharp discharges resembling ictal (seizure) discharges (Fig. 15-16C). When diffuse delta slow waves are present, the distinction between EEG slow waves and pulse artifact may be difficult (Fig. 15-16D). Changing the head position slightly or relocating the electrode may eliminate the artifact (Video 15-5).

PACEMAKER ARTIFACT. Cardiac pacemakers produce high-voltage transients of very short duration, which are clearly artifactual in appearance. The ECG monitor in a dedicated channel is useful to document the artifacts (Fig. 15-17).

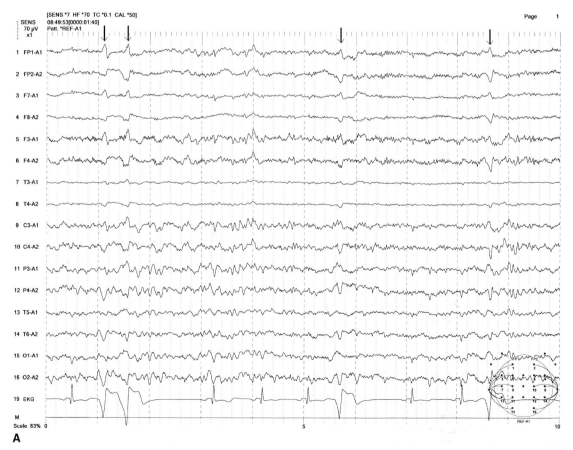

FIGURE 15-15 | Contamination of abnormal ECG onto the EEG tracing. In **(A)**, note the intermittent and irregular occurring of PVC (premature ventricular contraction) appearing as sharp transients (shown by *downward arrows*) on the EEG. Without ECG monitoring, this could be mistaken as abnormal epileptiform discharges. Note opposite polarity of PVC artifacts between A1 and A2 reference recordings, which provide some hint that these are ECG artifacts. **(B)** shows unusual contamination of a portion of the EKG complex (T wave) in the O2 electrode.

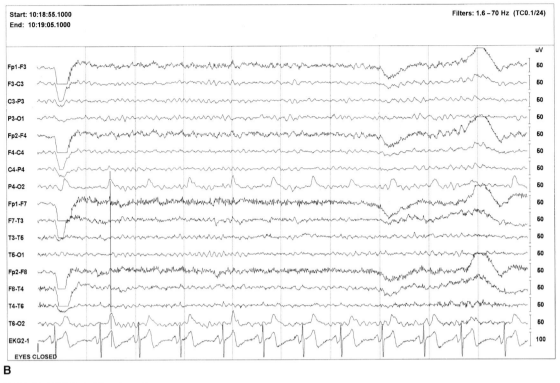

B

FIGURE 15-15 | (*Continued*)

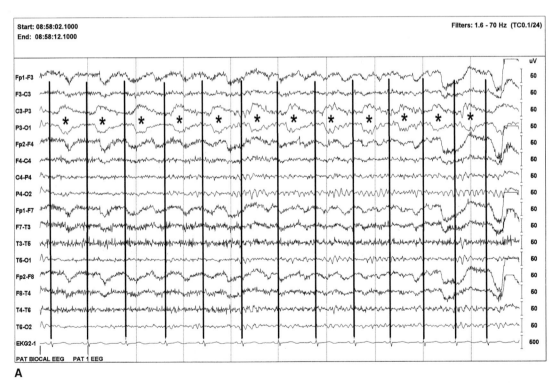

A

FIGURE 15-16 | Several examples of pulse artifacts showing variety of waveforms; typically appear as rhythmic delta activity on one or more channels; peak of each delta activity (shown by * mark) occurs about ½ second after the ORS complex **(A)**. When ECG rhythm is irregular, pulse artifacts follow the same rate and become irregular (shown by *arrows*) **(B)**. Sometimes, pulse artifacts appear as repetitive sharp discharges (a few examples are shown by *arrows*) **(C)**. When pulse artifacts appear mixed with diffuse delta slow waves, distinction between the delta and pulse artifacts could become difficult (each artifact is shown by *arrow*) **(D)**.

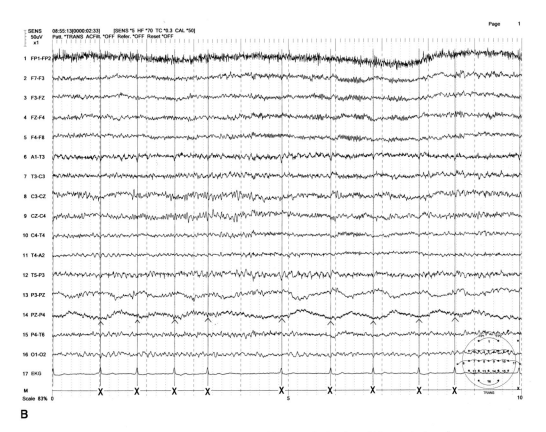

B

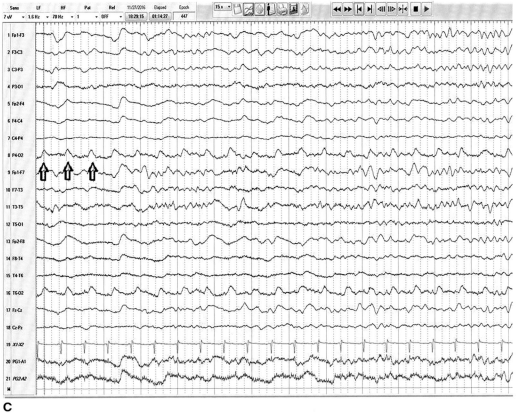

C

FIGURE 15-16 | (*Continued*)

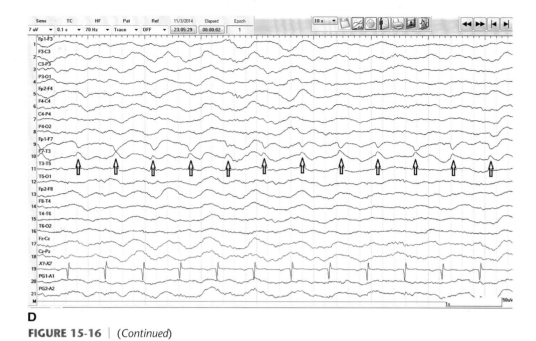

D

FIGURE 15-16 | (Continued)

Other Artifacts Related to Swallowing, Hiccups, and Sobbing

Swallowing is a common artifact producing short crescendo–decrescendo bursts of muscle artifacts, often together with a slow activity of glossokinetic origin (Fig. 15-18A and B). Chewing and sucking movements may cause rhythmic delta activity and, if necessary, can be monitored by electrodes placed over the jaw or near the lip.

The artifacts introduced by sobbing, sniffles, or hiccups may present problems since they often resemble spike wave or other paroxysmal discharges (Fig. 15-19). Each sob or hiccup must be annotated by the technologist. It should be noted that a baby may continue to sob even when the EEG shows stage II sleep.

Sweat Artifact

"Sweat artifacts" are generated from sweat gland potentials that are electrically negative. The potential is a DC-like slow frequency that causes slow-drifting deflections (Fig. 15-20A). This can be minimized by the use of a shorter time constant setting (Fig. 15-20B). However, it should be noted that using a shorter

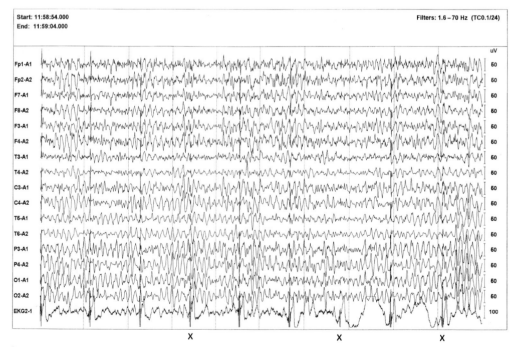

FIGURE 15-17 | An example of cardiac pacemaker artifact showing needle-like "spike" artifact on the EEG, coinciding with paced pulse just prior to QRS complex on ECG channel. Note the artifacts are intermittently "skipped" (marked by "x"). This is not due to lack of transmission but due to the short duration of the pacemaker pulse occurring in between digital sampling points, thus not sampled (see Chapter 3).

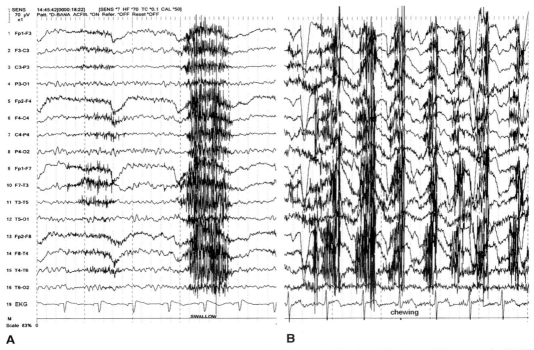

FIGURE 15-18 | An example of swallowing **(A)** and chewing **(B)** artifacts. Swallowing **(A)** shows diffuse muscle (EMG) artifact with crescendo–decrescendo sharp. Repetitive muscle artifacts representing chewing artifacts during eating **(B)**.

time constant or higher low-filter setting will also attenuate slow waves of cerebral origin (see Fig. 15-41A and B). Sweat artifacts occur randomly at any electrode without an organized potential field distribution, which aids to differentiate them from delta activity of cerebral origin.

Cooling the head, wiping the area with alcohol, and providing air conditioning to control the recording environment can reduce the artifacts.

BODY AND HEAD MOVEMENT ARTIFACTS

Any movements that change the impedance between electrode and scalp cause artifacts. Loose or high-impedance electrodes tend to produce artifacts even with slight movements. It is important to maintain low-impedance electrodes at <10 kΩ to minimize artifacts. Even with low-impedance and secure electrode placement, artifacts created by violent and rhythmic

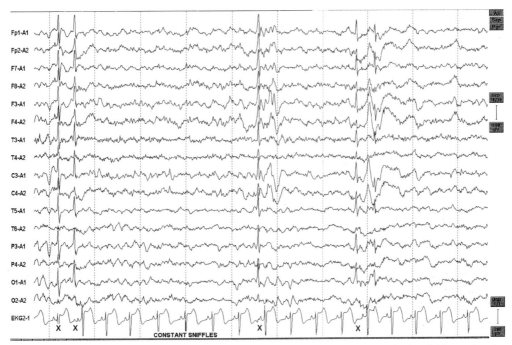

FIGURE 15-19 | An example of "sobbing" (*sniffle*) artifact (marked by "*x*") in a 2-year-old child. The child may continue to "sob" even in stage II sleep. Because the discharges mimic epileptiform spikes and their distribution and waveform may not be uniform, the technologist must note and document each "sob" or sniff artifact.

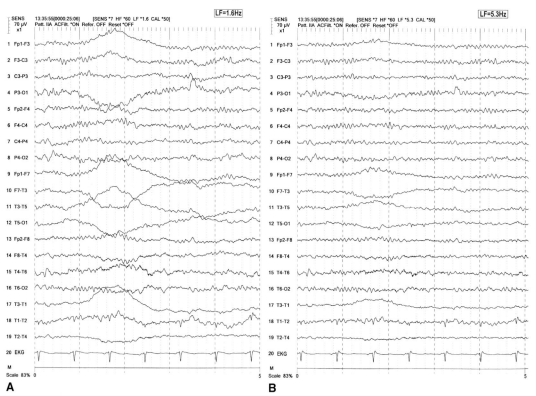

FIGURE 15-20 | An example of "sweat" artifact (sweat gland potential). Note slow-drifting potentials at F7, T3, T5, and O1 electrodes occurring randomly and independently among multiple electrodes **(A)**. The "sweat" artifacts can be minimized by using a shorter time constant or higher low-frequency filter **(B)**. (**A** and **B** are the same EEG samples.)

movements such as seen in pseudoseizures may mimic the seizure (ictal) event. Close scrutiny of the waveforms and their distribution often differentiate artifacts from EEG activity; the artifacts created by movement show double- or triple-phase reversal in sequential bipolar derivation, which is extremely rare in true EEG activity (see Video 13-9, see Fig. 15-23, see also Figs. 2-28, 2-29).

Respiration Artifact

The respiration artifact is a slow-rhythmic wave appearing synchronously with inhalation and/or exhalation, usually involving electrodes on which the patient is lying. Respiration artifacts are commonly seen during vigorous hyperventilation or gasping respiration obviously due to head movement (Video 15-6A). In patients with artificial ventilation in the ICU setting, however, artifacts associated with respiration vary considerably from repetitive slow waves to spiky discharges (Fig. 15-21A–D) and occur with even minor abdominal movement (Video 15-7). Some respiration artifacts may simulate periodic delta activity or periodic lateralized epileptiform discharges (PLEDs/LPD*). Respiration-related artifacts may also arise from bubbling of the accumulated moisture in the ventilation tube (Video 15-8). Also, the waveforms may vary from one respiration to another, which makes it more difficult to differentiate from periodically recurring EEG activity. Repositioning the head or respiration hose or clearing the moisture from the tube could eliminate the artifacts (see Video 15-8). Technologists must monitor respiration by visual observation or with commercially avail-

able devices. Also, careful video review may be needed to clarify the question.

Tremor Artifact

Patients with tremors in any part of the body may introduce rhythmic artifacts on one or more electrodes, usually those electrodes on which the patient lies. For example, patients with Parkinson's disease may produce 2- to 4-Hz rhythmic artifacts, which may be accompanied by myogenic (EMG) artifacts (Fig. 15-22, Video 15-9). The movements can be monitored by placing a pair of electrodes over the involved muscles and recording the associated EMG activity. Or, one may use an accelerometer that can register very quick movement.

Other Movement Related Artifacts

Various rhythmic or nonrhythmic artifacts occur, especially in the ICU setting, because of the variety of activities occurring around the patients' bed. These could be caused by patients themselves (Videos 15-10 and 15-11) or by others (Videos 15-12 and 15-13). Other artifacts may arise from mechanically moving devices (Video 15-14).

These artifactual potentials may resemble ictal activity or focal slow waves. However, careful analysis often reveals illogical or aberrant field distribution among neighboring electrodes, resulting in so-called "double"- or "triple"-phase reversals (Figs. 15-23 and 15-24, see also Figs. 2-28 and 2-29), which are rarely seen in genuine cerebral potentials (see Fig. 2-30).

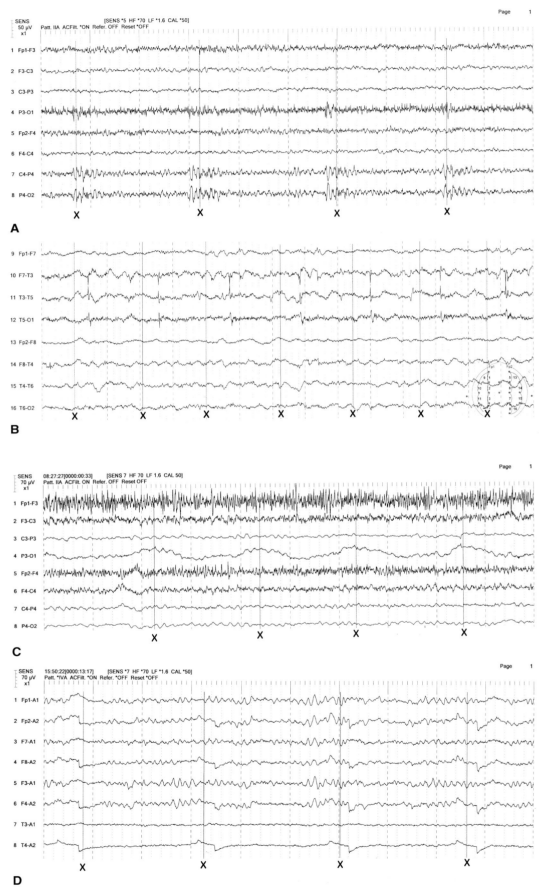

FIGURE 15-21 | **A–D:** Examples of various respiration artifacts. Note varieties of waveforms associated with respiration (marked by *"x"*). Some may mimic epileptiform activity, and technologist's notation and close scrutiny of video are important to distinguish them, because movement could be quite subtle (see Videos 15-7 and 15-8).

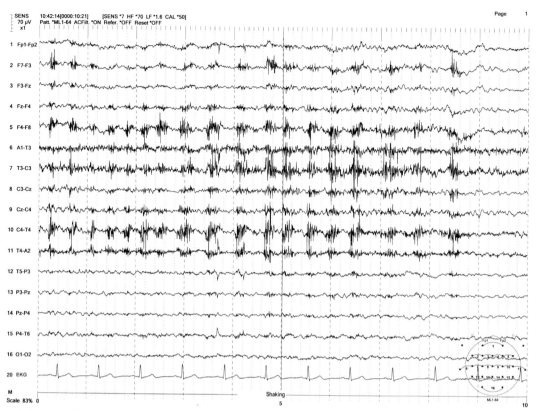

FIGURE 15-22 | An example of tremor artifact in a patient with Parkinson's disease. Note rhythmic muscle burst artifacts associated with delta waves of about 2 to 2.5 Hz (see Video 15-9).

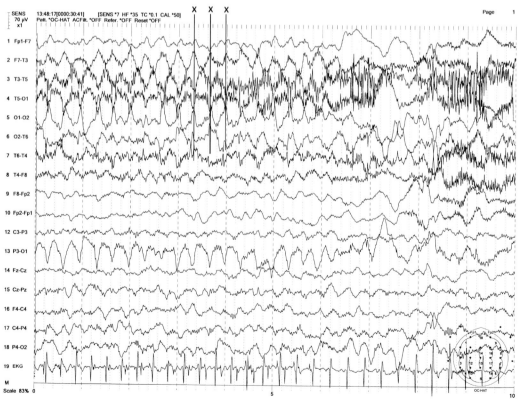

FIGURE 15-23 | An example of movement artifact induced by a mother patting her baby. Note rhythmic 3-Hz delta activity involving left temporal/occipital electrodes. The rhythmicity of the discharges resembles electrographic ictal (seizure) event. Proving this activity to be artifact is based on the double- or triple-phase reversals between channels 2 and 3 and 4 and 5 (examples are shown by "x").

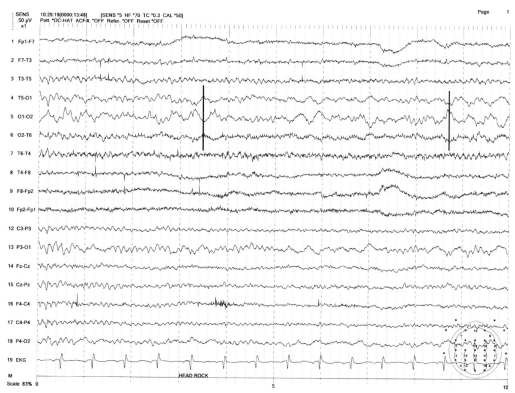

FIGURE 15-24 | An example of slow headshaking movement artifact. Note semirhythmic delta activity involving O1 and O2. The double-phase reversal between channels 4 to 5 (O1 electrode) and 5 to 6 (O2 electrode) supports the artifactual origin (examples are shown by *vertical lines*) (see also Fig. 2-29, Video 15-10).

NONPHYSIOLOGICAL ARTIFACTS/ELECTRICAL INTERFERENCE ARTIFACTS

Nonphysiological artifacts arise from external sources such as electrodes, EEG instrument, or other electrical devises in the vicinity or attached to the patient.

Interfering Artifacts from Medical Devices

The electrical devices attached to the patient can produce various interfering artifacts which usually consist of fixed frequency and rhythmicity specific to the instrument or device. Because the external interference likely affects all electrodes equally, it will be canceled out if all electrodes are of low impedance and well balanced. Thus, the artifacts tend to appear selectively in the channels of high-impedance or unbalanced electrodes. Two examples (one by an unknown devices and the other from dialysis machine) are shown in Videos 15-15 and 15-16.

60-Hz Artifact

Electrostatic 60-Hz interference is inescapable in any recording environment, but in normal recording condition, it is effectively canceled by the differential EEG amplifier. If, however, unequal electrode impedance between the pair of electrodes exists, 60-Hz artifact will be readily introduced (Fig. 15-25A). If 60-Hz artifact appears in one or a few channels, check the impedance of the involved electrodes (see also Fig. 15-34). High impedance of the ground electrode is another common technical fault that will introduce 60-Hz artifact, generally in all recording channels. Check the ground electrode impedance if the artifact is widespread.

The source of a 60-Hz interference may be a device with AC power near the patient (Video 15-17) or from an adjacent room including rooms located above or below. In order to minimize 60-Hz interference, keep electrode wires bunched close together and avoid placing the AC power cable or devise close to the patient or input cable or head box.

Sixty-hertz artifact can be easily recognized by its sinusoidal waveform and exact frequency. These artifacts can be eliminated, in most cases, with the use of a "notch" filter (see "Notch filter," Chapter 2) (Fig. 15-25B). Although the use of a 60-Hz notch filter does not affect much in EEG interpretation, the presence of a 60-Hz artifact indicates the existence of some technical problem; it should be used only when the 60-Hz artifact cannot be eliminated by all other measures. Conversely, the notch filter can be used to verify if the artifact in question is 60 Hz or not: if the notch filter cannot eliminate or minimize the artifact, it is unlikely to be 60-Hz artifact.

Electrode Artifacts

Electrodes with changing properties of electrode paste and skin conductance may produce artifacts. The discharge simulates spikes or sharp waves and is commonly referred to as "electrode pop." The electrode pop is not caused by high-electrode impedance but by an electrically unstable electrode, by drying electrolyte, or by slight mechanical instability that changes the electrode contact with the skin. Poorly chlorided silver–silver chloride electrodes tend to produce frequent "popping." The waveform often has a fast-rise and slow-decay phase resembling a calibration signal (Fig. 15-26A).

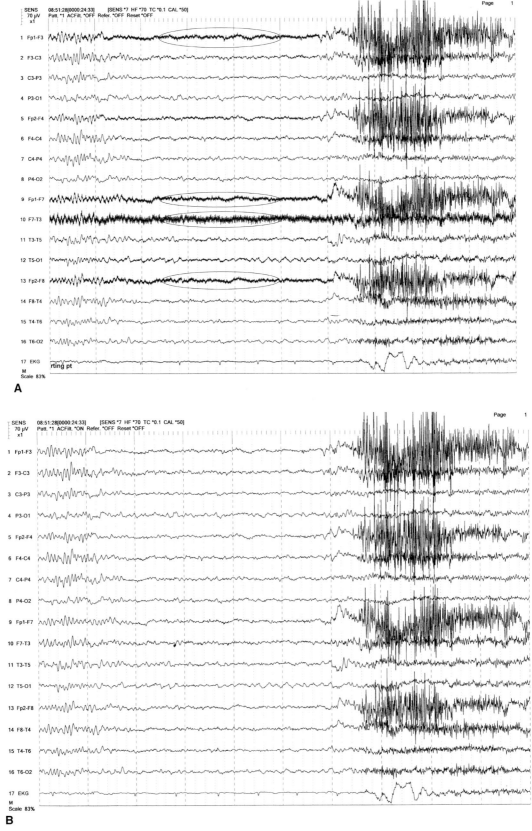

FIGURE 15-25 | An example of 60-Hz artifact in channels 1, 9, 10, and 13 due to high impedance in Fp1, F7, and Fp2 (shown by *oval circle*) **(A)**. Notch filter (60-Hz filter) selectively eliminates 60-Hz activity, not affecting muscle artifacts **(B)**. (**A** and **B** are the same EEG samples.)

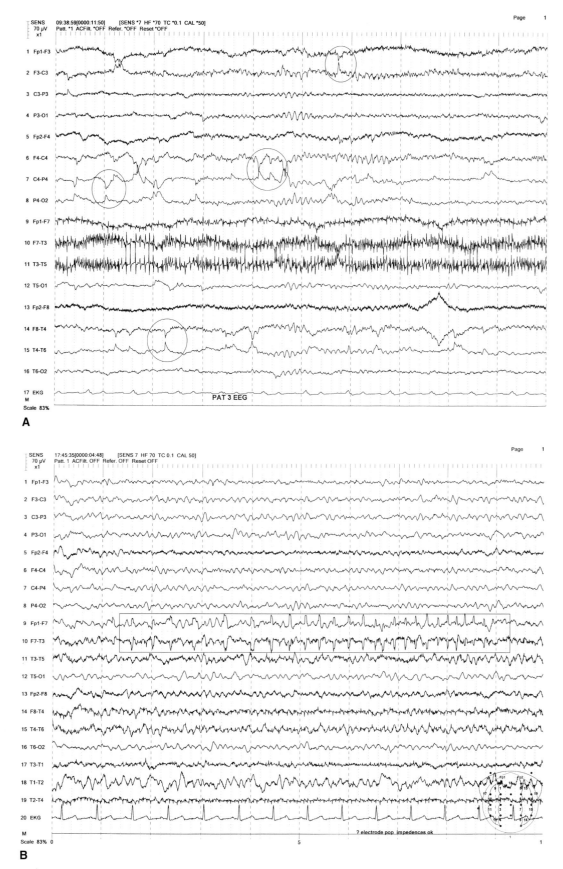

FIGURE 15-26 | An example of electrode "pop" arising from multiple electrodes. Pops appear randomly at F3, C4, P4, and T4 (shown in *circles*). The waveforms vary but typically resemble a calibration waveform **(A)**. Sometimes, "pops" appear in a repetitive fashion with progressively changing frequency (shown by *rectangular box* in **B**). This mimics the onset of an electrographic ictal (seizure) event. Limited to a single channel distinguishes "pop" artifacts from ictal or EEG activity.

Repetitive electrode pops may mimic a progressive focal ictal discharge with progressively changing waveform and frequency (Fig. 15-26B). These electrode pop artifacts can be differentiated from cerebral potential by the appearance in a single electrode without concomitant involvement in other electrodes.

Electrostatic Artifacts

When recording an EEG, especially when using high sensitivity, movement of people near the patient may generate artifacts of electrostatic origin. The artifacts consist of a burst of various frequencies and waveform. The technologist must note the recording of each movement around the patient's bed. Capacitive artifacts occur by moving or stepping on the input cable. These artifacts are easily elicited, especially when electrode impedances are high.

High-Frequency Noise

Radio, microwave, telephone, or hospital paging system may induce high-frequency noise, especially in the intensive care unit or operating room where the patient is connected to electronic devices using radio frequencies. Although the EEG amplifier attenuates much of the activity faster than 70 Hz, high-frequency noise may appear as second- or third-order harmonic frequencies. Another source of high-frequency noise arises from the EEG instrument itself and may be problematic when recording with high sensitivity such as in ECS recording. High-frequency deep brain stimulation used for the treatment of Parkinson's disease or dystonia has been popularized in recent years. The high-frequency noise totally obscures EEG activity but may be effectively eliminated by using a lower high-frequency filter setting (Fig. 15-27A and B). When a lower high-frequency filter setting is used, however, one can trust only slower-frequency activity; fast-frequency activity may still be partially present and mimic beta activity or spike discharges (Fig. 15-27B, see also Figs. 15-39A and B and 15-40A and B).

Technical Pitfalls and Errors

Recording EEG requires systematic and multiple stages of preparation. A variety of recording parameters must be set correctly and according to laboratory protocol for reliable recording. Any mistake or omission in preparation may lead to serious errors in interpretation. An astute technologist is able to identify the problem and correct the errors should this occur during the recording.

The following should be checked systematically:

1. Is the input cable securely connected to the EEG instrument (see Fig. 2-1)? Even if the EEG instrument is not connected to the patient (open air recording), the EEG may show a variety of electrical waves, mimicking seemingly realistic EEG activity (Fig. 15-28A). Shaking the electrodes (open wires) rhythmically or flailing the hand in front of the headbox alters the EEG pattern and can even make "seizure-like" discharges (Fig. 15-28B). Careful analysis of the EEG, however, usually reveals illogical pattern, waveforms, or distribution of the activities.

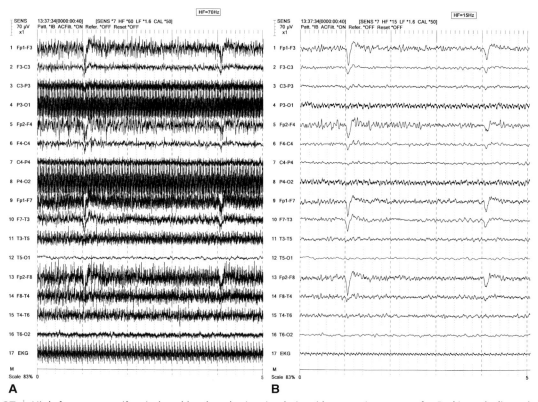

FIGURE 15-27 | High-frequency artifact induced by deep brain stimulation (therapeutic measure for Parkinson's disease). The artifacts totally obscure EEG activity **(A)**. Lowering the high-frequency filter from 70 to 15 Hz revealed the basic background activity, though the artifacts were not totally eliminated **(B)**. (**A** and **B** are the same EEG samples.)

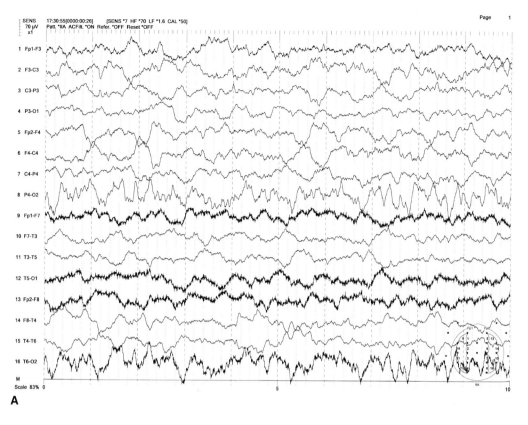

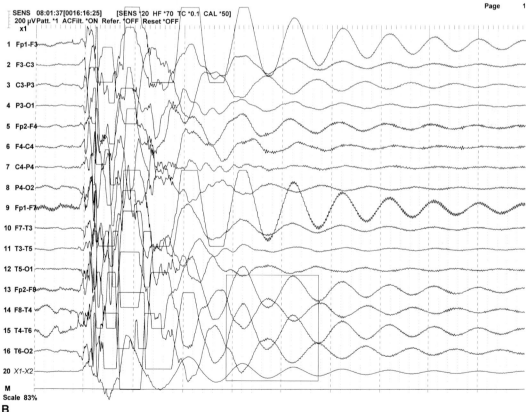

FIGURE 15-28 | EEG patterns recorded *without* connecting to the patient. The recording showed irregular and varieties of frequency activities, which at a glance appear "genuine" EEG activity, though the distribution of the patterns are random and not logically organized **(A)**. Shaking electrode wires rhythmically created the discharges resembling polyspike wave followed by rhythmic delta activity. The clue to determining that this is an artifact is their illogical field distribution of the delta activity showing a triple-phase reversal at F8, T4, and T6 **(B)** (example is shown in *box*).

2. Is each electrode correctly plugged into its designated site on the head board? This mistake will result in peculiar, unusual, or illogical potential field distribution. For example, reversing Fp1 and F3 electrodes will result in illogical distribution of eye potentials (Fig. 15-29A and B). A few other examples of this similar mistake are shown in Figures 15-30A and B and 15-31A–D.

3. Are all channels set with the same recording parameters (filter and sensitivity settings)? If a filter or sensitivity setting in one channel is different from others, the EEG activity from this channel will be disproportionately different from other channels (Figs. 15-32A and B and 15-33A and B).

4. Is each electrode's impedance sufficiently low (preferably <5 kΩ, at least <10 kΩ)? One electrode's impedance that is high compared to others tends to cause 60-Hz artifact, ECG, or head and cable movement artifacts (Fig. 15-34). Also it can create a so called "ground recording" in which the ground electrode acts as a recording electrode, replacing the electrode of high impedance. As a result, EEG activity arising from the region of the ground electrode (wherever it is placed) will be recorded. An example of these erroneous distributions created by a high impedance electrode is shown in Figure 15-35. In order to avoid this problem, all impedances should be balanced, preferably within 5 kΩ of each other. If the impedance of the ground electrode is high, all channels can be contaminated by 60 Hz.

5. Are preprogrammed montage settings correct? If the montage is incorrectly programmed, there may be erroneous amplitudes or illogical potential field distribution (Fig. 15-36A and B).

6. Is the sweep speed appropriate? Conventional sweep speed is 10 seconds for a full screen view. If the display is unknowingly set at 5 seconds, frequency falsely appears to be slower (Fig. 15-37A and B). Conversely, a slower sweep speed (15 seconds/page) gives a false impression that the frequency is faster than the actual frequency (Fig. 15-38A and B).

7. Is filter setting appropriate? The judicious use of filter settings helps reveal the cerebral activity hidden by various artifacts. For example, excessive muscle artifacts obscuring EEG can be minimized by effectively lowering the high-filter setting (see Fig. 2-12A and B). However, one should be cautious in interpreting the EEG because filtered muscle can mimic beta activity (Fig. 15-39A and B) or polyspike discharges (Fig. 15-40A and B). Raising the low-filter setting is useful to eliminate or minimize slow-wave artifacts such as sweat gland potential or respiration artifact (see Fig. 15-20A and B). But one should be aware that this also attenuates or eliminates slow waves of cerebral origin (Fig. 15-41A and B).

8. Is the sensitivity appropriate? When EEG shows exceedingly large amplitude activity obscuring the waveforms and/or distribution of the activity of interest, decreasing the sensitivity helps reveal true waveforms (Fig. 15-42A and B). However, this may eliminate small but potentially significant activity. Conversely, increasing the sensitivity may enhance the appearance of underlying slow waves making the EEG "look" more abnormal (Fig. 15-43A and B).

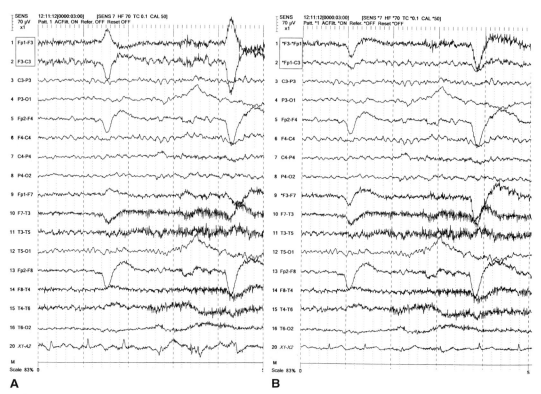

FIGURE 15-29 | An example of plugging electrode into the wrong jack of the headbox. The EEG showed eye potential (eye blink artifact) maximum at F3 (instead of Fp1) indicated by its phase reversal between channel 1 and channel 2. This is wrong for eye potential field (**A**). Correcting the mistake electronically resulted in normal eye field distribution (**B**). (**A** and **B** are the same EEG samples.)

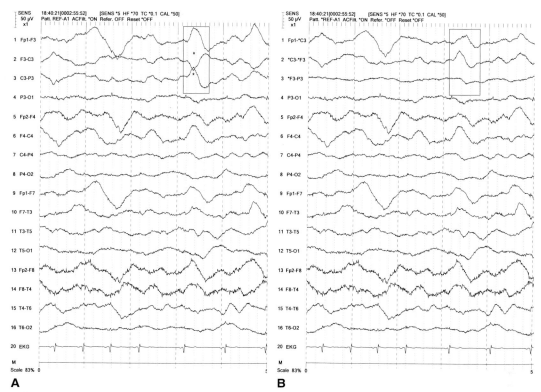

FIGURE 15-30 | Another example of a mistake by plugging electrodes into the wrong jack of the headbox. The EEG shows large ampli-tude delta slow waves with double-phase reversals between F3 and C3 (shown by * mark in the *box*), which are different from the cor-responding pairs on the right hemisphere **(A)**. This resulted from reversing F3 and C3 electrodes plug in at the headbox. Correcting the mistake electronically created the proper distribution of delta activity (shown by *box*) **(B)**. (**A** and **B** are the same EEG samples.)

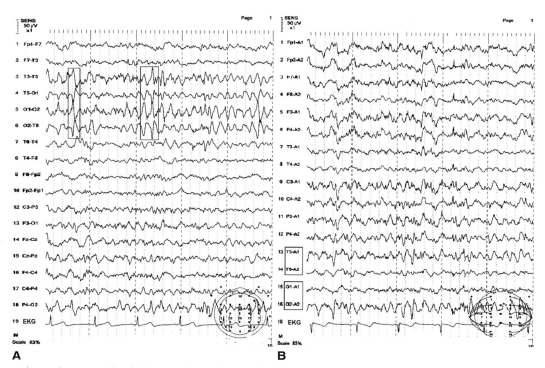

FIGURE 15-31 | Another example of plugging electrode into the wrong jack. This sleep EEG shows an unusual distribution of POSTs with triple-phase reversals (shown by *rectangular box*) **(A)**. Changing the montage to referential recording shows some clue that the amplitude distribution was illogical with greater amplitude activity at O2 and T5 than O1 and T6, respectively **(B)**. This was due to a reversal of T5 and O1 at the headboard. Correcting this reversal electronically resulted in symmetric amplitude between O1 and O2 and T5 and T6 in a referential recording **(C)** and normal distribution of POSTs **(D)**. (**A–D** are all the same EEG samples.)

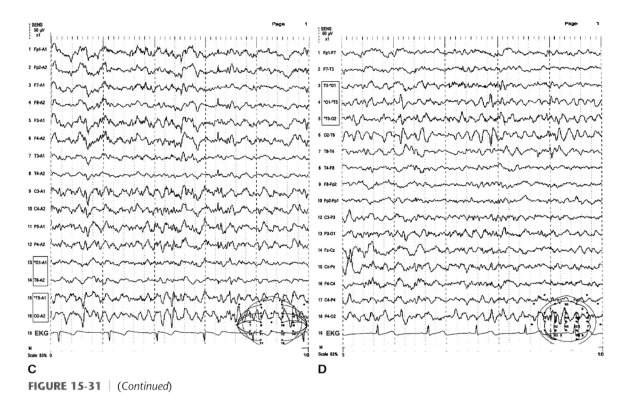

FIGURE 15-31 | (Continued)

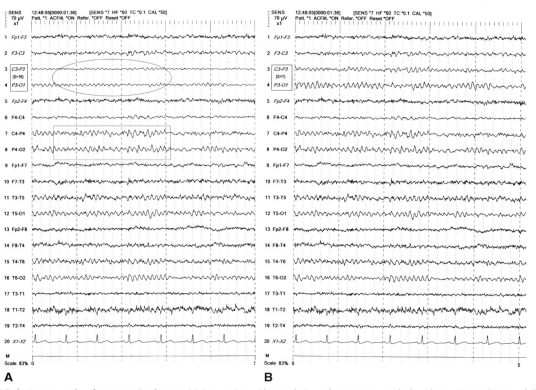

FIGURE 15-32 | An example of an error in the sensitivity setting. Channels 3 and 4 were recorded with $S = 10$ µV/mm, while the others were $S = 7$ µV/mm. Comparing homologous electrode pairs (shown by *oval circle and rectangular box*) gives a false impression that the alpha amplitude was depressed on the left **(A)**. Correcting the sensitivity setting showed a symmetric amplitude distribution **(B)**. (**A** and **B** are the same EEG samples.)

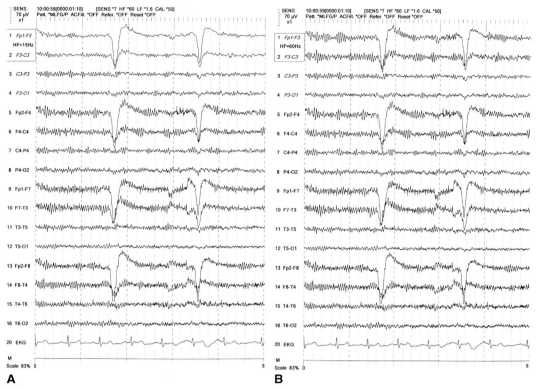

FIGURE 15-33 | An example of an error in filter setting. Channels 1 to 4 were recorded with a high-filter setting of 15 Hz, while the others were 70 Hz (shown by *box*) **(A)**. This gives a false impression that the beta activity is depressed on the left frontocentral region. Equalizing all filter settings at 70 Hz corrected the asymmetry **(B)**. (**A** and **B** are the same EEG samples.)

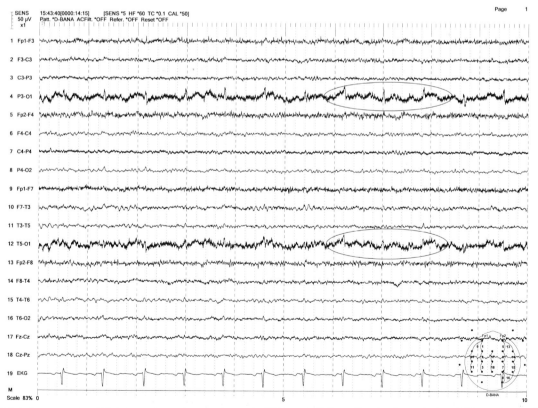

FIGURE 15-34 | An example of high impedance in one electrode. EKG and 60-Hz artifact in channels 4 and 12 are the result of unequal electrode impedance (high impedance in O1) (shown in *oval circle*).

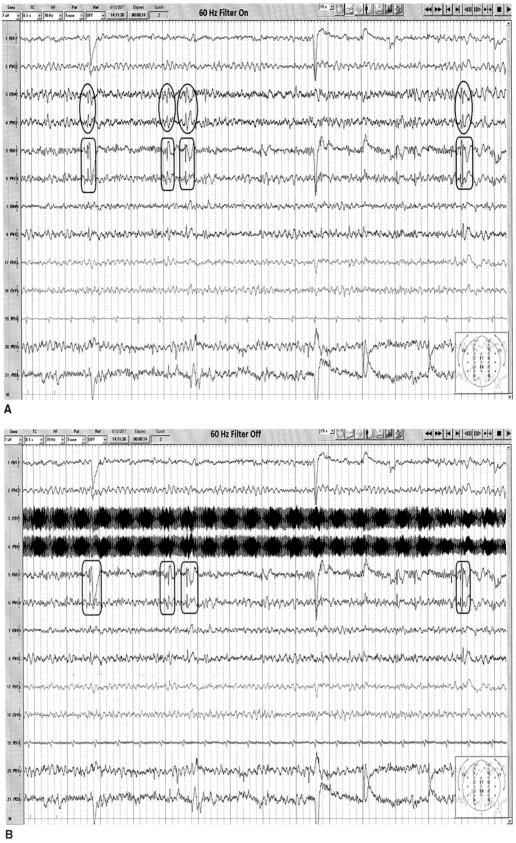

FIGURE 15-35 | The EEG (recorded with 60 Hz filter on) shows well defined and well localized spikes from right frontal region as shown in *rectangular boxes* **(A)**. Also this shows synchronous spikes at left parietal (P3) electrode (shown in *circles*). It is obvious that the distribution of spikes is illogical. This erroneous distribution occurred due to the high impedance of P3 electrode and in reality, P3 was replaced by ground electrode which was placed at Fpz. In a sense, Channels 3 and 4 are acting as C3-Ground (FpZ) and Ground (FpZ)-O1 recording, respectively, registering spikes from FpZ electrode. The same EEG sample provided the evidence of high impedance electrode at P3 by high amplitude 60 Hz artifact when recorded with 60 Hz filter off **(B)**. After correcting the P3 impedance, spikes are correctly localized at F3 electrode **(C)**.

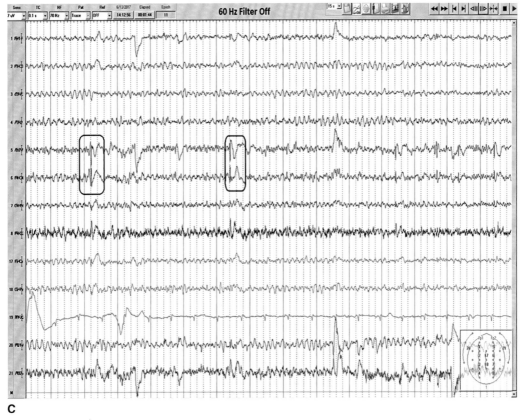

C

FIGURE 15-35 | (Continued)

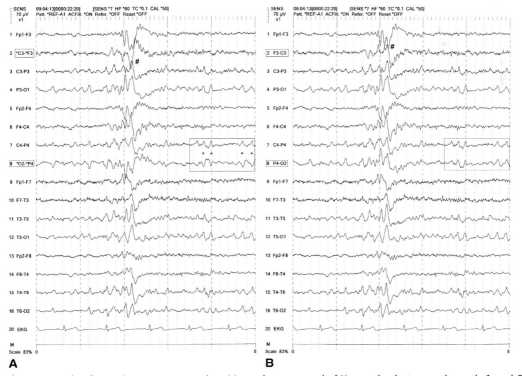

A   **B**

FIGURE 15-36 | An example of error in montage creation. Note phase reversal of K complex between channels 1 and 2 (shown by #
mark) and also POSTs at channels 7 and 8 with "negative" polarity (shown by *asterisk marks* in the *rectangular box*). These do not make
sense for normal distribution of K complex and POSTs **(A)**. These anomalous distributions and polarity were created by reversing an
electrode pair in channel 2 (C3 to F3 instead of F3 to C3) and in channel 8 (O2 to P4 instead of P4 to O2). Correcting the error showed
appropriate distribution and polarity of K complex and POSTs **(B)**. (**A** and **B** are the same EEG samples.)

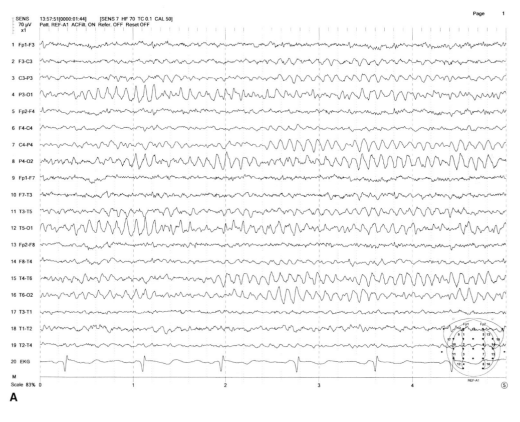

A

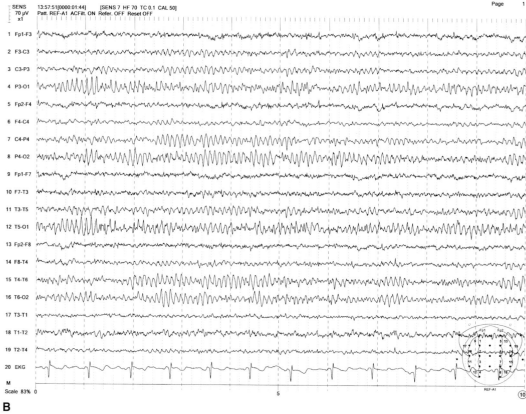

B

FIGURE 15-37 | An example of fast sweep speed (5 s/page) giving false visual impression that the background activity is "slow" **(A)**. Background frequency is obviously normal when viewed at conventional sweep speed (10 s/page) **(B)**. (First 5 seconds of EEG in **B** is the same as **A**.)

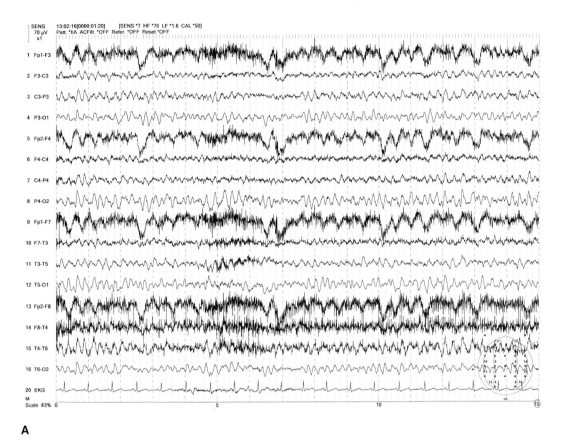

A

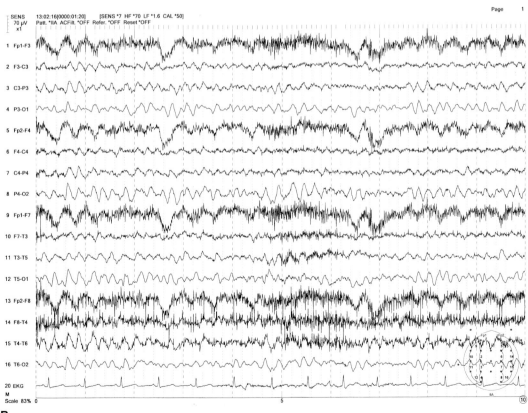

B

FIGURE 15-38 | An example of slow sweep speed (15 s/page) giving false visual impression that background activity is "normal" **(A)**, which is actually slow when viewed at conventional sweep speed (10 s/page) **(B)**. (First 10 s of EEG in **A** is the same as **B**.)

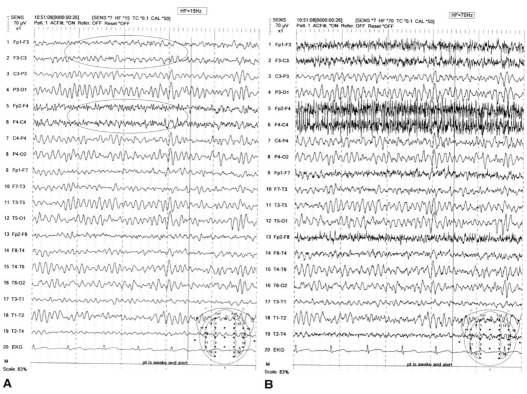

FIGURE 15-39 | An example of filtered muscle artifact. Note the asymmetric fast ("beta") activity at F4, but not at F3 when recorded with a high filter of 15 Hz (shown by *ovals* in **A**). This was actually asymmetric muscle artifact, which was evident with a high filter of 70 Hz **(B)**. (**A** and **B** are the same EEG samples.)

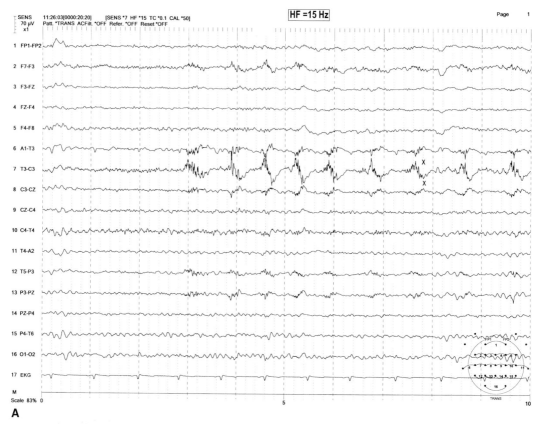

FIGURE 15-40 | An example of filtered muscle artifact. The figure shows repetitive "polyspike" discharges arising from left temporal region recorded with a high filter of 15 Hz **(A)**. Double-phase reversal (an example is shown by *"x" mark*) provides some clue that they are of artifactual origin. Changing the filter to HF 70 Hz **(B)** clarifies that they are muscle artifacts. (**A** and **B** are the same EEG samples.)

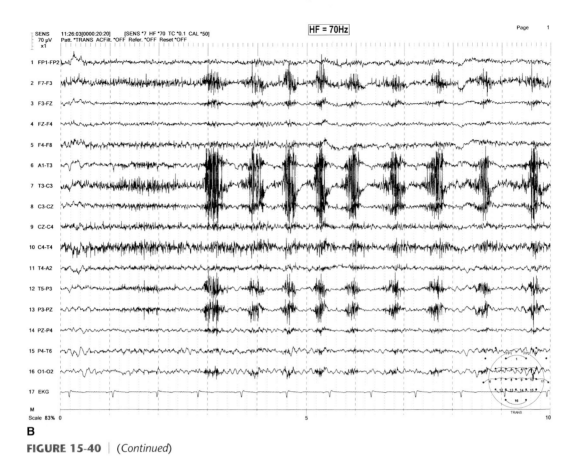

B

FIGURE 15-40 | (Continued)

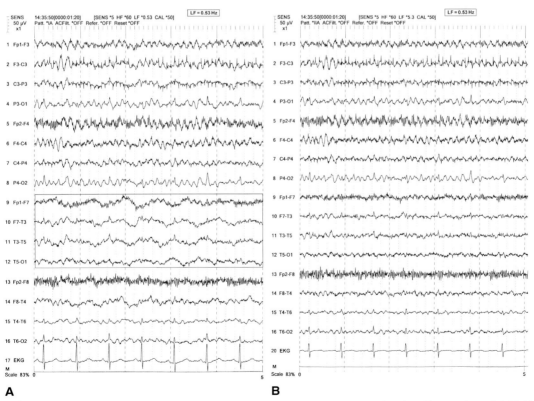

A   **B**

FIGURE 15-41 | An example of raising low-filter setting eliminating focal slow wave. With a low-filter setting of 0.53 Hz, focal delta activity over left temporal region is evident (see *rectangular box*) **(A)**. With a low-filter setting of 5 Hz, the above focal delta is hardly recognized **(B)**. (**A** and **B** are the same EEG samples.)

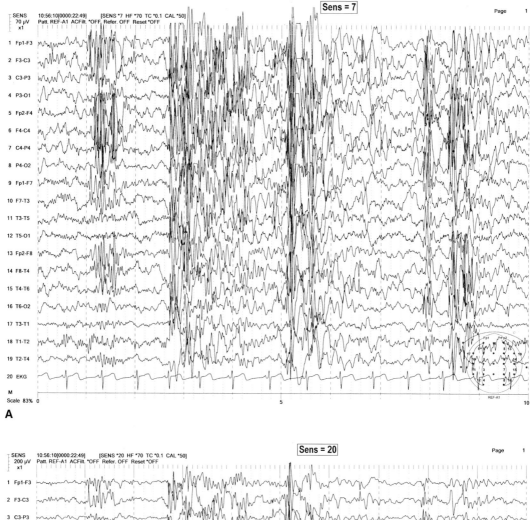

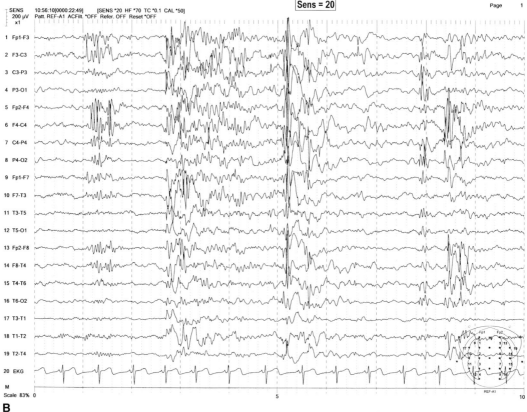

FIGURE 15-42 | An example of using sensitivity to aid in visualizing the details of waveforms and distribution. With a sensitivity of 7 μV/mm, high-amplitude polyspike and wave bursts obscure the focal nature of the discharge **(A)**. Lowering the sensitivity to $S = 20$ μV/mm makes the multifocal nature of these discharges more evident **(B)**. (**A** and **B** are the same EEG samples.)

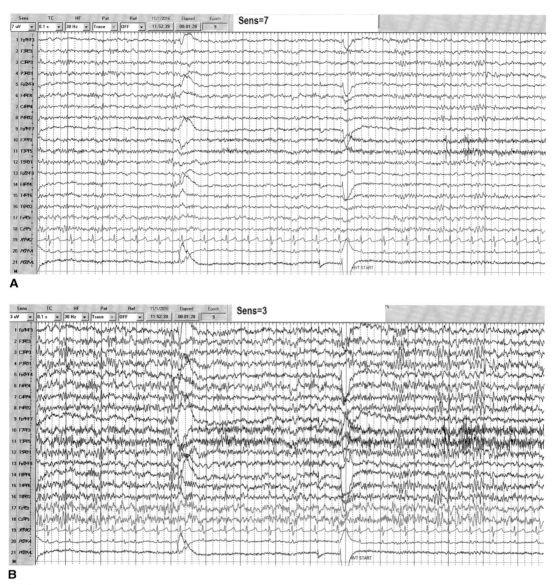

FIGURE 15-43 | An example to show how normal low-voltage EEG **(A)** seemingly changed to abnormal EEG containing excessive underlying theta–delta slow waves **(B)** by raising sensitivity from 7 **(A)** to 3 **(B)**.

9. Is the montage change appropriate? Depending on the field distribution of a given activity, certain montages may enhance the activity, while others may eliminate or minimize the activity (Figs. 15-44A and B and 15-45A and B). In some cases, an abnormality is visible in one montage but not in the other (Figs. 15-46A and B and 15-47A and B). Or, certain montages may give rise to false distribution or false asymmetry due to cancelation effect of bipolar montage (Fig. 15-48A and B). In some occasions, changing montages may help differentiate artifacts from genuine cerebral activity.

10. Are electrodes placed with accurate measurements? If there is an unequal electrode distance between two homologous electrode pairs, the amplitude from a pair of shorter interelectrode distance becomes smaller compared to that from the corresponding pair (Fig. 15-49). The reverse is true for longer interelectrode distance.

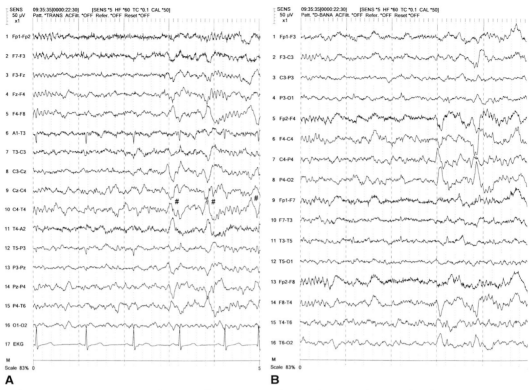

FIGURE 15-44 | An example of a montage change making a certain abnormality more distinct. This sleep EEG on a transverse montage showed a V wave, which is skewed to the right hemisphere evident by phase reversal at C4 (an example is marked by "#") **(A)**. The V-wave asymmetry became much more distinct on a longitudinal montage **(B)**. (**A** and **B** are the same EEG samples.)

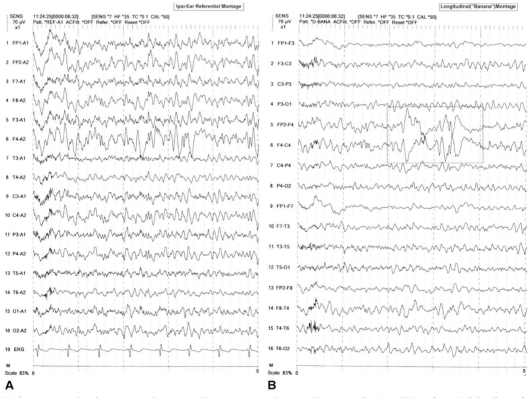

FIGURE 15-45 | An example of montage change making a certain abnormality more distinct. This referential (ipsilateral ear reference) shows relatively "subtle" focal delta with sharp discharges from right frontal (F4) region **(A)**. These focal discharges are much more distinct in longitudinal montage (shown by *rectangular box*) **(B)**. The patient had a history of craniotomy with burr hole nearby F4 electrode. (**A** and **B** are the same EEG samples.)

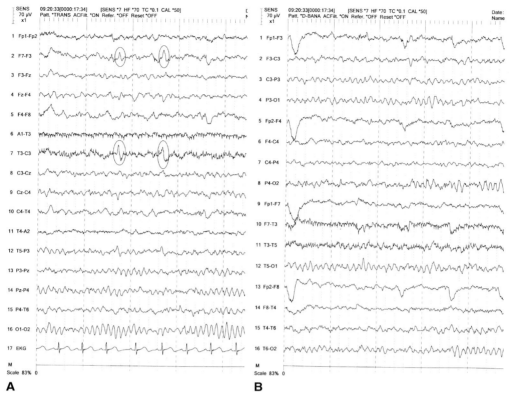

FIGURE 15-46 | An example of abnormal discharges shown in one montage but not in the other montage. The transverse recording showed intermittent sharp discharges from F7, T3, and T5 (shown by *ovals* in **A**). These discharges became totally obscured in longitudinal derivation **(B)**. This was due to a cancelation effect by a near equipotential field distribution of the sharp discharges at F7, T3, and T5. (**A** and **B** are the same EEG samples.)

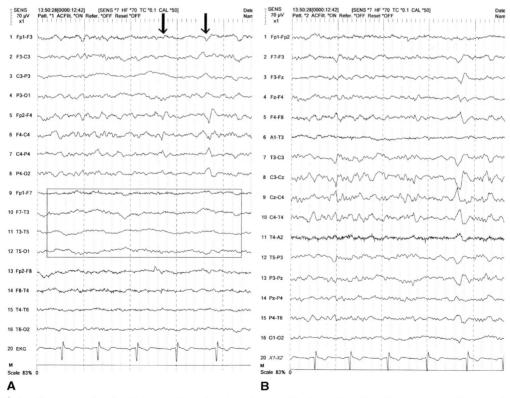

FIGURE 15-47 | Another example of certain montage showing abnormality but not in the other montage. The longitudinal montage showed delta activity over left temporal and parietal regions (shown by *rectangular box*) and depression of V waves on left parasagittal region (shown by *arrows*) **(A)**, but these asymmetries were hardly recognizable in the transverse montage **(B)**. (**A** and **B** are the same EEG samples.)

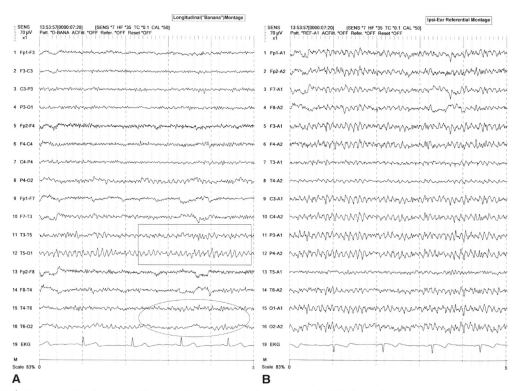

FIGURE 15-48 | An example showing false amplitude asymmetry and/or distribution of a certain activity by bipolar derivation. Longitudinal bipolar recording showed depressed alpha on the right as compared to the left posterior head region (shown in *rectangular box* and *oval circle*, respectively, in **A**). Referential recording with ipsilateral ear reference showed the symmetric amplitude of alpha rhythm between O1 and O2 but greater amplitude at T6 than T5 **(B)**. The greater amplitude difference between O1 and T5 resulted in the greater amplitude in T5 and O1 derivation, while the similar amplitude difference between T6 and O2 resulted in the smaller amplitude by cancelation in bipolar recording. (**A** and **B** are the same EEG samples.)

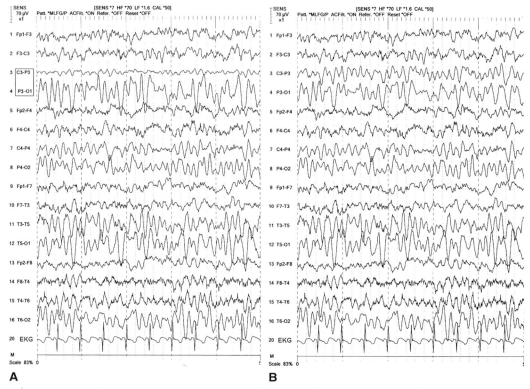

FIGURE 15-49 | An example of error in electrode placement. The longitudinal montage showed depressed activity in channel 3 as compared to homologous derivation (channel 7) **(A)**. This was due to P3 electrode placement error with shorter interelectrode distance between C3 and P3 (shown by *box*), as compared to the homologous electrode pair. Adjusting the electrode placement corrected the asymmetry **(B)**.

EEG of Premature and Full-Term Infants

THORU YAMADA, ELIZABETH MENG, and MICHAEL CILIBERTO

The EEG of premature and neonatal infants must be viewed from a different perspective than the EEG of adults or children because of the wide variation of "normal" EEG patterns in the neonate, especially in premature infants. The rapid progression of EEG maturation and a number of EEG patterns of uncertain clinical significance impose further difficulty in determining normality. Accurate interpretation of neonatal EEG has become increasingly important since many neonatal seizures occur without definite evidence of clinical seizures and also, even experienced clinical observers may have a difficulty in recognizing seizures in neonates.[1] This has led to an era of expanding use of EEG in the neonatal periods. The aim of this chapter is not to discuss the variations of premature EEG patterns in detail; only essential and well-established concepts will be described here. For further details, the reader should refer to several excellent review papers.[2-4]

Recording Techniques

Because of the smaller head size in children, fewer electrodes are generally used than in adult patients with whom the 10-20 system is typically used. American Clinical Neurophysiologic Society (ACNS) guidelines[5] recommend the following placement: Fp1 and Fp2 [or Fp3 and Fp4 (Fp3 is halfway between Fp1 and F3 and Fp4 is halfway between Fp2 and F4)], C3 and C4, T3 and T4, O1 and O2, A1 and A2, and Cz. A recording utilizing at least 12 channels should be used. For EEG recording, the use of low-frequency filter of 0.3 to 0.6 Hz or time constant of 0.27 to 0.33 second is recommended. The sensitivity is usually 7 μv/mm but might need to be adjusted either higher or lower depending on the case.

In order to assess waking and sleeping states (quiet and active sleep), respiratory movements and airflow, EKG, EOG, and submental EMG are routinely recorded. This has been facilitated by the ability of some software packages to interface with typical neonatal monitoring systems allowing the accurate acquisition of respiratory, pulse oximetry, and heart rate data. Besides recording EEG, additional channels are dedicated to respiratory movements by abdominal and/or thoracic strain gauges or impedance pneumogram and airflow by thermistors/thermocouples, EKG, EOG, and submental EMG. For EOG recording, low-frequency filter of 0.3 to 0.6 Hz would be adequate. For EMG recording, low-filter setting of 5 Hz and high filter of 70 Hz, and sensitivity of 3 μv/mm are used.

Commonly used montages (as recommended by ACNS) are shown in Table 16-1.[5] Recording montages should routinely include the vertex (Cz) electrode because significant EEG patterns characteristic for this age group (positive vertex sharp waves, negative vertex sharp waves, and electrographic seizures) may be detected only from this region. Unlike in older children and adults, multiple reviewing montages are typically not used with readers typically relying on a comprehensive bipolar montage with the addition of the aforementioned other leads.

The Role of Technologists

Besides gathering routine information for EEG recording (history, reason for referral, medication, state of consciousness, etc.),

TABLE 16-1 Neonatal Montages			
Channel	Montage A	Montage B	Montage C
1	Fp1-T7(T3)	Fp1-C3	Fp1-T7(T3)
2	T7(T3)-O1	C3-O1	T7(T3)-O1
3	Fp2-T8(T4)	Fp1-T7(T3)	Fp1-C3
4	T8(T4)-O2	T7(T3)-O1	C3-O1
5	Fp1-C3	Fp2-C4	Fp2-T8(T4)
6	C3-O1	C4-O2	T8(T4)-O2
7	Fp2-C4	Fp2-F8(T4)	Fp2-C4
8	C4-O2	T8(T4)-O2	C4-O2
9	T7(T3)-C3	T7(T3)-C3	T7(T3)-C3
10	C3-Cz	C3-Cz	C3-Cz
11	Cz-C4	Cz-C4	Cz-C4
12	C4-T8(T4)	C4-T8(T4)	C4-T8(T4)
13	ECG	ECG	ECG
14	Respiration	Respiration	Respiration
15	LOC-A1 or A2	LOC-A1 or A2	LOC-A1 or A2
16	ROC-A1 or A2	ROC-A1 or A2	ROC-A1 or A2
17	EMG	EMG	EMG

ECG, electrocardiogram; EMG, electromyogram; LOC, left outer cantus electrode; ROC, right outer cantus electrode (see Fig. 8-16).

it is imperative to note the gestational age (GA) (the time elapsed between the first day of the last menstrual period and the day of delivery) and chronological age (the time elapsed since birth). The term "conceptional age (CA)" has been used based on the day of conception. The American Academy of Pediatrics now recommends using postmenstrual age, not the day of conception for determining GA. For example, a baby whose EEG is recorded at 4 weeks after birth with a GA of 30 weeks at the time of birth is 34 weeks CA. A baby born at 38 to 40 weeks GA is a full-term baby. A baby born at or before 38 weeks GA is considered to be premature. And, a baby born after 40 weeks GA is postmature. The survival of infants born before 34 or 35 weeks GA was not common 30 years ago, but today, it is not uncommon for a 24- to 26-week-GA baby to survive.

Other relevant clinical information includes blood gas, body temperature, serum electrolyte, and current medications. Also, technologists should consult nursing staff concerning the patient's condition or any limitation in handing the baby.

The recording is preferably scheduled right after feeding time, since babies tend to sleep after feeding although an hour-long recording of most neonates should capture all stages of sleep and sleep–wake transitions. The technologist must observe the patient carefully throughout the recording and annotate the baby's movement or behavioral changes. The notation may include eye opening and closing, head position, hiccups, sucking, breathing patterns, etc. The technologist should also note any unusual behaviors such as tonic posturing, clonic movement, eye deviation, skin color change, and other vital signs including SaO$_2$ saturation, blood pressure, and respiratory changes (Video 16-1). It is also important for the technologist to observe and note the baby's state of consciousness. Routine use of video recording with EEG would be extremely helpful to correlate EEG findings with babies' various behaviors.

Except for extremely premature infants (23 to 24 weeks GA), wakefulness is simply determined by eye opening and sleep is determined by eye closure. It may be possible to determine clinically if a baby is in *active or quiet sleep*, because of corresponding rapid eye movement (REM) or non-REM sleep, respectively, by observing the baby's behavior. In *active sleep*, a baby may show a variety of facial, eyelid, arm, and leg twitches or body movements, sucking, or even crying. Under closed eyelids, REMs (rapid eye movements), predominantly in the horizontal direction, can be observed. Respiration becomes irregular, occasionally associated with apnea. The EEG during active sleep essentially consists of a low-voltage and continuous pattern, resembling quiet wakefulness (Fig. 16-1). In newborn infants, 50% of sleep time is active sleep, and sleep may start with active sleep directly from wakefulness. This pattern of active sleep onset may continue until about 4 months postterm, when *quiet sleep* becomes a prerequisite to entering active sleep. Also, the percentage of active sleep decreases rapidly to 20% to 25% of sleep time. In contrast to active sleep, quiet

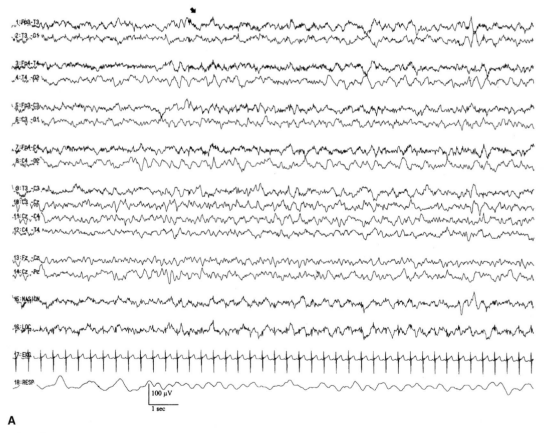

A

FIGURE 16-1 | Wakefulness **(A)** and active (REM) sleep **(B)** in a 41-week-CA infant. Both EEGs show continuous low to moderate amplitude and variably mixed frequency activity (*activité moyenne*). EEG patterns are similar in both states. The only distinctions are the absence of muscle tone and REM in REM (active) sleep, while muscle tone is maintained in awake state. (From Clancy RR, Bergqvist AGC, Dlugos DJ. Neonatal electroencephalography. In: Ebersole JS, Pedley TA, eds. *Current Practice of Clinical Electroencephalography*. 3rd Ed. Philadelphia, PA: Lippincott Williams & Wilkins, 2003:160–245, with permission.)

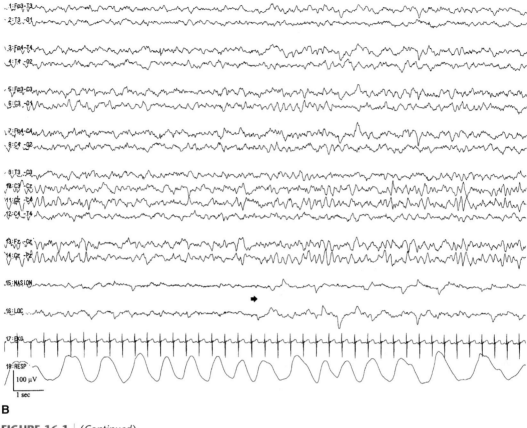

B

FIGURE 16-1 | (*Continued*)

sleep is characterized by few movements or twitches of face, head, limb, or trunk. Respirations are quiet and regular, without apnea. The EEG of quiet sleep consists of a variety of slow waves or bursts interrupted by a relatively low-voltage pattern representing *trace discontinue* (*TD*) (Fig. 16-2) or *trace alternant* (*TA*) (Fig. 16-3). It is important to capture quiet sleep because this may be the only state in which some EEG abnormalities become evident. The recording should include waking and all cycles of sleep including active and quiet sleep. Since active sleep occupies more than 50% of the sleep time in the neonate, a 1-hour recording will generally capture all states. After a satisfactory sleep record, the baby may be aroused while the recording continues. In order to capture all sleep stages and awake record, recording time for neonates should be at least 1 hour.

General Characteristics of Normal Neonatal EEG

The first step of neonatal EEG analysis is to examine the degree of continuity of EEG activity. The second step is to examine the synchrony of EEG activity between homologous cortical areas. The third step is to evaluate the various EEG patterns characteristic for neonates and, lastly, to determine whether these features are appropriate for the stated CA.

CONTINUITY VERSUS DISCONTINUITY

The EEG in a neonate less than 27 to 30 weeks CA is characterized by a discontinuous pattern, consisting of intermittent irregularly mixed bursts of theta–delta with sharp and fast activities interrupted by relative voltage suppression periods. There are two types of discontinuous patterns: one is *TD* (Fig. 16-2) and the other is *TA* (Fig. 16-3). Both patterns occur during all stages of sleep.[6] The TD pattern consists of very slow (0.3 to 1 Hz) delta bursts, which may be intermixed with 4- to 5-Hz theta activity, alternating with quiescent periods.[7,8] The length of this "flat" or inactive EEG may carry important diagnostic value; a flat period greater than 30 seconds carries a greater risk of nonsurvival, whereas a shorter inactive period tends to correlate with a favorable outcome.[9] However, some data suggest that longer periods of relative voltage suppression may be acceptable in CAs less than 28 weeks.[10] TD continues until 35 weeks CA and evolves to TA thereafter (Fig. 16-3, see also Fig. 16-14). TA consists of a variety of theta–delta waves mixed with fast and "spiky" or sharply contoured activities lasting 3 to 10 seconds followed by a relative suppression period of 5 to 10 seconds. Unlike TD, the inactive period of TA is not truly "flat" but consists of low-voltage activities of mixed frequency. The TA pattern is gradually replaced by slow-wave sleep toward full term and is completely replaced by 44 to 45 weeks CA (Fig. 16-4, see also Fig. 16-14).[11]

SYNCHRONY VERSUS ASYNCHRONY

Degrees of interhemispheric synchrony of the above described bursts differ depending on the CA. About 70% of the bursts during quiet sleep are synchronous at 31 to 32 weeks CA. Thereafter, synchronization increases to 80% at 33 to 34 weeks

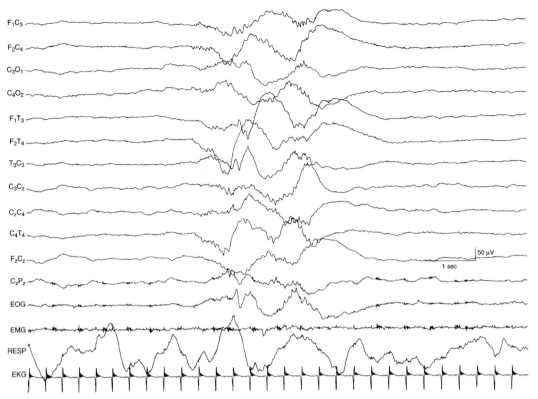

FIGURE 16-2 | EEG of trace discontinue (TD) in a 26- to 27-week-CA infant. A burst, consisting of large irregular delta with super-imposed fast activity, appears intermittently preceded and followed by periods of inactivity. Note overall symmetry of the burst but with some asynchrony between two hemispheres. (From Mizrahi EM, Hrachovy RA, Kellway P. *Atlas of Neonatal Electroencephalography*. Philadelphia, PA: Lippincott Williams & Wilkins, 2004, with permission.)

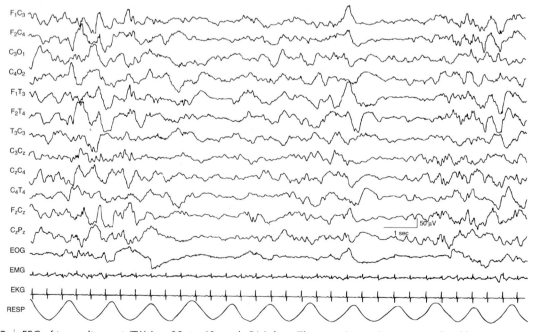

FIGURE 16-3 | EEG of trace alternant (TA) in a 38- to 40-week-CA infant. There are intermittent generalized bursts consisting of various frequency activities lasting several seconds followed by relative quiescent period during quiet (non-REM) sleep. Note the quiescent period is not as "flat" as in TD (see Fig. 16-2). (From Hrachovy RA. Development of the normal electroencephalogram. In: Levin KH, Luders HO, eds. *Comprehensive Clinical Neurophysiology*. Philadelphia, PA: WB Saunders, 2000, with permission.)

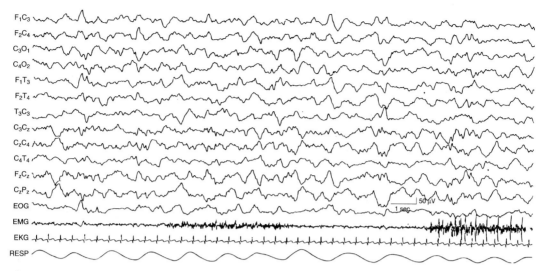

FIGURE 16-4 | EEG of continuous slow-wave sleep (CSWS) during quiet sleep in a 38- to 40-week-CA infant. EEG is dominated by relatively high amplitude continuous delta mixed with some theta and fast activities. Note the difference from TA (see Fig. 16-3), wherein slow waves are interrupted by relatively quiescent periods. (From Hrachovy RA. Development of the normal electroencephalogram. In: Levin KH, Luders HO, eds. *Comprehensive Clinical Neurophysiology*. Philadelphia, PA: WB Saunders, 2000, with permission.)

CA, 85% at 35 to 36 weeks CA, and 100% after 37 weeks CA.[5,8,12] Paradoxically, infants younger than 30 weeks CA may show more synchronized bursts with infants less than 26 weeks CA being mostly synchronous.[13] Persistent asynchrony after 37 weeks CA is considered to be abnormal.[12] Despite the presence of interhemisphere and intrahemisphere asynchrony, overall EEG activities between the two hemispheres should be symmetric. An abnormality is suspected if an amplitude asymmetry is consistently greater than 50%; the depressed side is abnormal in most cases.

ACTIVE VERSUS QUIET SLEEP AND WAKE EEG PATTERN

In early prematurity (before 30 weeks CA), no sleep stage distinction can be made; newborns show an atypical pattern with mixed characteristics of active and quiet sleep. EEG of active sleep consists of more or less continuous, relatively low amplitude (<100 μV), theta activity mixed with delta and some alpha and fast frequency activities (see Fig. 16-1B). After 30 weeks CA, continuity occurs only in active (REM) sleep. Active sleep is predominant until 34 weeks CA[14] (see Fig. 16-14). The wake EEG pattern closely resembles active sleep, consisting mostly of low amplitude (15 to 60 μV), mixed theta and delta rhythms, with intermingled or superimposed low-voltage alpha and beta activities. The high tonic EMG activity and eye opening help to distinguish awake from active sleep. Active sleep is characterized by (i) REMs; (ii) irregular respiration, often associated with apnea; and (iii) decreased muscle tone. Despite decreased muscle tone, phasic motor activities such as random muscle twitches, smiling, or grimacing increase in this state.

Quiet sleep emerges after 34 to 36 weeks CA, and at full term (40 weeks CA), active sleep and quiet sleep share an equal percentage of sleep[15] (see Fig. 16-14). During quiet sleep, the infant (i) lies quietly with only occasional startle-like movements, (ii) shows no eye movements, (iii) has regular respiration, and (iv) shows continuous tonic muscle activity in the

EMG channel. The EEG of quiet sleep is characterized by two types of activity; one is *high-voltage slow* (HVS) or *continuous slow waves* (CSW) and the other is TA.

The EEG pattern of TA consists of bursts of 3- to 10-Hz waves mixed with sharp, spike-like discharges lasting 3 to 10 seconds, separated by periods (5 to 10 seconds) of low voltage (see Fig. 16-3). HVS is characterized by 0.5- to 4-Hz delta–theta waves with amplitude reaching 200 V, mixed with low-voltage faster activity (see Fig. 16-4). After full term, quiet sleep progressively increases with concomitant decrease of active sleep, and by 8 months of age, active sleep occupies only 25% of total sleep time, which approximates the amount of REM sleep in an adult.

Specific Pattern Characteristic for a Premature Baby

DELTA BRUSH

The delta brush has also been called "*spindle-like fast*,"[11] "*brushes*,"[12] "*rapid bursts*,"[15] or "*ripple of prematurity*."[16] This pattern consists of a slow wave of 0.5 to 1.5 Hz with amplitude ranging from 100 to 250 μV with a superimposed, rhythmic 8- to 22-Hz activity of 40 to 70 μV amplitude[17,18] (Fig. 16-5). Delta brush appears as early as 27 weeks CA, mainly in the central areas and becomes most abundant at 32 to 34 weeks CA, appearing maximally in occipital and/or temporal, central areas (see Fig. 16-11). They are rare at full term and should not be present after 44 weeks CA. They are more common in quiet than in active sleep.

TEMPORAL THETA BURSTS

This pattern has also been called "*temporal sharp transient*"[17] or "*temporal sawtooth*."[7] It consists of brief bursts of rhythmic, sharply contoured 4- to 7-Hz theta bursts with amplitude of 150 to

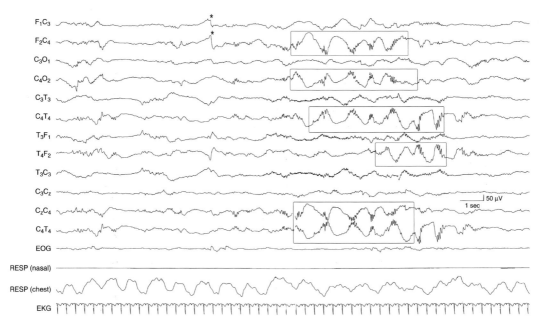

FIGURE 16-5 | Examples of delta brushes in a 34- to 35-week-CA infant. Delta brushes consisting of high amplitude delta with superimposed spindle-like fast activity are present mostly from right central region (*indicated in boxes*). Also note frontal sharp transients (encoches frontales) *indicated by star (') mark*. (From Mizrahi EM, Hrachovy RA, Kellway P. *Atlas of Neonatal Electroencephalography*. Philadelphia, PA: Lippincott Williams & Wilkins, 2004, with permission.)

200 μV located in temporal areas (Fig. 16-6). The appearance of this pattern is limited to very young premature infants (29 to 32 weeks CA), after which it rapidly diminishes (see Fig. 16-14).[18]

FRONTAL SHARP TRANSIENTS

This has also been called "*encoches frontales*."[19] It appears at 35 to 36 weeks CA and may persist until 2 months postterm.[20] These sharps are localized to frontopolar areas, appearing unilaterally or bilaterally, and are often asynchronous (Fig. 16-7).

They tend to appear more during the transition from active to quiet sleep. The waveform is quite sharp at 36 to 37 weeks CA but becomes more blunted with maturation and may persist until 44 weeks CA (see Fig. 16-14).

FOCAL SHARP WAVES AND SPIKES

The distinctions between "normal" and "abnormal" spikes or sharp waves are not always clear and stringent criteria have not been developed. In general, these "normal" spike or sharp waves

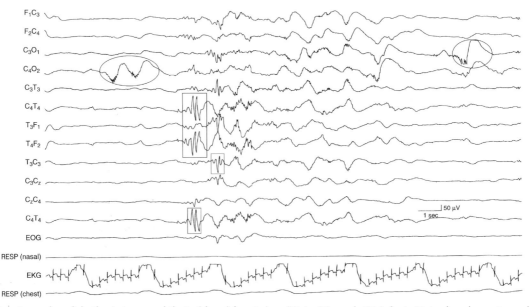

FIGURE 16-6 | Examples of rhythmic temporal theta (sharp) bursts in a 30- to 32-week-CA infant. Note sharply contoured theta bursts from T4 electrode (shown in *boxes*) at the onset of diffuse asynchronous delta bursts in this TD pattern. There are also asynchronous delta brushes at O1, O2, and T4 electrodes (examples are shown by *oval circle*) within the bursts. (From Mizrahi EM, Hrachovy RA, Kellway P. *Atlas of Neonatal Electroencephalography*. Philadelphia, PA: Lippincott Williams & Wilkins, 2004, with permission.)

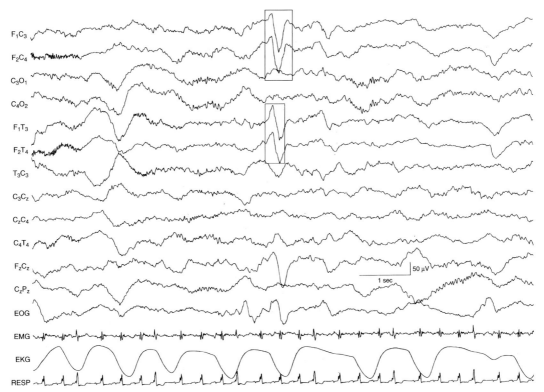

FIGURE 16-7 | Examples of frontal sharp transients (encoches frontales) in a 36- to 37-week-CA infant. Note broad sharp transients appearing synchronously at frontal electrodes (shown in *boxes*). (From Mizrahi EM, Hrachovy RA, Kellway P. *Atlas of Neonatal Electroencephalography*. Philadelphia, PA: Lippincott Williams & Wilkins, 2004, with permission.)

occur infrequently (generally at intervals >1 minute), singly, and randomly at midtemporal or central electrodes without consistent focal features or runs of recurrence. The waveforms are monophasic or diphasic with dominant surface-negative polarity. In premature infants, the discharges can occur in any state; in a term infant, they should "normally" be seen only in sleep. Runs of rhythmic discharges are considered to be abnormal irrespective of polarities, especially if not arising from the temporal region (Fig. 16-8). A discharge with positive polarity or polyphasic wave form is also abnormal (Fig. 16-9).

Normal EEG of Premature Neonates According to Conceptional Age

LESS THAN 27 WEEKS CA

The EEG patterns are invariably discontinuous (i.e., TD pattern). The bursts consist of various activities of delta (0.5 Hz) to slow beta (14 Hz) frequencies of 50 to 300 μV amplitude. The bursts last one to several seconds and are interrupted by an inactive or "flat" background lasting a few seconds to as long as 60 seconds. Bursts are synchronous. Differentiation between sleep and wakefulness cannot be made by EEG.

27 TO 29 WEEKS CA

The EEG patterns are invariably discontinuous (i.e., TD pattern). The bursts consist of various activities of delta (0.5 Hz) to slow beta (14 Hz) frequencies of 50 to 300 μV amplitude. The bursts last a few seconds to several seconds and are interrupted

by an inactive or "flat" background lasting a few seconds to as long as 30 seconds (Fig. 16-2). Some consider inactivity lasting more than 30 seconds to be abnormal.[9] Delta brush may be present within the bursts. The bursts in each hemisphere may

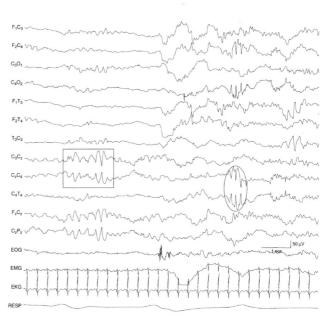

FIGURE 16-8 | Examples of abnormal midline (vertex) rhythmic theta bursts (shown in *box*) and central (C4) spike bursts (shown by *oval circle*) in a 35-week-CA infant with intraventricular hemorrhage. Both are negative polarity but runs of rhythmic discharges are abnormal. (From Mizrahi EM, Hrachovy RA, Kellway P. *Atlas of Neonatal Electroencephalography*. Philadelphia, PA: Lippincott Williams & Wilkins, 2004, with permission.)

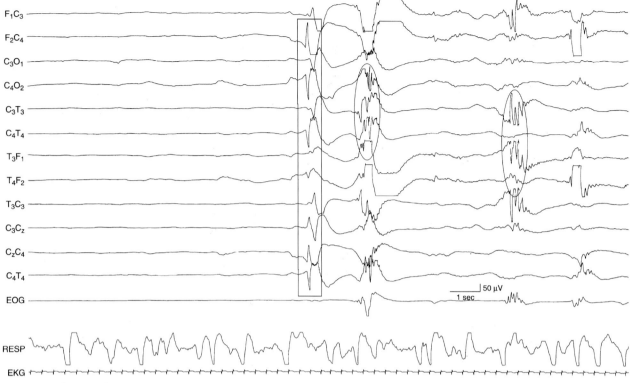

FIGURE 16-9 | Examples of surface-positive sharp wave at C4 electrode (shown in *box*) in a 29- to 30-week-CA infant with an intraventricular hemorrhage. Note also polyphasic spikes and sharp waves from central and temporal electrodes (shown in *circles*). (From Mizrahi EM, Hrachovy RA, Kellway P. *Atlas of Neonatal Electroencephalography*. Philadelphia, PA: Lippincott Williams & Wilkins, 2004, with permission.)

be strikingly synchronous. Awake, quiet sleep, or active sleep cannot be differentiated at this age. The EEG also shows an atypical stage of sleep with mixed characteristics of active and quiet sleep.

29 TO 31 WEEKS CA

Rudimentary active sleep may be identified starting at this CA. TD pattern persists, but the discontinuity is decreased with shorter epochs of inactive EEG activity during sleep. During stretches of the EEG, prominent slow delta bursts (<1 Hz) associated with superimposed fast activity (around 16-Hz activity) appear[12] (Fig. 16-10). Delta brush is characteristically asynchronous between the hemispheres. Other physiological patterns characteristic for this age are temporal theta bursts, temporal sharp transients,[16] or temporal sawtooth waves[8] (Fig. 16-10).

32 TO 34 WEEKS CA

Starting at this age, the differentiation between wakefulness, active sleep, and quiet sleep becomes possible, though active sleep occupies more than 50% of sleep time. The EEG becomes more continuous, especially during active sleep and the awake state, but still exhibits long periods of discontinuity in quiet sleep. Delta waves of high amplitude predominate posteriorly, often with bilateral synchrony. The spindle component of delta burst (delta brush) now has slower frequencies and predominates over the central, temporal, and occipital areas (Fig. 16-11; compare

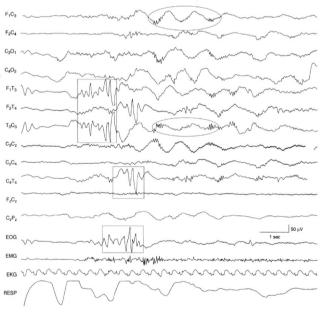

FIGURE 16-10 | Normal EEG in a 29- to 30-week-CA infant. Note temporal theta bursts from T3 and T4 (shown in *boxes*) independently and asynchronous delta brushes (shown in *circles*) from C3 and C4 electrodes. (From Mizrahi EM, Hrachovy RA, Kellway P. *Atlas of Neonatal Electroencephalography*. Philadelphia, PA: Lippincott Williams & Wilkins, 2004, with permission.)

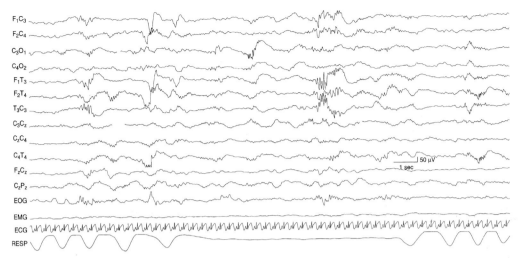

FIGURE 16-11 | Normal EEG in a 33-week-CA infant. Note abundant delta brushes with long durations from bilateral temporal regions and brief discontinuity of EEG pattern. (From Mizrahi EM, Hrachovy RA, Kellway P. *Atlas of Neonatal Electroencephalography*. Philadelphia, PA: Lippincott Williams & Wilkins, 2004, with permission.)

with Fig. 16-6). Up to this CA, delta brushes are still more common in the wake state and active sleep than in quiet sleep. The most characteristic EEG change at this CA is the increase of multifocal sharp transients appearing in waking as well as quiet and active sleep. TD continues to be the quiet sleep pattern.

34 TO 37 WEEKS CA

The differentiating characteristics of active and quiet sleep become more obvious. In active sleep as well as in the awake state, EEG activity becomes more continuous with relatively low to medium amplitude (20 to 100 μV) delta and theta waves (Fig. 16-12A).

Activité moyenne, meaning "average activity," can be seen at this age. This EEG pattern has less fluctuation in amplitude. Low-voltage beta rhythms are often present with anterior dominance.

The discontinuous EEG pattern (TD) persists in quiet sleep but becomes more like TA, in which the EEG inactivity between bursts consists of a low-voltage pattern instead of the "flat" tracing seen in TD (Fig. 16-12B). The inactivity between the two hemispheres may be quite asynchronous and may become more synchronous as the infant reaches term CA. Delta brush appears more in quiet sleep than in active sleep. Also, multifocal spikes diminish but frontal sharp transients persist or are even more frequent and of higher amplitude (see Fig. 16-7).

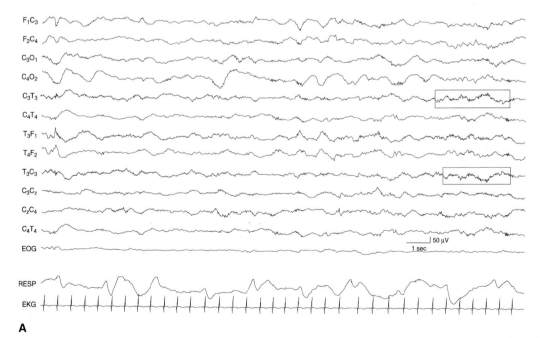

A

FIGURE 16-12 | EEG in a 34- to 35-week-CA infant, awake state and quiet sleep. Awake EEG shows more or less continuous EEG activity with intermittent delta brushes (examples are shown in *boxes*) **(A)**. Quiet sleep (non-REM sleep) shows prominent delta brushes (shown in *circles*) from right central and temporal regions with a period of discontinuity (shown by *horizontal line*) **(B)**. (From Mizrahi EM, Hrachovy RA, Kellway P. *Atlas of Neonatal Electroencephalography*. Philadelphia, PA: Lippincott Williams & Wilkins, 2004, with permission.)

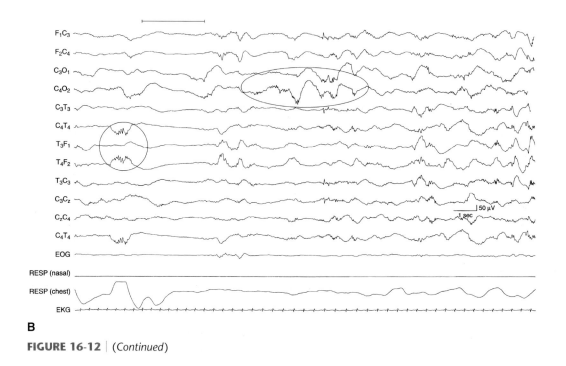

B

FIGURE 16-12 | (Continued)

38 TO 40 WEEKS CA

Cyclic changes of waking, quiet sleep, and active sleep are fully established. The EEG of awake and active sleep consists of a continuous low-voltage pattern, that is, *activité moyenne* (Fig. 16-13). In quiet sleep, TA may continue until 44 weeks CA. Delta brush starts to decrease but may continue until 44 weeks CA. Of total sleep time, about 50% is active sleep, 25% is quiet sleep, and the remaining 25% is indeterminate sleep, which constitutes mixed traits of active and quiet sleep. If the infant continues to sleep, the TA pattern eventually changes to continuous slow-wave sleep (CSWS) (see Fig. 16-4).

41 TO 44 WEEKS CA

In waking and active sleep, more stable and continuous EEG activities (*activité moyenne*) become the dominant pattern (see Fig. 16-1A and B), whereas delta brush gradually disappears by 44 weeks CA. There may be broad biphasic lambda waves

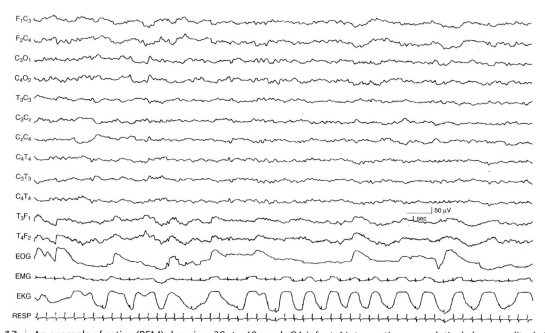

FIGURE 16-13 | An example of active (REM) sleep in a 38- to 40-week-CA infant. Note continuous, relatively low amplitude EEG activity with scarce delta waves, associated with REM, irregular respiration, and absence of muscle tone. (From Hrachovy RA. Development of the normal electroencephalogram. In: Levin KH, Luders HO, eds. *Comprehensive Clinical Neurophysiology*. Philadelphia, PA: WB Saunders, 2000, with permission.)

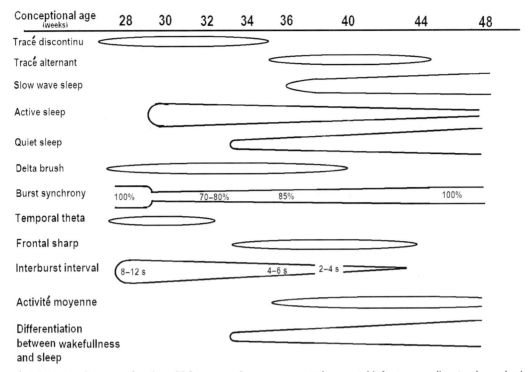

FIGURE 16-14 | Schematic diagram of various EEG patterns in premature and neonatal infants according to chronological age.

(see Chapter 7, Normal awake EEG; see also Figs. 7-27 and 7-28) in the occipital regions during eye-opening periods. In quiet sleep, slow-wave sleep gradually replaces the TA pattern and tends to appear only at the onset of quiet sleep. The bursts during TA are well synchronized between the two hemispheres. The suppression period in TA is brief, usually less than 2 to 4 seconds. CSWS progressively becomes the dominant pattern in quiet sleep.

Figure 16-14 summarizes various neonatal and premature EEG patterns by chronological age.

Abnormal EEG in Neonates

In evaluating the neonatal EEG, the first consideration is the presence or absence of characteristic EEG patterns appropriate for the stated CA. Deciding favorable or unfavorable prognosis from a single EEG is often risky. Serial EEGs are crucial in many cases. This is especially true for EEG abnormalities showing "*dysmaturity*" or "*dyschronism*," in which EEG patterns are immature for the stated GA or CA. Further, the abnormal EEG (e.g., the burst suppression pattern) could change rapidly within a few hours if the infant's physiological condition improves.

The abnormalities of neonatal EEG can be classified into the following three categories: (i) abnormalities of background activities and abnormal patterns, (ii) abnormalities in maturation and organization of states, and (iii) ictal abnormalities.

ABNORMALITIES OF BACKGROUND ACTIVITY AND ABNORMAL PATTERNS

Continuous Low-Voltage or Near-"Isoelectric" Pattern

This is characterized by more or less continuous cerebral activities less than 10 μV (Fig. 16-15). This prolonged "inactive"

EEG pattern is abnormal at any age. This low-voltage pattern should be differentiated from TD or TA in which the inactive period is rarely longer than 60 seconds.[13,21] Continuous low-voltage or near-isoelectric patterns indicate grave clinical conditions and may be seen or exacerbated by hypothermia, drug effect, severe asphyxia, massive intracerebral hemorrhage, gross congenital malformation of the brain, inborn metabolic syndromes (such as *nonketotic hyperglycemia*), or the *postictal state*.

Burst Suppression Pattern

The burst suppression pattern consists of periods of low-voltage EEG (<15 μV) interrupted by synchronous or asynchronous burst activity consisting of various mixtures of delta and theta slow waves and sharp transients lasting 0.5 to 5 seconds (Fig. 16-16). This pattern must also be differentiated from physiological TA or TD. In fact, it is often difficult to differentiate between them in a neonate younger than 32 to 33 weeks CA. The burst suppression pattern is often extremely discontinuous with interburst intervals as long as 30 minutes and fewer expected cyclic changes such as delta brush. Also, the burst itself does not have any age-related specific EEG patterns such as delta brush, temporal theta brush, or frontal sharp transients. When differentiation of active and quiet sleep becomes possible or EEG reactivity to a stimulus becomes apparent after 34 weeks CA, the burst suppression pattern can be differentiated by its unremitting and nonreactive pattern. After this age, the physiological TD pattern resembling pathological burst suppression appears only in quiet sleep. A burst suppression pattern is commonly seen in severe encephalopathy in both premature and full-term infants. If discontinuity occurs over the course of the whole hour-long study with little variability, this is a good indicator that this pattern may be present.

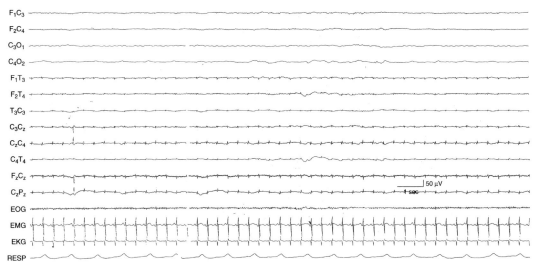

FIGURE 16-15 | Severely depressed EEG activity in a 37-week-CA infant with hypoxic–ischemic encephalopathy. (From Mizrahi EM, Hrachovy RA, Kellway P. *Atlas of Neonatal Electroencephalography*. Philadelphia, PA: Lippincott Williams & Wilkins, 2004, with permission.)

Amplitude Asymmetry between Two Hemispheres

Transitory or shifting asymmetry of background activity is a common finding in newborns and has no pathological significance. Persistent depression of all states in one hemisphere should be considered abnormal at any age, suggesting focal pathology such as prenatal or postnatal vascular accidents, tumor, porencephaly, congenital malformation, etc. (Fig. 16-17). Conversely, persistent and exceedingly high amplitude in one region (disproportionate to other regions) suggests focal abnormality. The voltage depression could be secondary to subgaleal or scalp edema or a technical problem from asymmetric electrode placement or electrode shunting (caused by sweat or smearing of electrode paste). If any of the above conditions exists, this should be noted by the technologist to avoid misinterpretation.

Significance of Sharp and Spike Discharges of Negative Polarity

Because sporadic sharp discharges, especially from frontal (*encoches frontales*), central, and temporal electrodes, are seen in "normal" premature babies, distinction between physiologic and pathologic sharp discharges is often difficult. The morphology, frequency, and location of the discharge can provide some distinction. The "innocent" discharges are more commonly sharp waves rather than spike waves (see Figs. 16-6 and 16-7). The pathologic spike or sharp discharges are more "spiky" (Fig. 16-18) and tend to occur more frequently (>2/min) than physiological discharges.[22] They also may occur in runs implying abnormality. Consistent unilateral or focal discharges, rather than randomly scattered discharges, imply abnormality. Polyphasic spikes are also abnormal (Fig. 16-19). Further, abnormal sharps and spikes

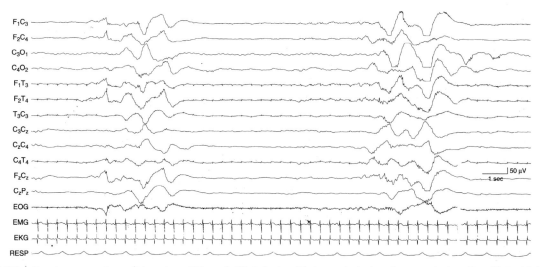

FIGURE 16-16 | Burst suppression pattern in a 37-week-CA infant with hypoxic–ischemic encephalopathy. Note high amplitude asynchronous delta bursts with superimposed fast activity interrupted by periods of inactivity. The degree of suppression is much greater than expected for TA pattern for a 37-week-CA infant. This could be normal in infants less than 32 weeks CA. (From Mizrahi EM, Hrachovy RA, Kellway P. *Atlas of Neonatal Electroencephalography*. Philadelphia, PA: Lippincott Williams & Wilkins, 2004, with permission.)

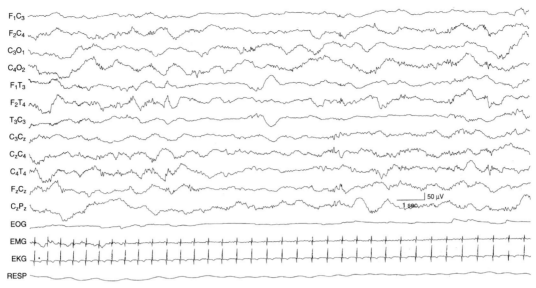

FIGURE 16-17 | Amplitude asymmetry with consistent depression on left hemisphere in a 35- to 36-week-CA infant with left frontoparietal intracerebral hemorrhage and intraventricular hemorrhage. (From Mizrahi EM, Hrachovy RA, Kellway P. *Atlas of Neonatal Electroencephalography.* Philadelphia, PA: Lippincott Williams & Wilkins, 2004, with permission.)

are often associated with abnormal background activity. During periods of discontinuity, abnormal sharp waves often occur at the end of bursts.

Positive Sharp Waves from Central, Vertex, and Temporal Regions

Positive sharp waves are broad-based surface-positive discharges (50 to 250 μV, 100 to 250 ms duration) appearing at the central regions unilaterally or bilaterally or at the vertex or temporal regions (Fig. 16-9). These occur singly or in brief runs. This has been reported mostly in premature babies and was first described by Cukier et al.,[24] who considered it a pathognomonic sign for *intraventricular hemorrhage.* As was originally described, central or vertex positive sharp waves have high sensitivity but low

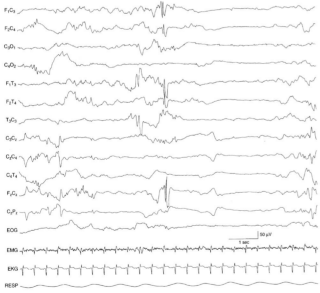

FIGURE 16-18 | Abnormal frontal spikes in a 38-week-CA infant with cerebral dysgenesis, congenital ventriculomegaly, and choroid plexus hemorrhage. The morphology of spike is much "spikier" than the "innocent" frontal sharp (encoches frontales) transients (compare with Fig. 16-7). Also note isolated spikes from T3 electrode. (From Mizrahi EM, Hrachovy RA, Kellway P. *Atlas of Neonatal Electroencephalography.* Philadelphia, PA: Lippincott Williams & Wilkins, 2004, with permission.)

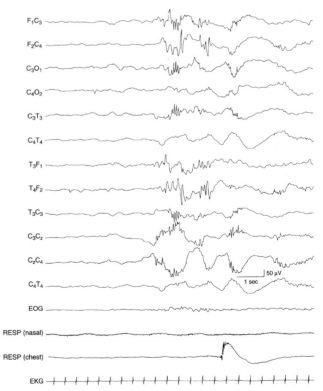

FIGURE 16-19 | Abnormal polyphasic spikes (polyspikes) arising from frontal and central regions independently in a 32-week-CA infant. (From Mizrahi EM, Hrachovy RA, Kellway P. *Atlas of Neonatal Electroencephalography.* Philadelphia, PA: Lippincott Williams & Wilkins, 2004, with permission.)

specificity for the diagnosis of intraventricular hemorrhage.[24] Further, their association with other conditions, including periventricular leukomalacia, meningitis, hydrocephalus, and asphyxia, has been reported.[25–30] Although the pattern is paroxysmal, it is unlikely to be epileptogenic activity and is better considered to be an electrographic sign of underlying structural brain damage. However, later studies have found that this may occur transiently in very young premature infants without pathological significance.[17] Their presence in babies of 32 weeks CA or older should be considered abnormal. Most of the above described positive sharp waves are from Rolandic (C3, C4) or vertex (Cz) regions. The positive discharges from temporal regions have received less attention but appear to share similar clinical correlates including *intraventricular hemorrhage*, *periventricular leukomalacia*, and *cerebral infarct*.[29]

ABNORMALITIES IN ORGANIZATION OF AWAKE AND SLEEP STATES AND EEG

Dysmaturity

Active and quiet sleep become clearly differentiated after 33 to 37 weeks CA, and cyclic changes between wakefulness and sleep stages are fully established after 38 weeks CA. The absence of cyclic changes in babies past 35 weeks CA, therefore, raises the suspicion of abnormality. Determining abnormalities in state organization, however, requires prolonged and/or serial EEG recording.

Within a week after birth, the normal full-term baby exhibits mostly a TA pattern during quiet (non-REM) sleep. As the baby matures, the TA pattern progressively diminishes, and by 4 weeks, a CSW pattern dominates. A TA pattern persisting after 8 weeks from full-term birth is probably a sign of delayed CNS maturation.[4]

Active (REM) sleep occupies about one half of total sleep time during the first 2 weeks after birth. It decreases to less than 25% of total sleep time by 8 weeks. Excessive amounts of REM in an infant beyond 2 months of age raises the suspicion of dysmaturity. Healthy near-term or full-term babies may go into REM at sleep onset. Persistence of REM-onset sleep for 4 to 6 weeks after full-term birth also raises the possibilities of CNS abnormality or delayed maturation. However, an increase or decrease of REM and non-REM sleep may be affected by multiple factors, such as polydrug exposure in the mother, and various perinatal factors such as seizures, birth weight, Apgar score, etc. Therefore, clinical significance and prognostic values for these REM/non-REM state deviations are still uncertain and must await further confirmation.

Sleep spindles may appear as early as 3 to 5 weeks postterm and should be present by 2 months. Sleep spindles at this age characteristically are very asynchronous, and the asynchrony remains till 1 year of age (see Fig. 7-42). They also may be prolonged compared to children and adults lasting 5 to 10 seconds. A delay in the emergence of sleep spindles past 8 weeks after term is abnormal and has been reported in trisomy 21[31] and in neonates with prenatal anoxic–ischemic insults.[4]

ICTAL ABNORMALITIES (IN PREMATURE AND FULL-TERM INFANTS)

In contrast to the EEGs of older infants and children whose interictal focal spike or sharp discharges are to establish a diagnosis of epilepsy, the presence of the "interictal" epileptiform discharges in neonates is not necessarily indicative of a seizure tendency. Additionally, if an infant has a seizure, the ictal activity may arise from areas other than those of the interictal spike or sharp discharges. In order to establish the diagnosis of seizure, it is important to record an ictal (clinical seizure) event by long-term EEG recording.

In a newborn, the majority of electrical ictal (seizure) activities are focal in onset and often well localized to a relatively small brain region and involve only one electrode, especially at onset. Generalized, bilaterally synchronous ictal onset is extremely rare. The discharges most commonly arise from the central and temporal regions and rarely from frontal areas. Ictal discharges may be unifocal or, more commonly, multifocal. Two independent ictal events from different brain regions can occur simultaneously or can overlap in time (Fig. 16-20A and B).

The morphology, amplitude, and frequency of seizure activity vary considerably from one patient to another and also from one seizure to the next within one recording epoch. A rhythmic or repetitive appearance of stereotyped activity of any frequency (delta, theta, alpha, and beta) could be an electrographic ictal event (Fig. 16-21). Some discharges progressively change in amplitude, frequency, and morphology (Fig. 16-22), while others begin and end abruptly without changing character (Fig. 16-23). Evolution of an ictal discharge from one area to another may sometimes be exceedingly slow. The waveforms are often "bizarre" and may be quite different from ictal discharges of adults or children. In fact, they often resemble artifacts arising from a single electrode (Fig. 16-24A–F). Amplitudes may also be quite low (10 to 25 μV) making them difficult to identify in the face of typical myogenic or EKG artifact. Careful analysis, repeated occurrence, and spread to other electrodes aid in distinguishing them from artifact. In some cases, recording from additional electrodes placed near the electrode of focal discharge is necessary to differentiate seizure activity from artifact.

In general, neonates with seizures associated with a normal EEG background pattern appropriate for CA have a lower risk of adverse outcome, whereas those whose seizure is associated with a moderately or severely abnormal background pattern tend to have worse outcomes.[32,33] Infants with multifocal ictal abnormalities associated with a low amplitude or periodic background pattern have much worse outcomes than those with unifocal ictal abnormalities or normal background pattern.[32] Long-term monitoring is validated by revealing a high incidence (>80%) of ictal discharges in patients who have abnormal background activity compared to those who have normal background activity.[34]

Clinical characteristics of neonatal seizures may also be quite different from seizures of adults or children. Many varieties of motor, autonomic phenomena, and behavior can be seen in clinical seizures. It should be noted that many clinically recognized seizures may not be associated with electrical ictal discharges. Conversely, an obvious electrical ictal event may not necessarily be associated with an appreciable clinical seizure. The clinical expression of some seizures may be extremely subtle, such as simple "eye opening." In such situations, it is necessary to repeatedly observe the same EEG change associated with the same clinical symptoms to confirm the seizure diagnosis.[35]

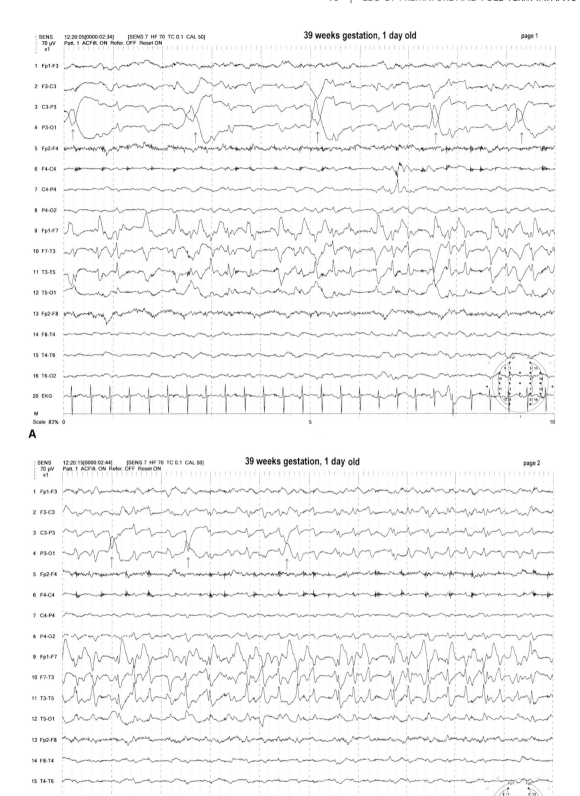

FIGURE 16-20 | An example of electrographic ictal (seizure) events showing two independent seizure activities within the same hemisphere [(**A**) and (**B**) are consecutive tracing]. Note rhythmic sharp discharges with progressively faster repetition rate from left temporal region, which progressively become faster rate, spreading to the parasagittal region. At the same time domain, recurrent large and broad sharp discharges from left parietal region appear independently, which progressively fade out (shown by *arrows*).

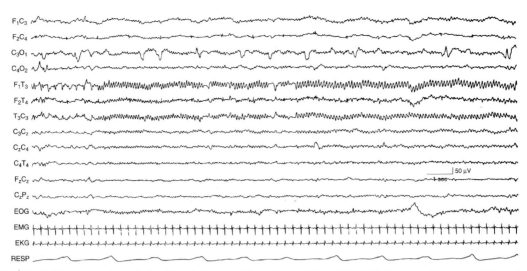

FIGURE 16-21 | Ictal discharges characterized by rhythmic alpha activity (10 to 11 Hz) that evolved from repetitive sharp discharges at T3 electrode in 38 weeks CA infant with pneumococcal meningitis. (From Mizrahi EM, Hrachovy RA, Kellway P. *Atlas of Neonatal Electroencephalography*. Philadelphia, PA: Lippincott Williams & Wilkins, 2004, with permission.)

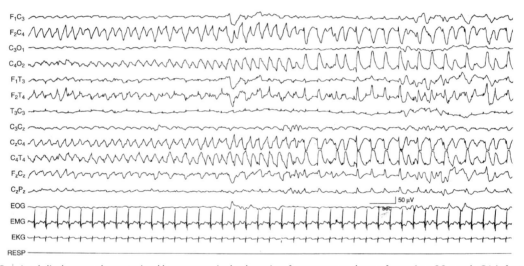

FIGURE 16-22 | Ictal discharges characterized by progressively changing frequency and waveforms in a 38-week-CA infant with hypoxic encephalopathy. The ictal onset consists of rhythmic, sharply contoured 3.5-Hz theta, arising from F2, C4 electrodes, which become progressively slower-frequency and greater amplitude activity including spikes as seizure evolves. (From Mizrahi EM, Hrachovy RA, Kellway P. *Atlas of Neonatal Electroencephalography*. Philadelphia, PA: Lippincott Williams & Wilkins, 2004, with permission.)

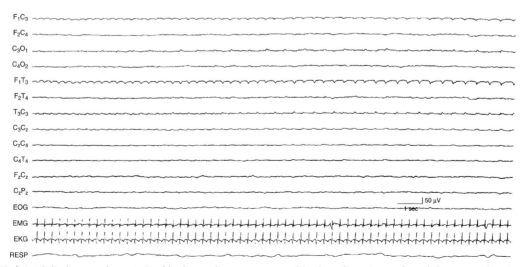

FIGURE 16-23 | Ictal discharges characterized by low-voltage monomorphic slow sharp waves from left temporal region with minimal frequency change in a 38-week-CA infant with hypoxic–ischemic encephalopathy. Note also severely depressed background activity. (From Mizrahi EM, Hrachovy RA, Kellway P. *Atlas of Neonatal Electroencephalography*. Philadelphia, PA: Lippincott Williams & Wilkins, 2004, with permission.)

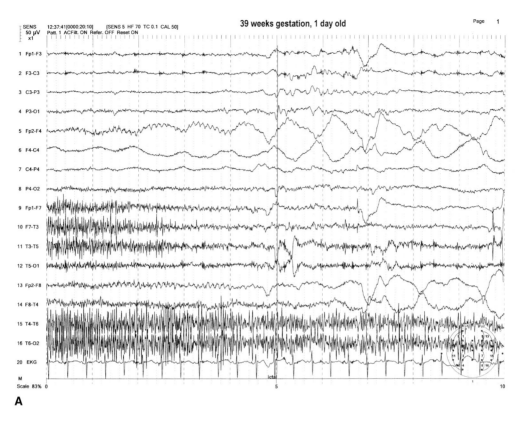

A

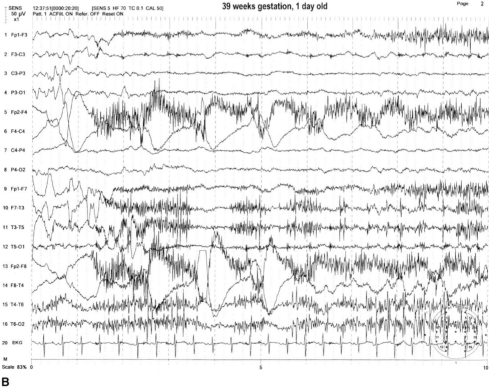

B

FIGURE 16-24 | Ictal discharges characterized by rhythmic delta waves at onset with progressively changing pattern as seizure activity evolve in a 39-week-CA infant (**A** to **D** are consecutive recordings). The ictal onset is rhythmic 1-Hz delta activity with superimposed 10-Hz alpha starting at F4 electrode (this appears as artifact but actually is not). The delta activity spreads to F8 electrode **(A)**. The delta activity then starts to fade **(B)** and become somewhat irregular **(C)**. Then, the rhythmic sharp and triphasic waves emerge from the right hemisphere **(D)** and become progressively faster frequency **(E)** and **(F)**. The waveforms of ictal onset represented by rhythmic delta appear to be "bizarre" and look like "artifact." However, repeated observation of the same onset and sequence of the event confirms that this is a genuine EEG activity as an ictal onset. Note that this is the same patient as in Figure 16-20A and B, which shows a different type of ictal event.

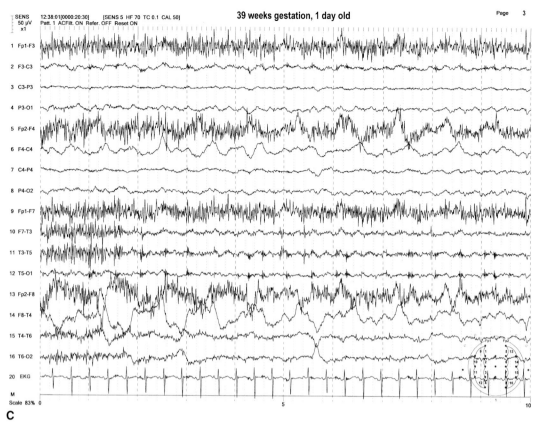

C

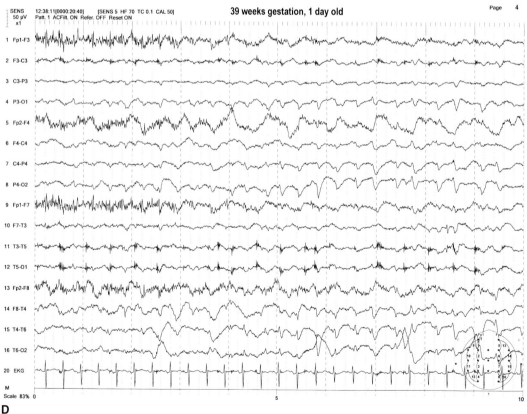

D

FIGURE 16-24 | (*Continued*)

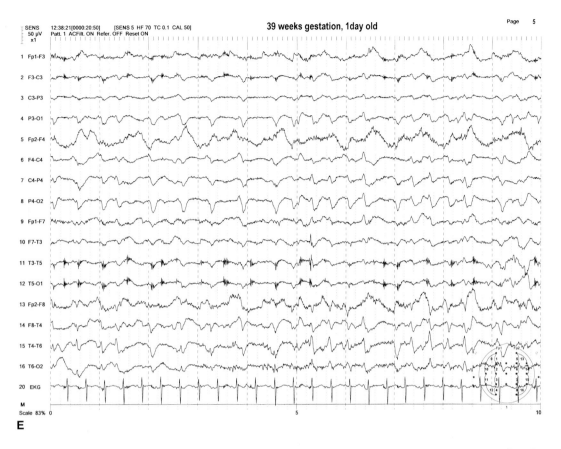

E

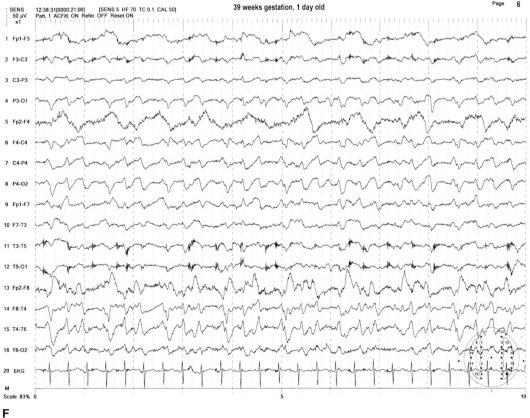

F

FIGURE 16-24 | (Continued)

References

1. Clancy RR. Prolonged electroencephalogram monitoring for seizures and their treatment. *Clin Perinatol* 2006;33:649–665.

2. Dreyfus-Brisac C. The electroencephalogram of the premature infant and full-term newborn. Normal and abnormal development of waking and sleeping pattern. In: Kellaway P, Petersen I, eds. *Neurological and Electroencephalographic Correlative Studies in Infancy.* New York: Grune and Stratton, 1964:186–207.

3. Tharp BR. Electrophysiological brain maturation in premature infants: An historical perspective. *J Clin Neurophysiol* 1990;7:302–314.

4. Lombroso C. Neonatal polygraphy in full-term and preterm infants: A review of normal and abnormal findings. *J Clin Neurophysiol* 1985;2:105–155.

5. Kuratani J, Pearl PL, Sullivan L, et al. American Clinical Neurophysiology Society Guideline 5: Minimal technical standard for pediatric electroencephalography. *J Clin Neurophysiol* 2016;33(4):320–323.

6. Dreyfus-Brisac C. The electroencephalogram of the premature infant. *World Neurol* 1962;3:5–15.

7. Clancy RR, Chung HJ, Temple JP. Neonatal electroencephalography. In: Spering MR, Calncy RR, eds. *Atlas of Electroencephalography.* New York: Elsevier, 1993:182.

8. Werner SS, Stockard JE, Bickford RG. *Atlas of Neonatal Electroencephalography.* New York: Raven Press, 1977.

9. Benda CI, Engel RCH, Zhang Y. Prolonged inactive phases during the discontinuous pattern of prematurity in electroencephalogram of very-low-birth weight infants. *Electroencephalogr Clin Neurophysiol* 1989;72:189–197.

10. Vecchierini MF, d'Allest AM, Verpillat P. EEG patterns in 10 extreme premature neonates with normal neurological outcome: qualitative and quantitative data. *Brain Dev* 2003;25(5):330–337.

11. Watanabe K, Iwase K, Hara K. Development of slow-wave sleep in low-birth weight infants. *Dev Med Child Neurol* 1974;16:23–31.

12. Lombroso C. Quantified electrographic scales in 10 pre-term healthy newborns followed up to 40–43 weeks of conceptional age by serial polygraphic recording. *Electroencephalogr Clin Neurophysiol* 1979;46:460–474.

13. Selton D, Andre M, Hascoët JM. Normal EEG in very premature infants: reference criteria. *Clin Neurophysiol* 2000;111(12):2116–2124.

14. Tharp BR, Cukier F, Monod N. The prognostic values of the electroencephalogram in premature infants. *Electroencephalogr Clin Neurophysiol* 1981;51:219–236.

15. Parmelee AH. Changes in sleep patterns in premature infants as a function of brain maturation. In: Minkowski A, ed. *Regional Development of the Brain in Early Life.* Oxford: Blackwell, 1967:459–480.

16. Dreyfus-Brisac C. Ontogenesis of sleep in human prematures after 32 weeks of conceptual age. *Dev Psychobiol* 1970;3:91–121.

17. Engel R. *Abnormal Electroencephalograms in the Neonatal Period.* Springfield, IL: Charles C. Thomas, 1978.

18. Lombroso CT. Normal and abnormal EEGs in full term neonates. In: Henry CE, ed. *Current Clinical Neurophysiology. Update on EEG and Evoked Potentials.* New York: Elsevier/North Holland, 1980:83–150.

19. Anderson CM, Torres F, Faoro A. The EEG of early premature. *Electroencephalogr Clin Neurophysiol* 1985;60:95–105.

20. Monod N, Pajot N. Le sommeil du nouveau-ne et du premature. I. Analyse des etudes polygraphiques (mouvements oculaires respiration et EEG chez le nouveau-ne a terme). *Biol Neonate* 1965;8:281–307.

21. Ellingson RJ. EEGs of premature and full-term newborns. In: Klass DW, Daly DD, eds. *Current Practice of Clinical Electroencephalopathy.* New York: Raven Press, 1979:149–177.

22. Hahn J, Monyer H, Tharp B. Interburst interval measurements in the EEGs of premature infants with normal neurological outcome. *Electroencephalogr Clin Neurophysiol* 1989;73:410–418.

23. Clancy RR. Interictal sharp EEG transients in neonatal seizures. *J Child Neurol* 1989;4:30–38.

24. Cukier F, Andre M, Monod N, et al. Apport de l'EEG au diagnostic des hemorragies intra-ventriculaires du premature. *Rev Electroencephalogr Neurophysiol Clin* 1972;2:318–322.

25. Clancy RR, Tharp BR. Positive rolandic sharp waves in electroencephalograms of premature neonates with intraventricular hemorrhage. *Electroencephalogr Clin Neurophysiol* 1984;57:395–404.

26. Marret S, Parain D, Jeannot E, et al. Positive rolandic sharp waves in the EEG of the premature newborn: A five year prospective study. *Arch Dis Child* 1992;67:948–951.

27. da Costa J, Lombroso CT. Neurophysiological correlates of neonatal intracranial hemorrhage. *Electroencephalogr Clin Neurophysiol* 1980;50:183–184.

28. Novotony EJ Jr, Tharp BR, Coen RW, et al. Positive rolandic sharp wave in the EEG of the premature infant. *Neurology* 1987;37:1481–1486.

29. Blume WT, Dreyfus-Brisac C. Positive rolandic sharp waves in neonatal EEG: Types and significance. *Electroencephalogr Clin Neurophysiol* 1982;53:277–282.

30. Chung H, Clancy R. Significance of positive temporal sharp waves in the neonatal electroencephalogram. *Electroencephalogr Clin Neurophysiol* 1991;79:256–263.

31. Ellingson RJ, Peters JF. Development of EEG and daytime sleep pattern in trisomy-21 infants during the first year of life: Longitudinal observations. *Electroencephalogr Clin Neurophysiol* 1980;50:457–466.

32. Sher MS. Seizures in the newborn infant: Diagnosis, treatment, and outcome. *Clin Perinatol* 1997;24:735–772.

33. Rowe JC, Holmes GL, Hafford J, et al. Prognostic value of the electroencephalogram in term and preterm infants following neonatal seizure. *Electroencephalogr Clin Neurophysiol* 1985;60:183–196.

34. Laroia N, Guillet R, Burchfield J, et al. EEG background as prediction of electrographic seizures in high risk neonates. *Epilepsia* 1998;38:545–551.

35. Murray DM, Boylan GB, Ali I, et al. Defining the gap between electrographic seizure burden, clinical expression and staff recognition of neonatal seizures. *Arch Dis Child Fetal Neonatal Ed* 2008;93(3):F187–F191.

Index

Note: Page numbers in *italics* denote figures; those followed by a "t" denote tables.